FUNDAMENTALS OF THE HISTOLOGY OF DOMESTIC ANIMALS

Alfred Trautmann
&
Josef Fiebiger

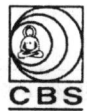

CBS

CBS Publishers & Distributors Pvt. Ltd.

New Delhi • Bengaluru • Chennai • Kochi • Mumbai • Pune
Hyderabad • Kolkata • Nagpur • Patna • Vijayawada

| Fundamentals of the Histology of Domestic Animals |

ISBN: 978-81-239-2692-6

First CBS Reprint: 2015

Published by:
Satish Kumar Jain for CBS Publishers & Distributors Pvt. Ltd.,
4819/XI Prahlad Street, 24 Ansari Road, Daryaganj, New Delhi - 110002
delhi@cbspd.com, cbspubs@airtelmail.in • www.cbspd.com
Ph.: 23289259, 23266861, 23266867 • Fax: 011-23243014
Corporate Office: 204 FIE, Industrial Area, Patparganj, Delhi - 110 092
Ph: 49344934 • Fax: 011-49344935
E-mail: publishing@cbspd.com • publicity@cbspd.com

Branches:
- *Bengaluru:* 2975, 17th Cross, K.R. Road, Bansankari 2nd Stage, Bengaluru - 70
  Ph: +91-80-26771678/79 • Fax: +91-80-26771680
  E-mail: cbsbng@gmail.com, bangalore@cbspd.com
- *Chennai:* No. 7, Subbaraya Street, Shenoy Nagar, Chennai - 600030
  Ph: +91-44-26681266, 26680620 • Fax: +91-44-42032115
  E-mail: chennai@cbspd.com
- *Kochi:* 36/14, Kalluvilakam, Lissie Hospital Road, Kochi - 682018
  Ph: +91-484-4059061-65 • Fax: +91-484-4059065
  E-mail: cochin@cbspd.com
- *Mumbai:* 83-C, Dr. E. Moses Road, Worli, Mumbai - 400018
  Ph: +91-9833017933, 022-24902340/41 • E-mail: mumbai@cbspd.com
- *Pune:* Bhuruk Prestige, Sr. No. 52/12/2+1+3/2,
  Narhe, Haveli (Near Katraj-Dehu Road Bypass), Pune - 411041
  Ph: +91-20-64704058/59, 32342277 • E-mail: pune@cbspd.com

Representatives:

- Hyderabad: 0-9885175004
- Nagpur: 0-9021734563
- Vijayawada: 0-9000660880
- Kolkata: 0-9831437309, 0-9051152362
- Patna: 0-9334159340

Printed at:
Neekunj Print Process, Delhi

Preface

IN THE English-speaking world the histology of domestic animals has always been taught without the aid of a textbook on the subject. The excellent textbooks of human histology, while furnishing a valuable background for the veterinary student, are deficient and often misleading in important particulars of animal histology. This is especially true of the digestive and genital systems and of the skin and its modifications. Even in the introductory discussions of the basic tissues it is desirable from the standpoint of the veterinary student to draw the examples from domestic animals.

This gap in our literature is hard to condone when we consider the importance of special histology to the study of veterinary physiology and pathology. It is even harder to understand in view of the fact that a histology of domestic animals has been published in German for more than sixty years and is now in its ninth edition. Wilhelm Ellenberger's *Fundamentals of Comparative Histology of the Domestic Mammals* appeared in 1888. It was a textbook based on a larger reference work—*Handbook of Comparative Histology and Physiology*—edited by Ellenberger. The third edition of the *Fundamentals* (1908) was augmented by material from a new three-volume *Handbook of Comparative Microscopic Anatomy of the Domestic Animals* (1906–1911), also edited by Ellenberger. After Ellenberger's death in 1928, his collaborator, Alfred Trautmann, brought out the sixth edition (1931) with the assistance of Josef Fiebiger. The title was changed to *Textbook of Histology and Comparative Microscopic Anatomy of the Domestic Mammals*. With the seventh edition in 1941, the histology of birds—mostly the chicken—was added. The last edition, published in 1949, was designated the eighth and ninth because the plates for the eighth edition were destroyed by bombing before publication, and it became necessary to revise the text while new plates were being prepared.

The adaptation of this book to the needs of the American veterinary student was a considerably larger task than simple translation. The material has been rearranged, and some of the more oppressive detail has been eliminated. Wherever it seemed necessary for clarity, the original text has been supplemented. When the text was at variance with ideas commonly accepted in this country, it became necessary to consult the literature and attempt to reconcile the differences. This was made somewhat difficult by the lack of a bibliography in the German edition, but ample bibliographical material on the histology of domestic animals is available in the reference works listed in the back of this book. Wherever it seemed advisable to give the authority for a statement, a footnote has been added. References to books repeatedly cited are given in abbreviated form in the footnotes, but complete bibliographical information will be found in the annotated list of references mentioned above. The appendix on microscopic technique has been omitted because the subject is usually taught in special advanced courses, for which several good books are available. The senior translator and editor assumes full responsibility for the text in its final form. Criticism will be gratefully received.

The illustrations are the same as those in the ninth German edition, with certain exceptions. The color plates of the blood cells and bone marrow cells were painted by Miss Pat Barrow from dry smears stained routinely by Wright's method. Figures 288 and 329 required redrawing because of labeling difficulties. Figure 354, showing the tracts of the spinal cord of the cat, is printed by courtesy of Dr. J. W. Papez. It first appeared in his *Comparative Neurology* (New York: T. Y. Crowell Co., 1929).

We wish to thank the firm of Oliver and Boyd, Ltd., Edinburgh, for permission to print a large portion of the table of blood counts prepared by H. H. Holman for Boddie's *Diagnostic Methods in Veterinary Medicine*. We also wish to acknowledge the assistance of the staff of Flower Library, of Drs. L. Z. Saunders, C. G. Rickard, John Bentinck-Smith, and A. V. Machado, all of the Department of Pathology, New York State Veterinary College, and of Dr. H. F. Parks, formerly of the Department of Zoology, Cornell University.

ROBERT E. HABEL
ERNST L. BIBERSTEIN

Ithaca, New York

Contents

PART TWO, SPECIAL HISTOLOGY: MICROSCOPIC ANATOMY

CONTENTS

CONTENTS

FUNDAMENTALS OF

The Histology of Domestic Animals

Introduction

WHEN examined under the microscope, the building materials of the animal body often exhibit a structure reminiscent of the products of the loom. For this reason they are called tissues,[1] and the study of these building materials is called histology.[2] Because it treats not only of the morphology, the structure, of the tissues but also of the microscopically visible life processes and evidence of life, histology is at the same time microscopic anatomy and physiology—microscopic biology.

The study of the tissues leads finally to the smallest elements in which the phenomena of life may still be observed—elements which must therefore be regarded as the anatomical and physiological units. These microscopic formations of living substance, where the scene of all life is laid, are called cells.

One of the most important physiological properties of cells is their ability, under certain conditions, to multiply, to reproduce. The simplest animals, the protozoa, consist of but one cell. All of the metazoa, even the most highly organized animals, grow from a single cell, the fertilized egg. From this, by repeated division (cleavage), are produced cells of apparently indeterminate character, the segmentation spheres or blastomeres.[3] In the course of development this cellular material is arranged in two layers, which form the wall of a hollow sphere and are called the outer germ layer (ectoderm) and the inner germ layer (entoderm). Between them appears a third layer, also composed of cells lying in direct contact with each other, the middle germ layer (mesoderm). Certain cell masses derived from the mesoderm are called mesenchyme.[4]

The whole organism of the animal is derived by a series of transformations from the three germ layers. In the development of the tissues (histogenesis) the descendants of the three germ layers form associations of cells having definite characteristics of form and structure that fit them for specific functions. Gradually, with the appearance in each of these cell groupings of typical substances that come from the cells and are deposited between them, the different tissues are completed. A

---

[1] Fr. *tisser* to weave.
[2] Gr. *histion* tissue.
[3] Gr. *blastos* germ, and *meros* part.
[4] Gr. *mesos* middle, and *enchyma* that which is poured in.

tissue is therefore an association of similar cells with similar powers, together with the interstitial substance.

The germ layers and the mesenchyme each give rise to certain specific tissues; for example, the whole group of connective tissues comes from the mesenchyme. On the other hand, one type of tissue may have several different origins: the epithelia are derived from all three germ layers; smooth musculature, usually of mesenchymal origin, may exceptionally come from the ectoderm, and so on. The tissue concept is used without regard for definite spatial limitations; the latter apply only to the organs, by which we mean parts of the body with definite form, function, and structure, made up of one or more tissues. Organs that perform a common task are grouped into systems for descriptive purposes.

Because the tissues and the cells themselves can exhibit individual functions, it follows that a simple tissue, as long as it occurs with a definite form and boundaries, must be regarded as an organ (e.g., cartilage).

The science of histology, in addition to the study of the cells and tissues as such, is also concerned with the manner in which individual tissues take part in the structure of the different organs. Therefore, histology may be divided into a general and a special part. The former, histology in the narrow sense, comprises the knowledge of the cells and tissues; the latter, microscopic anatomy, deals with the finer structure of the organs.

PART ONE

GENERAL HISTOLOGY

I

The Animal Cell

AS EARLY as 1665 Hooke discovered in a vegetable tissue (cork) spaces which he called cells. Gradually the universal distribution of cells throughout the plant kingdom came to be recognized. In 1839 Schwann showed that the animal body as well is composed of such "cells" and their products. At that time cells were regarded as vesicles consisting of a firm skin (cell membrane) and a fluid content (cell sap). It was known that the vesicle contained a circumscribed body, the cell nucleus, which in turn contained a still smaller corpuscle, the nucleolus. It was not until later that the living cell substance was discovered and its importance recognized. Von Mohl gave it the name of protoplasm.[1] Max Schultze showed that the membrane was not an essential part of the cell. The meaning of the term cell was thus transferred from the wall to the contents. Flemming introduced the terms karyoplasm[2] and cytoplasm[3] to distinguish the protoplasm of the nucleus from that of the rest of the cell, or cell body.

A. THE STRUCTURE OF THE CELL

A cell is considered to be a discrete mass of living substance, which is at once the performer of the vital functions and the structural unit of all tissues. It is the elementary organism. Despite the great variation in cellular structure, there are three components that may be recognized in almost every cell: (1) the cytoplasm, (2) the nucleus, and (3) the cell center.

1. The Cytoplasm

The cytoplasm consists of protoplasm—a semiliquid mass of varying, usually viscous, consistency and slightly alkaline reaction. It swells but does not dissolve in water. It is usually described as a highly complex colloidal system of various proteins, carbohydrates, fats, and lipids in all stages of dispersion in water or fatty substances. The present conception of the architecture of protoplasm is that of a submicroscopic framework of long protein molecules (macromolecules, polypep-

[1] Gr. *protos* first, and *plasma* the thing formed: that which was formed first.
[2] Gr. *karyon* kernel.   [3] Gr. *kytos* hollow vessel, cell.

tide chains) held together by cross linkages and permeated by the more fluid constituents. Between the two phases there is probably a constant exchange of the materials involved in the great chemical activity of the cell. This network may make either a sol or a gel, depending on the degree of folding of the protein chains and the strength of the cross linkages. Where the chains are oriented together in an orderly array, the structure becomes birefringent (doubly refractive) and may show visible fibrils (p. 62). Any stimulus that causes a folding of the protein chains or an increased molecular aggregation will decrease the birefringence and cause a rearrangement of the material, or change of shape, which may be described as a contraction.[4] In addition to the colloids, we find crystalloids (mineral salts) either in solution or as crystals.

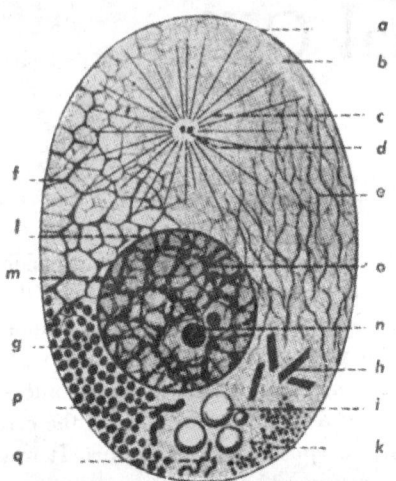

Living protoplasm appears under the microscope as a clear fluid in which are embedded certain filamentous or granular structures, visible because they are more strongly refractive to light (i.e., they appear bright with dark outlines). When permanent, stained preparations of cells are made, the protoplasm is coagulated in the process and forms an artificial pattern, which varies with the technique of fixation, the kind of cell, and the physiological state of the cell at the instant of death. Previous concepts of the actual structure of protoplasm were based on the stained coagulation patterns, which were described as filamentous (Figs. 1,e; 2), spongy or reticular (Figs. 1,f; 3), and granular (Fig. 1,g). Inasmuch as these

Figure 1. Diagram of a cell. The upper part of the cell shows the filamentous and reticular structure of protoplasm. *a*, cell membrane; *b*, ectoplasm; *c*, aster; *d*, centriole; *e*, filamentous mass; *f*, walls of honeycomb in reticular protoplasm; *g*, granules; *h*, crystals; *i*, fat globules; *k*, pigment granules; *l*, nuclear membrane; *m*, karyoplasm with *n*, nucleolus, and *o*, chromatin; *p*, lecithin, *q*, mitochondria.

fixation patterns are fairly constant in cells of the same kind fixed by the same technique, they have some value as a means of identification.

Organoids. These are permanent features of cytoplasmic differentiation, which vary with the kind of cell. They include mitochondria, fibrils, the Golgi apparatus, and, according to some authors, the cell center.

Mitochondria[5] are minute granular or filiform cytoplasmic structures, usually demonstrable only by means of special techniques. They are concerned with the secretory activity of the cell. Some of the enzymes are associated with them.

Fibrils occur in many cells. They are prominent characteristics of nerve, muscle, and certain kinds of epithelium.

[4] Rudolf Höber et al., *Physical Chemistry of Cells and Tissues* (Philadelphia: Blakiston, 1945), p. 447.
[5] Gr. *mitos* thread, and *chondros* cartilage.

The internal reticular apparatus (Fig. 5), discovered in nerve cells by Golgi, is of importance in the life of the cell. It is demonstrable by special techniques in almost all cells. It occurs in the cytoplasm as a network of anastomosing strands (or canals) in a perinuclear or polar position. Lipoids seem to take part in its make-up. As an organ of the cell, the Golgi apparatus appears to participate actively in the work of the cell, especially secretion.

Also worthy of note are the intracellular secretory canaliculi (intracellular secretory capillaries, Fig. 44,*c*).

Cellular Inclusions. These do not take part in the vital processes as permanent constituents of cytoplasm but merely occur in it as inert particles or products of metabolism. The inclusions may be fat, protein, yolk granules, glycogen, pigment granules, and secretory granules. The granules may be so numerous as to give a

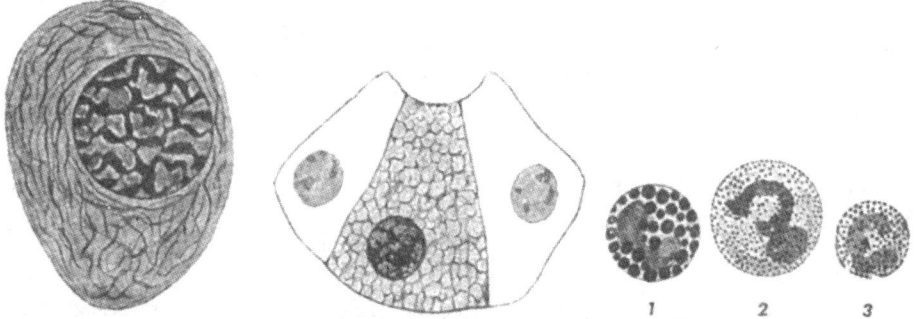

Figure 2 (left). Chondrocyte from the head of the femur of a salamander larva, showing filamentous structure of the cytoplasm.

Figure 3 (center). Cell from the deep gland of the third eyelid of a pig, showing the foamy (reticular) structure of the cytoplasm.

Figure 4 (right). Cells (leukocytes) with coarse and fine granules. *1*, from the horse; *2*, from the ox; *3*, from the pig.

fine or coarse granular appearance to the whole cell (Fig. 4). The nature of the granules cannot always be determined. In glandular and epithelial cells, they are usually secretory (e.g., zymogen, mucus, fat, keratin); sometimes we are dealing with coloring matter (pigment granules). Besides granular forms, we may also encounter fibrillar inclusions, droplets of fluid (mistakenly called vacuoles), crystals, and, finally, independent cells (bacteria, blood corpuscles). (See Figs. 1,*h, i, k;* 7.)

Coloring matter, pigment, is often present in cytoplasm. The red pigment hemoglobin[6] is found in solution in the cytoplasm of the red blood cells. It is related to the bile pigment, which is dissolved in bile. Melanin[7] occurs in the form of brownish-black granules, notably in the connective tissue cells of the uveal tract of the eye and provides protection against excessive light. Inclusions of melanin granules in the more deeply situated epidermal cells and in the hair cells produce a brown or black coloration of the skin and hair. The pigment fuscin,[8] a variety of melanin,

[6] Gr. *haima* blood, and globin, a protein.

[7] Gr. *melas* black.

[8] L. *fuscus* brown.

occurs in the form of delicate rods and needles in the pigmented epithelial cells of the retina. Lipofuscin granules, which are associated with fatty substances, are found in striated muscle fibers and nerve cells. Lipofuscin has been called the wear-and-tear pigment.

Outer Limit of the Cell Body. Usually there is an outer zone of relatively dense, clear cytoplasm called ectoplasm, which blends into the softer interior endoplasm without a distinct boundary. The *plasma membrane* or surface layer of the cytoplasm is too thin to be visible (100–200 Å[9]). It acts selectively to permit the passage of some solutes and to retain others; i.e., it is differentially permeable. The plasma membrane can be demonstrated by microdissection to have some resistance and elasticity. When it is punctured at one point, a new membrane is soon formed by the underlying cytoplasm.

Not to be confused with the plasma membrane are the *visible cell membranes*, or pelliculae, which are relatively rare in animal tissues. They are products of cytoplasmic secretion or differentiation and have staining properties and physical characteristics that differ from those of the cytoplasm which they surround. A membrane that covers only one end of the cell, usually the free pole, is called a cuticula.

2. The Nucleus

The nucleus is a living structure which occurs, usually singly, in every cell. It is a sharply outlined body located more or less centrally in the cytoplasm. It may change its location and shape, but is originally spherical or ovoid. Sometimes the shape of the cell influences that of the nucleus. Irregularly shaped (polymorphic) nuclei also occur. The nucleus is commonly more refractive than the cytoplasm and gives a different reaction to many chemicals. It is easily stained by certain dyes. The nuclear material (karyoplasm) contains, among other substances, certain phosphorus-containing compounds characteristic of nuclei, called nucleoproteins. Nucleus and cytoplasm are intimately related; the nucleus exhibits variations in structure in accordance with the physiological state of the cell. Upon experimental removal of the nucleus, the residual cell fragment may live for some time but finally dies, whereas a fragment that contains a nucleus has the capacity to regenerate itself. The isolated nucleus is not viable.

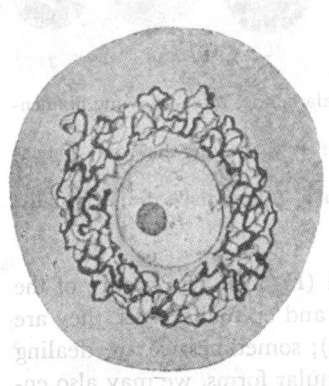

Figure 5. Golgi's internal reticular apparatus in a neuron from the ganglion of the trigeminal nerve (70×). Section through the center of the cell.

In some cells the nucleus is so pale or obscured by cytoplasmic inclusions that it can be demonstrated only by special techniques (the addition of acetic acid, staining, etc.). In other cells (e.g., those of the epidermis or the erythrocytes) the nucleus is lost during the life of the cell. On the other hand, some masses of cyto-

---

[9] A, an angstrom unit or 10^{-7} mm.

plasm contain several nuclei. These are formed either by the fusion of originally separate cells (syncytium) or by failure to separate into individual cells in spite of continuous multiplication of nuclei and growth of cytoplasm (plasmodium). Both forms may be called polykaryocytes or giant cells. We also speak of syncytial cell associations where cells are interconnected by cytoplasmic processes (cytoplasmic bridges) to form a network.

In the stained nucleus, and less clearly in the living nucleus, one is able to distinguish the nuclear membrane and the nuclear sap, in which are found chromatin and nucleoli.

The *nuclear membrane* (Fig. 1,*l*) is always present, except in dividing nuclei. It exhibits characteristic staining properties and resistance to chemical reagents.

The *nuclear sap* (karyolymph) is a proteinaceous substance of gelatinous consistency and homogeneous appearance *in vivo*. In it we find a material that is easily and deeply stained by certain dyes. It is called *chromatin*[10] (karyotin, Fig, 1,*o*) and occurs in the form of threads, grains, and clumps. The "linin network" seen in some preparations is an artefact. Chromatin is composed of nucleoproteins containing thymonucleic acid. The chromatin threads are actually chromonemata[11] (see p. 15) distorted by fixation. During cell division, the chromonemata are coiled and impregnated with a chromatin matrix to form the short, thick chromosomes.[12] Between cell divisions, the matrix disappears from all except the heterochromatic parts of the chromosomes, which remain stainable as the chromatin "clumps" of the interphase nucleus. Interphase is a better term than resting for the nondividing nucleus, which is actively engaged in the work of the cell.

The *nucleoli* (Fig. 1,*n*) occur in the nuclear sap as strictly defined, usually spherical, easily stained structures. They are usually 1 to 5 in number and are composed of nucleoproteins containing ribonucleic acid. Their size and number increase in physiologically active cells. During mitosis they disappear, but are visible again in the final phase of division. Nucleoli must not be confused with clumps of chromatin.

The Cell Center. This structure varies according to the type and activity of the cell. In the cytoplasm of most cells we are able to demonstrate two minute (usually less than 1μ[13]) granules, which are called centrioles or, collectively, the diplosome (Fig. 1,*d*). They are closely adjacent to each other and often close to the nucleus. Surrounding the centrioles is a clear ellipsoid of dense cytoplasm, the centrosome. During cell division, the centrosome is in turn surrounded by a larger clear area (centrosphere) and a radial figure called the aster (Fig. 1,*c*). The centrioles play an important part in cell division and probably also in other cell movements. (See spermiogenesis, p. 264.)

Cell Size. Mammalian cells are microscopic. Their diameter as a rule ranges from 3 to 20 μ. The largest cells are the egg cells, which reach a size of 100 to 200 μ. In birds, they attain a diameter of several centimeters. The diameter of the smallest cells (lymphocytes) is 3 to 5 μ.

---

[10] Gr. *chroma* color.   [11] Gr. *nema* thread.   [12] Gr. *soma* body.
[13] The Greek letter μ denotes a micron or 0.001 mm. or 10,000 Å.

Cell Shape. The basic shape of the cell is spherical. Through unequal growth and the influence of external factors, such as pressure and traction, older cells usually assume a different final form which is characteristic of the kind of cell involved. Thus we distinguish cuboidal, prismatic, polygonal, columnar, conical, stellate, fusiform, squamous, and fiber cells.

The shape of the nucleus often reflects that of the cell on a smaller scale: a spherical cell would have a spherical nucleus. In fusiform cells the nucleus is often elongated to such an extent that one speaks of a rod-shaped nucleus.

B. VITAL PHENOMENA OF THE CELL

The life of the cell, which depends upon the integrity of its protoplasm, manifests itself in metabolism, independent movement, irritability (reaction to external stimuli), and reproduction. While the first three of these occur essentially within the cytoplasm, it is the nucleus that plays the most important role in reproduction. It exerts a directing influence on the other functions as well.

1. Metabolism

Metabolism comprises:

a. The intake and assimilation of solid and liquid substances and their elimination by cellular secretion and excretion.

b. The intake of oxygen, oxidation within the cells, and elimination of carbon dioxide (respiration).

The products eliminated by the cell either find their way to the outer world or are deposited between the cells as intercellular substance. The assimilated material serves either to replace used-up components of the cell or to add to the living substance, resulting in growth.

2. Movement

Movement is visible either as currents of granules within the cytoplasm (protoplasmic streaming) or as changes in external shape. The latter may be achieved by contraction, ameboid movement, and ciliary or flagellar motion. The streaming of granules in the cytoplasm differs from Brownian movement, an irregular oscillation of particles suspended in liquid. Brownian movement is caused by the impact of surrounding molecules and is not a phenomenon of life.

a. *Contraction* may occur in any kind of cell, but it is usually understood to mean the shortening of elongated cells.

b. In *ameboid motion*, the cell is seen to progress by extending temporary processes of cytoplasm called pseudopodia.[14] When one of these adheres to a point of support, the rest of the cell flows into it. According to the contractility theory of amebism, the outer, denser layer of cytoplasm (plasmagel) contracts in the posterior portion of the cell and forces the softer interior plasmasol out through the plasmagel at one point. The peripheral layer of the resulting pseupododium then gels, and the cell contracts to its original shape in a new location.

The cytoplasmic processes may engulf small particles and draw them into the

---

[14] Gr. *pseudos* false, and *podes* feet.

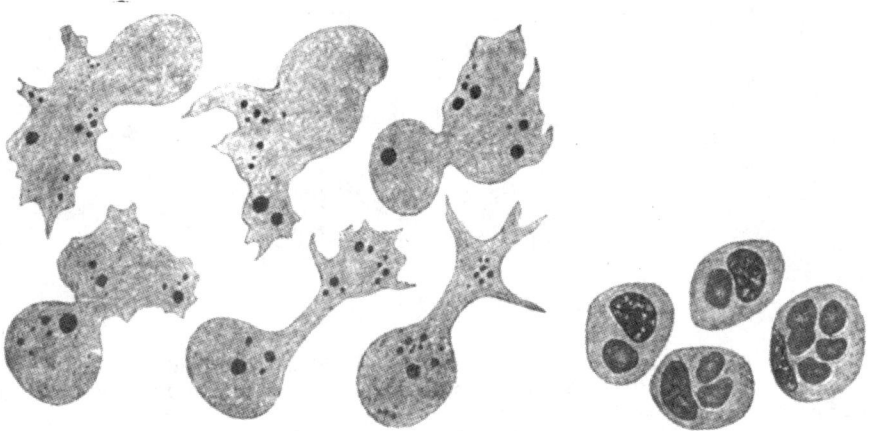

Figure 6 (left). Leukocytes in ameboid motion. The black particles are India ink which had been injected 24 hours previously into the dorsal lymph sac of a frog.
Figure 7 (right). Phagocytes with engulfed red blood cells, from a lymph node of a monkey.

cell. This phenomenon is called phagocytosis,[15] and a cell with the ability to ingest particulate matter is a phagocyte (Fig. 7). This property is found primarily in neutrophilic leukocytes. Phagocytes in the animal body play an important part in bacterial disease by ingesting live bacteria and rendering them harmless by enzyme action. Phagocytes have the property of storing dyes (e.g., carmine) injected into the living animal. (See *reticulo-endothelial system*, p. 37.)

c. *Ciliary or flagellar movement* is a regular beat exhibited by permanent thread-like cytoplasmic processes of certain cells.

3. Irritability

Irritability of the cell is manifested by its reaction to external influences. These stimuli are partly of a chemical, partly of a physical, nature and may evoke movement, metabolic processes (such as assimilation and elimination), and cell growth. They may also serve to intensify, diminish, or abolish these phenomena. Certain stimuli attract or repel free cells (positive and negative taxis or tropism). Among these responses are chemotaxis, hydrotaxis, phototaxis, galvanotaxis, and rheotaxis.

Cells of epithelial tissues rest with one surface (base) on a layer of connective tissue, which provides nourishment, while the opposite cell surface is freely exposed to external influences. As a result of adaptation, the two ends or cell poles differ in appearance. The free, or animal, pole is specialized for the higher functions of the cell. Here we find cilia or sensory hairs, cuticular structures, etc. The basal, or vegetal, pole serves mainly to anchor and nourish the cell and exhibits a less differentiated character. Only in rare instances does it bear processes that act as adhesive organs. The contrast between the two ends of the cell is called polarity and persists even after the epithelial cell has lost its direct relation to a free surface; thus pigment found in stratified epithelia occurs predominantly at the animal pole.

---

[15] Gr. *phagein* to eat.

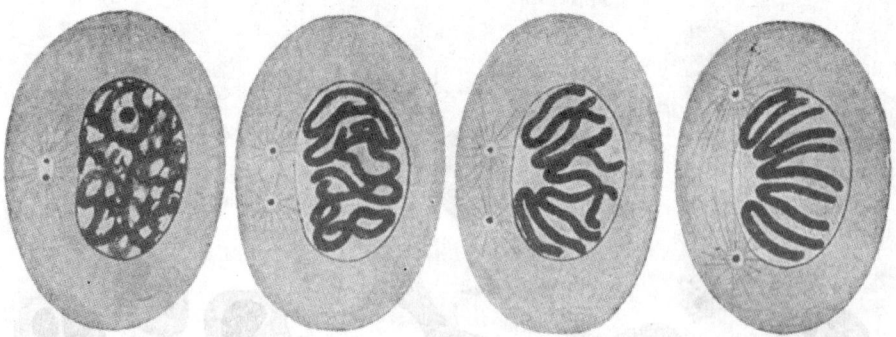

Figure 8 (extreme left). Cell, about to divide, with centrioles and aster.
Figures 9, 10, 11 (from left center to right). Successive stages of prophase. The centrioles are moving apart, while the central spindle is forming.

4. Reproduction

Reproduction, or cell multiplication, is the only source of living cells. We know of no instance of spontaneous generation. The idea that cells could originate only from other cells was advanced by Remak and later formulated by Virchow in the axiom, *omnis cellula e cellula*. Cell multiplication is probably the most important activity in the life of the cell, but it is limited to a definite age range. It is accomplished, with few exceptions, by an equal division of the nuclear material and cytoplasm, called *mitosis*. The division of the cytoplasm immediately follows that of the nucleus, It occurs so rapidly that it is complete before the nuclei of the two daughter cells have attained the "resting state." Mitosis has little or no disturbing influence on the metabolism of substances previously absorbed by the cell. Intensive cellular activity, accumulation of metabolic products, differentiation, and growth hinder cell division, while a decrease in the work of the cell favors it. Conversely, mitosis checks cell growth.

Mitosis (karyokinesis, indirect cell division) exhibits a regular sequence of events, which are usually grouped into four different phases: prophase, metaphase, anaphase, and telophase.

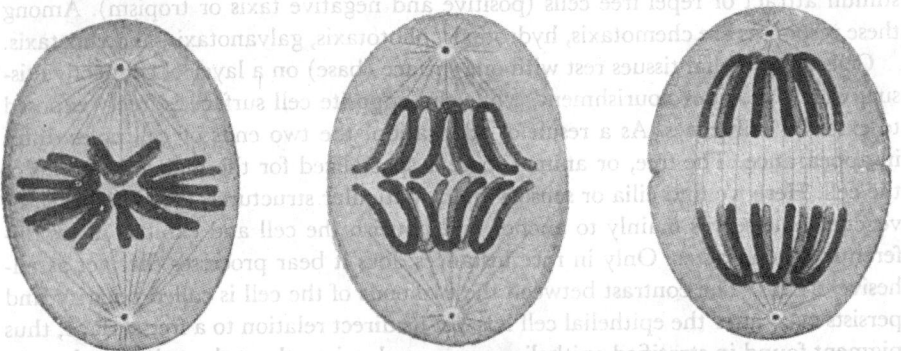

Figure 12 (left). Metaphase. The chromosomes are in the equatorial plate.
Figure 13 (center). Early anaphase. The daughter chromosomes are moving toward their poles.
Figure 14 (right). Late anaphase.

Prophase. Cells about to divide assume a more nearly spherical shape. Their cytoplasm becomes more strongly refractive and later separates into an outer layer and a light, almost liquid inner portion. The spherical nucleus enlarges, and long slender intertwined double filaments become visible (Fig. 18). These are the *chromosomes*, the main carriers of heredity. Their number is constant for each species: 2 or 4 in the roundworm of the horse, 48 in man, 60 in the horse and ox, 40 in swine.

The chromosomes become progressively shorter and thicker with the accumulation of a chromatin matrix and the coiling of the chromonemata. The *chromonema* is a long thin protein filament beaded with thickenings called chromomeres, which give the thymonucleic acid reaction and are probably the carriers of the genes. In the interphase nucleus, each chromosome is represented by two identical chromonemata closely associated in loose spirals. In prophase, each chromonema of the

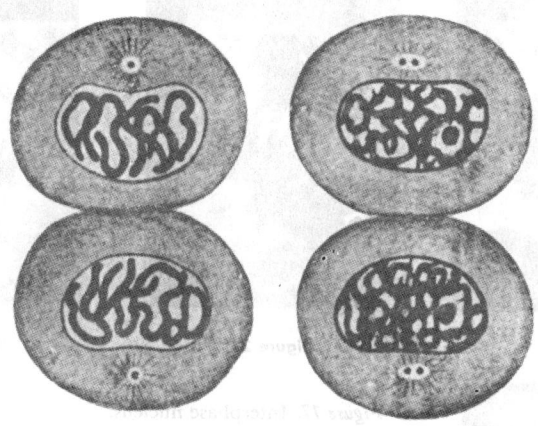

Figure 15 (left). Beginning cytokinesis, the division of the cytoplasm. *Figure 16 (right).* Cell division completed.

pair coils and accumulates a matrix to form a *chromatid*. The two **chromatids,** closely apposed and parallel, are the identical halves of a chromosome. In late prophase, the chromonema in each chromatid splits in anticipation of the next mitosis.

Meanwhile the nucleoli have disappeared; and the centrioles have moved into the vicinity of the nucleus. The now ellipsoid centrosphere exhibits distinct radiations by this time. These spread out toward the periphery of the cell and are called the aster (Fig. 8). Soon the centrioles move apart, and each is surrounded by its own aster (Fig. 11). As the two centrioles separate, a bundle of fibrils appears between them. With increasing distance between the centrioles, these fibrils become longer and finally form the central *spindle* (Figs. 11, 12). The two centrioles migrate around the nucleus until they reach diametrically opposite points, which will be the poles of the daughter cells. The karyoplasm becomes less viscous, and the nuclear membrane disappears. The spindle moves into the center of the cell, and the chromosomes move toward the equatorial plane of the spindle.

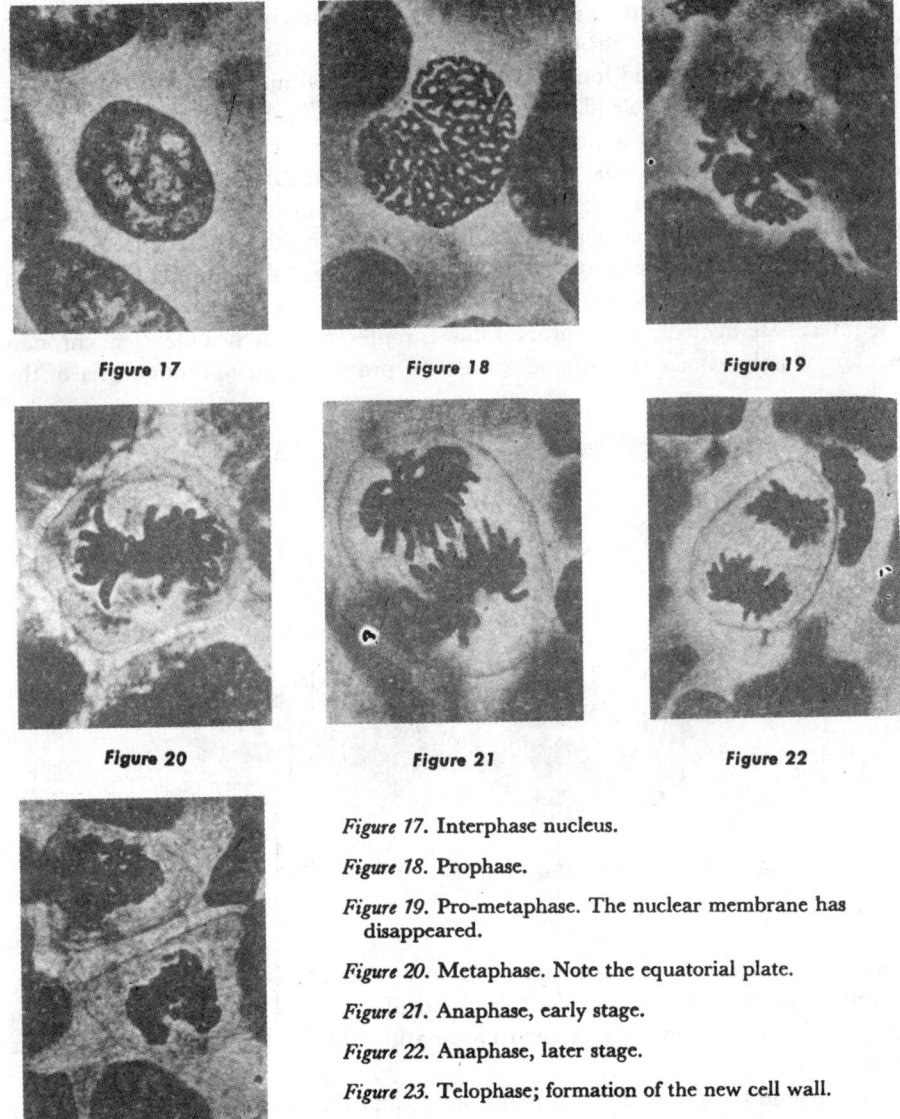

Figure 17

Figure 18

Figure 19

Figure 20

Figure 21

Figure 22

Figure 17. Interphase nucleus.

Figure 18. Prophase.

Figure 19. Pro-metaphase. The nuclear membrane has disappeared.

Figure 20. Metaphase. Note the equatorial plate.

Figure 21. Anaphase, early stage.

Figure 22. Anaphase, later stage.

Figure 23. Telophase; formation of the new cell wall.

Figure 23

Metaphase. This is a short period when the chromosomes are all arranged around the spindle in the *equatorial plate* (Figs. 12, 20). Specialized portions (kinetochores[16]) of the further shortened and clearly double chromosomes appear to be attached to the spindle fibers. The kinetochore is always in the same position on the same chromosome, but in different chromosomes it may be at one end or it may divide the chromosome into equal or unequal limbs to produce a V or a J

---

[16] Gr. *kinein* to move, and *choros* spot, place.

shape. The free ends of the chromosomes stick out toward the edge of the equatorial plate.

Anaphase. This is the process of equal distribution of the halves of the chromosomes to the prospective daughter nuclei (Fig. 13). The kinetochores of each pair of chromatids separate and move toward the poles of the spindle as though they were being pulled. The free ends of the chromatids are the last to separate as they become daughter chromosomes. The centrioles move still farther apart along the longitudinal axis of the spindle (Fig. 14). Between the separated chromosomes the spindle persists, and some stainable debris may mark the equatorial plate. As the chromosomal groups approach their respective centrioles, the stage is set for the organization of the daughter nuclei (Figs. 14, 21, 22).

Telophase. In this phase the chromosomes aggregate more closely; and, as they absorb water, swell, and lose their matrix, their outlines gradually become blurred. The cell body is divided by an annular furrow which deepens until it constricts the cytoplasm into two halves at the level of the equatorial plate (Fig. 15).

Following cytoplasmic division, the daughter nuclei are transformed into interphase nuclei by the reappearance of the nuclear membrane, the nucleoli, and the typical chromatin pattern. The spindle disappears and the centriole is now double. Occasionally the centriole remains single until the next cell division. The duration of mitosis in warm-blooded animals is one-half to one hour.

In this context we should mention the salivary chromosomes of the larvae of *Chironomus* and other Diptera (Fig. 24). These four giant chromosomes are visible in the interphase nucleus. According to some authorities their great size is the result of longitudinal division of the chromonemata without subsequent separation, while the cross bands or discs are stainable aggregates of chromomeres. They are of great value in genetic research because of the ease with which the parts may be identified.

Amitosis is a rare form of cell division in which the nucleus divides directly without the appearance of chromosomes. This division is preceded by that of the nu-

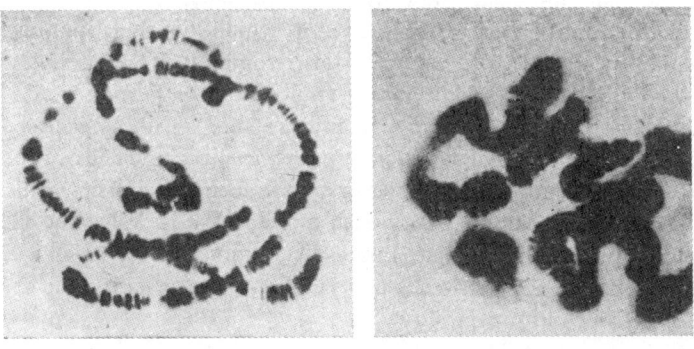

A   B

Figure 24. Giant chromosomes from the salivary gland of a *Chironomus* larva. *A*, 150×; *B*, 350×. At the higher magnification, the bands are clearly visible only on those parts of the chromosomes that are in focus.

cleolus. Amitosis was formerly thought to be more common, but improved techniques have revealed mitotic figures in almost all cases of true cell division in the higher animals.

In *budding* or sprouting, nuclear division may be either indirect, as in the formation of the polar bodies of the ova, or direct, as in the megakaryocytes of bone marrow, which show budding of the nuclei without cytoplasmic division.

The cell divisions which produce the mature sex cells are of a special and important kind, and the process is called *meiosis*[17] (pp. 264, 284). In fertilization, two cells, the spermatozoon and the ovum, each of which possesses only half the usual number of chromosomes, combine to form one cell, the fertilized ovum. Fertilization is followed by the division of the ovum, referred to as cleavage (p. 3), which gives rise to the body cells. All of these possess the full complement of chromosomes, which serve to transmit hereditary characters from parents to offspring, from mother cells to daughter cells.

The *life history* of cells varies greatly. Some have only a short life span, as is the case with many epithelial cells. Others, as nerve cells and ovocytes, live a long time. After the juvenile cells have attained their full growth, they may either keep their cellular nature or lose it and become fibers, reticula, tubules, platelets. Or they may change only their appearance and chemical composition or surround themselves with a membrane. The youthful cells are tender, motile, and lack a membrane (i.e., they are protoblasts). Later many lose their motility owing to the formation of a tougher, firmer cytoplasmic structure. Old cells frequently lose their nuclei. Other conspicuous alterations within the cytoplasm, such as keratinization and mucoid or fatty changes, are frequent indications of the imminent death of the cell.

The *death of the cell* is a normal phenomenon in the animal body. Cells characterized by intensive metabolism (e.g., glandular cells) die off comparatively rapidly. The first evidence of dying is observed in the nucleus. It shrinks, assumes jagged contours, and loses its structure. The chromatin is clumped into a compact, spheroid mass, and stains uniformly dark (pyknotic[18] nucleus). The nucleus and chromatin soon break up into a number of fragments, which lose their staining properties and subsequently dissolve (karyolysis[19] and chromatolysis, respectively). The remains of the cytoplasm dissociate into granules or fatty substance and are sometimes phagocytosed. Cells often cornify and are shed as horny scales. Some cells are destroyed in the process of secretion (e.g., sebaceous gland cells). Wherever cells die, replacement is immediately provided by the formation of new cells. Once removed from the animal body, cells perish more or less rapidly, but ciliated cells, smooth muscle fibers, and cardiac muscle fibers may live for as long as 24 to 48 hours. Some cells survive for weeks in serum and may even divide and grow in that medium (tissue culture).

---

[17] Gr. *meiosis* diminution, from *meion* less.
[18] Gr. *pyknos* dense.   [19] Gr. *lyein* to dissolve.

II

The Epithelial Tissues

The Structure of Animal Tissues

A TISSUE is an association of cells with the interstitial substance they produce. The cells are alike in form and function and specialized for the per-
formance of a definite task.

The cell is the starting point of all histogenesis. It absorbs substances, processes
them, and deposits them either within itself or on its surface. Many of the original
properties of the cell are lost during histogenesis; others become more pronounced.
As it assumes definite tasks, the cell undergoes morphological changes (structural
adaptations) associated with the division of labor and loses its embryonic versatil-
ity as it takes on its characteristic traits.

The building stones of tissues are the cells. They also produce all the other building material. In the germ layers of the embryo they lie in contact with each other,
forming the most primitive kind of tissue. In the formation of definitive tissues they
produce the *intercellular substances* that are deposited between the cells. These intercellular substances may occur in very small quantity, as in epithelial tissues, where
they form a thin layer of *cement* between the cells. On the other hand, they may predominate over the cellular elements, as in connective tissues (p. 33). In the latter
case, the intercellular substance is composed of *amorphous ground substance* (matrix)
and *fibers*, the formed elements.[1] Insofar as the amorphous ground substance serves
to unite the fibers, it may also be called cement.

The intercellular substances may be products of cell secretion or cell metamorphosis. That elaborated by the connective tissue cells represents a special form of
the living substance. It participates, along with the cells, in the metabolic processes
and may even be capable of further independent differentiation.

In the early stages of histogenesis, the cells are in direct contact with each other,
sometimes without visible cell boundaries. Such a structure is called a syncytium.
With the deposition of the intercellular substances, this intimate relation is lost,

---

[1] Isidore Gersh and H. R. Catchpole, The Organization of Ground Substance and Basement
Membrane and Its Significance in Tissue Injury, Disease, and Growth, *Am. J. Anatomy 85* (1950):
457–522.

except for the cellular processes that traverse the intercellular substance and connect the cells in certain tissues.

Tissues are classified mainly by morphological criteria as follows:

1. Epithelial tissues
2. Connecting and supporting tissues
3. Muscular tissues
4. Nervous tissues
5. Blood and lymph, which may be considered tissues with liquid intercellular substances. When coagulated they resemble connective tissues.

In general, the tissues can only be delimited morphologically. From the functional viewpoint, it is inconceivable that epithelium could exist without connective

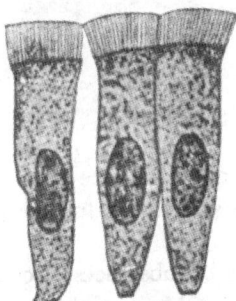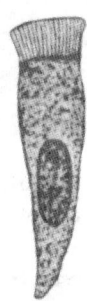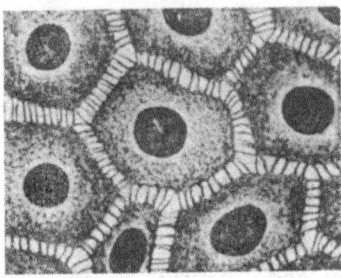

Figure 25 (left). Isolated columnar epithelial cells showing heavy cuticular border in the small intestine of a dog (700×).

Figure 26 (right). Epithelial cells with intercellular bridges; stratified squamous epithelium from the esophagus of a pig.

tissue, muscle without connective tissue and nerves, or nerves without connective tissue.

We must keep in mind that the customary morphological and functional classification of tissues is one-sided and often contradictory. Thus the epithelia are characterized by morphological features exclusively, while physiologically and embryologically they differ greatly among themselves. The supporting tissues, derived from mesenchyme, have a common embryological background, but they diverge widely in morphology and function. Muscular tissues are alike in function but not in form or origin. Nervous tissues are embryologically, but not morphologically, identical.

Epithelial Tissues

The epithelial[2] tissues consist of closely adjacent cells held together by small amounts of intercellular substance. The surface and protective epithelia are sheet-like cell associations which form thin and tender or thicker and more resistant covering membranes. These clothe all free external and internal body surfaces and

---

[2] Gr. *epi* on, and *thele* nipple. This kind of cellular arrangement was first observed on the nipple. Later the term was applied to all tissues of this type. *Thele* also means wart or papilla, and according to another derivation the term was originally restricted to the cell layers on top of the papillae of stratified squamous epithelium (Fig. 36).

furnish a protective cover for deeper-lying structures. They may at the same time perform such work as absorption and secretion, as well as other functions (e.g., those of pigmented or ciliated epithelium). Epithelium also occurs as glandular epithelium, the main component of glands, and as sensory epithelium. The latter is composed of highly specialized cells in the sensory organs.

The epithelial cells are relatively large. In the fresh state they may be light and transparent or granular and turbid. Their sharp boundaries are usually formed only by a layer of ectoplasm. Their variety of form, determined by adaptation to prevailing conditions of pressure around the cell, is accounted for by the consistency of their cytoplasm. It is generally soft, but at the same time greatly extensible and elastic, and therefore capable of continuous changes in shape. All epithelial cells

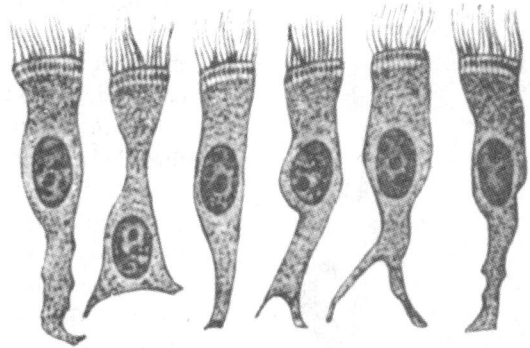

Figure 27. Isolated ciliated columnar cells from the trachea of a dog.

exhibit polar orientation; i.e., they possess a free pole and a basal pole. Their more or less flat lateral walls often serve in the exchange of nutrients. The free pole of the cell frequently bears a *cuticular border*[3] (p. 10 and Fig. 25). Sometimes the cells undergo a horny transformation. The cell surface is either smooth or marked by bulges and hollows. It is often covered with delicate cytoplasmic processes that run from cell to cell as *intercellular bridges* (Fig. 26). The intervening unoccupied intercellular spaces or clefts contain a fluid which plays an important part in the nourishment of the cell. In the upper strata of thick epithelia, the bridges are stretched farther and are more distinct because the intercellular clefts contain greater quantities of tissue fluid than they do in thinner epithelia or the basal layers of thick epithelia. Here the cells can obtain their nutriment from underlying tissues. The nucleus of epithelial cells usually lies in the basal portion of the cell, where the most favorable conditions for nourishment prevail. The Golgi apparatus is present in most epithelial cells and in all glandular cells. It is usually in the distal portion of the cell.

Epithelial cells are classified according to their shape as *squamous* or *columnar*. The former are wider than they are high, the latter higher than wide. An inter-

---

[3] L. *cutis* skin. This and similar uses of the term border are well-established misnomers. The cuticula is actually a layer; it appears as a border only in sections.

mediate form is represented by the *cuboidal* cells, which are of about equal width and height. *Ciliated epithelial cells* (Figs. 27; 28,*g*) are a special kind which bear on their free surface delicate, hairlike cytoplasmic processes of equal length. About fifty cilia are found on each of the cells. They show a vigorous beat directed toward the exterior. This motion occurs in waves resembling those caused by wind in a field of grain. The ciliary current thus generated is capable of expelling particulate matter (e.g., dust particles from the trachea). This activity is characteristic of true cilia (kinocilia) as opposed to the similar, but immobile, stereocilia.[4] Every cilium ends proximally in a basal corpuscle (Fig. 27), which is said to give origin to the ciliary beat. It is strongly refractive and is found in the cuticular border which is generally present, or immediately below it. Sometimes filamentous, conically converging structures (ciliary roots) run from the basal corpuscles past the nucleus to the basal part of the cell. Related to the stereocilia are the *brush borders*, which consist of fine, short rods on the distal end of the cell. Some epithelial cells present a striated appearance (basal filaments) in their proximal portion. According to the arrangement of the cells, we distinguish simple (single-layered) and stratified (many-layered) epithelia. The latter are classified according to the cell shape found in the surface layer.

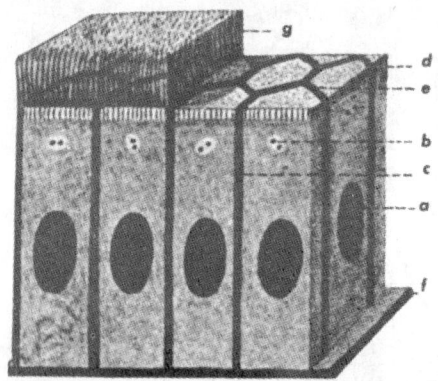

Figure 28. Simple columnar epithelium (schematic). *a*, nucleus; *b*, centriole; *c*, cement; *d*, terminal bar in cross section; *e*, terminal bar pattern, surface view; *f*, basement membrane; *g*, cilia.

Between the epithelial cells there is a presumably viscous material, the *intercellular cement*. This occurs in such small quantities that it has little effect on the form of the tissue, but it does serve to bind the cells together as mortar binds bricks. It differs chemically from the cells, coagulates upon death, and may then be dissolved by chemical reagents (30 percent alcohol, dilute chromic acid) that do not affect the cells so isolated. Treatment with silver nitrate followed by exposure to light stains the cement brown while the cells remain unstained. At the free surface or just under the cuticula, the intercellular substance of columnar epithelium usually shows a special staining reaction in the so-called *terminal bars* (Fig. 28,*d,e*). These are narrow strips of a relatively firm material that act as a frame around the free pole of the cell, sealing off the intercellular spaces from the surface. The terminal bars are interconnected and in a surface view form a network (Fig. 28,*e*). In sections perpendicular to the surface they appear as dots.

Epithelium is usually separated from the underlying connective tissue by a glassy, apparently homogeneous *basement membrane* (Figs. 28,*f*; 36,*b*) to which the cells adhere. It is a product of the underlying connective tissue, and can be demonstrated

---

[4] Gr. *stereis* rigid.

by proper techniques to contain a fine latticework of reticular fibers (p. 35). Occasionally, rootlike cytoplasmic processes reach into the underlying tissue.

Pigment may be formed and deposited in epithelial tissues. Sometimes leukocytes (wandering cells), nervous tissue, and occasionally blood capillaries appear. Worn-out cells are continuously replaced.

A. SURFACE AND PROTECTIVE EPITHELIA

According to the morphology and the stratification of the cells epithelia may be classified as follows:

1. Simple epithelium
$\begin{cases} \text{a. Squamous} \\ \text{b. Cuboidal} \\ \text{c. Columnar} \end{cases}$

2. Stratified epithelium
$\begin{cases} \text{a. Squamous} \\ \text{b. Columnar} \\ \text{c. Transitional} \end{cases}$

3. Pseudostratified epithelium

1. Simple Epithelium

(a) **Simple squamous[5] epithelium** (Figs. 29–31) consists of flat, scalelike, usually irregularly polygonal cells. Their borders are usually wavy, but sometimes

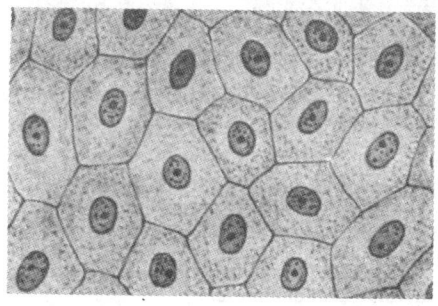

Figure 29 (left). Simple squamous epithelium from the lens of a cat (Zietzschmann); surface view. Note the straight cell boundaries (325×).

Figure 30. Simple squamous epithelium from the lens of a dog; a vertical section.

they are straight. They occur in a single layer. In a lateral view one sees little more than a line in which the nuclei appear as slight thickenings (Fig. 30). The cytoplasm is homogeneous and transparent or, rarely, granular.

OCCURRENCE. This type occurs in the epithelium of the rete testis, the inner wall of the membranous labyrinth of the ear, the epithelium of the lens, the parietal layer of Bowman's capsule, and the descending limb of Henle's loop in the kidney. There are three types of epithelium which are simple squamous morphologically, but have received other designations in recognition of their embryological origin: (1) *Mesothelium* covers the serous membranes (pleura, pericardium, and peritoneum; Fig. 31). It is formed from the mesoderm and is originally columnar. In the embryo it bears flagella which may persist on the flattened cells after birth. Unlike other epithelia, mesothelium destroyed in the adult can be replaced by fibroblasts. Conversely, in inflammation, mesothelial cells change into fibroblasts. (2)

---

[5] L. *squama* scale.

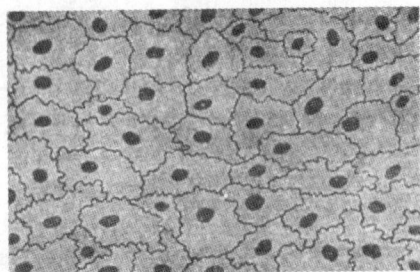

Figure 31. Surface view of a simple squamous epithelium (mesothelium) from the mesentery of a horse. Note the irregular cell boundaries, blackened by silver nitrate.

Endothelium lines the blood and lymph vascular system (Fig. 54,*a**). It is derived from mesenchyme. (3) *Mesenchymal epithelium* is a catchall term for the remaining simple squamous epithelium derived from the mesenchyme; it lines the subdural and subarachnoid spaces, the perilymphatic spaces of the ear, and the anterior chamber of the eye.

The *pigmented epithelium* of the retina (Figs. 32, 33) is intermediate in height between squamous and cuboidal epithelium. The cytoplasm of its hexagonal prismatic cells contains brown or black rods of pigment (fuscin) which permit the non-pigmented nucleus to shine through as a round light spot. Where the cells face the rods and cones of the retina, they bear fringelike processes (Fig. 33).

(b) Simple cuboidal epithelium (Fig. 34) consists of somewhat higher cells with straight contours. They are short prisms with four or more sides. They appear square in sections perpendicular to the surface, and may be ciliated.

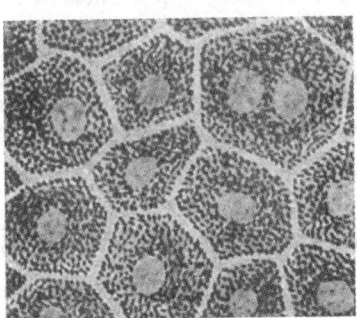

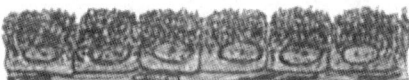

Figure 33. Vertical section through the pigmented retinal epithelium of a sheep.

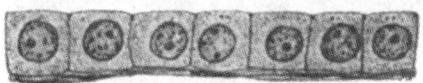

Figure 34. Cuboidal epithelium from the thyroid gland of a horse.

Figure 32 (left). Surface view of the pigmented retinal epithelium of a dog (320×). At the top, right, is a large cell with two nuclei. The pigment is in the form of crystalline rods. The nucleus shows up as a light spot in the cell.

OCCURRENCE. This type is found on the chorioid plexuses, in many glands and their excretory ducts, in the lateral parts of the anterior epithelium of the lens, in the neighborhood of the maculae and cristae staticae, in the organ of Corti, and in the germinal epithelium.

(c) Simple columnar epithelium (Figs. 28, 35) consists of cylindrical, prismatic, or pyramidal cells that are higher than they are wide. The ovoid nucleus is usually found in the basal half of the cell, while the centrosome lies near the free end.

The free surface often bears cilia or a cuticular border (Figs. 25; 35,*A,a*). The

---

* Fig. 54 is on p. 51.

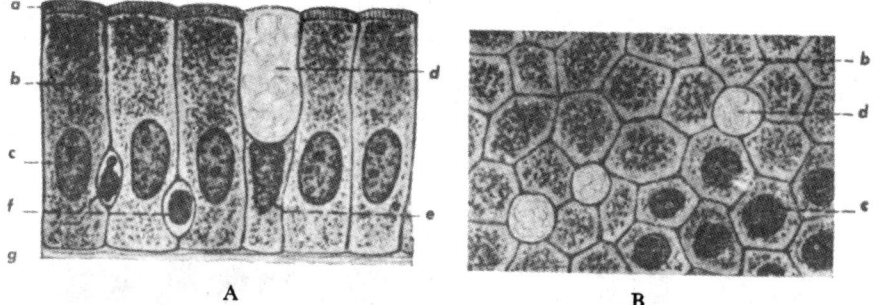

Figure 35. A, longitudinal section and, B, cross section through the simple columnar epithelium of an intestinal villus of a donkey. a, cuticular border; b, cytoplasm; c, nucleus; d, goblet cell with e, its nucleus; f, nuclei of leukocytes (wandering cells); g, basement membrane.

latter may be given a striated appearance by fine perforating canaliculi, which in turn are invaded by cytoplasmic processes. The cell often adheres to its base by means of delicate anchoring processes. The columnar cells are not rigid structures but are capable of changing their height according to the pressure to which they are subjected.

OCCURRENCE. This type occurs in the mucosa of the gastrointestinal tract, in many excretory ducts of glands (kidney, accessory sex glands), in the gall bladder, and in some of the sensory epithelia.

Ciliated simple columnar epithelium is found in the oviduct, the head of the epididymis, the small bronchi, the paranasal sinuses. The simple columnar epithelium of the uterus is ciliated at certain times. A special type of ciliated columnar epithelium is found in the ependyma of the cerebral ventricles and the central canal of the spinal chord.

2. Stratified Epithelium

(a) **Stratified squamous epithelium** (Figs. 36, 37) derives its name from the flattened cells of its surface layer. It forms membranes up to several millimeters thick.

The basal layer, resting upon the basement membrane, is composed of soft columnar cells (stratum cylindricum, Fig. 36,c) with an oval nucleus (Fig. 38,a,b). Occasionally these cells send delicate processes into the underlying tissue. The cells in the middle layers are polyhedral with a spherical nucleus (Fig. 36,d). They show evidence of the pressure they exert on one another in the form of ridges and furrows (Fig. 38). Here we also find cells with processes that are inserted between other cells (Fig. 38,d). Upon isolation all cells in the middle layer exhibit fine rod- or thornlike processes on their surface. They are therefore called prickle cells (stratum spinosum, Figs. 26; 36,d). These spines are broken intercellular bridges. They serve as a good example of connections between epithelial cells. Often, as in skin epithelium, cytoplasmic strands called tonofibrils run through the processes. They may extend through several cells and are considered to be supporting structures. They probably develop as a result of tension in the cytoplasm.

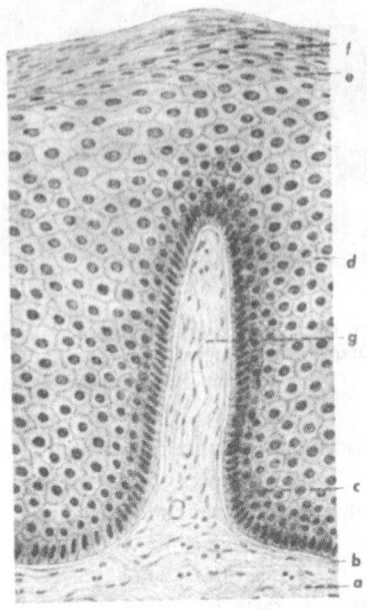

Figure 36 (left). Stratified squamous epithelium from the stomach of a horse. a, subepithelial connective tissue of the mucosa; b, basement membrane; c, deepest, columnar, cell layer (stratum cylindricum); d, intermediate cell layers (prickle cells); e and f, superficial flat cells; g, a mucosal papilla.

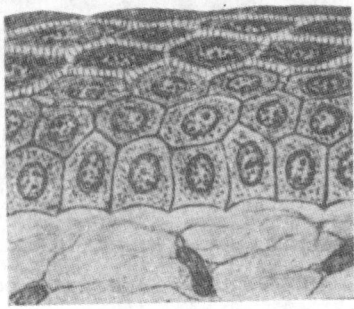

Figure 37. Stratified squamous epithelium without papillae, from the pharynx of a dog.

The cells of the superficial layers (Figs. 36,e,f; 38,f) are always greatly flattened and contain a flat nucleus. Generally the cells cornify, forming the stratum corneum as the deeper layers are pushed toward the surface and are exposed to the drying action of the air. They are then scaled off (desquamated) either singly or in groups forming grossly visible scales. The nuclei are no longer visible. (See skin, p. 335.)

The cells of stratified squamous epithelia are not rigid but yield to pressure and show resilience on bending, etc. From the vascular connective tissue base, conical protuberances called papillae (Figs. 36,g; 126) extend into the epithelium. The papillae contain capillary loops and are important in the nutrition of the epithelium.

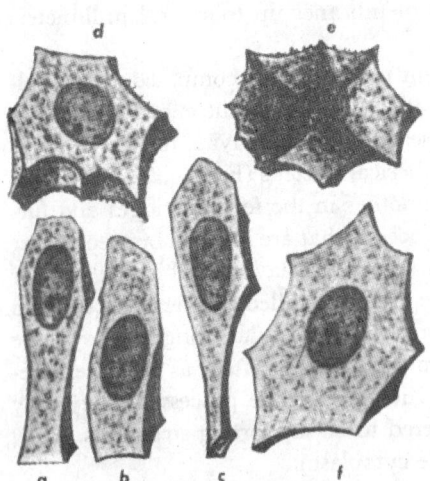

Figure 38 (left). Isolated cells from the stratified squamous epithelium of the cornea of a horse (700×). a,b,c, columnar cells from the basal layer; d,e, cells from the intermediate layer (d, lateral; e, basal view); f, flattened cell from the most superficial layer (surface view).

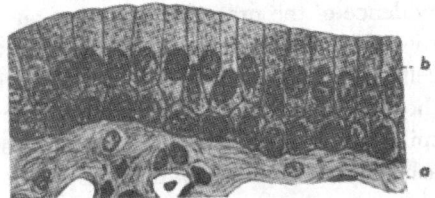

Figure 39. Two-layered columnar epithelium. a, subepithelial connective tissue; b, epithelium.

The papillae in the aggregate constitute the papillary body. Papillae are lacking when there are but few cell layers present (Fig. 37).

OCCURRENCE. This type of epithelium may be found wherever the body surfaces are exposed to severe mechanical or chemical insult: the epithelium of the skin (epidermis), digestive tract from the mouth to the secretory portion of the stomach, anal canal, anterior surface of the cornea, bulbar conjunctiva, lacrimal canaliculi, vaginal vestibule, glans penis, and elsewhere.

(b) Stratified columnar epithelium (Figs. 39; 41,*b*) is characterized by columnar cells in the top cell layer; underneath are found conical cells with the apex directed toward the surface, fusiform cells, and other forms that fill the spaces be-

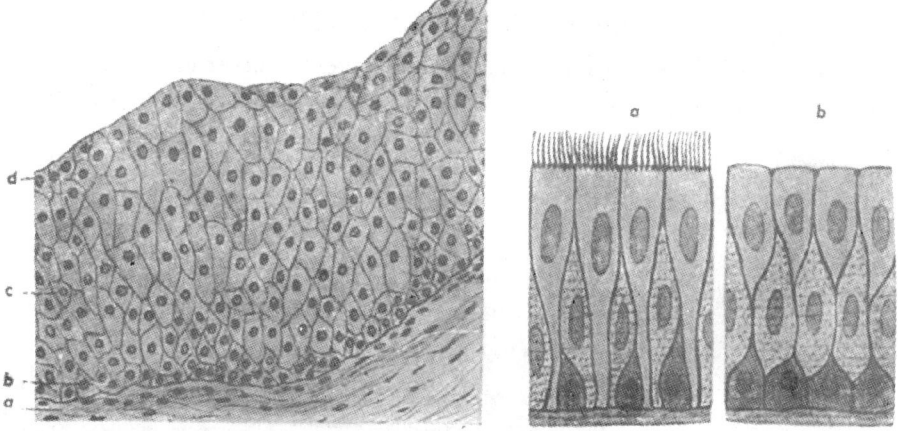

Figure 40 (left). Transitional epithelium from the ureter of a horse. *a,* subepithelial connective tissue; *b,* deepest, *c,* intermediate, *d,* superficial, cell layers.

Figure 41 (right). a, pseudostratified ciliated epithelium (schematic); *b,* stratified columnar epithelium (schematic).

tween the tapering ends of the superficial layer. Under these are one or several layers of polyhedral cells which adhere—with or without the help of basal processes—to the basement membrane.

OCCURRENCE. This type occurs in the larger excretory ducts of some glands and in the epithelium of the palpebral conjunctiva of horses and carnivores.

(c) Transitional epithelium (Fig. 40) is intermediate between stratified squamous and stratified columnar epithelium. The deeper layers resemble those of stratified columnar epithelium. The surface cells are very extensible and variable in shape. In addition to the columnar, there are cuboidal or flat (bricklike) cells. The latter are never as flat as the cells of stratified squamous epithelium; they vary in height according to the state of distention of the organ they line (Figs. 305, 306). These cells often possess a layer of thickened ectoplasm on their free surface. A basement membrane is apparently lacking in this type of epithelium. Capillaries from the highly vascular connective tissue base frequently reach out between the more deeply situated epithelial cells.

OCCURRENCE. Transitional epithelium is found in the excretory passages of the urinary system.

3. Pseudostratified Epithelium

All cells in this type of epithelium adhere to a common base, but not all of them extend to the free surface (Fig. 41,a). Their nuclei lie in different planes. As some cells are joined to the epithelium by threadlike processes only, it is often difficult to differentiate between pseudostratified and stratified columnar epithelium. The former is usually ciliated.

OCCURRENCE. Pseudostratified epithelium occurs in the respiratory region of the nasal cavity, larynx, trachea, large bronchi, epididymis.

B. GLANDULAR EPITHELIUM

Many epithelial cells do not merely form a protective cover for the underlying tissues. They elaborate substances which are not incorporated in the tissues, but

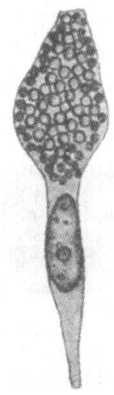

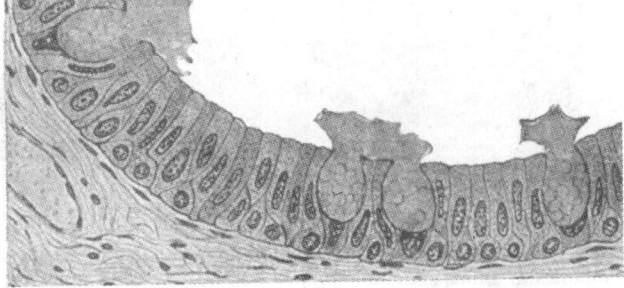

(After Zipkin.)　　　　　*Figure 43.* Goblet cells (blue) in an epithelial membrane.

find other uses as *secretions* or are eliminated as useless *excretions*. This sort of activity characterizes gland cells. They are found either singly between the nonsecretory cells of protective epithelia as unicellular glands, or they form more or less extensive associations as multicellular glands. The glands are usually displaced by growth from the surface to a deeper position. Thus they acquire excretory ducts lined with epithelium and opening on the surface at the point where the gland started on its downward growth.

Many glandular cells contain granules that are considered the precursors of the actual secretion (Fig. 173). These granules enlarge, become more or less liquefied, and emerge on the free surface (external secretion, Fig. 43), while the cell reverts to the depleted condition. During the formation and accumulation of its secretory constituents the cell increases in volume. Formation, storage, and extrusion of secreta may be demonstrated in favorable histological preparations. In the case of internal secretion (p. 137), the glandular products are borne away by the blood or lymphatic system. The mitochondria probably play an important part in granule formation. Only special techniques will render the granules visible.

The *unicellular glands* occur as goblet cells in the intestinal, respiratory, and conjunctival epithelium, where their mucous secretion fulfills important protective functions (Figs. 35,*d;* 42; 43; 452,*g;* 453,*e*). The distended, goblet-like distal part of the cytoplasm usually tapers basally to a slender stem, which contains the nucleus surrounded by undifferentiated cytoplasm. The remaining cytoplasm consists of a varying quantity of pale mucigenous granules (secretory granules), which lie embedded in a small amount of matrix. These are the forerunners of the mucous secretion, but because of their instability they are rarely seen as granules in histological preparations. Absorption of water causes a confluence of the granules followed by the extrusion of a flocculent mass of mucus at the free cell pole (stoma).

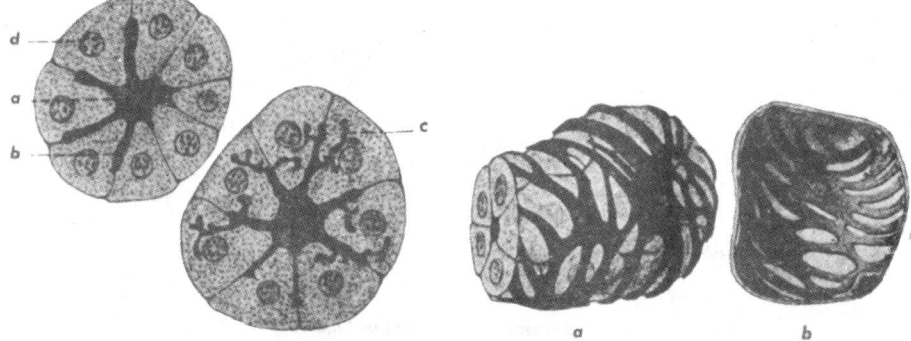

Figure 44 (left). Cross sections of glandular tubules showing secretory canaliculi. *a,* lumen of the gland; *b,* intercellular, and *c,* intracellular, secretory canaliculi; *d,* secretory cells.

Figure 45 (right). Secretory end-pieces with basket cells. *a,* end-piece, outside view; *b,* basement membrane of an end-piece, inside view with secretory cells removed.

Multicellular glands are rarely confined to the thickness of the covering epithelium as intra-epithelial glands. They usually grow into the underlying tissues, thereby gaining a larger surface area and greater secretory capacity. In this way is formed a system of interconnected cavities, which vary in shape and width and are lined or filled with epithelial cells. These tunnel-like spaces may lose all connection with the surface and become ductless or *endocrine*[6] glands like the thyroid or adrenal (p. 137). If they maintain their outside communication, they are called *exocrine* glands. In the latter case, the secretory activity is often confined to those cells that lie near the blindly ending portions of the gland. They absorb substances from the blood, process them, and pour the finished product into the lumen of the gland. From here the secretion is transported to the outside (to the skin or a visceral lumen) via the excretory duct.

In some glands delicate, unlined canaliculi branch off from the lumen. These may either extend into the cells as intracellular secretory canaliculi (Fig. 44,*c*), or they may pass between the cells as intercellular secretory canaliculi or capillaries (Fig. 44,*b*). They may be simple or branched. Special techniques are required to render them visible.

---

[6] Gr. *endon* within, and *krinein* to secrete.

The glandular epithelium is separated by a basement membrane from the surrounding connective tissue. Inside of the basement membrane of some glands there are star-shaped, interconnected basket cells or elongated smooth muscle cells (myoepithelial cells, Figs. 45; 392*), which surround the terminal portions of the gland. Their contractions are believed to aid in the emptying of the end-pieces. Around the basement membrane is a fibroelastic connective tissue sheath containing blood capillaries, nerves, and sometimes smooth muscle fibers (Fig. 170). Between this sheath and the basement membrane there are frequently lymph spaces or one continuous lymph space.

Glands are classified according to the shape of the lumina of their terminal portions and the arrangement of their ducts as follows:

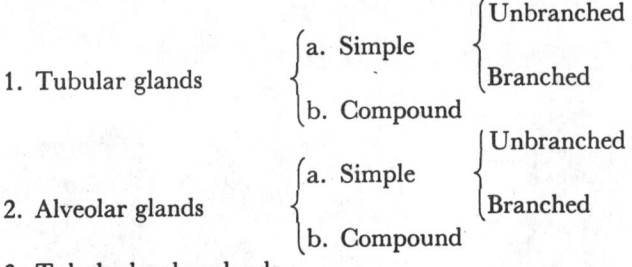

1. Tubular glands   a. Simple   Unbranched / Branched   b. Compound

2. Alveolar glands   a. Simple   Unbranched / Branched   b. Compound

3. Tubuloalveolar glands

* Fig. 392 is on p. 297.

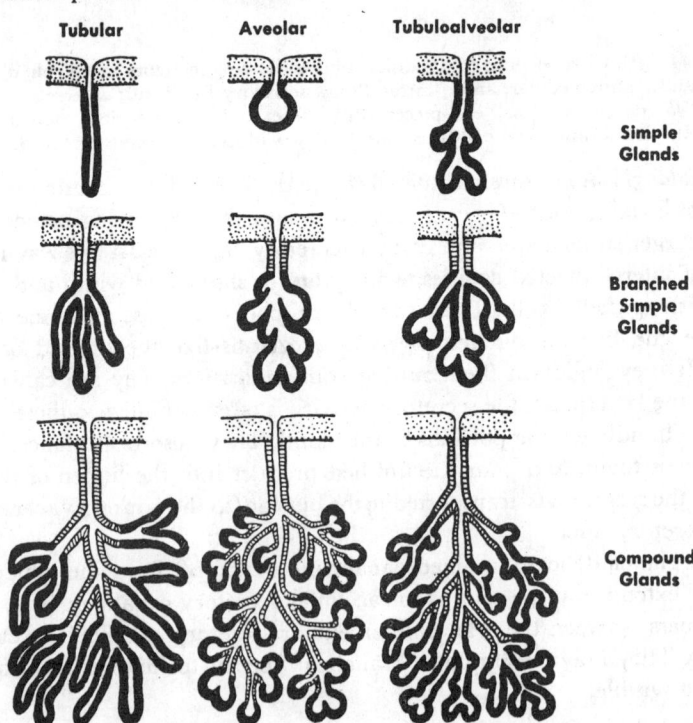

Figure 46. Diagram of the various types of glands

Simple glands (Fig. 46) have either no excretory duct or one that is unbranched. Compound glands have branched excretory ducts.

Tubular glands (Fig. 46) are characterized by the cylindrical shape of their end-pieces. They may be coiled into a tight knot (Fig. 47). Alveolar glands have more or less spherical or hemispherical terminal portions with a saclike lumen (Figs. 46, 48). A spherical end-piece with a narrow lumen is called an acinus.

Tubuloalveolar glands (Fig. 46) are mixed forms having both kinds of end-pieces, or tubular secretory portions with lateral and terminal alveoli.

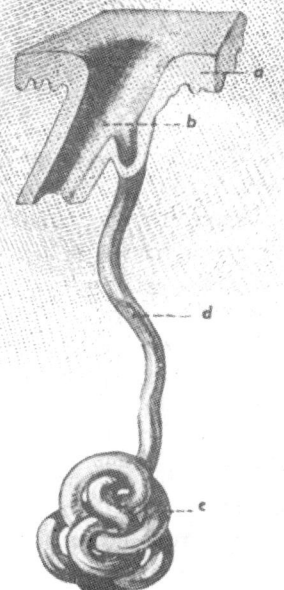

Figure 47 (left). Tubular skin gland, a stereogram. *a*, epidermis; *b*, neck of hair follicle; *c*, secretory end-piece; *d*, excretory duct.

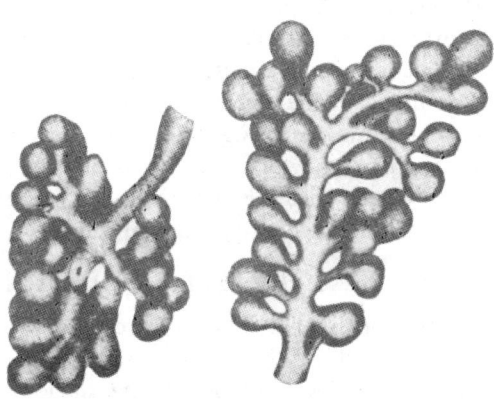

Figure 48. Alveolar glands.

Secretory cells are classified on the basis of their secretions as serous, mucous, or mixed (mucoserous). (See also p. 000.) *Serous glands* contain only epithelium that elaborates a watery albuminous secretion. *Mucous glands* consist of epithelium that produces mucus, a cohesive, slimy fluid. A *mixed gland*, finally, is one that contains both kinds of cells. These may be present in the same end-piece or in separate end-pieces or lobules. There are also cells that produce different kinds of secretions in succession (e.g., in the bulbo-urethral gland).

Examples of serous glands are the parotid, the pancreas, and the liver. The small glands of the oral cavity are mostly mucous. The mandibular and sublingual salivary glands are of the mixed type.

Glands are also distinguished by the morphological changes involved in the secretory process. We recognize three types: merocrine, apocrine, and holocrine glands.[7] Where secretion leaves the glandular cell essentially intact, we speak of *merocrine glands*. Here secretion merely involves the extrusion of secretory products. In cells of the *apocrine* type the distal part of the cell is thrown into the secretion

---

[7] Gr. *meros* part, *holos* whole, *apo* away from, and *krinein* to secrete.

(as in the mammary gland). *Holocrine* glands are those whose secretion consists of dead cells, for example, the sebaceous glands. Other glands (the testis and ovary) produce live cells.

The excretory ducts of glands consist of an elastic connective tissue sheath, which may also contain muscle fibers, and of an epithelial lining, often composed of non-secreting cells. The shape of the cells varies with the size of the ducts. The small ducts generally show a cuboidal type of epithelium, while simple, double, or stratified columnar epithelium is found in the larger ones.

The terminal branches of the ducts end in one or several secretory end-pieces. These, with the terminal branch, make up a primary lobule. When several primary lobules are joined to form a larger group by the confluence of their efferent ductules into one larger branch, a secondary lobule is formed. This process may go on with a resulting formation of tertiary lobules, etc.

The interstitial connective tissue of glands is usually sparse within lobules, and in the vicinity of capillaries it has the characteristics of reticular connective tissue. It is more abundant between lobules. At the periphery it blends into the capsule of the gland. The interstitial connective tissue contains excretory ducts, nerves, and numerous blood vessels. The latter form an extensive capillary net next to the basement membrane (Fig. 122). The nerves here are extremely delicate, non-medullated fibers which may surround the basement membrane or penetrate it and end on the cells themselves. In the former case they are said to form an epilemmal, in the latter, a hypolemmal[8] plexus.

C. SENSORY EPITHELIUM (NEUROEPITHELIUM)

The neuroepithelial cells act as receptors for stimuli from the outside. They are elongated structures that stand close together on their base. As a rule they exhibit a fusiform swelling that contains the nucleus. The free end is equipped with cuticular appendages in the form of small rods or hairs, and the basal end or cell body is in contact with nerve fibers. The olfactory cells are an exception in that their basal end is continuous with the axis cylinder of a nerve fiber. This indicates that the olfactory cells are actually nerve cells. The neuroepithelial cells are variously arranged in the different sense organs. They either form a continuous layer of adjacent vertical cells, or they occur singly or in groups between ordinary, usually columnar, epithelial cells so that every sensory cell or every group of sensory cells is surrounded by one or more layers of supporting cells.

OCCURRENCE. The neuroepithelial cells occur in taste buds, the olfactory epithelium, the cristae and maculae staticae, the organ of Corti, and the retina.

THE DERIVATION OF EPITHELIA. The epithelial tissues are derived from all three germ layers. They develop into their definitive forms according to their arrangement within the organism, their functions, and the stimuli to which they are exposed.

---

[8] Gr. *epi* upon, and *hypo* below; *lemma* sheath.

III

The Connecting and

Supporting Tissues

IN CONTRAST to the epithelia, the connecting and supporting tissues are almost always separated from free surfaces. They serve to fill interstices, to encapsulate organs, to connect parts and maintain their relative positions, and to furnish support and security. They form the passive locomotor organs and the attachments of the active locomotor organs. In accordance with their mechanical function, they are sometimes very soft (loose connective tissue), sometimes firm but still cleavable (cartilage), sometimes hard as stone (bone). These differences in firmness, hardness, and elasticity are dependent on the nature of the intercellular substance secreted by the cells. The connective tissues consist of (1) cells and (2) intercellular material, the latter of which in turn is composed of (a) fibers and (b) amorphous ground substance (matrix). The term amorphous is used here to mean formless as seen with the ordinary light microscope. It is probable that the ground substance has a definite submicroscopic structure. The intercellular substance usually predominates over the cellular elements. In exceptional cases it is less prominent and its function is assumed by the cell membranes or the cellular substance itself.

The intercellular material yields glue or related substances when boiled, and in the youthful state contains much mucin. All connective tissues develop from the mesenchyme, are often continuous with each other, and often substitute for each other in different species. Neuroglia (the supporting tissue of the central nervous system), derived from ectoderm, is an exception.

We distinguish (a) connective tissue proper, (b) adipose tissue, (c) cartilage, and (d) bone, with which perhaps the dentin should be included.

A. CONNECTIVE TISSUE PROPER

The cell masses which split off or grow out from the epithelial association of the middle germ layer and give rise to the connective tissues are called mesenchyme. All the mesenchymal tissue is continuous, whereas the primordia of the organs are separate. The continuity of the mesenchyme holds the body together, and this characteristic is maintained through all the later development. Through the pathways of the mesenchymal system every part of the body is accessible from every other part. For this reason, the mesenchymal tissue becomes the carrier of all the conduction systems: vessels, nerves, and ducts. While some constituents of the mesenchyme (e.g., cartilage, bone) remain in an indifferent stage and only later begin their tissue-building functions, one part differentiates early into embryonic connective tissue (Fig. 49). This consists of stellate, branched, spindle-shaped cells with relatively large nuclei, poor in chromatin. The cytoplasmic processes anas-

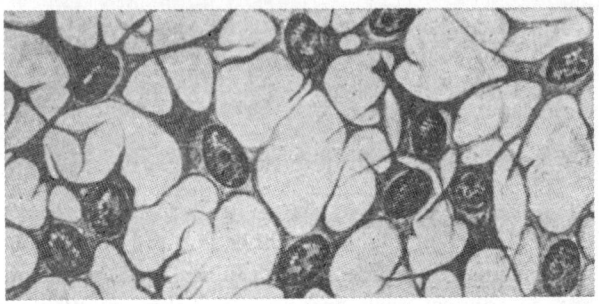

Figure 49. Embryonic connective tissue, from 12-mm. pig fetus.

tomose so that the embryonic connective tissue may be regarded as a reticular syncytium, the meshes of which are filled by a soft, viscous, interstitial substance (intercellular or ground substance).

From the embryonic connective tissue, which in embryos and fetuses covers the whole body under the ectoderm and fills all the spaces between organs, all other forms of connective tissue develop. In the process the cells undergo changes, and fibrillar structures appear in the intercellular substance. We distinguish collagenous, elastic, and reticular fibers.

Collagenous Fibers (Figs. 54,*f**; 57,*a*). They consist of very fine fibrils (0.3–0.5 μ thick), which are smooth, unbranched, and usually wavy. The fibrils are always united by a mucoid cement into bundles (fibers), which, in contrast to fibrils, may branch. The collagenous fibers usually unite to form strands and trabeculae. They are pale (i.e., only slightly refractive), very slightly extensible, and possessed of great tensile strength. (The Achilles tendon, for example, can withstand 6 kg. per sq. mm.) When boiled, they yield glue, whence the term collagenous.[1] Their principal constituent is the protein collagen. In dilute acids and alkalies they swell and gradually dissolve. They stain red with eosin and van Gieson's stain, blue with Mallory's stain.

Elastic Fibers (Figs. 54,*g**; 57,*b*,*c*). They may be very fine or very thick (18 μ). They are highly refractive (bright with dark borders). They branch but do not form bundles. The ends are often curved like a shepherd's crook. They are often mixed, singly or as nets, with collagenous fibers. They may be selectively stained

---

[1] Gr. *kolla* glue, and *gennan* to produce.   * Fig. 54 is on p. 51.

brown with orcein, dark blue with resorcin-fuchsin. They are elastic; i.e., they are extensible and return after stretching to their former length. Elastic fibers and their principal constituent, the protein elastin, are resistant to boiling, acids, and alkalies.

Reticular Fibers (Fig. 53). The name of these fibers is derived from their presence in reticular connective tissue (see p. 36), and from the fact that they branch and anastomose, as collagenous fibers are not supposed to do. They vary in thickness, but are usually very fine; they form no bundles, but lattice-like networks. They are more resistant to boiling, acids, and alkalies than collagenous fibers, but resemble the latter in their reactions to Mallory's stain. According to Plenk, they are precollagenous fibers. With Bielschowsky's silver solution they stain black and are therefore called argyrophil[2] fibers.

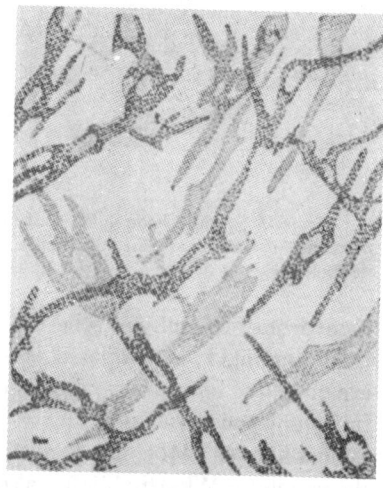

Figure 50. Pigment cells from the stratum suprachorioideum of the horse. The nuclei of the individual cells appear as light areas.

OCCURRENCE. The reticular fibers are incorporated in the finer structure of many organs. They are joined by the collagenous fibers, with which they may be continuous. Reticular fibers are found in lymphatic tissue and in the interstitial tissue of various glands, e.g., in endocrine glands. They are also distributed along the liver sinusoids and the capillaries of the kidney. By the Bielschowsky method, certain membranes that were formerly considered to be homogeneous have been demonstrated to consist of a feltwork of argyrophil fibers, e.g., the basement membrane of the epidermis and the glands, the membranelles (sheaths) of smooth muscle fibers, the sarcolemma of striated muscle, and the fat cell membrane.

The gelatinous fluid ground substance which fills the intercellular spaces in embryonic connective tissue remains as a mucoid, amorphous, totally displaceable mass in the other forms of connective tissue. It forms membranes with the invested fibers in loose connective tissue and constitutes the scanty cement that binds the fibrils into fibers. According to the arrangement and nature of the intercellular substance or of the cells, the following kinds of connective tissue are recognized:

1. Embryonic. Homogeneous ground substance predominates.
2. Reticular.
3. Fibrillar. Fibrillar intercellular substance predominates.
4. Elastic.

1. Embryonic Connective Tissue

This is described on p. 34.

In *mucous connective tissue* (Fig. 51), which represents the next stage of develop-

---

[2] Gr. *argyros* silver, and *philein* to love.

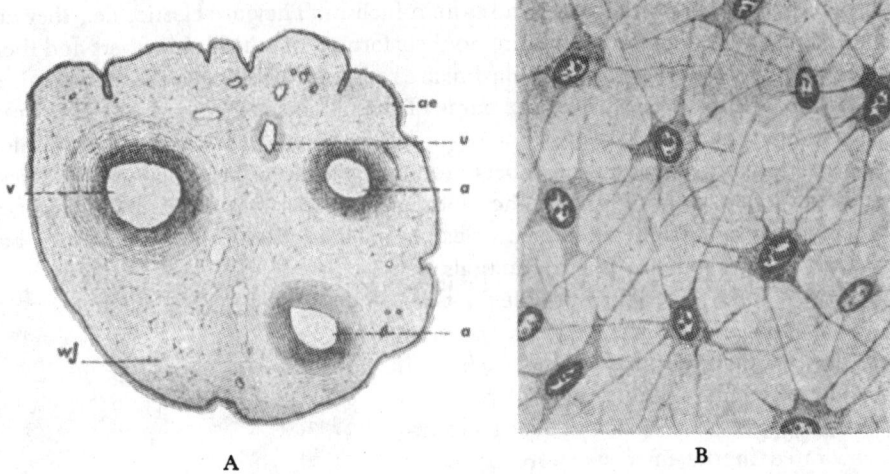

A   B

Figure 51. Section through the umbilical cord of a pig. *A: ae*, amnion epithelium; *a*, umbilical arteries; *v*, umbilical vein; *u*, urachus; *wj*, Wharton's jelly. *B:* Wharton's jelly, greater magnification.

ment from mesenchyme, the fibrillar intercellular substance has not yet become predominant. It is composed of a gelatinous, mucous ground substance in which are embedded fine wavy collagenous fibers and stellate or rounded cells connected by cytoplasmic processes.

OCCURRENCE. Mucous connective tissue is found in the umbilical cord around the vessels, as Wharton's jelly, also in embryos in place of the future perilymphatic spaces of the inner ear. The omasal papillae contain a tissue of similar structure, as does the supporting lamella in the comb and in the wattles of the chicken.

A related tissue in the adult is the *pigmented connective tissue* of the eye (Fig. 50). It consists of branched connective tissue cells with lobulated, often coarse, processes and yellow-brown to black pigment granules. The cells anastomose. The nucleus is free of pigment and is seen as a light spot under certain conditions. There are also bundles of collagenous fibrils.

OCCURRENCE. The pigmented connective tissue is present in the chorioid, ciliary body, iris, and sclera, and scattered in the skin.

2. Reticular Tissue

Reticular tissue presents a wide- or narrow-meshed network of reticular cells united in a syncytium (Fig. 52). The arrangement resembles that of mesenchymal cells. The reticular fibers (Fig. 53), produced by the cells and occurring mostly in the cytoplasmic network, serve to support and lend firmness to the syncytium. The fibers, which pass through the cell processes, are usually entirely surrounded by cytoplasm, but often appear to lie on the surface. The presence of elastic and collagenous fibers in the reticulum has been reported.

One form of reticular tissue never occurs alone but always from its first appearance contains in its meshes other mesenchymal derivatives, the lymphocytes. These

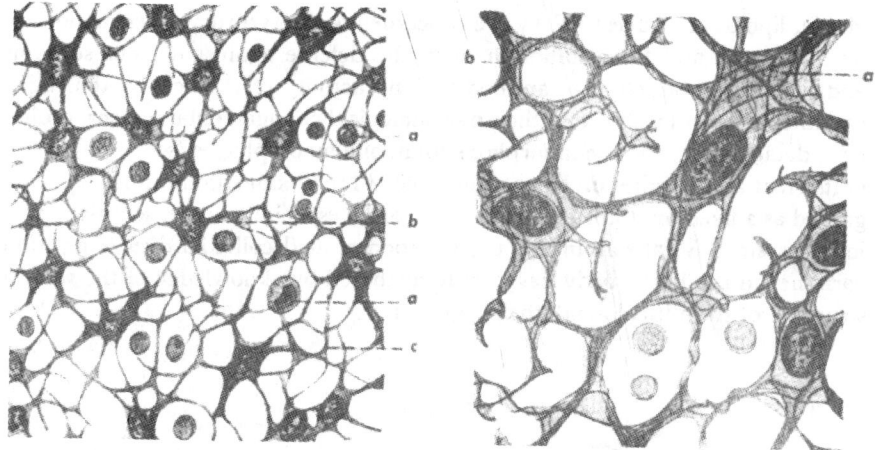

Figure 52 (left). Reticular tissue from a mesenteric lymph node of the horse. Most of the lymph cells have been shaken out of the section. *a*, lymphocytes and (below) macrophage; *b*, reticular cell; *c*, netlike connections of the reticular cells. The fibers in the reticulum are not represented.

Figure 53 (right). Reticular fibers in reticular cells; demonstrated by silver methods. *a*, reticular cell with intracellular reticular fibers; *b*, meshes of the reticulum.

cells, which are not attached to the tissue, occur at first sparsely, but later in such masses that they obscure the reticulum. The latter can be seen only after removal of the lymphocytes by brushing, shaking or selective staining. This mixed tissue of sessile reticular cells, which produce the fiber network, and the loosely embedded lymphocytes is called *lymphatic tissue*.[3] The reticular cells can usually be recognized only by their nuclei, which are larger and stain lighter than the lymphocyte nuclei.

OCCURRENCE. Reticular tissue forms the finer framework of whole organs, such as lymph nodes, solitary and aggregated lymph nodules, tonsils, spleen, and bone marrow; it is also found in the thymus, intestinal mucosa, conjunctiva, and elsewhere. Where the reticular fibers form a latticework around the end-pieces of glands, muscle fibers, or capillaries, the reticular cells lie on the outside of the lattice.

The close relationship apparent in certain organs between reticular and certain special endothelial cells, not only in cytoplasmic and fibrillar connections but also in functional similarities, has led to the designation *reticulo-endothelial system*. To this system belong the lining cells of the sinuses of the lymph nodes; the sinusoids of the spleen, bone marrow, and liver; and the reticular cells of the splenic pulp and the other lymphatic tissues (lymph nodes, tonsils, and lymph nodules). They are intimately related and form the reticulo-endothelial system in the narrow sense. They are distinguished by their phagocytosis of erythrocytes, foreign particles, bacteria, and protozoa, and by their storage of colloidal substances (hemo-

---

[3] Lymphatic tissue is also called lymphoreticular, adenoid, cytogenic, cytoblastic, lymphoid, and lymphadenoid.

globin, lipoids, and dyes).[4] They are concerned with erythrocyte destruction, with iron, vitamin, and fat metabolism, with the defense against noxious substances, and with the production of antibodies. The activity of the cells of the reticulo-endothelial system is shown in their morphological changes, enlargement, proliferation, detachment, and metamorphosis to mobile macrophages (see p. 39). Because of its great adaptability under the influence of functional stimuli, it is less to be regarded as a fixed anatomical concept than as an especially labile, sensitive, physiological system. Vital staining by the injection of acid colloidal dyes (e.g., lithium carmine) in the living body has greatly furthered our knowledge of the work and structure of the reticulo-endothelial system.

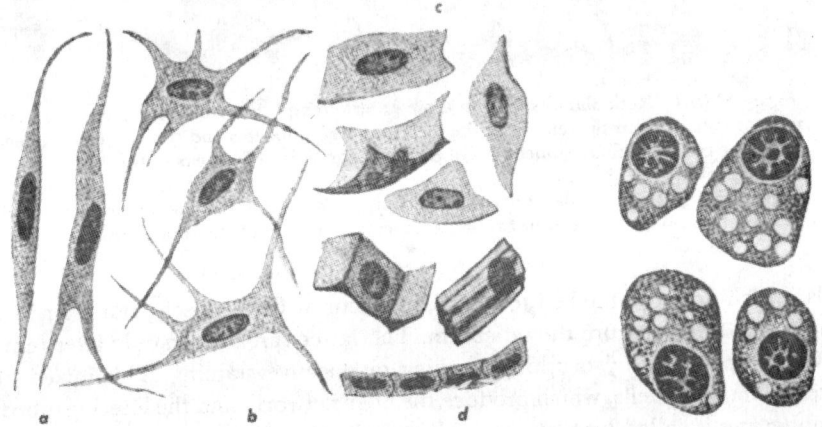

Figure 55 (left). Fibroblasts. *a*, spindle-shaped; *b*, stellate; *c*, flat, some bent; *d*, tendon cells arranged in rows.
Figure 56 (right). Plasma cells. The nuclear pattern is typical.

3. Fibrillar Connective Tissue

In fibrillar connective tissue the intercellular substance with its collagenous fibrils predominates over the cells. The extremely fine collagenous fibrils are held together by small amounts of amorphous cement to form longitudinally striated fibers. The fibroblasts (Fig. 55) lie on these bundles of fibrils (Fig. 57,*a*). The collagenous bundles are always accompanied by elastic fibers (Fig. 57,*b*), which may predominate in numbers, forming a special tissue. (For their characteristics see p. 34.)

The following kinds of cells occur in fibrillar connective tissue:

The fixed connective tissue cells, *fibroblasts*[5] (Figs. 54,*c**; 55) with their elliptical, chromatin-poor nuclei are usually greatly flattened and conform in shape to the

---

[4] Other mesenchymal cells (histiocytes, splenocytes, and monocytes) show a similar storage and are therefore included in the reticulo-endothelial system in the broad sense.
[5] L. *fibra* fiber, and Gr. *blastos* germ, bud.   * Fig. 54 is on p. 51.

course of the fibers. They may be curved or sharply bent, sometimes with ragged, veil-like processes that connect the fibroblasts with each other. They lie immediately upon the bundles of fibrils and often form complete sheaths around them. The fibroblasts produce the fibrous intercellular substance.

Histiocytes (Fig. 54,*d**) are thin, often multiform cells which resemble fibroblasts and are considered by some authors to be formed from them as a result of irritation. Histiocytes, however, have sharper outlines and stain better than do fibroblasts; they possess abundant granular cytoplasmic inclusions, and their nuclei are richer in chromatin. Above all, they have the power of phagocytosis, and for this reason they are also called fixed macrophages.[6] They store foreign substances, for example, intravitally injected dyes (neutral red), in the form of granules. They are considered to be "resting wandering cells," which may resume their wanderings upon suitable stimulation. They are found principally in the subcutaneous tissue and mesentery, where they are especially numerous near the small blood vessels. They have great significance in the defense activities of the body.

Lymphocytes continually pass from the blood vessels into the connective tissue and thence into, or through, the epithelia.

Coarsely granular *acidophil leukocytes* (granulocytes, p. 91) wander out of the blood vessels. They are especially numerous in the intestinal mucosa.

Mast cells (Fig. 54,*b**) resemble the coarsely granular, basophil leukocytes of the blood (oval cell body, rounded nucleus, basophilic water-soluble granules), but are not identical with them. They are found only in loose connective tissue, often in rows along the vessels. In spite of their name (Ger. *mästen*, to fatten) they have nothing to do with nutrition. Perhaps they produce the mucin of the ground substance; their granules sometimes give a mucoid reaction. They have been associated with the production of heparin.

Plasma cells (Fig. 56) are round or polyhedral cells with an eccentric nucleus and a large amount of cytoplasm. In the fixed and stained nucleus the chromatin is arranged about the periphery like the spokes of a wheel. The cells resemble the lymphocytes, from which they are derived. The cytoplasm has a mottled appearance and is basophilic, except for an unstained area at one side of the nucleus. Plasma cells are usually found under conditions of increased metabolism, for example, in the intestinal wall during digestion and in inflammatory processes. Degenerating plasma cells contain spherical acidophil bodies in the cytoplasm.

Fibrillar connective tissue may be subdivided into loose, membranous, regular fibrous, and irregular dense connective tissue.

a. Loose Connective Tissue

Loose connective tissue (Figs. 54*, 57) has no definite outward form. It is a displaceable substance which forms the gliding, mobile layers of the body. The collagenous fibers and trabeculae (Fig. 57,*a*) run a wavy course, cross, and interweave. Loose connective tissue is always traversed in all directions by abundant

---

[6] Gr. *makros* large, and *phagein* to eat. * Fig. 54 is on p. 51.

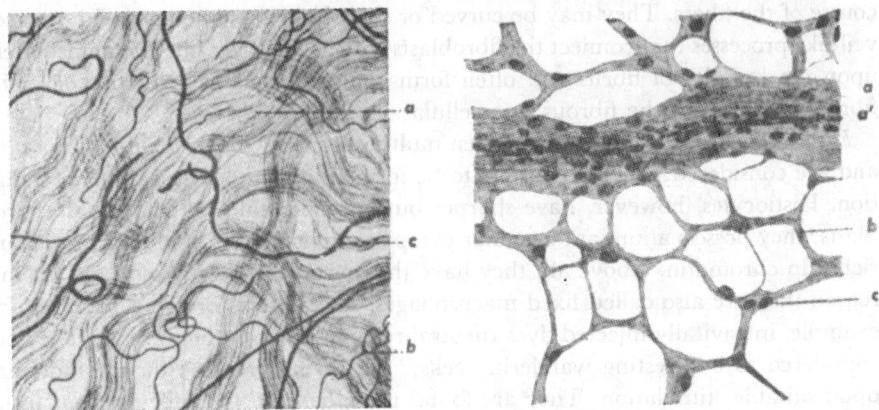

Figure 57 (left). Loose connective tissue. a, collagenous trabecula; b, thin, and c, thick, elastic fibers.

Figure 58 (right). Connective tissue from the omentum of the cat. a, thick trabecula with a', capillary; b, trabeculae; c, fibroblasts.

elastic fibers (b,c). All the cells described on pp. 38–39 are included in its structure. In addition, fat cells (p. 44) occur in varying numbers. It invades the organs as interstitial tissue and serves as a filling and connecting mass between neighboring organs and body parts, as well as between the larger divisions (lobes) of the organs. As inter- and intraparenchymatous connective tissue, it forms the binding substance in muscles, nerves, and glands. The interparenchymatous connective tissue of the organs invades them from their connective tissue capsules and separates the divisions of the parenchyma (bundles and lobules), enclosing each in a more or less firm sheath. The delicate framework of bundles of fibrils inclosing the tissue elements of the organs is the intraparenchymatous connective tissue.

The interstitial tissue is a continuous framework, the trabeculae of which are formed of collagenous fibers and carry the vessels and nerves. The trabeculae cross in all directions and form a network. The amorphous ground substance combines with the fiber nets to form membranes enclosing tissue spaces (tissue lacunae) with small amounts of tissue fluid. When air is introduced (e.g., into the subcutis), these small clefts are distended to vesicular spaces (emphysema). This occurs in wounds. In the same way, blood stasis can cause the accumulation of fluid in the tissue spaces (hydrops, edema, or anasarca). This characteristic gave rise to the old terms areolar tissue or cellular tissue; in the latter term cell has its original meaning of any small space surrounded by walls. (Compare with cellulitis.) The looseness of the tissue depends upon the size of the tissue spaces.

In addition to the mechanical function (maintenance of form), which is an attribute of the fibrous components, loose connective tissue also has important metabolic functions to perform. The exchange of metabolites between the capillaries and the various cells of the organs takes place through the connective tissue covering the capillaries. The tissue fluid which mediates this exchange is a component of the intercellular substance of the connective tissue. The connective tissue is also important to the water economy of the body. The water in the organism is continually passing back and forth between the blood and the tissues (intercellular substance). The cells of the connective tissue (histiocytes and wandering cells), with the blood, are concerned with the defense against noxious substances in the organs. This is one of the most important functions of connective tissue, which reacts rapidly to irritants. Finally, the loose connective tissue plays a role in regeneration. All the connective tissues repair defects with the products of the fibroblasts. Strong mechanical demands on the connective tissue cause a reduction in the cells other than fibroblasts and a greater development of the intercellular structures.

b. Membranous Connective Tissue

In membranous connective tissue the bundles of fibrils of different sizes, crossing each other in various directions, are spread flat. They are accompanied by a close network of elastic fibers. The cellular elements are the same as in loose connective tissue. The lamina propria of the serous membranes (p. 102) is composed of membranous connective tissue in which the elastic nets form a layer on both sides of the fibrous sheet.

The connective tissue of the greater omentum (Fig. 58) is a variation in which the fiber bundles surround large or small holes in a lacelike structure. Flat fibroblasts lie on the bundles, which are accompanied by elastic fibers and may be covered by very delicate membranes containing circular reticular fibers. Vessels run in the thicker trabeculae. Omentum and serous membranes are covered by simple squamous epithelium (mesothelium).

A further variation is found in the arachnoid, where the fiber bundles do not run in one plane but in all directions. The surface of the trabeculae is covered by an incomplete layer of flat cells.

c. Regular Fibrous Connective Tissue

Regular (tense, stretched) fibrous connective tissue is developed under conditions of mechanical stress of the fibrous intercellular substance. It is distinguished by its tensile strength and by the regular arrangement of its fiber bundles. It is usually poor in elastic tissue. Fibroblasts of shapes characteristic of the various organs are almost the only cells present (Figs. 55,d; 59,b; 60,b).

OCCURRENCE. It forms the ligaments, tendons, aponeuroses, and certain deep fasciae.

The tendons (Figs. 59, 60), like the ligaments, are composed of parallel, tautly stretched bundles of fibrils, the primary tendon bundles (tendon fibers). Between them lie the rows of fibroblasts or tendon cells. These are flat, polygonal, stellate, or fusiform, usually have winglike processes, and are marked by many pressure grooves and ridges from the embedded fibers. The nuclei are elongated and often resemble those of smooth muscle cells. The tendon cells lie in anasto nosing tissue spaces, which they almost fill (Fig. 60,b). A number of primary bundles unite to form secondary and these to form tertiary bundles. The tendons are covered super-

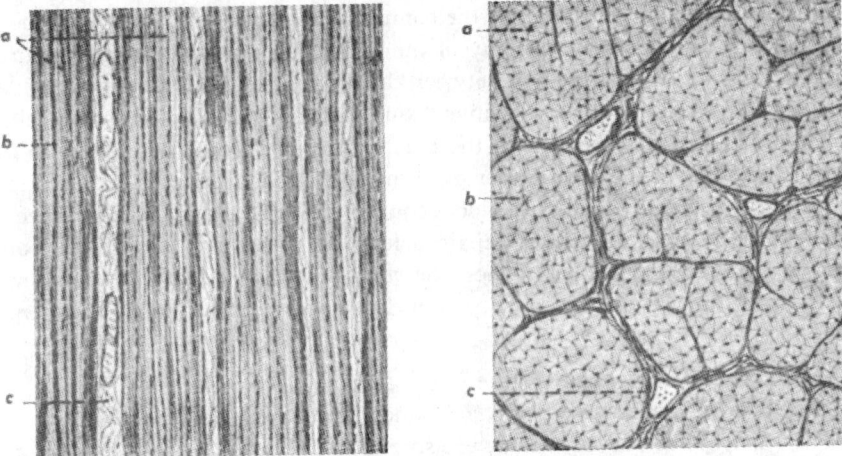

Figure 59 (left). Longitudinal section through a tendon of the horse. *a*, tendon bundles; *b*, nuclei of tendon cells; *c*, peritenonium internum with blood vessels.
Figure 60 (right). Cross section of a tendon of the horse. Labeled as in Fig. 59.

ficially by loose connective tissue (peritenonium[7] externum), except where the tendon sheaths occur. From the peritenonium externum, processes (peritenonium internum) invade the tendon and clothe the bundles as interfascicular tissue. The latter contains elastic fibers, fat cells, and occasionally cartilaginous structures.

The blood vessels form a well-developed vascular net in the peritenonium, but they are lacking inside the bundles. The lymph vessels are distributed similarly. The tendon fibers are richly supplied with sensory nerve fibers, which end in tendon spindles and terminal corpuscles. The functional demand on the tendons has a profound influence on the nature and the course of their fibers.

Aponeuroses are flat, sheetlike tendinous structures in which groups of parallel fibers sometimes cross at right angles.

Lamellar connective tissue is seen in the fibrillar intercellular substance of lamellar bone, where the parallel fibers of one lamella take a different direction from those of the neighboring lamellae. The perineurium and the lamina propria of the cornea have a similar structure.

d. Irregular Dense Connective Tissue

Irregular dense connective tissue forms the remaining fibrous membranes, which are characterized by a feltwork of interwoven fibers and trabeculae. Examples are fasciae, periosteum, perichondrium, connective tissue capsules of many organs (tunicae albugineae and tunicae fibrosae), sheaths of the blood vessels and nerves, synovial membranes, bursae, sclera, and corium. When the fasciae serve as muscle covering, they are rich in elastic fibers; when they act as tendons, they have an aponeurotic structure.

The tendon sheaths consist of two cylinders, which are continuous with each

---

[7] Gr. *tenon* tendon.

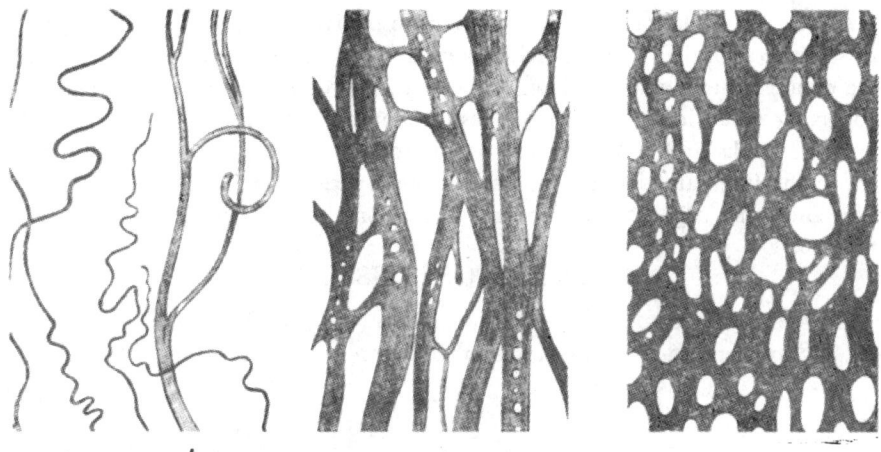

a   b

Figure 61 (left). Elastic fibers. *a*, unbranched fibers; *b*, branched fibers.
Figure 62 (center). Elastic fibers arranged in a net, from the pulmonary artery of a horse (350×).
Figure 63 (right). Fenestrated elastic membrane (350×).

other at the ends of the sheath. Between them is a space filled with synovial[8] fluid. The wall of the outer cylinder is a tough fibrous coat joined by loose connective tissue to the synovial membrane lining the space. The synovial membrane bears flat cells of connective tissue origin and vascular villi. This membrane is reflected over the tendon, fuses with it, and forms the inner cylinder of the tendon sheath.

In the subtendinous bursae, the outer layer of the wall, which is attached to the surrounding tissues, is composed of dense connective tissue. The inner surface is lined by a synovial membrane. In the places where the flat lining cells are lacking, there is usually compact connective tissue mixed with cartilage cells. The subcutaneous bursae have walls of thickened fibrillar connective tissue, from which trabeculae extend across the cavity. (For the structure of joint capsules, see p. 56.)

4. Elastic Tissue

Elastic fibers, unlike collagenous fibrils, do not form bundles; they often branch (Fig. 61,*b*); and in addition to woven textures they form characteristic fine or coarse nets by anastomosis (Fig. 62). At the intersections where the fibers fuse, there are often weblike expansions.

OCCURRENCE. As thick elastic fibers, it is the main constituent of certain ligaments (ligamentum nuchae, ligamenta arcualia, or flava, liga-

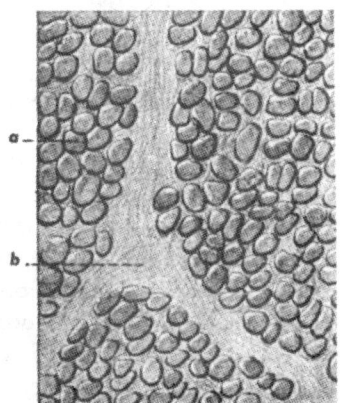

Figure 64. Cross section of the dried ligamentum nuchae of the horse; unstained. *a*, cross sections of coarse elastic fibers; *b*, connective tissue that holds the individual elastic fibers together.

---

[8] Gr. *syn-* together, and L. *ovum* egg. Synovial fluid resembles egg white in viscosity and cohesiveness.

menta vocalia, and ligamentum suspensorium penis). In these structures the fibers are stretched parallel and are held together by loose connective tissue (Fig. 64). The elastic ligaments are yellow. In general, a pronounced yellowish color in a supporting tissue indicates a high elastin content. Elastic tissue also appears as elastic networks and as fenestrated or continuous elastic membranes (lamellae), e.g., in the large arteries. Elastic tissue plays a large part in the structure of the lungs and other organs. It also occurs in the form of nodules, as in the epiglottis of the ox.

B. ADIPOSE TISSUE

Adipose tissue is composed mostly of fat cells (Fig. 65). These are spherical, 60–80 μ in diameter. The cytoplasm is displaced by a large fat globule, so that it forms

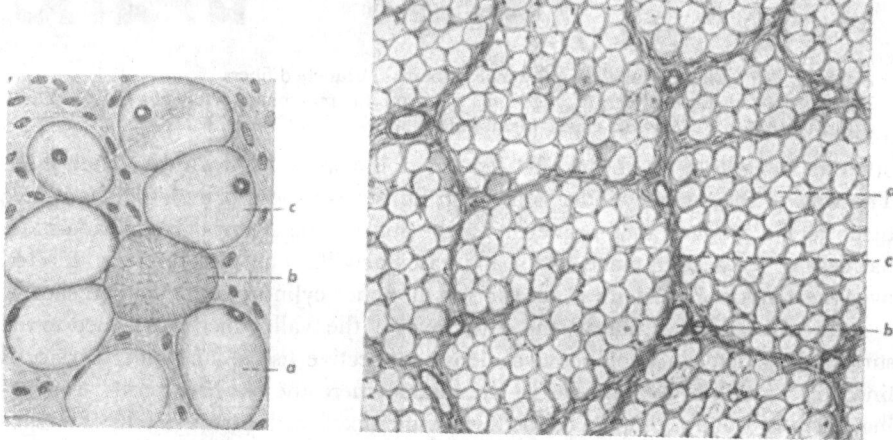

Figure 65 (left). From the adipose tissue (panniculus adiposus) of a pig. a, fat cells (signet ring form); b, fat cell with margarin crystals; c, fat cell with cavity in the nucleus.
Figure 66 (right). Adipose tissue from the fatty cushion of the stifle of a donkey. a, fat cells; b, blood vessel; c, connective tissue framework.

only a thin peripheral layer. In the region of the elliptical, parietal, often flattened nucleus, there is a somewhat thicker layer of cytoplasm (signet ring form, Fig. 65,a). In addition, each fat cell possesses a fine membrane of reticular fibers.

In fresh preparations the nucleus is usually invisible. In stained sections many nuclei show a space that represents a fat-filled cavity (Fig. 65,c). Fat stains black with osmic acid, red with Sudan III and scarlet red. The fat is extracted by the fat solvents used in embedding, so that only the empty cells are seen in paraffin and celloidin sections. In the dead animal, tufted margarin crystals are often found in the fat cells (Fig. 65,b).

Fat cells may occur singly or in groups anywhere in the connective tissue. When they are aggregated in large masses like bunches of grapes, they are the main constituent of adipose tissue, which is rich in nerves and vessels (Figs. 65, 66). This tissue is regularly encountered in certain regions of the body (the fat organs). The cell groups are of various sizes; the microscopic ones are called primary lobules and, when avascular, fat islands. In large deposits of fat, a number of primary lobules are united by loose connective tissue to form secondary lobules, and the latter may form larger tertiary lobules, and so on.

In severe starvation the fat in the cells is reduced to small droplets. There remains in the flattened cells a pale cytoplasmic mass mixed with mucoid fluid (serous fat cells).

OCCURRENCE. Adipose tissue serves as a supporting substance that is elastic under pressure, and as a protective, insulating, contour-building, filling, and structural material. In well-nourished animals, it is especially abundant in the subcutis (panniculus adiposus) and in the mesentery, also on and around very mobile or sensitive organs and those which must be protected from chilling. Fat plays an important structural role in and around joints and in the foot pads and digital cushions of animals. Fat is formed in the involution of the thymus. It is absent in the cranium, eyelids, scrotum, and skin of the penis and clitoris. It occurs in very small amounts in the ear, nose, and lips. In lean animals fat is found only in the orbits, around the kidneys, in the mesentery, bone marrow, and vertebral canal, along the nerves and arteries, and in the lyssa of the tongue.

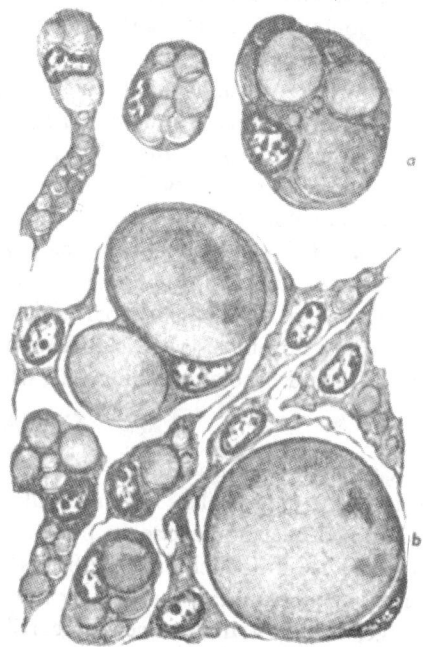

Figure 67. Development of fat cells in the subcutis; stained with Sudan (900×). a, single cell; b, cell group from a lobule.

DEVELOPMENT OF THE CONNECTIVE TISSUE. Connective tissue arises from the middle germ layer through the mesenchyme (p. 34). A part of the mesenchymal cells are to be regarded as producers of the collagenous fibrils and are therefore called fibroblasts. The fibrils probably form by association and parallel orientation of long molecules of protein (p. 8) secreted by the cells. There is a question as to whether this takes place within the cytoplasm or in the intercellular substance. In areas of great concentration of actively fibril-producing cells, extensive organs of fibrillar connective tissue are developed. In these formed connective tissues, e.g., tendons, the division into primary, secondary, and tertiary fiber bundles is always apparent. When there are only a few scattered fibroblasts of moderate activity, the more delicate membranes, or large or small irregular formations of loose connective tissue are developed.

It is probable that the elastic fibers are also produced by fibroblasts. The development of elastic fibers may prevail over the production of collagenous fibrils, so that gradually the collagenous fibers and the cells come to form the minor, almost unnoticeable portion of the whole structure, as in the ligamentum nuchae. The elastic fibers appear homogeneous from the beginning.

Adipose tissue develops very late in ontogenesis, for the fetus must reach a high stage of development before it can store reserve material for nutritional purposes. Previous to that, all available nutrients are used in the formation of the organs. In restricted areas, where the fat bodies are to form, the mesenchyme in the vicinity of the blood vessels takes on a reticular character. The individual cells store fat, which first appears as single droplets. These coalesce finally to one large globule (a univacuolar fat cell, Fig. 67). The cytoplasm forms a thin layer around the fat globule, which presses the nucleus to the periphery. Fat storage in the cells of reticular tissue is particularly evident in the transformation of red to yellow bone marrow. Fat cells may also come from fibroblasts.

In poultry, there is much yellow, plurivacuolar adipose tissue, in which many fat droplets lie around the central nucleus, as in embryonic fat cells. The "hibernating gland" on the necks of rodents is also of this type of adipose tissue, but is brown in color.

Pigmented connective tissue cells are also derived from the undifferentiated mesenchymal cells. It is assumed that there is a division of labor among the mesenchymal cells which separate from the parietal layer of the mesoderm, some becoming fibroblasts with elaboration of intercellular substance, some becoming fat cells, and others becoming cells which produce intracellular pigment granules.

C. CARTILAGE

Cartilage is composed of an abundant intercellular substance and the encapsulated cartilage cells. The intercellular substance, which is firm but flexible, is composed of a homogeneous mass and fibrillar elements. It may have a hyaline appearance, in which case the fibrils are masked, or it may contain visible elastic or collagenous fibers, bundles, or networks. Therefore we distinguish hyaline cartilage, elastic cartilage, and fibrocartilage.

1. Hyaline Cartilage

The cartilage cells fill completely the cavities they occupy in the intercellular substance (Figs. 68–70). They may be spherical, oval, half-spherical, or flattened into a lens shape. They are usually surrounded by a closely applied capsule (Figs. 68; 69,b), which, however, is sometimes invisible. The capsule is a differentiation of the intercellular substance produced by the cells. The cells have a soft, delicate cytoplasm, which contains granular or threadlike mitochondria and inclusions of glycogen, fat, and, rarely, pigment. The nucleus is spherical, contains nucleoli, and may occasionally be double. The Golgi apparatus is well developed. The cells shrink easily on fixation, become wrinkled, and no longer fill their cavities.

The daughter cells derived from one mother cell are often associated in *isogenous groups* (Fig. 69,c). After new ground substance appears between the daughter cells, their common origin may still be recognized by their proximity, by the fact that their apposed surfaces are flattened, or by a common capsule around the individual capsules. Near the free surface of the cartilage, the cells are often flattened and lie parallel to the surface in layers. Farther within the cartilage the cells are more rounded, and in the deepest portions they are often arranged in rows perpendicular to the surface (Fig. 70).

The intercellular substance (Figs. 68,c; 69,f) is very firm and elastic, has a bluish-white translucent appearance, and seems to be homogeneous throughout like ground glass. However, after maceration with 10 percent NaCl, KMnO₄, baryta water, lime water, or trypsin, a fibrillar structure becomes visible. The intercellular substance is composed of a feltwork of fine collagenous fibrils permeated by a mucoid cement. Because the fibrils and the interfibrillar ground substance have the same refractive index, the fibrils are invisible, masked. Hyaline cartilage con-

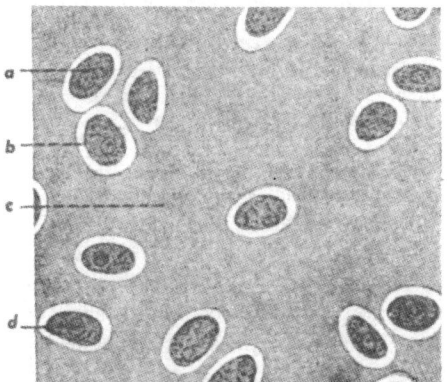 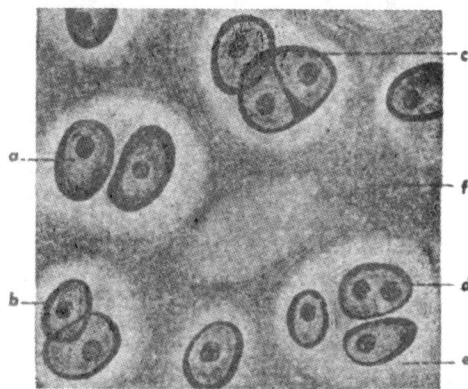

Figure 68 (left). Hyaline cartilage from the hock of a calf; unstained (700×). *a*, cartilage cell; *b*, capsule; *c*, hyaline intercellular substance; *d*, nucleus of a cartilage cell.

Figure 69 (right). Hyaline cartilage from the hock of a calf; hematoxylin-eosin (700×). *a*, cartilage cell; *b*, capsule; *c*, isogenous cell group; *d*, dividing cell; *e*, cell zone; *f*, intercellular substance with fine fibrils.

tains a great deal of water (costal cartilage of calf, 75 percent), and shrinks on drying to a horny translucent mass. With prolonged boiling, cartilage yields chondrin (cartilage glue), which contains among other things chondroitin-sulfuric acid, the cause of the basophilia of the ground substance (which stains dark blue with hematoxylin). The intercellular substance immediately surrounding the capsules has a different staining reaction, forming a halo or cell zone which often includes a whole group of cells (Fig. 69,e).

In many cartilages, e.g., costal cartilages, there are areas in the hyaline intercellular substance where one can see fibers without the use of reagents. They often radiate from one point. Such areas present an asbestos-like appearance to the naked eye. In old age, cartilage often loses its elasticity through calcification.

With the exception of the articular cartilages, the hyaline cartilages are surrounded by a dense connective tissue membrane which blends with the cartilage. This *perichondrium* (Fig. 70,a) plays an important role in the growth and regeneration of cartilage. Because the cartilage itself is avascular, it is nourished by diffusion

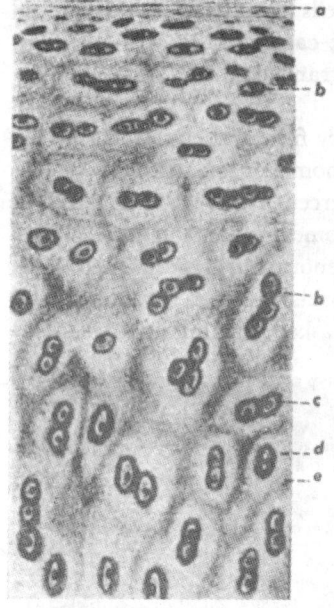

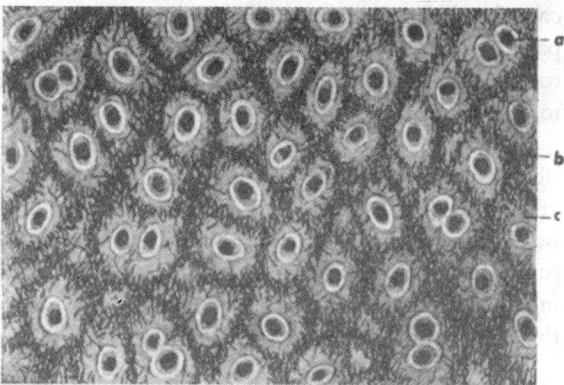

Figure 70 (left). From a costal cartilage of a calf (110X). *a*, perichondrium; *b*, cartilage cell with capsule; *c*, dark inner cell zone; *d*, light outer cell zone; *e*, intercellular substance between cell zones.

Figure 71 (right). Elastic cartilage from the third eyelid of the horse. *a*, cartilage cell; *b*, elastic fibers; *c*, hyaline intercellular substance.

from the perichondrium. The development of blood vessels in the cartilage is always a sign of beginning calcification or ossification. This process begins early in the costal cartilages—at six months in the dog, forming a core of spongy bone by two years of age.

OCCURRENCE. Hyaline cartilage is found in articular cartilages; in the thyroid, cricoid, and the base of the arytenoid laryngeal cartilages; in the cartilage of trachea and bronchi; in the cartilages of the nose; and in the primordia of most of the bones during development.

2. Elastic Cartilage

Elastic cartilage (Fig. 71) is characterized by a network of fine or coarse elastic fibers in the otherwise hyaline intercellular substance. The fiber networks vary in density in different cartilages. The fibers gradually become fewer and thinner as they extend into the perichondrium. The cartilage cells are spherical or flattened, often occur in groups, and are surrounded by a distinct capsule. Elastic cartilage is more flexible than hyaline. It contains very few collagenous fibers and is more or less yellow in color.

OCCURRENCE. This type occurs in the epiglottis, the corniculate and cuneiform cartilages of the larynx, the auricular cartilages, the cartilage of the third eyelid, part of the cartilage of the Eustachian tube, and part of the arytenoid cartilage.

3. Fibrocartilage

In fibrocartilage the intercellular substance contains bundles of collagenous fibers, which sometimes run parallel, sometimes form an irregular texture. The cells lie in thick capsules between the fibers, singly or in groups or rows. Fibrocartilage often merges gradually into connective tissue or hyaline cartilage.

OCCURRENCE. This is found in articular discs and menisci, intervertebral discs, marginal parts of the articular cartilages and synchondroses, accessory cartilage of the patella, and cartilaginous parts of the tendons and tendon sheaths.

DEVELOPMENT. Cartilage can develop directly from indifferent mesenchymal cells (chondroblasts) or by the transformation of another tissue, e.g., perichondrium. Embryonic cartilage arises from a syncytium of cells lying close together without cell boundaries. The boundaries become distinct with the secretion of a capsule around each cell. As growth continues, the outer layer of the capsule changes to hyaline intercellular substance, which at first forms only a thin-walled framework around the cells (cellular or precartilage) but increases in amount as it pushes the cells farther apart. Cartilage growth may be *interstitial* by cell division followed by the formation of new intercellular substance or it may be *appositional* by the transformation of the deepest layer of perichondrium into cartilage.

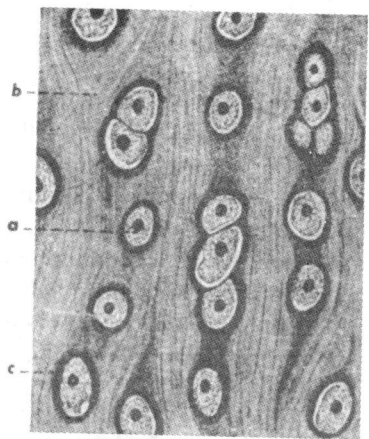

Figure 72. Fibrocartilage (cartilage of the third phalanx of the horse). *a*, cartilage cell; *b*, collagenous fibers; *c*, basophilic cell capsule.

Fibrocartilage shows collagenous bundles as early as the cellular cartilage stage. The fibers of elastic cartilage develop on the surface of the cell rows and are at first very fine. They exhibit an independent growth, becoming thicker and splitting off new fibers.

Other Forms of Supporting Tissue. In addition to cartilage and bone, there are other, relatively soft, tissues that have a supporting function. One example is adipose tissue, composed of elastic cellular sacs filled with fat. Similar to fat cells are the cells of the vesicular supporting tissue in the notochord (chordoid type). They are large saclike cells with a strong membrane, parietal nucleus, and a fluid, nonfatty content, which presses the cytoplasm to the wall. The cell fluid is under strong pressure (turgor) and, because of the close contact of the cells, lends firmness and resistance to the tissue. The cells are held together by an elastic and collagenous notochordal sheath to form a flexible supporting rod.

Chondroid tissue is composed of glassy, translucent, elastic cell bodies, which maintain a constant form. The nucleus is spherical. Between the cells are collagenous fibers and a thin interstitial substance arranged like a honeycomb. In contrast to cartilage cells, chondroid cells do not shrink. The tissue has a cartilaginous consistency. It occurs mostly in lower animals, but is also found in birds and mammals, e.g., in tendon attachments, sesamoid bones of the cat, and tuber calcanei of the calf. It is closely related to fibrocartilage.

D. BONE

1. Osseous Tissue

Osseous tissue is the principal constituent of the bones. It is composed of intercellular substance and bone cells which lie in cavities called lacunae.

The hardness and rigidity of the osseous tissue are properties of its *intercellular substance*, which is rich in calcium salts. The latter increase with age at the expense of the organic material. The intercellular substance exhibits an almost uniformly dense structure and contains closely compressed bundles of collagenous fibrils. An apparently homogeneous binding substance, in which the inorganic material is deposited, binds the bundles together and also appears in small quantities between the individual fibrils. The delicate bundles of fibrils, 1–3 μ in thickness, form lay-

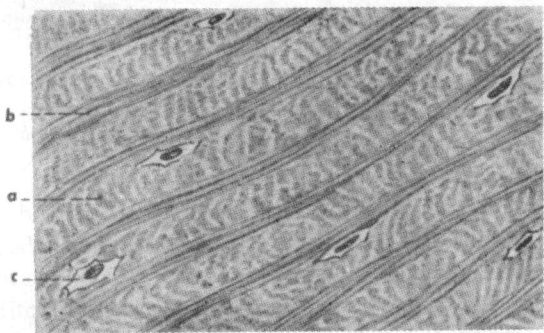

Figure 73. Cross section of bone lamellae from a decalcified long bone. *a*, lamella in which the fibers are cut across; *b*, lamella in which the fibers are cut longitudinally; *c*, bone cell.

ers, the *lamellae* (Fig. 73). The binding substance is also found between lamellae, and they are held together by bundles that run obliquely from one to the other. The bundles within each lamella are parallel to each other, but their direction varies from one lamella to the next. For this reason, in sections the lamellae appear alternately striated and punctate (Fig. 73).

In addition to this fine-fibered or lamellar bone of the adult mammal, there is also a coarse-fibered texture found in the bone of fetuses, in which the fibril bundles are thicker and form no lamellae, or only indistinct ones. The bundles are interwoven in an irregular fashion. It occurs in only a few places in the adult, e.g., at the sutures and the attachments of tendons.

At certain places in lamellar and coarse-fibered bone we find coarse *Sharpey's fibers* (perforating fibers) penetrating the intercellular substance from the periosteum. They may be calcified or uncalcified, and they represent bundles entrapped during the development of the outer layers of bone (p. 55).

The lacunae, which usually lie between but may lie within the lamellae, are greatly flattened like the cells they contain (Figs. 75,*c;* 76; 77,*b,c,d;* 78,*c;* 79,*e*). They are connected by many fine, sinuous, branched *canaliculi* (Figs. 76; 77,*b,d*),

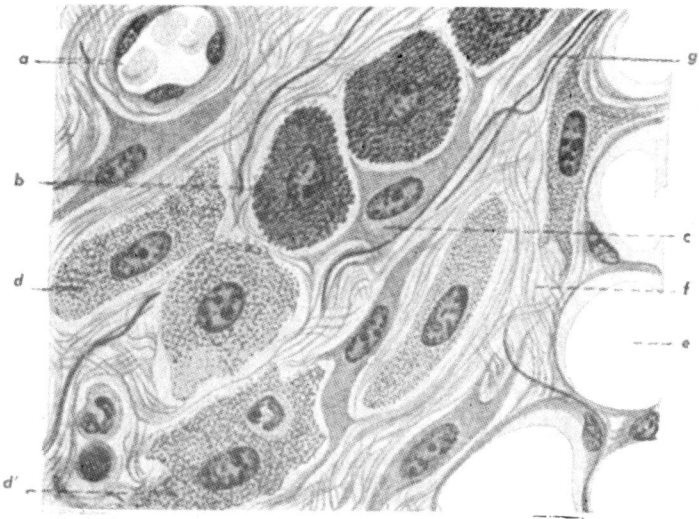

Figure 54. Subcutaneous connective tissue of a rat intravitally injected with lithium carmine; hematoxylin-eosin (600×). *a*, capillary; *b*, mast cell; *c*, fibroblast; *d*, histiocyte with stored lithium carmine; *d'*, histiocyte with phagocytosed granulocyte; on the left, granulocyte and lymphocyte; *e*, fat cell; *f*, loose fibrillar connective tissue; *g*, elastic fiber.

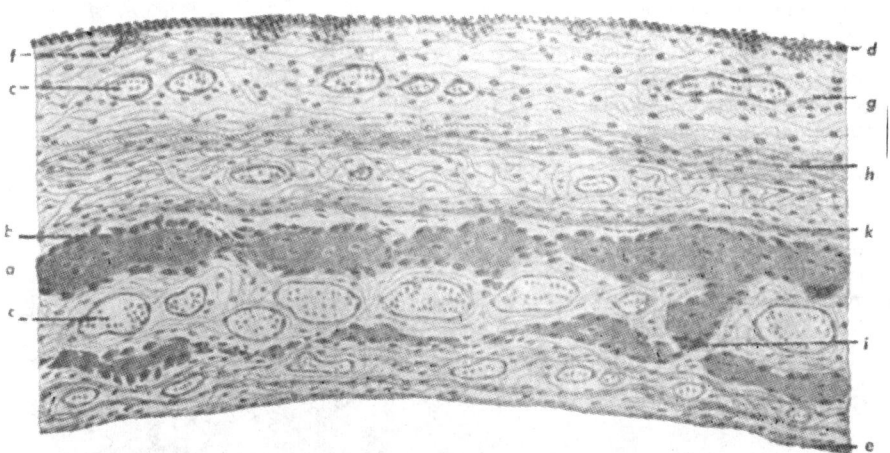

Figure 81. Frontal section through the roof of the cranium of a pig embryo of 5.5-cm. crown-rump length; ossification of the parietal bone; hematoxylin-eosin. *a*, bone trabecula; *b*, osteoblasts; *c*, blood vessel; *d*, epidermis; *e*, endosteum; *f*, hair bud; *g*, corium; *h*, cutaneous muscle; *i*, osteoclast; *k*, periosteum.

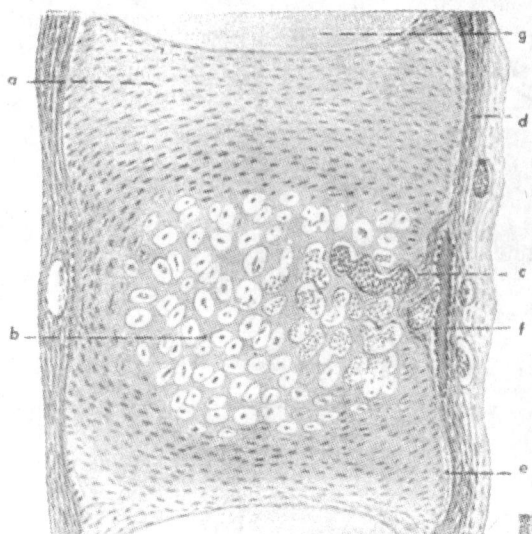

Figure 82. Sagittal section of the body of a vertebra of a newborn rat (60×). *a*, hyaline cartilage with flattened cells; *b*, cartilage with enlarged cells; *c*, periosteal bud with many blood vessels; *d*, fibrous layer of the periosteum (perichondrium); *e*, osteoblastic layer of the periosteum; *f*, perichondral bone; *g*, intervertebral disc.

Figure 83. Sagittal section through the digit of a fetal pig of 14 cm. crown-rump length (about 10 weeks old); hematoxylin-eosin (25×). *A*, phalanx I; *B*, distal half of the metacarpus; *a*, hyaline cartilage of the distal epiphyses; *b*, columnar cartilage; *c*, calcified cartilage; *d*, perichondral bone collar; *e*, cartilaginous primordium of a sesamoid bone; *f*, osteoblasts; *g*, blood vessels; *g′*, periosteal bud; *h*, periosteum; *m*, primary bone marrow; *n*, primordia of tendons; *o*, mesenchyme; *p*, epidermis; *p′*, hair bud; *r*, joint cavity. *This area is represented at greater magnification in Fig. 84.

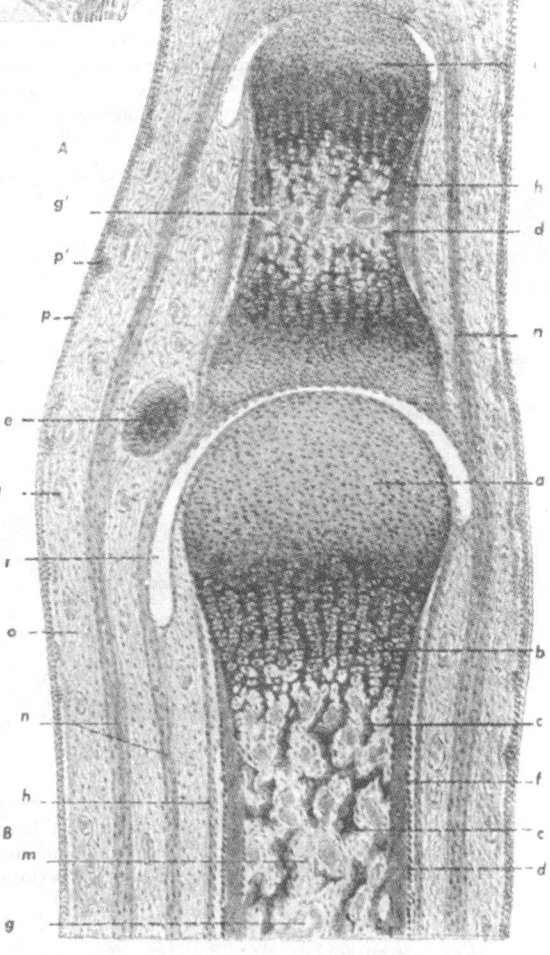

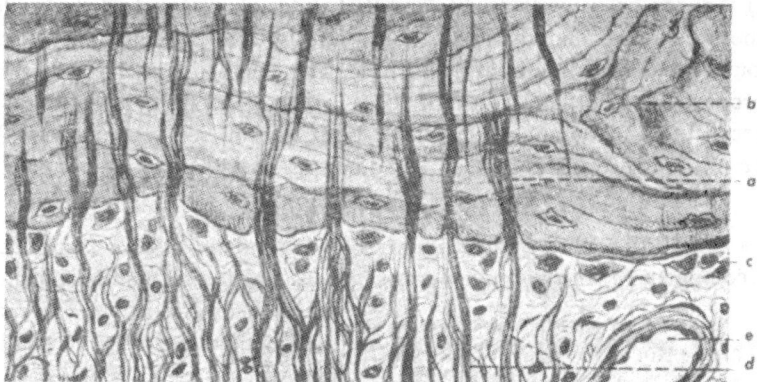

Figure 74. Sharpey's fibers in the wall of the alveolus of a tooth. The fiber bundles of the alveolar periosteum are continued into the bone as Sharpey's fibers. *a*, Sharpey's fibers; *b*, bone cell; *c*, osteoblasts; *d*, fiber bundles of the alveolar periosteum; *e*, blood vessel. (After Kopsch.)

which pass between the fibrils of the intercellular substance. The whole tissue is thus penetrated by a network of fine canals, which are of great importance to its nutrition.

The *lacunae* are 18–40 μ long, 8–15 μ wide, and 4–8 μ thick. The walls of the lacunae and the canaliculi are especially resistant and may be isolated from the rest of the tissue by treatment with hydrochloric acid and by other methods. We can therefore speak of capsules or sheaths of the lacunae and canaliculi.

The bone cells, *osteocytes* (Figs. 73,*c*; 75), in the lacunae are flattened like pumpkin seeds. Many processes extend from them into the canaliculi and serve, at least in young osseous tissue, to connect the cells. The finely granular cytoplasm surrounds a flattened nucleus. In old bone the cells lose their processes and their nucleus; the cytoplasm undergoes fatty degeneration and may be resorbed. In such cases the lacunae contain only granular masses of debris.

The inorganic substance in osseous tissue makes up about two thirds of its dry weight and is composed mostly of calcium carbonate and calcium phosphate. Bone may be decalcified by treatment with acids, leaving a cartilage-like elastic mass

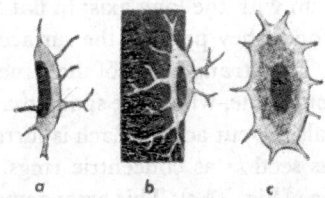

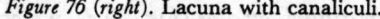

▼ *Figure 75.* Bone cells. *a*, isolated; *b*, half surrounded by intercellular substance; *c*, in a lacuna.

Figure 76 (right). Lacuna with canaliculi.

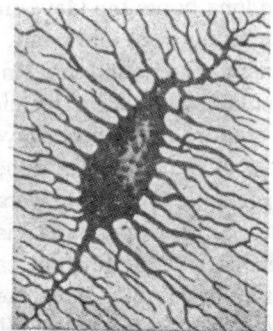

(ossein) that can be cut with a knife and that yields glue when boiled. The form of the bone is retained after decalcification, and also after calcination, i.e., the destruction of the organic material by burning. The calcined bone has lost its elasticity, a property of the organic substance; it is brittle.

A special modification of osseous tissue is the dentin (see *teeth*, p. 170). The cementum of the teeth is true coarse-fibered osseous tissue.

2. Bones as Organs

Bones (Fig. 86) have a basic structure of two kinds of osseous tissue: the substantia compacta (*a*) in the outer part or cortex, and the substantia spongiosa (*b*)

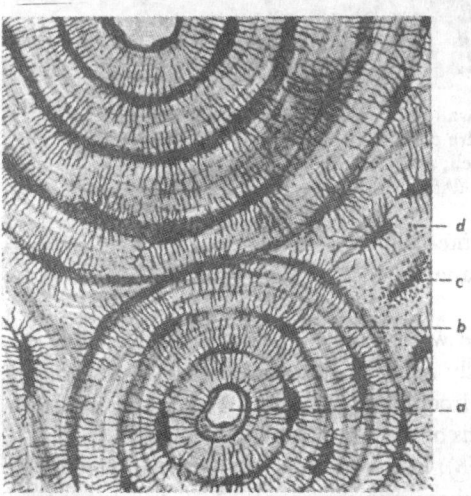

Figure 77. From a cross section of the metacarpal bone of the horse. *a*, Haversian canal; *b*, lacuna with canaliculi; *c*, lacuna below the plane of section; *d*, canaliculi cut across. (After Lungwitz.)

in the central portion. The spaces in the spongy bone are filled with bone marrow, as is the marrow cavity of the long bones (*c*). The ratio of compact to spongy bone is not everywhere the same. In the shafts of long bones the compact substance predominates; in the epiphyses and in short bones, the spongy substance. Either type may prevail in the flat bones. Many skull bones are entirely compact.

The surface of the bones is covered by a fibrous membrane rich in vessels and nerves, the periosteum, which gives way to a cartilaginous covering at the articular ends.

Besides the lacunae and canaliculi, the compact bone also contains a system of larger canals, the *Haversian canals*, 20–100 μ in diameter (Figs. 77; 78,*a*; 79,*c*), which conduct vessels and nerves. They form, by multiple transverse and oblique anastomoses, a network that penetrates the entire compact substance and opens in many places on the external surface and in the marrow cavities of the bone. In long bones the Haversian canals run with the long axis; in flat bones they usually radiate from one point; in short bones they parallel the surface but some run in one direction and some in the other. The arrangement of the lamellae is best seen in cross sections from the middle of a long bone, where the spongiosa is lacking. In such sections most of the Haversian canals are cut across. Each is surrounded by a number of lamellae that appear in cross section as concentric rings. They are called special lamellae or Haversian lamellae (Fig. 79,*c*). This arrangement of concentric tubes (8–15 per canal) is chiefly responsible for the great rigidity of bone. The lamellae surrounding one canal comprise a *Haversian system* or osteon, the unit of structure of compact bone. Adjacent Haversian systems are united by a cement substance, and the spaces are filled by *interstitial lamellae* (Fig. 79,*d*), which are the

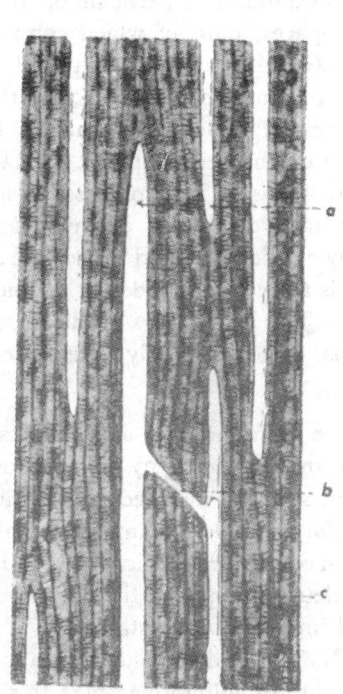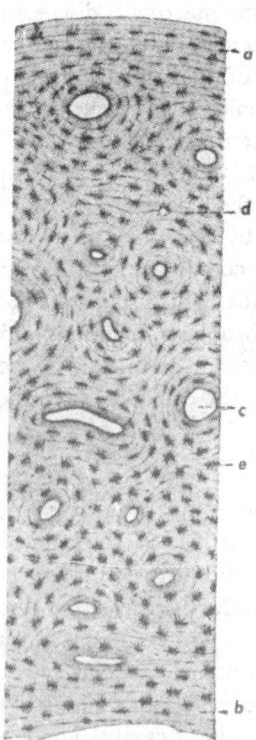

Figure 78 (left). From a longitudinal section through the diaphysis of a long bone (70×). *a,* Haversian canal; *b,* Volkmann's canal; *c,* lacuna.

Figure 79 (right). Cross section through the cortex of the diaphysis of a long bone (100×). *a,* outer; *b,* inner basic lamellae; *c,* cross section of an Haversian canal surrounded by its special lamellae; *d,* interstitial lamellae; *e,* lacunae.

remnants of Haversian systems partially destroyed in the reconstruction of the bone (p. 60). Next to the surface and around the marrow cavity are the outer and inner basic or *circumferential lamellae* (Fig. 79,*a,b*). The inner lamellae are always lacking at the ends of the marrow cavity, where they are replaced by spongy bone. They may be absent elsewhere as well.

Spongy bone is composed of thick and thin trabeculae, of which only the thicker have Haversian systems. In the thin trabeculae of the spongiosa, the lamellae are parallel to the surface, as are the most superficial lamellae of the thick trabeculae.

The basic and interstitial lamellae contain, in addition to Haversian canals, others which have no lamellar systems. These are *Volkmann's canals* (Fig. 78,*b*). They have many connections with the Haversian canals and conduct the perforating vessels from the outer surface and from the marrow cavity.

The outer basic and the adjacent interstitial lamellae contain collagenous *Sharpey's fibers* (Fig. 74), often accompanied by elastic fibers. These disappear toward the interior. Tendons and ligaments are continued into the bone at their insertions by Sharpey's fibers.

The bone marrow is discussed on p. 135.

Avian bones, with certain exceptions such as those of the pelvic limb, are hollow. In place of the marrow they contain air spaces, most of which communicate through holes in the cortex with the air sacs (p. 243) and thus with the lungs.

Periosteum. The bones are covered by a fibrous membrane called the periosteum. It is thickest at the points of attachment of tendons and ligaments because a part of their connective tissue passes over into the periosteum. It is attached to the bone by Sharpey's fibers and by the blood vessels. It is composed of an outer relatively coarse adventitia, rich in nerves and vessels, and an inner layer, the fibroelastica, which has few vessels but many elastic fibers and round and spindle-shaped fibroblasts. In young animals there is a layer of rounded or cuboidal cells (osteoblasts) on the inside of the periosteum. The bone grows in thickness by the activity of the osteoblasts. In the aged animal these occur only in restricted areas.

3. Joints

The bones may be connected by movable or immovable articulations. In an immovable joint, or *synarthrosis*, the bones are connected by collagenous fibers, bone, or cartilage. In the latter, fibrocartilage is usually involved. The cartilaginous joints (synchondroses) may be complex, as, for example, the intervertebral articulations. In the intervertebral discs we have an outer fibrous ring with an admixture of cartilage, which merges into a pulpy nucleus (a vestige of the notochord). The nucleus contains vacuolar cells in a mucoid intercellular substance.

The movable joints, *diarthroses* (Fig. 83,r*), have articular surfaces, a joint capsule, and a joint cavity. The *articular surfaces* are usually formed by a thin layer of hyaline cartilage (fibrocartilage in the temporomandibular joint), which is united with the bone by a layer of calcified cartilage. The perichondrium is lacking on the friction surface. In the articular cartilages of the limbs of the horse and ox there are depressions lined by connective tissue, the synovial fossae. The *joint capsule* is composed of an outer layer of dense connective tissue of varying thickness, the stratum fibrosum, and a closely attached *synovial membrane*, the stratum synoviale. The latter contains collagenous and elastic fibers, and on the side next to the joint cavity, a great many fibroblasts. These cells do not completely cover the surface of the synovial membrane; there are areas where the fibers are exposed. The membrane is rich in blood vessels, occasionally lies in folds, and bears villous processes, which may be vascular or filled only with a mucoid substance. The *joint cavity* contains the *synovia*, a clear, yellowish, cohesive fluid containing protein, mucin, fat droplets, cells, cellular debris, and salts.

4. Bone Development (Osteogenesis)

The development of osseous tissue, ossification, is dependent upon the appearance of rounded connective tissue cells, the osteoblasts,[9] which develop very late in ontogenesis, multiply rapidly, and produce a fibrous substance. They have a dense basophilic cytoplasm and an eccentric nucleus. At first they lie in a single

---

[9] Gr. *osteon* bone, and *blastos* germ.

* Fig. 83 is on p. 52.

layer upon the still uncalcified intercellular substance, with short processes reaching into it (Figs. 75,*b;* 80,*b*). Then as they surround themselves with intercellular substance (Fig. 80,*a*), they become deeply embedded bone cells, osteocytes. They are now star-shaped and often connected by their processes. On the surface of the osseous tissue so formed, new osteoblasts develop from the connective tissue cells, and the process is repeated as long as the bone grows. Therefore, bone growth is primarily by apposition. There is probably a small amount of interstitial growth in the early stages, as shown by the increase in the distance between cells..

The development and growth of bone are accompanied by destructive processes associated with peculiar multinucleate giant cells, the *osteoclasts*.[10] These are finely granular cytoplasmic masses of various shapes, bulky, oval, or flat, with as many as twelve nuclei, each with a nucleolus. On the side toward the bone they often show a striated border, which has been regarded as evidence of their destructive activity (Fig. 84,*o**). Another characteristic suggestive of bone destruction is their frequent presence in grooves known as Howship's lacunae. Cells of the same kind (chondroclasts) are associated with the destruction of cartilage.

Osseous tissue does not develop until the parts to be protected and supported have already reached a rather advanced stage of development. Its function is performed at first by connective tissue and cartilage, which are only gradually, and in part postnatally, replaced by bone. This sequence of development has certain advantages. The embryo, with its protected location and restricted movements, has little use for a complete bony skeleton, which would be disagreeable ballast because of its weight and a hindrance to parturition because of its rigidity. Moreover, because bone grows only by apposition, therefore slowly, it cannot keep up with the rapid growth of the other parts of the embryo as well as cartilage, which also has interstitial growth, is not calcified, and is flexible.

According to their development, bones may be divided into (a) membrane bones and (b) bones that develop from cartilage models. To the membrane bones belong those of the sides and roof of the cranium and most of the facial bones. All the rest are preformed in cartilage.

a. Intramembranous Ossification

At certain points in the mesenchyme, osteoblasts appear and form trabeculae of osseous intercellular substance (Fig. 81,*a**). As the bony trabeculae join one another, a macroscopic point of ossification is formed, usually in the middle of the future bone. From this point, ossification proceeds in one plane toward the periphery by the formation of radially arranged anastomosing trabeculae. The coarsely porous plate of bone thickens later with the production of trabeculae perpendicular to the surface and connected with each other. The membrane bones of the roof of the cranium grow by apposition on the outer surface, while on the inner surface a simultaneous resorption of bone makes room for the growing brain. In the process of ossification collagenous fibers are enveloped so that the membrane bone is at first coarse-fibered; but it is later resorbed, except for small remnants

---

[10] Gr. *klan* to break.   * Fig. 81 is on p. 51 and Fig. 84 on p. 89.

at the sutures, and replaced by lamellar, fine-fibered bone. By the thickening of the surface layers, the inner and outer tables and the intervening spongy diploë are differentiated.

b. Development of Bones Preformed in Cartilage

The cartilage models, which are miniatures of the future bones, are not simply changed to bone but are destroyed and replaced by spongy bone and marrow (endochondral ossification); at the same time a coat of bone is formed on the surface by perichondral ossification, which later produces the greater part of the bone. Thus strength is maintained through all stages of development, an important requirement for long bones. There is also an independent ossification of the epiphyses. The actual formation of osseous tissue is the same as in intramembranous ossification. Short cylindrical bones, e.g., the phalanx of a pig, are well adapted to the study of bone development (Fig. 83*).

(1) **Endochondral Ossification.** In the middle of the diaphysis the cartilage cells begin to absorb fluid and swell up with a corresponding decrease in intercellular substance. At the same time small granules of calcium salts are deposited in the intercellular substance, forming a chalk-white center of calcification. Previous to this, a perichondral collar of bone is formed on the outside of the cartilage by osteoblastic tissue (see below; see also Figs. 82,*f**; 83,*d**). A vascular, conical, periosteal bud penetrates the spongy collar into the calcification center and dissolves the intercellular substance. The walls of the capillaries apparently have the same action in the resorption of bone and calcified cartilage as that attributed to the osteoclasts, which are said to develop from endothelium. The cartilage cells fall out of their cavities and die or mingle with the invading tissue. The latter is composed of vessels, branched mesenchymal cells, osteoblasts, and chondro- or osteoclasts, and forms the primary bone marrow, which fills the primordial bone cavity (Figs. 83*; 84,*m**; 85,*e*). The osteoblasts spread over the recessed walls of the cavity in a continuous layer and deposit on the calcified cartilage a fine-fibered osseous intercellular substance which is at first uncalcified. The calcified cartilage stains deep blue with hematoxylin, while the newly formed bone stains red with eosin.

Because the bone-collar prevents the cartilage from growing in thickness, the cartilage cells multiply in longitudinal rows (cartilage columns, Fig. 83,*b**) and assume a bread-loaf shape by mutual compression. The cells are separated by thin transverse partitions and the columns by thicker strips of intercellular substance. This cartilage transformation extends toward the end of the bone as far as the edge of the periosteal collar and is limited by a sharp transverse line. The deposition of calcium salts extends to the same line (zone of provisional calcification). Beyond the line the cartilage cells are still in groups.

Meanwhile the progressive destruction of the cartilage continues. The partitions in the columns are destroyed first, followed by the more resistant intercolumnar strips. In the recesses vacated by the cartilage cells, the osteoblasts deposit endochondral bone, forming spongy trabeculae within which cartilage can still be seen

---

* Figs. 82 and 83 are on p. 52 and Fig. 84 on p. 89.

(Figs. 83*; 84,c*; 85,b), a characteristic which distinguishes endochondral from perichondral bone. The trabeculae are also separated from the perichondral bone by an incomplete layer of calcified cartilage, the endochondral boundary line.

The mesenchymal cells of the primary bone marrow, which fills all of the excavated spaces, have changed in the meantime to branched reticular cells. Lymphoid cells (hemocytoblasts) appear between them and multiply rapidly, forming myelocytes and erythroblasts, the progenitors of the granular leukocytes and the erythrocytes (p. 92). Larger veins develop. The primary bone marrow has become red, hemopoietic bone marrow.

(2) **Perichondral Ossification.** In long bones, this begins in the middle of the diaphysis near the center of calcification and before endochondral ossification, thus reducing the danger of fracture at the point of destruction of the cartilage. The mesenchymal cells on the inner surface of the perichondrium change into osteoblasts and begin to form the bone cortex

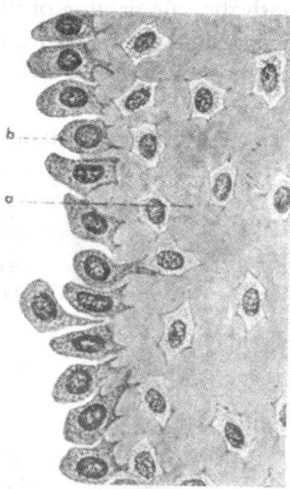

Figure 80. A piece of diaphysis from a fetal pig, showing the formation of bone by osteoblasts. a, intercellular substance between osteocytes; b, osteoblasts.

upon the cartilage (Figs. 82,e,f*; 83*; 84,d*). The vascularity of the perichondrium is greatly increased at this time. The bone collar becomes wider, keeping pace

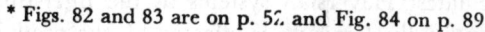

* Figs. 82 and 83 are on p. 57 and Fig. 84 on p. 89.

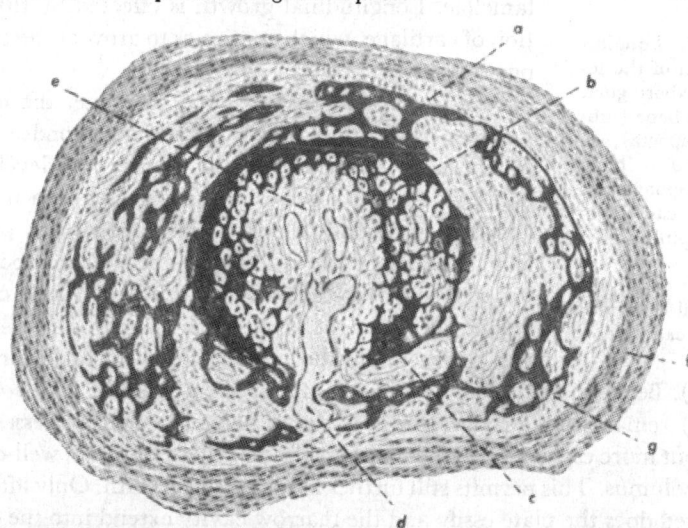

Figure 85. Cross section of the radius of a fetal pig (70×). a, perichondral; b, endochondral bone; c, calcified cartilage; d, blood vessel; e, primary bone marrow in the marrow cavity; f, fibrous; g, osteogenous layer of the periosteum.

with the calcification of the cartilage toward the epiphyses. It incorporates many collagenous fibers from the perichondrium, which give it the character of coarse-fibered bone (p. 50). With the addition of new lamellae, it increases in thickness in the middle, while the edges remain thin and sharp. In addition to simple appositional growth, the diaphysis increases in thickness by another method. Along the

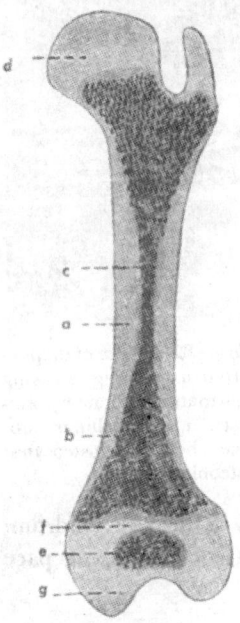

Figure 86. Longitudinal section of the femur of a newborn goat. *a*, periosteal bone (substantia compacta); *b*, endochondral bone (substantia spongiosa); *c*, marrow cavity; *d*, proximal epiphysis; *e*, ossification center in the distal epiphysis; *f*, epiphyseal cartilage; *g*, articular cartilage.

course of the longitudinal vessels, the osteoblasts build bony troughs which close over the vessels to form wide tubes, the Haversian spaces (Fig. 85, near *g*), containing osteoblasts, connective tissue, and a blood vessel. By the deposition of successive layers of bone on the inner walls of the tube, concentric Haversian lamellae are produced until the space is reduced to a Haversian canal with only room enough for the blood vessel.

The spongy lamellae in the diaphyses do not last long. They are resorbed in the presence of osteoclasts, which can be seen in Howship's lacunae on the lamellae (Fig. 84,*o**). This process enlarges the marrow cavity until finally the perichondral bone itself is being resorbed from the inside. In the cortex, however, the rate of resorption is exceeded by new growth on the exterior and by internal reconstruction. In the latter process, the tunnels formed by the resorption of bone around the blood vessels are constantly refilled with new Haversian systems. The old bone remains between the latest Haversian systems as the interstitial lamellae. Longitudinal growth is effected by the production of cartilage, which continues to grow at the ends without restriction.

Finally the end-pieces of the cartilage, the epiphyses, undergo ossification, mostly of the endochondral type. An independent *epiphyseal center* of ossification develops (Fig. 86,*e*), which has a grayish appearance and a mortar-like consistency. Usually blood vessels have already penetrated from the surface; they destroy the cartilage. Spongy bone is produced by osteoblasts. A thickened bone cortex develops later, but the layer of cartilage on the distal end of the bone remains throughout life as the articular cartilage (Fig. 86,*g*). Between the epiphysis and the diaphysis, a plate of *epiphyseal cartilage* (Fig. 86,*f*) remains for a longer time. It shows active growth processes on both surfaces, but more especially on the diaphyseal side, where there are well-developed cartilage columns. This permits still further longitudinal growth. Only after growth is completed does the plate ossify and the marrow cavity extend into the epiphysis. This process, part of which occurs after birth, results in the early formation of rigid

---

* Fig 84 is on p. 89.

articular ends on the bones without interfering with longitudinal growth. Ossification of the short and flat bones is like that of the epiphyses.

In the carnivora and man, the epiphyseal centers do not form until the time of birth, and the young are unable to walk for some time. The ungulata, which can stand and walk immediately after birth, have all of their centers of ossification developed at term, a condition which corresponds to that in man at the time of puberty.

The diaphysis of the long bones also shows many developmental processes in postnatal life. The surface is roughened by unclosed vascular grooves, and the osseous tissue is still mostly coarse-fibered. Growth is so extensive that the bones of the newborn would fit into the marrow cavities of the adult. Resorption and reconstruction produce newly formed Haversian systems composed entirely of fine-fibered bone. The end of the growth period is marked by the deposition of internal and external basic lamellae, which provide smooth surfaces. The internal resorption and reconstruction of bone continues at a restricted rate throughout life. The postnatal changes sometimes alter the external form of the bone.

IV

Muscular Tissue

MUSCULAR tissue consists of elongated cells called muscle cells or muscle fibers. They are characterized by their ability to respond to nervous stimuli by contraction. This property depends on the presence of certain organoids, myofibrils, which lie embedded in the sarcoplasm. We distinguish smooth and striated muscle fibers.

A. SMOOTH MUSCLE

Smooth muscle tissue consists of elongated cells that are tapered at both ends and lack a visible membrane (Figs. 87, 89). Their oblong or rod-shaped nuclei are located in the middle of the cell. In cross section they are round or elongated, or polygonal when closely packed. Their surface is smooth, and their ends·are sometimes divided into two or more branches. Their length ranges from 15 to 200 μ (up to 0.5 mm. in the gravid uterus) and their thickness from 4 to 7 μ.

The cytoplasm consists of longitudinal *myofibrils*[1] up to 1 μ thick and of an undifferentiated interstitial substance called *sarcoplasm*.[2] In the latter we often find, especially near the nucleus, rows of extremely fine granules in addition to occasional inclusions of glycogen or pigment granules. Because of their fibrillar structure the muscle fibers appear longitudinally striated. The fibrils are densely packed and decrease in number toward the tapering ends of the cell. They are uniformly birefringent.

It becomes necessary at this point to clarify some terms frequently used in describing the *refractive properties* of fibers. Objects seen with the ordinary light microscope are often said to be highly refractive or strongly refractive. This means that they have a higher index of refraction than the surrounding medium and appear bright with sharp dark borders when the microscope is properly focused. The appearance is altered by changing the focus.

Strong refraction, which is observed with the ordinary microscope, should not be confused with double refraction or birefringence, which is studied with the polarizing microscope. Birefringence is not dependent upon the refractive index but

---

[1] Gr. *mys* muscle.   [2] Gr. *sarx* flesh.

upon the parallel orientation of molecules within the substance (p. 8). When a birefringent crystal or fiber is examined in the polarizing microscope between crossed Nicol prisms, it glows with a‾ soft light in a dark field. It separates the polarized light received from the lower prism into two parts (constituting double refraction), one of which is polarized in a different plane and passes through the upper prism. Birefringent substances are also called *anisotropic* because they do not have the same optical properties in all directions.

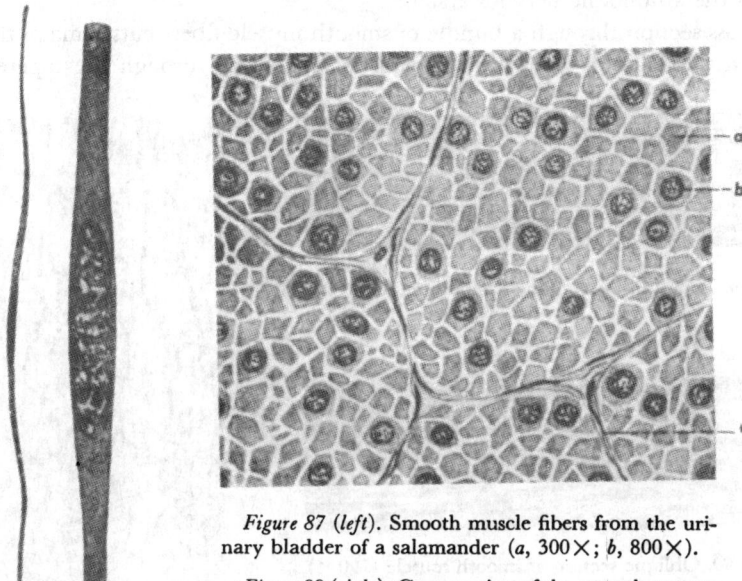

Figure 87 (left). Smooth muscle fibers from the urinary bladder of a salamander (*a*, 300×; *b*, 800×).

Figure 88 (right). Cross section of the smooth musculature from the stomach of a horse. *a*, cross section through a fiber; *b*, nucleus of a muscle fiber; *c*, interstitial connective tissue.

An *isotropic*, singly refracting, or nonpolarizing substance is one that transmits light vibrating in any plane. Therefore, it does not change the plane of polarization of the light received from the lower Nicol prism. When the upper prism is crossed, the field is entirely dark. Isotropic substances have a disorderly or folded molecular structure. Glass and unstretched fresh elastic fibers are examples of isotropic, but strongly refractive, material.

The nucleus is 15–20 μ thick. It is usually located in the middle, rarely toward one end, and exhibits a characteristic cross striation (Fig. 87,*b*) caused by a peculiar, presumably spiral arrangement of its chromatin. The nucleus may shorten or elongate, and sometimes during contraction it appears spiraled or compressed from end to end. The diplosome lies near the long side of the nucleus.

Smooth muscle fibers are either dispersed through the connective tissue or form bundles united by loose connective tissue in muscular sheets. The cells within these bundles are all oriented in the same direction. They are ensheathed and bound together by delicate *membranelles*, which contain many elastic and reticular fibers. Nets of elastic fibers are especially well developed around the sheaths of muscle fibers at the ends of the bundles, e.g., on the arrectores pilorum of the skin. Smooth muscle tissue often resembles regular connective tissue, but may be distinguished from the latter by the many rod-shaped nuclei within the fibers (Fig. 89).

Smooth muscle tissue is rich in blood and lymph vessels, which form dense networks with elongated meshes in the muscle sheets (Fig. 91). Its motor innervation is from the autonomic nervous system.

A cross section through a bundle of smooth muscle fibers cuts some of the fibers through the middle, where the nucleus is, and some through the tapered ends.

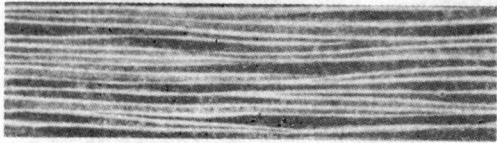

Figure 89. Longitudinal section of smooth muscle (790×)

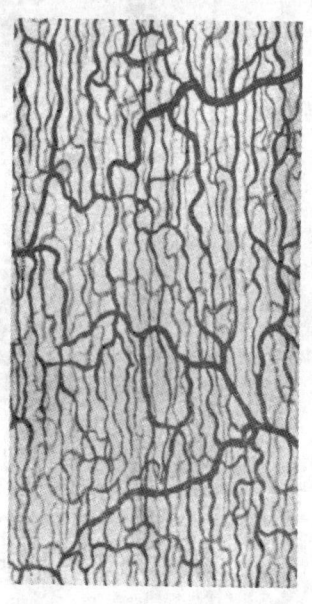

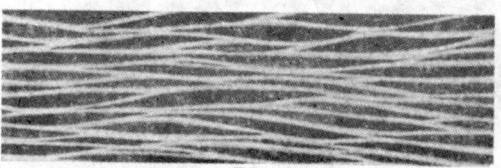

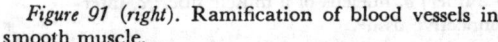

Figure 90. Oblique section of smooth muscle (790×).

Figure 91 (right). Ramification of blood vessels in smooth muscle.

Therefore the fibers appear as polygons of various sizes. Only the larger ones show a nucleus (Fig. 88). In oblique sections the fibers appear fusiform (Fig. 90). The cross striations seen in some stained longitudinal sections of smooth muscle sheets are contraction waves or fixation artefacts caused by shrinkage. In ordinary hematoxylin-eosin preparations the smooth muscle fibers assume a reddish-violet tinge.

Smooth muscle is not under voluntary control. Its contractions are slow but sustained.

OCCURRENCE. Isolated fibers and bundles are found in the skin and mucous membranes, in the spleen, lymph nodes, corpora cavernosa, tunica albuginea testis, etc. Smooth muscle sheets (tunicae musculares) occur in the walls of the gastrointestinal tract, bronchi, trachea, uterine tube, uterus, vagina, ductus deferentes, renal pelvis, ureters, urinary bladder, urethra, many excretory ducts of glands, blood and lymph vessels, and in the broad ligament and accessory glands of the genital tract. They also make up the ciliary and iridial muscles of the eye. In the muscle sheets the interstitial connective tissue is sometimes delicate (as in the intestinal wall), sometimes well developed (as in the ureter). The muscle cells that are found on the end-pieces of tubular skin glands and salivary glands have an epithelial origin and are called myoepithelial cells.

DEVELOPMENT. Like the connective tissue cells, most smooth muscle cells are mesenchymal derivatives. Some of them, however, arise from ectoderm (e.g., those of the skin glands and the iris) and entoderm (muscles of the primitive bronchi). Primitive connective tissue cells retain throughout life their ability to differentiate into smooth muscle cells. Thus smooth muscle can be continually replaced, repaired, and increased in amount.

B. STRIATED MUSCLE

Striated muscle includes skeletal and cardiac muscle. Here the myofibrils in the fibers, in contrast to those of smooth muscle, do not have a uniform structure, but

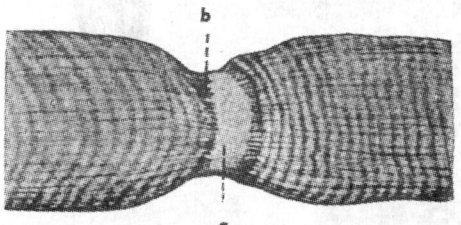

Figure 92. Piece of a freshly isolated skeletal muscle fiber. The contents (*b*) are torn apart. The sarcolemma (*a*) is intact.

are differentiated into segments which differ in refractive properties and cause a cross striation of the whole fiber.

1. Skeletal Muscle

By teasing apart a piece of skeletal muscle it is possible to isolate the striated muscle fibers (Figs. 93,*a;* 97). These are cylindrical in shape, are round or slightly flattened in cross section, and become thinner toward the ends. The ends may be pointed, blunt, clubbed, rounded off, or split into two or more branches, as in the musculature of the tongue, eyes, and esophagus. The fibers are larger than those of smooth muscle. Their length averages from 1 to 5 cm. but may be 12 cm. and even more, while their width is 10 to 150 μ—usually 20 to 50 μ. The width depends upon species, individual, stage of nutrition, age, size, and especially the function of the particular muscle; there are thick-fibered and thin-fibered muscles. Both kinds of fibers may occur side by side in the same muscle. Each muscle fiber must be considered a syncytium consisting of a membrane, its contractile contents, and the nuclei of the fibers.

The membrane of the muscle fiber, the *sarcolemma*, is thin (1 μ), transparent, and apparently structureless and shows great resistance to acids, alkalies, and mechanical insult. It forms a complete tube tightly adherent to the contents of the fiber (Figs. 92; 95,*B,a*). The sarcolemma may be demonstrated by mechanical rupture,

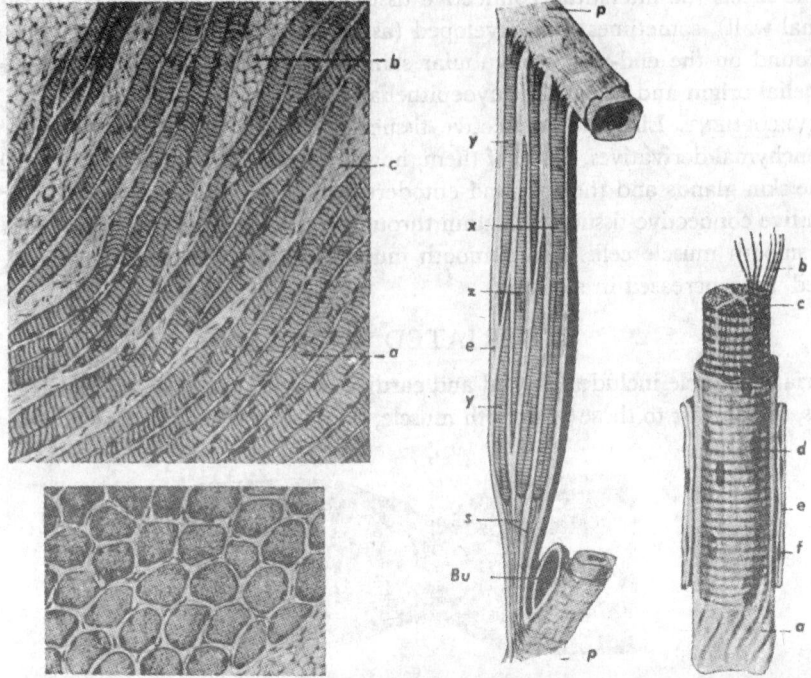

Figure 93 (upper left). Longitudinal section through striated muscle fibers of a horse. *a*, muscle fibers; *b*, adipose tissue; *c*, connective tissue.

Figure 94 (lower left). Striated muscle fibers from a horse, showing peripheral nuclei in the cross sections of the fibers, and intervening connective tissue.

Figure 95 (right). Striated muscle, schematic. (After Braus.)

A: Muscle between two bones. The size of the muscle fibers is disproportionately large. Muscle fiber *x* arises from the periosteum *P* and is inserted by means of a tendon on the bone; *y* ends within the muscle; *z* has both ends within the muscle. *e*, epimysium; *s*, tendon fibers; *Bu*, subtendinous bursa.

B: A muscle fiber under higher magnification. *a*, sarcolemma; *b*, myofibrils; *c*, Cohnheim's field; *d*, a nucleus of the muscle fiber; *e*, endomysium of the muscle fiber; *f*, connective tissue nucleus.

the addition of water, or staining. Silver impregnation shows the presence of reticular fibers. The sarcolemma has more than a simple mechanical function; it is of metabolic importance as the dividing membrane between the tissue fluid and the sarcoplasm.

The *cross striations* of the muscle fibers become evident even under low magnification (Fig. 93). These are caused by the alternation of more and less refractive zones ("transverse discs," Figs. 95, 97). In the polarizing microscope one disc appears doubly refractive or anisotropic and is called the A disc, while the other is singly refractive or isotropic and is called the I disc. In the relaxed fiber the A discs are stained more deeply than the I discs (Fig. 96). The lighter I discs are divided into two equal segments by a thin, dark (anisotropic) line, the intermediate or Z disc. Similarly, the dark A disc may be bisected by a light zone containing a poorly visible middle or M disc. Contraction supposedly occurs in the A disc. This may shorten the muscle to one tenth of its length. Under favorable conditions (as in insect muscles) one may distinguish on either side of the Z disc a birefringent line called the accessory or N disc. The Z, N, and M discs are highly variable, especially during contraction. In the contracted fiber there is a reversal of striation, i.e., the I disc stains darker than the A disc. The polarizing properties are not reversed, however.

Actually the muscle fibers consist of separate longitudinal fibrils, 1 μ in thickness, called myofibrils (Figs. 95,b; 96; 97,c). These products of cytoplasmic differentiation are contractile and are surrounded by an interstitial substance, the sarcoplasm. The fibrils often occur in groups (Fig. 95,B,b). Treatment with alcohol, picric acid, or chromic acid brings out the longitudinal striations more clearly and finally causes separation of the fibrils. The cross striations of the muscle fiber arc caused by the segments of its myofibrils, identical segments lying in the same transverse plane or disc (Fig. 97). The Z disc traverses the entire thickness of the fiber, including the sarcoplasm in the interfibrillar space, and attaches to the sarcolemma. It is said to hold the myofibrils in position. The portion of a myofibril lying between two Z bands is called a *sarcomere*. The greater development and specialization of the myofibrils probably accounts for the increased speed and magnitude of contraction in striated as opposed to smooth muscle fibers. In the horse and pig the cross striations are wide and prominent, but in ruminants the abundance of sarcoplasm emphasizes the longitudinal striae.

The *sarcoplasm*, which occurs between myofibrils or groups of myofibrils, contains granules of varying sizes called sarcosomes, sometimes also fat droplets. Glycogen and the wear-and-tear pigment, lipofuscin, may also be present. Sarcoplasm varies in amount in different muscle fibers. We distinguish therefore white muscle fibers, which are poor in sarcoplasm, and red ("muddy") muscle fibers, which carry an abundance of sarcoplasm. A cross section of a light fiber (Fig. 98,a) shows a uniform stippling caused by a uniform distribution of myofibrils and sarcoplasm throughout the plane of section. In the red fibers, however, the fibrils are grouped into bundles or muscle columns which in cross section appear as round or angular areas, known as Cohnheim's fields. Within these the myofibrils are visible as dots. The sarcoplasm is scanty between the individual fibrils, but more abundant between the muscle columns. Therefore it appears in cross sections as a network, which becomes especially conspicuous where great concentrations of sarcoplasm occur (Figs. 95,B,c; 98,b). The color of the red fibers is probably due to the presence of muscle hemoglobin and cytochrome in the sarcoplasm. These fibers, moreover, are richer in sarcosomes, smaller in diameter, more abundantly supplied with blood vessels, and more plainly striated longitudinally than the pale muscle, in which the cross striations are more pronounced. The two kinds of fibers also differ physiologically. The white fibers contract more rapidly and more vigorously, but they tire sooner than the dark fibers. The dark fibers occur principally in highly active muscles that are called upon to perform steadily, e.g., respiratory, eye, masticatory, and tongue muscles. In most muscles the ratio of light to dark fibers is in proportion to the

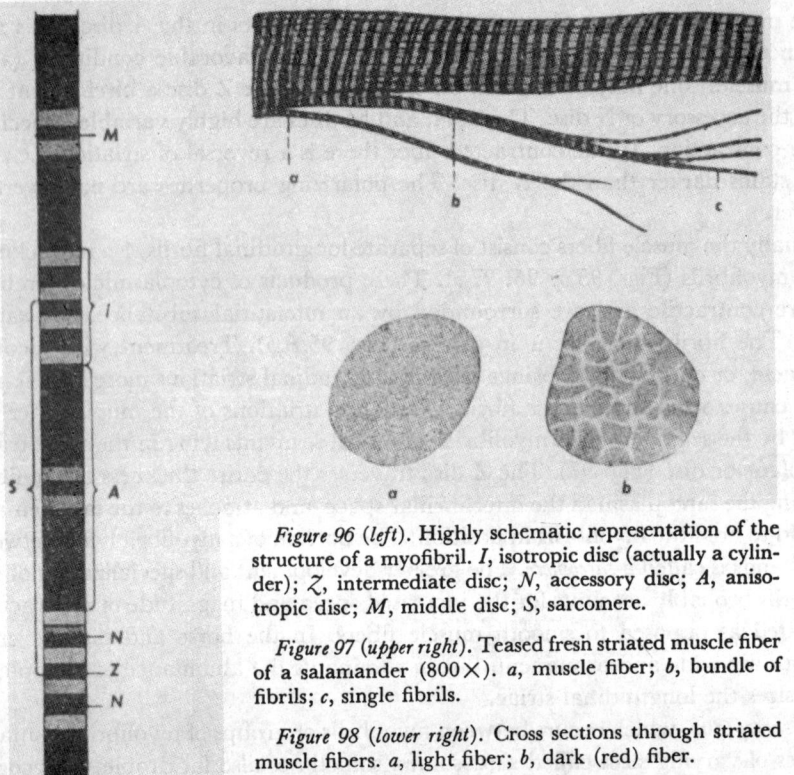

Figure 96 (*left*). Highly schematic representation of the structure of a myofibril. *I*, isotropic disc (actually a cylinder); *Z*, intermediate disc; *N*, accessory disc; *A*, anisotropic disc; *M*, middle disc; *S*, sarcomere.

Figure 97 (*upper right*). Teased fresh striated muscle fiber of a salamander (800×). *a*, muscle fiber; *b*, bundle of fibrils; *c*, single fibrils.

Figure 98 (*lower right*). Cross sections through striated muscle fibers. *a*, light fiber; *b*, dark (red) fiber.

amount of work that the muscle does. In some animals, muscles with only one kind of fibers are found. Examples of muscles with light fibers are the vastus intermedius, adductor longus, and biceps femoris of the rabbit and the flight muscles of the chicken. Examples of the dark-fibered or red muscles are the semitendinosus and soleus of the rabbit and the leg muscles of the chicken. In Thoroughbred horses, white muscles are more abundant than in cold-blooded horses. The pig has many light-colored muscles.

The nuclei of muscle fibers are oval and somewhat flattened. Their longitudinal axis runs parallel to the direction of the muscle fiber (Figs. 93; 95,*B,d*). They appear vesicular and have one or two nucleoli. Sarcosomes occur near their ends. Nuclei occur in great numbers in every muscle fiber. In mammals they usually have a peripheral location directly under the sarcolemma. They may be easily demonstrated in cross sections of fibers (Fig. 94). In fibers that are rich in sarcoplasm the nuclei are often more centrally located.

OCCURRENCE. In the skeletal muscles, skin muscles, extrinsic muscles of the eye and ear, in the tongue, pharynx, esophagus, larynx, and in the ciliary and sphincter pupillae muscles of birds.

DEVELOPMENT. With the exception of the head and neck muscles derived from branchial arches, the voluntary striated muscles originate from the mesodermal

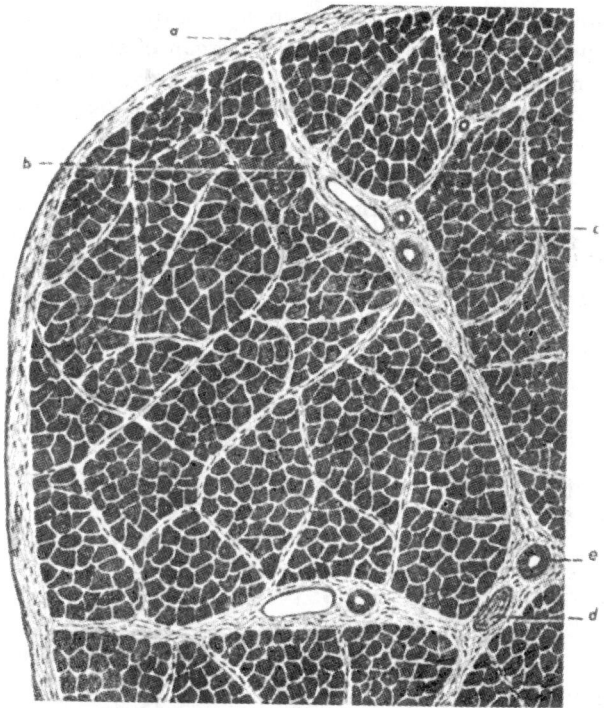

Figure 99. Cross section through a part of a striated muscle of a dog. *a*, epimysium; *b*, perimysium; *c*, muscle fibers surrounded by endomysium; *d*, nerve; *e*, blood vessel.

segments or somites. The myoblast that develops into a striated muscle fiber is a spheroidal or columnar cell with undifferentiated cytoplasm, no visible membrane, and only one nucleus. As the nucleus of each myoblast undergoes numerous mitotic divisions, the cytoplasm grows in length without dividing. Thus a multinucleated fiber-like structure is formed. Other investigators believe the muscle fiber to be a syncytium formed secondarily by many originally separate cells. Still others favor a combination of the two methods. The idea that the mitochondria give rise to myofibrils is no longer generally accepted. The myofibrils first appear as thin threads in the peripheral cytoplasm of the early myoblast. They proceed to form bundles, first around the periphery of the cell and later in the interior of the cytoplasm. The fibrils continue to form until the fiber is filled with them. Each fibril develops a series of thickenings at regular intervals. These are responsible for the striated effect of the mature muscle fiber. The fibrillar cytoplasm originally lacks a cell membrane. The sarcolemma does not appear until an advanced stage of development. Some of the nuclei lie close to the sarcolemma, while the remainder lie in the interior of the cytoplasm. As the fibrils develop in the more central cell portions, the nuclei are crowded toward the periphery. Striated muscle fibers multiply in the embryo by longitudinal division, preceded by active nuclear multiplication. Thereafter, growth occurs only by increase in the size of the fibers.

Skeletal Muscles as Organs. Muscles are formed by the combination of a great number of muscle fibers. Every muscle is an organ of special function. It is enveloped by a smooth sheath of connective tissue, which contains elastic fibers and occasionally adipose tissue. It is called the *epimysium* (Fig. 99,a). From this capsule, laminae of varying thicknesses are given off toward the interior. They unite to form a continuous framework, the *perimysium*, which separates the fiber bundles (*b*). The perimysium in turn gives off delicate membranes containing argyrophil fibers which envelop the individual muscle fibers as *endomysium* (*c*). The reticular fibers in this latticework are continuous with those of the sarcolemma and those surrounding the blood capillaries.

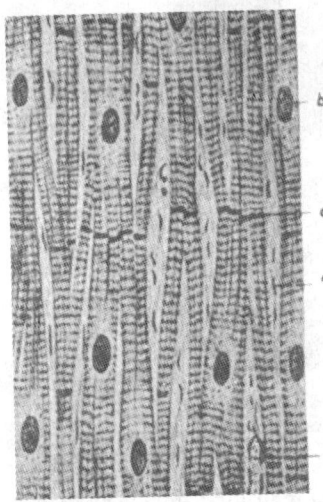

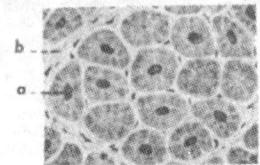

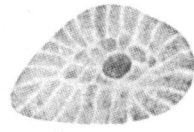

Figure 100 (*left*). Longitudinal section through cardiac muscle fibers. *a*, intercalated disc; *b*, nucleus; *c*, nucleus of a·connective tissue cell; *d*, blood vessel.

Figure 101 (*center*). Cross section through cardiac muscle fibers. *a*, nuclei of muscle fibers; *b*, connective tissue.

Figure 102 (*right*). Cross . section through a cardiac muscle fiber under high magnification.

Blood vessels are very numerous and ramify in the perimysium. The capillaries form meshes which are elongated in the direction of the fibers. The veins have many valves. There are only a few lymph vessels, which run next to the blood vessels. The nerves have somatic motor, sensory, and autonomic fibers. At least one motor nerve ends on each muscle fiber at its motor end plate (Fig. 374). Sensory fibers end in muscle spindles (Fig. 366). The connection of muscles to tendons, through which the muscle pull is transmitted, may be accomplished by the continuity of the endomysium with the tendon tissue. The sarcolemma is also tightly attached to the tendon. Myofibrils have been observed to penetrate the sarcolemma and blend into the tendon fibrils (e.g., muscles of the tongue, the rectus abdominis of the frog, and muscle fibers in the dorsal fin of the sea horse).

2. Cardiac Muscle

The fibers of cardiac muscle resemble those of skeletal muscle in being transversely and longitudinally striated. They are distinguished, however, by the central location of their nuclei and the numerous communicating branches which form a network of narrow meshes (Fig. 100). Both main and connecting fibers exhibit transverse, steplike *intercalated discs*. These are more strongly refractive and stain dark with hematoxylin (Fig. 100,a). The nature and function of the intercalated discs are in doubt. The myofibrils pass through them. They may be greatly thickened Z discs forming part of the framework supporting the cardiac muscle fibers.

The cross striations of cardiac muscle fibers are closer together than those of skeletal muscle. The longitudinal striations are usually very distinct. The myofibrils are grouped into round, polygonal, or ribbon-shaped bundles. In cross section they often present a characteristic radial structure (Figs. 101, 102). There is an abundance of sarcoplasm, especially in the immediate vicinity of the nuclei. It contains sarcosomes, glycogen, brownish-yellow pigment granules, and, in the case of carnivores, ruminants, and pigs, also fat droplets.

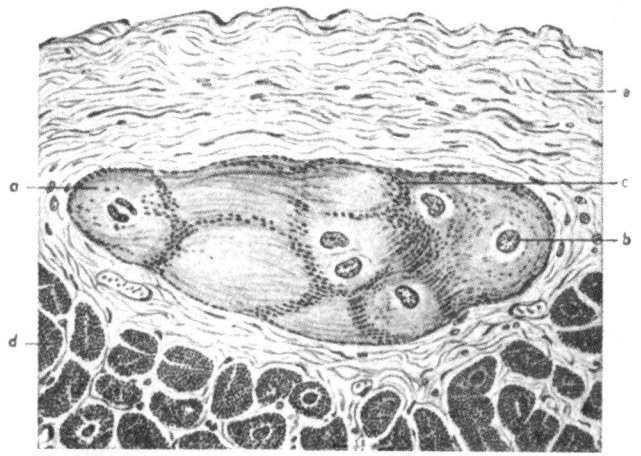

Figure 103. From a section through the heart of a sheep (250×). *a*, Purkinje fiber; *b*, nucleus; *c*, contractile fibrils in the peripheral layer of a Purkinje fiber; *d*, cardiac muscle fibers (cross section); *e*, endocardium.

The centrally located nuclei are larger but less elongated than those found in skeletal muscles. Their shape is ovoid, with the long axis running parallel to the course of the fibers (Figs. 100,*b;* 101,*a*).

Only a very thin sheath, comparable to the one that envelops smooth muscle fibers, serves as a sarcolemma. It also contains argyrophil fibers. Blood capillaries are found between fibers and intertwine with them. At the point where the papillary muscles blend into the chordae tendineae and at the openings of the heart there occur fibers that end in single points or in bifurcations.

Under the endocardium of the heart chambers specialized gray anastomosing cords are seen. These *Purkinje fibers* are a syncytium of specialized impulse-conducting cells. They are connected with the cardiac muscle fibers and surrounded by a sheath, which is continued on the cardiac fibers. In the peripheral portion of a Purkinje fiber there are striated contractile fibrils. The nuclei are central, sometimes paired, and surrounded by granular sarcoplasm. The Purkinje fibers and the sinoatrial and atrioventricular nodes, which have a similar structure, make up the impulse-conducting system, which co-ordinates the heart beat (p. 116).

OCCURRENCE. Cardiac muscle cells are found in the muscular wall of the heart and to a variable extent in the proximal portions of the vena cava cranialis and caudalis and the pulmonary veins.

DEVELOPMENT. The heart muscle fibers are derived from splanchnic mesoderm. In early embryonic life they are syncytial and resemble the smooth muscle cells. No striated fibrils are present at this stage even though the heart is already beating. Not until later do the striated fibrils develop in the cytoplasm, first, as in the case of skeletal muscle, in the periphery, then in the interior. The nucleus remains in the center of the cell. Intercalated discs appear late.

V

Nervous Tissue

THE work of the nervous tissue consists mostly of reception, conduction, and transmission of stimuli. The most important elements are the nerve cells or ganglion cells. These are equipped with processes that vary greatly in number, distribution, and length. Frequently one of the processes is very long. It is these long processes, usually surrounded by special sheaths, that form the nerve fibers of the nerves. They end in a terminal arborization called the telodendron.[1] The cell body and all its processes constitute a unit, the neuron. The neuroglia forms the special supporting and covering substance of the nervous tissue.

A. NERVE CELLS

OCCURRENCE. Nerve cells occur in the gray matter of the brain and spinal cord (central nervous system, C.N.S.), the eye, the ear, and the olfactory mucosa, in the ganglia of the cranial and spinal nerves and the sympathetic trunk, and singly or grouped in macroscopic or microscopic ganglia in and on many organs.

Processes. Nerve cells are characterized by their processes as well as by their location. Two types of processes may be distinguished, dendrites and axons.

The *dendrites*[2] or cytoplasmic processes (Figs. 105,*b;* 106,*a,b,c,d*) receive stimuli from the exterior or impulses from fibers of other nerve cells and conduct them toward the cell body. They have a broad origin from the cell body and divide into many fine divergent branches, which end in the vicinity of the cell, often in a thick feltlike tangle. Their area of distribution is sometimes very large. The thicker dendrites contain in their cytoplasm bundles of fine parallel fibrils. The surface of many dendrites is covered by small spines or nodules (varicosities, gemmules) considered by some authors to be synaptic (p. 76) organs. The wide distribution of the dendrites increases the capacity for absorption of nutrients and for the reception of impulses from the terminal expansions of adjacent axons.

The *axon* (axis cylinder) is almost always single (Figs. 105,*c;* 106,*Ax*). It conducts

---

[1] Gr. *telos* end, and *dendron* tree.
[2] The dendrites are not stained by the usual methods. They can be demonstrated by the chrome-silver impregnation method of Golgi.

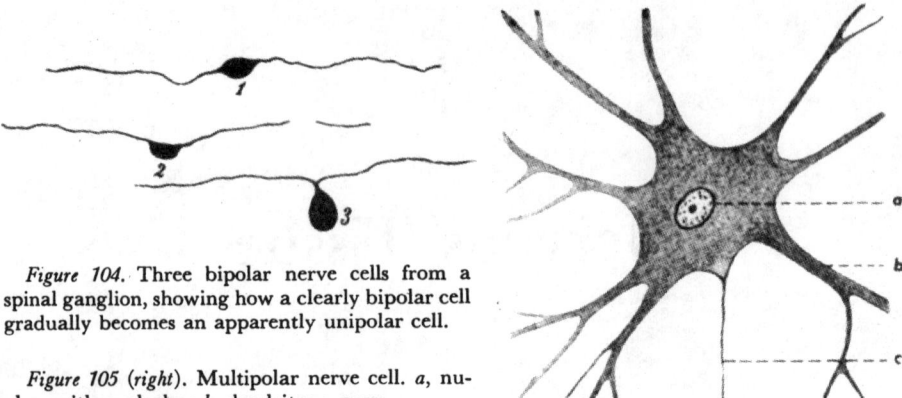

Figure 104. Three bipolar nerve cells from a spinal ganglion, showing how a clearly bipolar cell gradually becomes an apparently unipolar cell.

Figure 105 (right). Multipolar nerve cell. *a,* nucleus with nucleolus; *b,* dendrite; *c,* axon.

impulses away from the cell body. It is usually long, thinner at its origin than the dendrites, and homogeneous in appearance; it has a smooth surface. As a rule it arises from a small cone (axon hillock) on the cell body, tapers rapidly, and then continues at a uniform thickness.

According to the number of processes on the nerve cell but without regard for the kind of process (axon or dendrite), we distinguish the following types:

1. *Unipolar nerve cells* (Figs. 104,*3;* 359) are found in the cerebrospinal ganglia. Their unipolarity is only apparent. In the embryo they are bipolar, but during development the origins of the two processes approach each other until they are fused for a short distance. This produces a unipolar cell with a T-shaped process. The peripheral branch, corresponding physiologically to a dendrite, conducts peripheral stimuli to the cell body (sensory or afferent nerve fiber). The other branch conducts the impulse from the cell body farther into the central nervous system. Both branches have the morphology of an axis cylinder.

2. *Bipolar nerve cells* (Fig. 104,*1,2*) occur in the vestibular and spiral ganglia of the acoustic nerve, in the retina, and in many parts of the C.N.S. They have two processes, one conducting toward the cell body and the other conducting away from it.

3. *Multipolar nerve cells* (Figs. 105–107, 360) comprise the majority of all cells in the C.N.S. and are the chief cells of the sympathetic ganglia. Only one of the many processes conducts impulses away from the cell body. This is the axon, which often extends for great distances, either into the C.N.S. or, in the case of the motor or efferent cells, out of the C.N.S. to end on a muscle fiber or glandular epithelium.

Cells are classified also on the basis of the length of the processes. The Golgi type I (Fig. 108) has a long process which gives off fine, branching collaterals on its course within the C.N.S. and which in many cases emerges as the axis cylinder of a peripheral nerve fiber (Fig. 110,*3*). Cells of the Golgi type II (Fig. 109) have a short axon that ends near the cell body in fine branches without forming a nerve fiber. The terminal branches of the axon are called the neuropodium (Fig. 109,*n*). Type II cells occur only in certain restricted areas of the brain and cord.

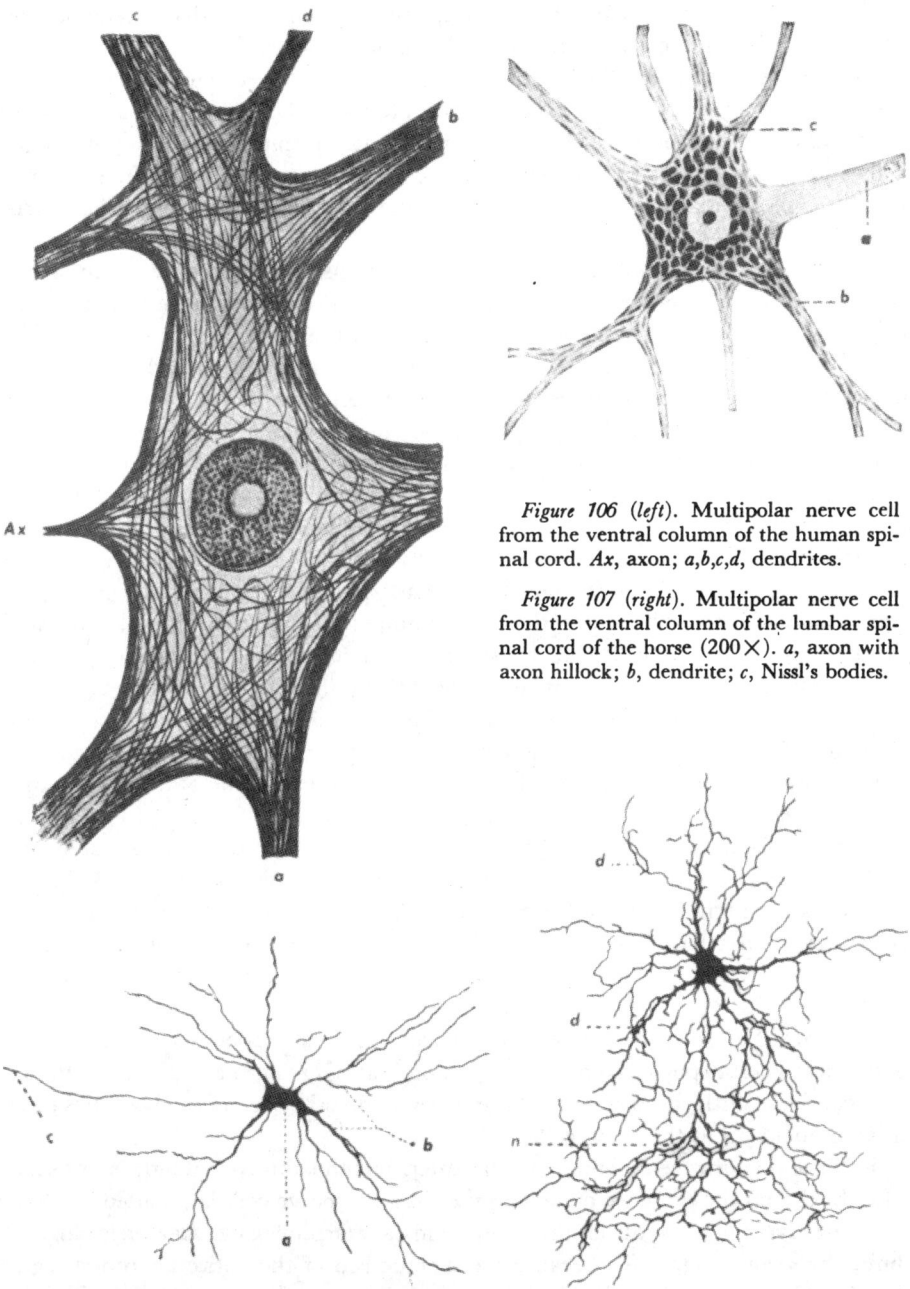

Figure 106 (left). Multipolar nerve cell from the ventral column of the human spinal cord. *Ax,* axon; *a,b,c,d,* dendrites.

Figure 107 (right). Multipolar nerve cell from the ventral column of the lumbar spinal cord of the horse (200×). *a,* axon with axon hillock; *b,* dendrite; *c,* Nissl's bodies.

Figure 108 (left). Nerve cell of the Golgi type I. *a,* cell body; *b,* dendrites; *c,* axon. (Golgi impregnation.)
Figure 109 (right). Nerve cell of the Golgi type II. *d,* dendrites; *n,* axon with neuropodium. (Golgi impregnation.)

Nerve cells vary in size from the smallest, which are no bigger than a lymphocyte (4 μ), to much larger cells which may be 150 μ in diameter.

The form of the nerve cells is also quite variable and depends upon the number, the type, and the manner of origin of the processes. Unipolar cells are usually spherical or pear-shaped, while bipolars are elongated, spindle-shaped. Multipolar cells have an irregular star-shaped, polygonal, or pyramidal form. In the cerebrum the pyramidal form predominates, in the cerebellum the spherical or pyriform.

Cytoplasm. The cytoplasm (perikaryon) contains *fibrils* that pass through the cell body from one process to another. They occasionally form networks in the peripheral cytoplasm, and there is often a tangle of fibrils around the nucleus. The fibrils were formerly regarded as the carriers of the nervous excitation, but they probably serve only to strengthen the nerve cell processes. Most physiologists accept the membrane theory of nerve impulse conduction—that the impulse is an electrical disturbance propagated along the plasma membrane of the neuron.

Between the fibrils lie particles of basophilic material called *Nissl's bodies* or tigroid granules (Fig. 107). They are stained only by special methods. Nissl's bodies appear in the proximal portions of the dendrites, but the axon hillock remains free of them. They are found in varying form, number, and arrangement, depending on the type and functional status of the cell. In unipolar spinal ganglion cells they are dustlike; in multipolar cells they form rods and clumps; in sympathetic ganglion cells, granules. Because the number decreases significantly in overexertion, disease, and old age, it may be assumed that they play an important role in metabolism and are used up during strong demands on the cell. The chemical nature of Nissl's bodies suggests a nuclear origin, and the term cytochromatin has been applied to them.

The cytoplasm also contains granular or rod-shaped mitochondria, fat droplets, and pigment granules. The pigment occurs as melanin in certain cells (as in the substantia nigra of the midbrain), and as yellowish lipoid material (lipofuscin), which accumulates in the cell body with advancing age and is taken as a sign of decreasing functional capacity. A Golgi apparatus is also demonstrable in nerve cells.

Nucleus. The spherical, sharply contoured nucleus is poor in chromatin and appears as a light spot. Oxychromatin predominates, giving the nucleus an affinity for acid dyes. With the exception of the ovocyte, no other cell of the body has such a large nucleolus as the nerve cell.

Embryonic nerve cells contain a cell center, but the ability to divide is lost soon after birth and the presence of a cell center in adult nerve cells is disputed.

The nerve cell with all its processes forms a morphological and physiological unit, the *neuron* (Fig. 110). Because the metabolism of the entire neuron is regulated by the nucleated cell body, the processes die when they are separated from it.

The nerve impulse is transmitted from one neuron to another through the *synapse*,[3] the point of contact between the axon termination of one neuron and the

---

[3] Gr. *syn* together, and *aptein* to touch.

cell body or dendrite of another. Transmission through the synapse is always in one direction, from the axon of the first neuron to the cell body or dendrites of the second. The bulk of the histological and physiological evidence indicates that there is no protoplasmic continuity from one neuron to the other across the synapse. According to the chemical theory of synaptic transmission, the impulse in the axon causes the liberation at the synapse of acetylcholine, which initiates an impulse in the second neuron. The acetylcholine is then destroyed by an enzyme, cholinesterase. According to the electrical theory, the second neuron is stimulated by a flow of current caused by the arrival of the nerve impulse at the axon termination. A third possibility is that the electrical and chemical changes that have been observed are two essential parts of the same process of transmission.[4]

B. NERVE FIBERS

A nerve fiber is composed of an axis cylinder and its sheaths. The axis cylinder arises as an axon (in sensory ganglia also as a dendrite) from a nerve cell body which acts as its trophic center. It receives a myelin sheath while it is still in the central nervous system (Figs. 110,2; 111,c; 112,b). As it emerges from the C.N.S., a second sheath is added, the neurilemma or sheath of Schwann (Figs. 110,1; 112,c). The myelin sheath is lacking as a rule in nerve fibers that arise from the cells in the autonomic ganglia (Remak's fibers).

The *axis cylinder* (Figs. 112,a; 113,a) appears homogeneous in the fresh state but, when examined by certain techniques, shows longitudinal striations. It may have a diameter as great as 10 μ. It is composed of neurofibrils (Figs. 111,a; 113,a) continuous with those of the cell body. They are somewhat interwoven in the axis cylinder and embedded in a soft watery mass, the axoplasm (Fig. 111,b). In cross sections the fibrils appear as dots. The axis cylinders of sensory and motor fibers show no structural differences.

In the region of the constrictions of Ranvier (p. 79; Figs. 111,d; 112,e; 113,e), a ringlike concentration of cement substance on the axis cylinder can be demonstrated by the silver nitrate method. This often takes the form of a biconical swelling. The axis cylinder is also stained black for a short distance on either side of the cement ring, and the two dark bands form Ranvier's cross.

On the basis of the number and kind of sheaths present, four kinds of nerve fibers are distinguished as follows:

(a) Myelinated with neurilemma
(b) Myelinated without neurilemma
(c) Unmyelinated with neurilemma
(d) Unmyelinated without neurilemma

Different portions of the same fiber may belong in any of these groups (Fig. 110). For example, the cerebrospinal nerve fibers arise as naked axis cylinders (c); they receive a myelin sheath while still in the C.N.S. (2) and a neurilemma

---

[4] Herbert S. Gasser et al., *Symposium on the Synapse* (Springfield, Ill.: C. C Thomas, 1939), pp. 399, 440.

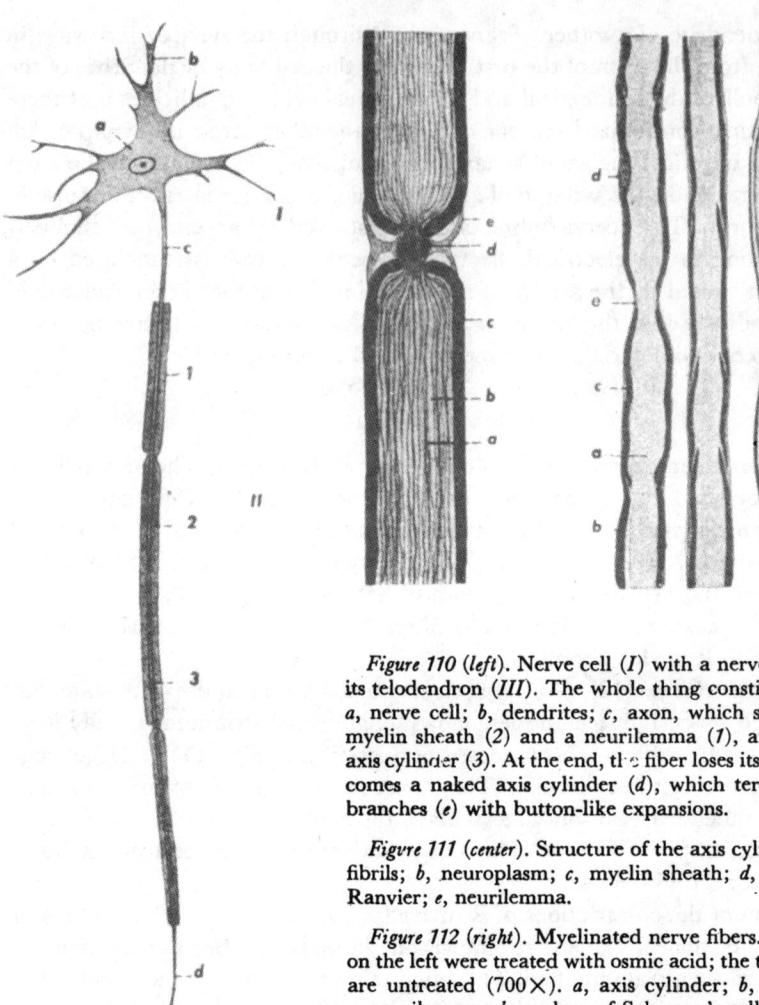

Figure 110 (left). Nerve cell (*I*) with a nerve fiber (*II*) and its telodendron (*III*). The whole thing constitutes a neuron. *a*, nerve cell; *b*, dendrites; *c*, axon, which soon acquires a myelin sheath (*2*) and a neurilemma (*1*), and becomes an axis cylinder (*3*). At the end, the fiber loses its sheath and becomes a naked axis cylinder (*d*), which terminates in fine branches (*e*) with button-like expansions.

Figure 111 (center). Structure of the axis cylinder. *a*, neurofibrils; *b*, neuroplasm; *c*, myelin sheath; *d*, constriction of Ranvier; *e*, neurilemma.

Figure 112 (right). Myelinated nerve fibers. The two fibers on the left were treated with osmic acid; the two on the right are untreated (700×). *a*, axis cylinder; *b*, myelin sheath; *c*, neurilemma; *d*, nucleus of Schwann's cell; *e*, constriction of Ranvier; *f*, myelin bulging out of the sheath.

where they emerge from the C.N.S. (*1*). Near their termination they lose first the myelin, then the neurilemma, and end as naked axis cylinders (*d*).

(a) Myelinated nerve fibers with neurilemma make up the great mass of all the fibers in the cerebrospinal nerves (with the exception of the olfactory and optic nerves). They also occur with a very thin myelin sheath in the sympathetic trunk, which is mostly composed of unmyelinated fibers. In the fresh condition they are cylindrical threads 1–20 μ in diameter with a smooth surface. Inside the glistening homogeneous myelin is a darker streak, the axis cylinder. The myelin

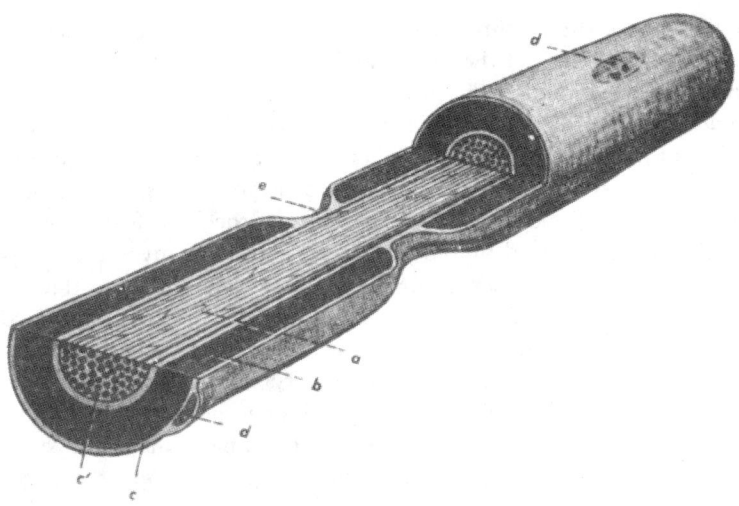

Figure 113. Myelinated nerve fiber, schematic. *a*, axis cylinder; *b*, myelin; *c*, neurilemma; *c'*, inner layer of the neurilemma, the existence of which is disputed; *d*, nucleus of a neurilemmal (Schwann's) cell; *e*, Ranvier's constriction.

gives the fibers their white appearance. It also causes the double contours seen when myelinated fibers are examined by transmitted light. At regular intervals the myelin sheath is interrupted by *Ranvier's constrictions* or *nodes* (Figs. 111,*d*; 112,*e*; 113,*e*). Finally, on the surface of the fiber are nuclei belonging to the neurilemma, which is barely visible in the fresh state.

The *myelin sheath* (Figs. 110,2; 111,*c*; 112,*b*; 113,*b*) may reach a thickness of 3 μ. It is not a continuous cylinder but is divided by Ranvier's constrictions into segments about 1 mm. in length (Fig. 110,2). It is a semifluid, strongly refractive, glistening, fatlike mass, composed of cholesterol, other lipids, and neurokeratin. It is easily and rapidly coagulated into clumps, which give the fiber a granular appearance (Fig. 112, *right*). At the same time, it swells out of the torn ends of the fibers (Fig. 112,*f*), forms cloudlike masses, and becomes paler. Treatment with osmic acid blackens the myelin sheath (Figs. 111; 112, *left*). Boiling alcohol and ether extract the fatty substances, leaving a network of coarse and fine trabeculae extending from the neurilemma to the axis cylinder. This neurokeratin framework is probably a fixation product representing the protoplasm which pervades the myelin and is a part of the surrounding neurilemma cell. Fixed nerve fibers also show the "clefts" of Lantermann (Fig. 112, *left*), usually described as incisions in the myelin sheath resulting from shrinkage in fixation. It is possible that they represent funnel-shaped protoplasmic partitions extending from the neurilemma to the axis cylinder.[5]

---

[5] A. A. Maximow and William Bloom, *A Textbook of Histology*, Fig. 163.

The significance of the myelin sheath is unknown. It is thought to have a great influence on the irritability of the nerves and to insulate them from the irritating substances in the tissue fluid of the surrounding connective tissue.

The *neurilemma* or sheath of Schwann (Figs. 112,*c*; 113,*c*) is composed of a continuous layer of Schwann's cells, neuroglial elements that have wandered out of the central nervous system and assumed a special form. These cells produce the myelin, which their cytoplasm closely surrounds. In the fresh fiber, the existence of the neurilemma is betrayed by the fact that it allows the myelin to escape only

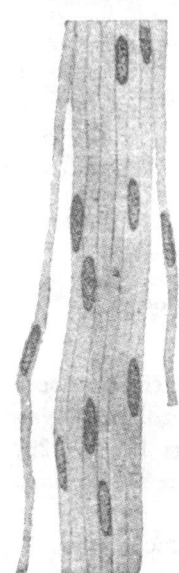

at points of rupture. It is usually less than 1 μ thick. On its inner surface are elongated ellipsoid nuclei surrounded by a small amount of cytoplasm. At Ranvier's constrictions, where the myelin is lacking, the neurilemma is closely applied to the axis cylinder. Here the cytoplasm is the only insulation between the axis cylinder and the surrounding connective tissue. It also connects adjacent segments. In every segment between constrictions there is usually one neurilemmal nucleus (i.e., one Schwann cell; Figs. 112,*d*; 113,*d*). In the newborn, the segments are considerably shorter (average 0.3 mm.) than in the adult. Only at Ranvier's constrictions can the exchange of metabolites for the axis cylinder take place easily. There is a constriction of Ranvier at the origin of every branch from a myelinated nerve fiber.

The neurilemma occurs only on peripheral nerves.

(b) **Myelinated fibers without a neurilemma** have no constrictions of Ranvier. In fibers isolated with 0.1 percent osmic acid, the myelin collects in drops, giving the fibers a varicose appearance. The thickness varies from 1 to 20 μ. To this group belong the myelinated fibers of the C.N.S. and the optic nerve. Each fiber is surrounded by neuroglia, which corresponds to the neurilemma of a peripheral nerve fiber.

Figure 114. Unmyelinated nerve fibers from the splenic nerve of the dog (700×).

(c) **Unmyelinated fibers with a neurilemma,** or Remak's fibers (Figs. 114; 360,*g*), form the bulk of the fibers of the autonomic nerves; they also occur singly in the cerebrospinal nerves. They are thin (1–10 μ) and surrounded only by a neurilemma. The neurilemmal nuclei in these fibers are longer, narrower, and much more numerous than in the myelinated fibers. At both ends of the nucleus there is a small amount of cytoplasm. The neurofibrils are thicker than in other nerve fibers and lie in groups.

(d) **Unmyelinated fibers without neurilemma,** the so-called naked axis cylinders, form the beginning and the end of the myelinated fibers, as well as fibers which remain naked axis cylinders throughout their courses. They occur in the central nervous system, in the olfactory nerves, and to some extent in the autonomic system.

C. THE NEUROGLIA[6] (GLIA)

The neuroglia forms the supporting substance of the C.N.S. and at the same time serves as a nutritive, protective, and isolating tissue. In the form of glial membranes and satellite cells, it separates the nervous elements from the vascular and connective tissues. In this way extraneous stimuli are kept away from the sensitive nervous tissue.

The neuroglia may be classified as follows:

Ependyma

Neuroglia proper

  Astrocytes

  Oligodendroglia

  Microglia

Capsule or satellite cells of peripheral ganglia

Schwann's cells

The *ependyma*[7] (Figs. 115, 346) is composed of a single layer of columnar cells which line the ventricles of the brain and the central canal of the spinal cord. They often bear motile cilia on the free end. At the basal end they extend deep into the brain or cord substance as long branched ependymal fibers, but, because these are not made visible by the usual staining methods, the ependyma looks like an epithelium.

The *astrocytes* are cells with much cytoplasm and many processes. According to the length of the latter, they are described as short-rayed (protoplasmic) and long-rayed (fibrous) astrocytes (Fig. 116,*A,B*). The short-rayed type forms a thick felt-work in the gray matter of the brain and cord. The long-rayed type does not branch so freely and is found mainly between the nerve fibers of the white matter of the C.N.S. The processes of the astrocytes contain fibers that pass through or lie in close apposition to the cell body (Fig. 117). The fibers, which are only demonstrable by special

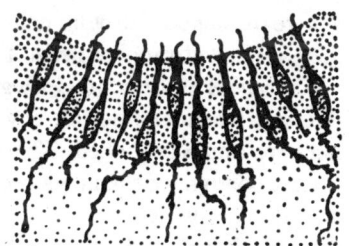

Figure 115. Ependymal cells of the central canal of the spinal cord.

methods, probably also occur separately, free from the cells. The short-rayed astrocytes have few fibers, the long-rayed have many. The glia cells, which are probably connected with each other, form with their processes and fibers a fine feltwork, in the meshes of which the neurons are embedded. In many areas of the central nervous system, these meshes contain no nerve cells but only the finest branches of their processes. This fine network is called the neuropil[8] or synaptic field. In other regions, the neuroglia is almost the only tissue present (e.g., in the substantia gelatinosa centralis; see *spinal cord*, p. 317).

The *oligodendroglia*[9] cells are smaller than the astrocytes. They have a spherical nucleus and few processes with less branching. They occur in columns along the

[6] Gr. *neuron* nerve, and *glia* glue.

[7] Gr. *ependyma* wrap.

[8] Gr. *pilos* felt.

[9] Gr. *oligos* few, and *dendron* tree.

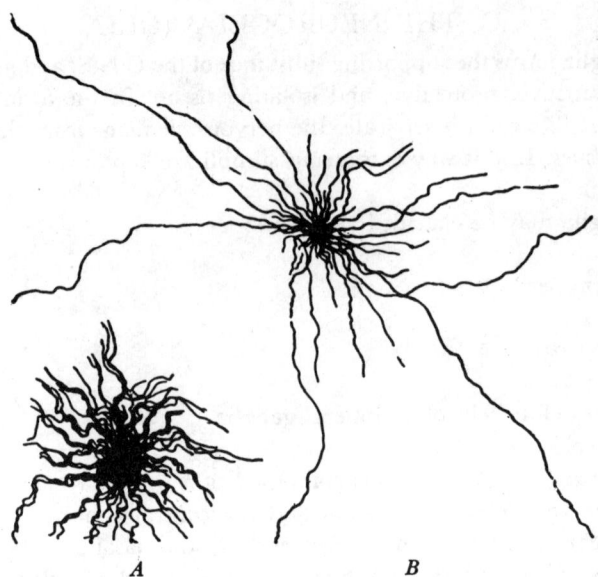

Figure 116. A, short-rayed (protoplasmic) astrocyte from the epiphysis of a horse; B, long-rayed (fibrous) astrocyte from the red nucleus of a horse. (Golgi impregnation.)

nerve fibers and are considered to have the same function as Schwann's cells. Where the oligodendroglia cells lie close to the nerve cell bodies in the gray matter, they are called satellite cells. They also lie next to small blood vessels in the C.N.S.

The *microglia* cells of Hortega are fewer in number and have a small, darkly staining, irregular nucleus, covered with a thin layer of cytoplasm. The few processes are much branched. These cells are highly motile and phagocytic.

DEVELOPMENT OF THE NERVOUS TISSUE. The nervous tissue is derived from the neural tube, which develops early from the ectoderm. The indifferent epithelial cells which form the neural tube gradually undergo extensive changes in form and location. Some of the cells are differentiated into *neuroblasts*, the forerunners of the nerve cells, while others become *spongioblasts*. The latter, outstripping the neuroblasts in development, form the neuroglia, of which the ependyma is the most primitive form. The ependymal cells are recognized by their position next to the lumen of the neural tube. As the lining of the cerebral ventricles and the central canal of the spinal cord, they represent vestiges of the originally epithelial primordium of the neural tube. Their connection with the rest of the glial framework is through their basal processes. The astrocytes differentiate

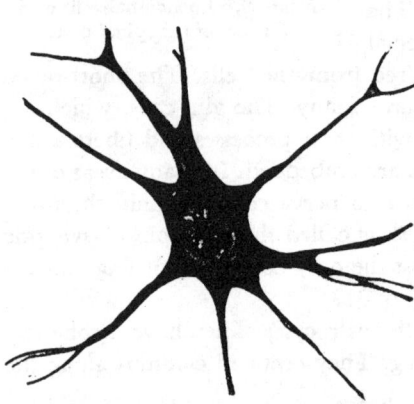

Figure 117. Fibrous astrocyte from the human spinal cord.

later than the ependymal cells, lose their contact with the lumen, and form cells with long or short processes, according to the kind of nervous tissue in which they are located. The oligodendroglia is also derived from spongioblasts, but the microglia develops from mesodermal cells which migrate into the C.N.S.

At first the neuroblasts are nested close together. From the small ends of their pear-shaped cell bodies grow slender primary processes, the future axis cylinders. These may grow to other parts of the neural tube, or they may leave the tube to grow out through the mesoderm to some peripheral structure, becoming associated in common nerve trunks as they go. The shape of the neuroblast changes with the increase of cytoplasm and the development of secondary processes, the dendrites, which sprout into the adjacent interstices of the glial framework. The neurofibrils appear early in the substance of the cell body and the processes.

The *sheaths* of the peripheral nerves are formed by glia cells that migrate out of the C.N.S. These develop into Schwann's cells and produce the myelin sheath. Fine glial fibers are also found on the surface of the so-called naked axon endings.

VI

Blood and Lymph

A. BLOOD

BLOOD is the nutritive fluid that carries to all parts of the body the substances required for growth, maintenance, and energy. It also carries the waste products of the life processes to the organs that dispose of them. It is composed of the fluid plasma and the formed elements—the red and white corpuscles and the platelets. The blood may be regarded as a tissue closely related to connective tissue. The intercellular substance is the plasma, composed of water, proteins, and salts and carrying a multitude of nutritional and regulatory substances, as well as waste products. It is colorless in thin films, yellow or gray in large quantities. The plasma coagulates or clots whenever it comes in contact with anything other than the living, healthy endothelium of the vessels. In coagulation, the protein fibrinogen, which is normally dispersed in the plasma, is caused to aggregate into fine strands of fibrin. The fibrin forms a tangled mass that traps most of the blood cells and shrinks to form a clot. The fluid expressed from the clot is called serum.

1. Erythrocytes[1]

The red blood corpuscles (Figs. 118,a–h; 119; 121,a*) are soft, flexible, and elastic. They are discoid or elliptical, depending on species, and undergo constant changes in shape in the blood stream. The discs (Figs. 118; 119,c) are concave on both surfaces with a thick rounded margin. When the focal plane of the microscope is lowered, the margin is dark and the center light. When the focus is raised, the light and dark portions are reversed (Fig. 118,b,c). These nonnucleated biconcave discs are found in all mammals except the Tylopoda (camel, llama; Fig. 120,4), where they are elliptical rather than round. In addition to the biconcave erythrocytes, mammals also have concavo-convex bell- or bowl-shaped forms (Fig. 118,e).

Birds, reptiles, and fish (except cyclostomes) have elliptical nucleated erythrocytes, which are larger and biconvex (Figs. 119,a,b; 120,1,2,3).

In preparations of fresh blood, the erythrocytes are often arranged like rolls of

---

[1] Gr. *erythros* red.   * Fig. 121 is on p. 90.

coins (rouleaux) as a result of surface attraction (Fig. 118,a). This does not occur in the blood of swine.

Erythrocytes appear homogeneous when examined in the living state or by ordinary staining methods. The surface layer is an invisible, selectively permeable, lipoid plasma membrane (p. 10). The more fluid interior contains hemoglobin, lipids, and salts. Individual living erythrocytes have a pale yellowish-green color caused by the hemoglobin contained in them. When several of them are superimposed, they appear red. The normal mature erythrocyte is eosinophilic, i.e., it stains red with the usual blood techniques.

When supravitally stained with brilliant cresyl blue, some erythrocytes show granules or a network of fibrils. Such cells are called reticulocytes. They occur most often in guinea pigs, rabbits, poultry, and newborn animals. They are considered to be immature erythrocytes and have considerable significance in anemia.

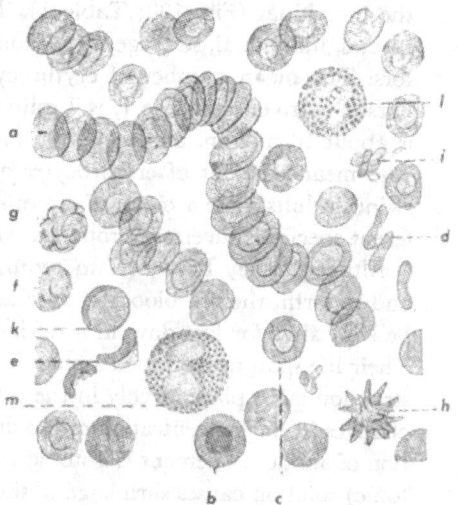

Figure 118. Formed elements of human blood, unstained (700×). a, erythrocytes in rouleau; b, erythrocyte with the focus raised; c, with the focus lowered; d, on edge; e, bell-shaped erythrocyte; f, erythrocyte in beginning crenation; g, mulberry form; h, thorn apple form; i, platelets; k, lymphocyte; l,m, granulocytes.

Howell-Jolly bodies are nuclear remnants which stain deeply with basic dyes.

The size of the erythrocytes varies in different species, and also in the blood of

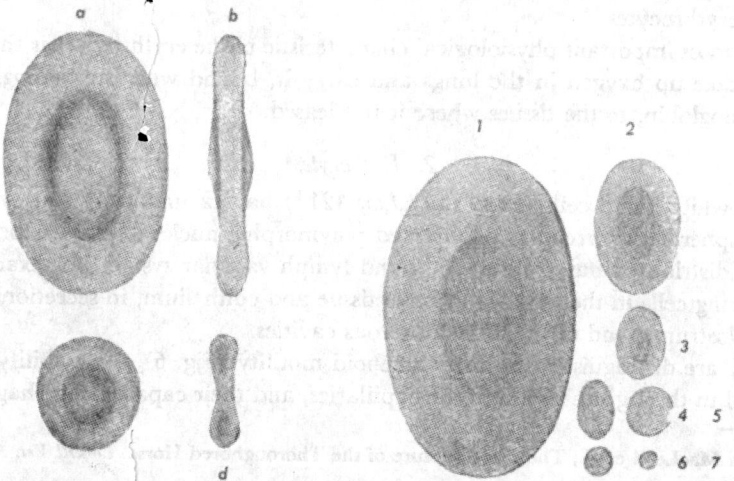

Figure 119 (left). a, avian erythrocyte; b, in profile; c, mammalian erythrocyte; d, in profile.

Figure 120 (right). Size relationships of different erythrocytes. 1, proteus; 2, frog; 3, chaffinch; 4, llama; 5, man; 6, goat; 7, musk ox.

the individual (Fig. 120; Table 1). The number of erythrocytes varies with the species, individual, sex, age, condition, time of day, work, altitude, and other factors. The mean number of erythrocytes per cubic mm. of blood in .adult draft horses, as given in Table 1, is 7 million, while the mean for Thoroughbred mares is about 10 million, and for adult Thoroughbreds other than mares, 11 million.[2] The mean number of erythrocytes given in the table for swine includes young swine. Adults have a mean of 7.4 million. The number of erythrocytes in the different species is inversely proportional to their size.

Although they have certain requirements for oxygen, moisture, temperature, and so forth, the red blood corpuscles are remarkably tenacious of life. They may be kept alive for five days in a refrigerator, but they cannot live without oxygen. Their life span in the blood stream has been estimated at one to four months. Destruction takes place largely in the spleen and liver. They are strongly affected by changes in the concentration of the fluid in which they are suspended. A salt solution of about 0.9 percent is isotonic with normal blood plasma. A stronger (hypertonic) solution causes shrinkage of the cells (crenation), with the formation of surface projections (mulberry or thorn apple forms, Fig. 118,g,h). The same effect is seen when blood is allowed to stand in contact with the open air; the evaporation of water concentrates the plasma. In weaker (hypotonic) solutions or water, the erythrocytes swell and give up their hemoglobin to the surrounding fluid (hemolysis). The colorless, spherical "ghost" or stroma that remains is difficult to see and eventually dissolves. The previously opaque red blood becomes a transparent red and is said to be "laked."[3]

Hemolysis is also caused by many chemical agents, serum of another species, serum of an incompatible blood group, bacterial toxins, and certain snake venoms. Another phenomenon caused by incompatible serum is agglutination or clumping of the erythrocytes.

The most important physiological characteristic of the erythrocytes is their ability to take up oxygen in the lungs and carry it, bound with the hemoglobin as oxyhemoglobin, to the tissues where it is released.

2. Leukocytes[4]

The white blood cells (Figs. 118,k,l,m; 121*) have a uniformly soft cytoplasm and a spherical or irregularly lobulated polymorphic nucleus. The leukocytes are widely distributed outside the blood and lymph vascular system; for example, as wandering cells in the loose connective tissue and epithelium, in secretions (saliva and colostrum), and in the fluids of serous cavities.

They are distinguished by their ameboid motility (Fig. 6), their ability to pass out and in through the walls of the capillaries, and their capacity for phagocytosis

---

[2] John MacLeod et al., The Blood Picture of the Thoroughbred Horse. Cornell Vet. 37 (1947): 305–313.

[3] From lake, a pigment, or lac, a resinous substance containing a scarlet dye.

[4] Gr. leukos white.   * Fig. 121 is on p. 90.

Table 1. Means and Standard Deviations of Normal Blood Counts

	Erythrocytes		Leukocytes				
	Millions per mm.³	Diam. in micra	Thousands per mm.³	Percentages			
				Lympho.	Mono.	Neutro.	Eosino.
Man	5	7.5	9	20	5	72	2
Horse (Holman)	7 ±0.7	5.6	9 ±1.6	29 ±11	5 ±2.5	58 ±12	7 ±3.5
Ox (Holman)	6 ±1.3	5.6	8 ±2	52 ±15	7 ±4	30 ±10	10 ±7
Sheep (Holman)	11.5±1.8	4.3	9.2±3.1	68 ±10	3 ±2.7	24 ±9	4 ±4.5
Goat	17.3	3.1	12	57	2.2	35	5.8
Swine (Holman)	5.6±0.7	6	14.7±4.5	38 ±13	4 ±2	53 ±11	4 ±2
Dog (Holman)	6.1±1	7.3	11.3±3.3	20 ±5.4	4 ±3	74 ± 7	2 ±2
Cat (Holman)	7.2±1	6.2	17.2±6.6	33	2.5	59	5
Guinea pig	5	7	12	45	6	40	8
Rabbit (Wirth)	4–6	6.6	8	55	2.5	40	1.5
Chicken (Olson)	2.9±0.54	12.2×7.3	19.8±9.6	62.5±11	9.4±3.7	24.4± 9.4	1.9±1.6

The figures given after ± are standard deviations. About two thirds of all normal individuals will fall within the range of one standard deviation on either side of the mean. Two standard deviations on either side of the mean will include about 95 percent of normal individuals. The values given for man, goat, and guinea pig are from the German edition. Sources of the other values are:

H. H. Holman, "Clinical Hematology," in George F. Boddie's Diagnostic Methods in Veterinary Medicine (Edinburgh: Oliver and Boyd, 1946), p. 320.

Carl Olson, Variations in the Cells and Hemoglobin Content in the Blood of the Normal Domestic Chicken, Cornell Vet. 27 (1937): 235–263.

David Wirth, Grundlagen einer Klinischen Hämatologie der Haustiere, 2d ed. (Vienna: Urban and Schwarzenberg, 1950), p. 124.

(p. 13 and Fig. 7). The form of the cells is continually changing but it is spherical in the resting condition. The size varies within wide limits (4–20 μ).

On the average, there are 8,000–12,000 leukocytes per cubic mm. of blood, but this is subject to great variation with species, sex, age, stage of digestion, and other factors. In dogs, cattle, rabbits, and chickens, the total leukocyte count is higher in the young than in the old. For example, the mean for cattle given in the table is 8,000, but a count of 12,000–15,000 is normal in young cattle. In guinea pigs and swine, the young animals have lower leukocyte counts than the a ults. In sheep and horses, there is no significant change with age. The count va ies i different blood vessels. In the splenic artery the ratio of white to red is 1: 00; in the splenic vein it is 1:100. The leukocytes are not uniformly distributed in the flowing blood, but keep close to the walls of the vessels.

The leukocytes in the blood come from several sources. We distinguish the lymphocytes, derived from the lymphatic organs; the monocytes, of disputed origin (p. 95); and the granulocytes, from the bone marrow.

a. Lymphocytes

Most of the lymphocytes are about 10 μ in diameter. They range from 5 to 15 μ. They are characterized by a relatively large nucleus, which is rich in chromatin and therefore easily stained. In some preparations the chromatin is arranged in clumps around the periphery like the spokes of a wheel. The nucleus is usually spherical, but is often bean-shaped, especially in larger lymphocytes. It is surrounded by a thin layer of basophilic cytoplasm (Figs. 118,k; 121,b*). There is usually a lighter zone around the nucleus, and large, dark-red azurophil granules often appear, especially in the ox and horse. Lymphocytes have a peculiar rolling motility. The percentage of lymphocytes (see Table 1) is higher in the young of most species than in the old.

Outside the vascular system, the lymphocytes are found as wandering cells in many different organs. They form the main mass of the parenchyma of lymphatic tissue. In the literature of pathology they are sometimes called round cells.

b. Monocytes

These cells (Fig. 121,c*) often have a diameter of 16 μ or more in blood smears. They have abundant, weakly basophilic, gray-blue cytoplasm, which often shows pseudopodia. No light-staining zone occurs around the nucleus. When azurophil granules are present in monocytes, they are much finer than they are in lymphocytes. The large nucleus is usually indented on one side and therefore appears kidney-shaped or horseshoe-shaped. Clover-leaf forms appear in the ox and horse. The nucleus does not stain so intensely as does that of a lymphocyte, and the chromatin structure is more delicate. It is difficult to differentiate some (young?) monocytes from large lymphocytes. This probably accounts for the wide variation in the normal monocyte counts given in the literature. Monocytes show good motility and, in extravascular situations, marked phagocytosis. They may be grouped with the other large phagocytes as macrophages (see *histiocytes*, p. 39).

c. Granulocytes, Polymorphonuclear Leukocytes

The granulocytes (Fig. 121,d,e,f,g*) have an irregularly lobulated nucleus, the segments of which are often connected only by thin filaments. This may give the false impression that the cell is multinucleate. In domestic mammals the granulocytes are larger than the erythrocytes (10–15 μ). Their ameboid motility is greater than that of the lymphocytes.

The cytoplasm contains coarse or fine granules which are distinguished by their affinity for certain dyes in the complex stains (Wright's, Giemsa's) used on blood smears. These so-called neutral stains are mixtures of compounds in which the only acid radical, or anion, is eosin (red), but the cations are several different basic-dye groups.[5] One of these is the common basic dye, methylene blue. The others, methylene violet and the azures, are oxidation products of methylene blue which are also basic but which give highly specific staining reactions in various shades of purple,

---

[5] H. J. Conn, *Biological Stains* (5th ed.; Geneva, N.Y.: Biotech Publications, 1946), pp. 26, 90–96, 181–191.

* Fig. 121 is on p. 90.

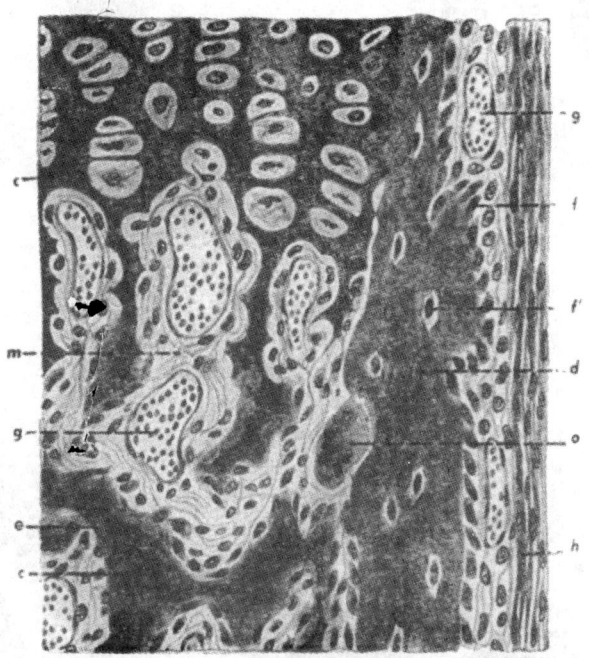

Figure 84. Longitudinal section through the meta-carpus at the * in Fig. 83 (p. 52); hematoxylin-eosin (350×). *c*, calcified cartilage; *d*, perichondral bone; *e*, osseous intercellular substance; *f*, osteoblasts; *f'*, osteocyte; *g* (*left*), blood vessel in primary bone marrow (*m*); *g* (*right*), periosteum with blood vessels; *h*, tendon primoridum; *o*, osteoclast with a striated border on the right in a Howship lacuna.

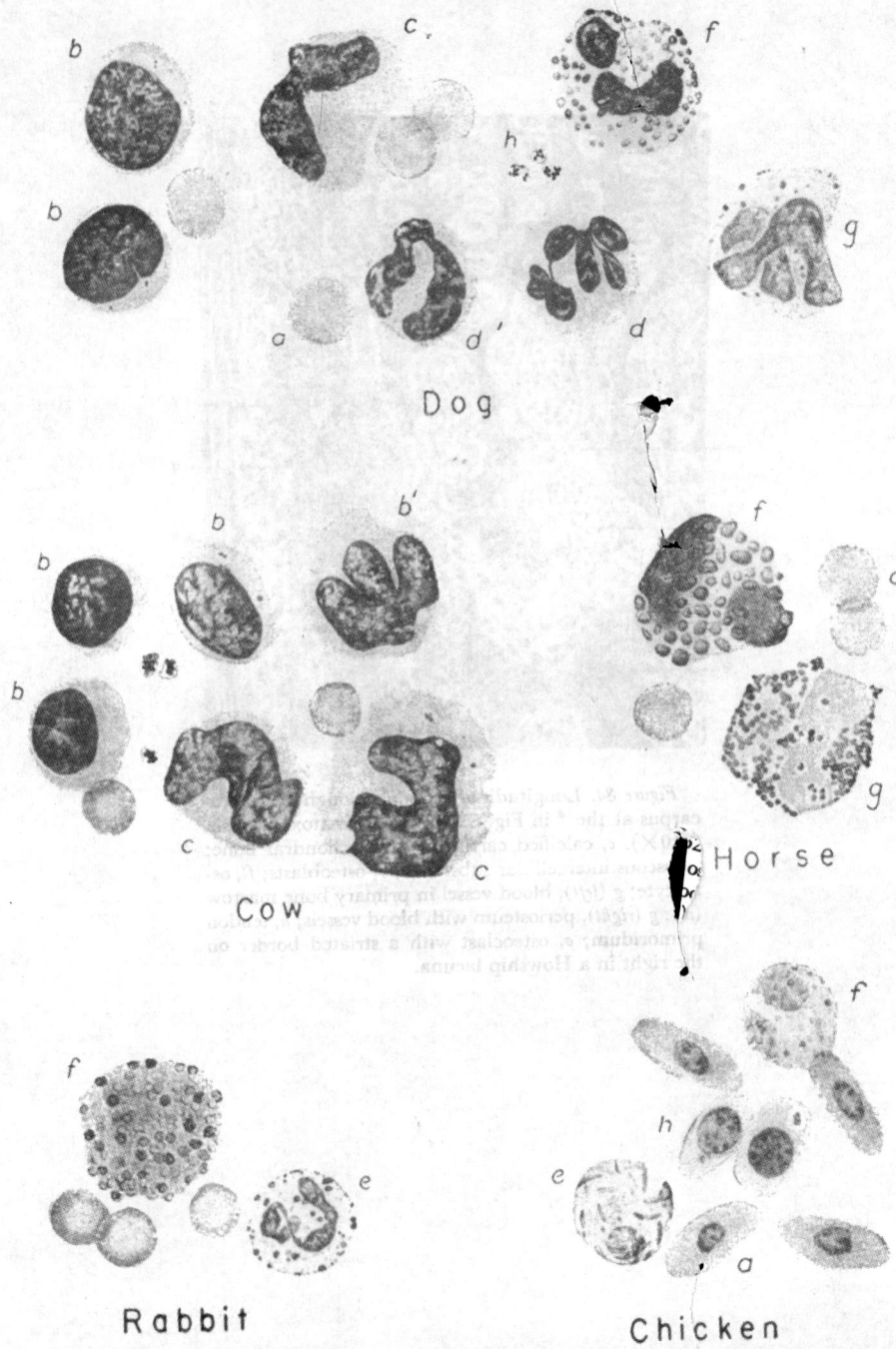

Figure 121. Blood corpuscles, Wright's stain (1300×). *a*, erythrocyte; *b*, lymphocyte; *b'*, intermediate type; *c*, monocyte; *d*, neutrophil; *d'*, band cell; *e*, heterophil; *f*, eosinophil; *g*, basophil; *h*, thrombocytes.

violet, or lilac. According to the staining qualities of the granules, the granulocytes are classified as follows:

(1) Neutrophils (Fig. 121,*d*). A slender, curved, sausage-like or segmented nucleus is characteristic. In counting neutrophils, the band cells (*d'*), which are younger forms, are distinguished from those with segmented nuclei. The cytoplasm has a fine dustlike granulation which is stained light purple or lilac by the common blood stains (neutral stains).

In the rabbit, guinea pig, and chicken, the cells that correspond to neutrophils are called heterophils (*e*). They have granules that stain red but are not the same as those of the eosinophil granulocytes. The heterophil granules of the rabbit and guinea pig are round or rod-shaped, and are smaller than the eosinophil granules, which are all round. In the chicken, the heterophil granules are large, elongated, and bright red, whereas the eosinophil granules are round and brick red.

Neutrophils have an average diameter of 12 μ. They are outstanding for their ameboid motility and phagocytosis.

In man, horse, swine, dog, and cat, the neutrophils are the commonest leukocytes in the blood. In ruminants, laboratory rodents, and chickens, the lymphocytes are predominant. Neutrophils are also found as wandering cells in the tissues especially in inflammations, where they form the pus cells. Here the filaments between the lobules of the nucleus break and the cells become polynuclear (i.e., they have a clover-leaf form).

(2) Eosinophils (Acidophils, Fig. 121,*f*). The nucleus of an eosinophil is coarser than that of a neutrophil and has only two or three lobes when mature. The cytoplasm is filled with coarse refractive granules, which have an affinity for the acid aniline dyes, e.g., eosin. They are especially large in the horse. The cells have a diameter of 10–15 μ. They occur in normal tissues as well as in the blood. Their numbers are increased in parasitic diseases.

(3) Basophils (Fig. 121,*g*). These rare cells make up about 0.5 percent of the leukocytes, except in chickens, in which they average 2 percent. They have a coarse polymorphic nucleus and rather sparse, coarse, basophilic granules in the cytoplasm. The granules are water-soluble, in contrast to those of the other granulocytes, and therefore often appear blurred. The size is about 10 μ. Apparently phagocytosis is lacking. Basophils are sometimes called hematogenous mast cells, but they are not identical with the mast cells of the connective tissue (see p. 39). Transitional forms between lymphocytes and granulocytes occur.

3. Platelets (Thrombocytes)[6]

In mammals these are small biconvex discs which appear spindle-shaped when seen on edge (Fig. 118,*i*). They are about 3 μ in diameter and colorless. They contain azurophil granules, but no nucleus. They have slight motility. The number of platelets per cubic mm. of blood is about 250,000–500,000, but they are difficult to count and reports differ widely.

Outside the vessels, the fragile platelets agglutinate in clumps, become granular.

---

[6] Gr. *thrombos* clot.

and form the coagulation centers and junctions of the fibrin net. They are said to be produced by segmentation of the cytoplasm of the megakaryocytes in the bone marrow.

The birds have true, nucleated thrombocytes, which resemble the erythrocytes but are shorter and have a round nucleus, a slightly basophilic cytoplasm with one or two dark granules, and, occasionally, vacuoles. They number about 100,000 per cubic mm.

Chylomicrons or elementary granules are fat droplets seen in the blood by dark-field illumination. They are easily demonstrated in herbivora, and increase greatly in other animals after a fatty meal. Blood dust or hemokonia are still smaller particles of proteins or lipids. They are in part the products of disintegration of the cellular elements.

4. Blood Formation (Hemopoiesis)

The first site of blood formation is outside the embryo, in the area vasculosa of the wall of the yolk sac. Here, between the extraembryonic splanchnic mesoderm and the entoderm, the blood islands develop. These are solid masses of mesenchymal cells, united by cellular strands to form a network. They become differentiated to the extent that the outer cells join to form the tubular wall of the blood vessels, while the inner cells are separated by the secretion of plasma between them and become the primitive blood cells, which multiply rapidly by mitosis. Formation of primitive blood cells also occurs for some time by the detachment of cells from the vascular wall (endothelium). Hemoglobin is soon formed in most of the cells, which become primitive erythrocytes, ceasing to divide but retaining their nuclei. These cells die out during embryonic life. They do not form definitive erythrocytes. Other primitive blood cells remain as colorless, proliferating hemocytoblasts. The yolk sac vessels become continuous with vessels that arise in the body mesenchyme, and a closed vascular system with circulating blood is quickly developed.

Blood formation is soon transferred from the yolk sac to the body of the embryo, where it is continued by the body mesenchyme, endothelium, liver, spleen, thymus, lymph nodes, and finally the bone marrow. The formed elements of the blood, with the probable exception of the lymphocytes, are not capable of regeneration.

The *hemocytoblasts* or stem cells are large ameboid cells with a large pale spherical nucleus containing a fine chromatin structure and one or more nucleoli. The cytoplasm is basophilic (Fig. 156,b). They arise from the mesenchyme and endothelium in the embryo, and occasionally from primitive connective tissue cells in postnatal life. All the definitive blood cells develop from stem or blast cells with the same characteristic appearance, although there is considerable disagreement as to whether they are actually identical. As they mature and differentiate, the chromatin structure becomes coarser and the nucleoli disappear. The nucleus grows smaller, takes a darker stain, and in granulocytes becomes segmented. The cytoplasm acquires the characteristics of the erythrocyte or leukocyte. According to the unitarian theory of hemopoiesis, adopted arbitrarily in this discussion for

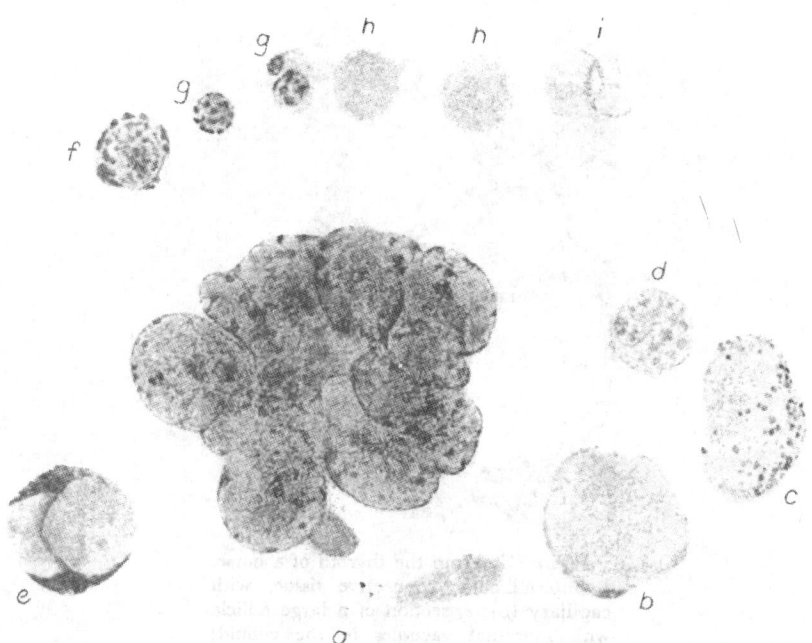

Figure 156. Selected cells from a smear of the bone marrow of the dog (Wright's stain, 1300×). *a*, megakaryocyte with phagocytosed cells; *b*, hemocytoblast; *c*, eosinophil myelocyte; *d*, neutrophil metamyelocyte; *e*, proerythroblast in division; *f*, basophil erythroblast; *g*, polychromatophil erythroblasts; *h*, polychromatophil erythrocytes; *i*, mature erythrocytes.

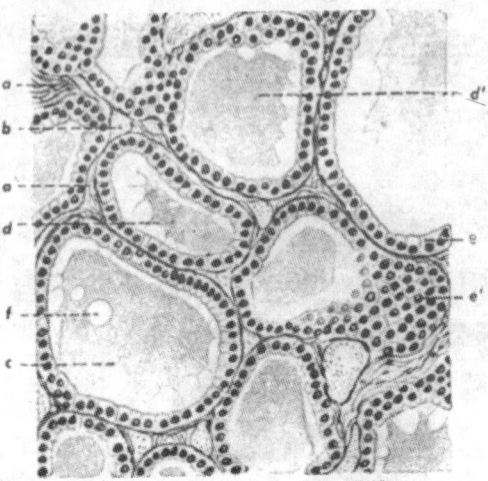

Figure 157. From the thyroid of a horse. *a,* interfollicular connective tissue, with capillary (b); *c,* section of a large follicle with marginal vacuoles in the colloid; *d,* small follicle; *d',* follicle with obliquely cut wall (above); *e,* follicular epithelium; *e',* tangential section of follicle wall; *f,* vacuole in colloid.

the sake of simplicity, the erythrocytes, lymphocytes, monocytes, and granulocytes are all descended from essentially identical cells, the hemocytoblasts. The large cells of the germinal centers of the lymphatic tissue (see p. 121) are hemocytoblasts. They do not appear in the normal blood and are not to be confused with the large lymphocytes, which have a condensed nucleus. The unitarians hold that the lymphocytes can revert to the primitive hemocytoblastic condition.

The unitarian view is by no means universal, however. Many hematologists prefer to distinguish lymphoblasts, monoblasts, and myeloblasts according to the type of cell with which they are associated. In this system, the myeloblasts are the stem cells of the bone marrow which give rise to the erythrocytes and granulocytes —the myeloid elements of the blood.

In postnatal life, the development of erythrocytes proceeds from the hemocytoblast through a series of erythroblasts in the red bone marrow. The nuclei of the erythroblasts have a circular outline and contain coarse angular clumps of chromatin, which give them a checkered appearance. The earliest stages have basophilic cytoplasm, but, when the eosinophilic hemoglobin begins to appear, the cytoplasm stains purplish or lilac, a reaction which has given rise to the term polychromatophil. The cytoplasm of more advanced erythroblasts is fully eosinophil, the nucleus is darker, and the size of the cell is about equal to that of the erythrocyte (normoblast). In the final stage, the mitotic multiplication ceases and the nucleus becomes pyknotic, i.e., shrunken, dense, and structureless. After the loss of the nucleus, probably by extrusion, the new erythrocyte is delivered to the blood stream. A revision of the nomenclature of the cells of the hemopoietic series has recently been proposed.[7]

Few granulocytes are found in the blood of the fetus. In the adult, they develop in the bone marrow from myelocytes, which are in turn descendants of the hemocytoblasts. The myelocytes have a large round or oval nucleus with coarser chromatin than the hemocytoblast. The cytoplasm contains increasing numbers of specific granules. The cells are therefore designated eosinophil, neutrophil, or basophil myelocytes. After a number of generations of mitotic reproduction, the myelocytes lose the capacity for cell division, and the nucleus becomes indented or horseshoe-shaped. These forms are called metamyelocytes or juveniles. In further stages of maturation of the granulocyte, the nucleus becomes a curved band and finally segments into lobules connected by filaments.

The lymphocytes are produced in the lymphatic tissue by proliferation of hemocytoblasts and large lymphocytes.

Monocytes, in the unitarian view, arise by transformation of the lymphocytes in the sinusoids of the spleen, liver, and bone marrow. Others derive them from the lining cells of the sinusoids or from monoblasts in the bone marrow.

B. LYMPH

The blood does not come in direct contact with the cells everywhere in the body. In the tissues the cells are bathed in tissue fluid, which is continuously renewed

---

[7] Committee for Clarification of the Nomenclature of Cells and Diseases of the Blood and Blood-forming Organs, Condensation of the First Two Reports, *Blood 4* (1949): 89–96.

from the blood in the capillaries. The lymph originates where the tissue fluid, laden with catabolic products, enters the lymph capillaries. It flows through the lymph vessels into the venous system. On the way it passes through the lymph nodes, where it is filtered and receives an admixture of lymphocytes. It is an opalescent, colorless or light yellow, coagulable fluid. It is composed of lymph plasma, a variable number of leukocytes—mostly lymphocytes—and fat droplets. A few erythrocytes appear occasionally in the main trunks of the lymphatic system. Chyle is formed in the lymph vessels of the villi in the small intestine. In addition to the components of lymph, chyle contains absorbed food substances, especially fat. On a fatty diet, the large numbers of fine fat droplets give the chyle a milky-white appearance. For this reason the intestinal lymphatics are sometimes called lacteals.

PART TWO

SPECIAL HISTOLOGY: MICROSCOPIC ANATOMY

VII

Introduction

A. GENERAL ORGANOLOGY

JUST as the cell represents the building stone of the tissues, so the tissues are the building stones of the organs. Organs are nearly always composed of several types of tissues, which combine and interpenetrate each other. The framework of the organs consists of supportive tissues containing vascular and nervous components. The meshes of this framework house the parenchyma,[1] on which the special function of the organ depends. A parenchyma may be absent, in which case the entire organ consists of nothing but vascularized and innervated connective tissue (e.g., ligaments). Despite the wide variation of organs in regard to form, structure, and function, the same basic architectural plan is found in all of them. The component parts of a parenchymatous organ may serve to illustrate this point:

(1) **Supporting Tissue.** Most organs are enveloped by a connective tissue capsule (Fig. 122,e'), which contains elastic fibers and often smooth muscle fibers, and conducts vessels and nerves. It gives off strands (trabeculae[2]) or membranous processes (septa) to the interior of the organ. These ramify extensively and form an interstitial framework, or stroma, which will vary in arrangement from one organ to another but will follow a basic pattern. We usually recognize a coarse interstitial framework whose trabeculae or septa are designated as interparenchymatous, interlobar, interlobular, perivascular, pericanalicular, etc. There is a finer meshwork also, the intraparenchymatous connective tissue, which has received various designations—e.g., intralobular, intertubular (Fig. 122,f), perialveolar, and interalveolar—according to the structure of the organ in which it occurs. In its meshes lie the parenchymatous elements, arranged in a manner characteristic of the particular organ.

(2) **Parenchyma.** In the framework the parenchymatous cells occur either

---

[1] Gr. *para* beside, and *enchyma* that which is poured in. The term has persisted from the ancient belief that the essential substance of an organ was cast in its framework by coagulation of the blood.

[2] L. *trabecula* small beam or bar. What appears in section to be a band of connective tissue is often the cut edge of a membrane.

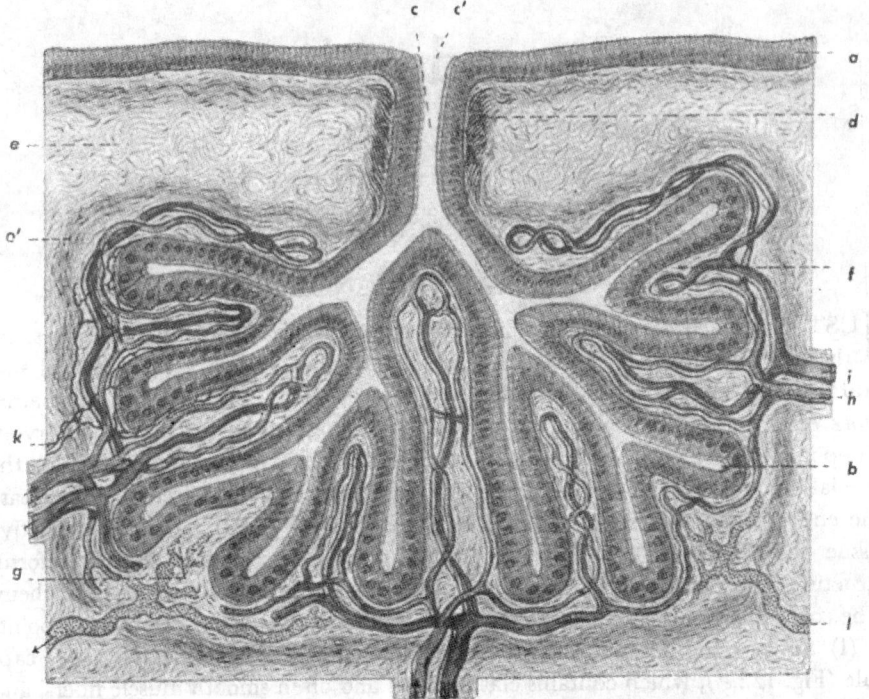

Figure 122. Diagram of the structure of an organ (branched tubular gland). *a*, epithelium; *b*, tubular secretory end-piece; *c*, excretory duct with opening (*c'*); *d*, smooth muscle in wall of duct; *e*, subepithelial connective tissue; *e'* fibrous gland capsule; *f*, delicate intraparenchymatous connective tissue; *g*, tissue spaces; *h*, arteries of the gland; these form capillary nets which flow into veins (*i*); *k*, nerves of the gland showing their ramification on two end-pieces; *l*, lymphatics draining the tissue spaces (*g*).

singly or in groups, in close relationship to the capillaries. They have a definite arrangement in cords, tubules (Fig. 122,*b*), clusters, or hollow spheres. Together with the intraparenchymatous connective tissue, capillaries, and nerve endings, they make up the parenchyma of the organs.

(3) **Vessels.** All organs with very few exceptions contain blood and lymph vessels. The arteries (Fig. 122,*h*) ramify in the interstitial connective tissue and finally form capillary nets, from which the veins emerge. The capillaries lie more or less directly apposed to the parenchymatous cells. They anastomose with each other and form networks of varying patterns. These occur not only in the parenchyma but also in the capsule, the interstitial connective tissue, and the walls of the larger vessels and ducts. Thus we differentiate between intraparenchymatous and interparenchymatous capillary beds. In some organs (liver and lungs) these two capillary regions have separate afferent vessels: those to the parenchyma are said to carry the functional blood supply; the others carry the nutritive blood supply. The shape and size of the meshes in the capillary network have a definite relation to the shape and arrangement of the tissue elements as well as to the function of the organ. The capillaries unite to form small veins, which usually accompany the arteries (Fig. 122,*h,i*).

Besides the lymph vessels proper (Fig. 122,*l*) most organs show, especially in their connective tissue, intercommunicating tissue spaces. These are filled with tissue fluid, which finally enters the lymphatics and becomes lymph. Lymphatic nodules are also present in many organs.

(4) **Nervous Elements.** In the organs we find nerves, nerve fibers with their · endings, nerve cells, and ganglia. The larger branches of the nerves usually run with the vessels. The nerve cells and ganglia lie along the course of the nerves.

B. THE ANIMAL MEMBRANES

The development of the animal body from germ layers makes it understandable that many cells and tissues occur in sheetlike arrangements or membranes. Membranes of different composition combine in layers to form separate organs or take part in their formation. Often they form the walls of hollow organs, especially tubes.

1. Simple Membranes

(a) Homogeneous (structureless) membranes: the capsule of the lens. Formerly the sarcolemma and the hyaline and basement membranes underlying the epithelia were classified under this heading. Later investigations, however, indicate that these consist to a large extent of a feltwork of very delicate reticular fibrils.

(b) Elastic membranes: the tunicae elasticae of blood vessels.

(c) Cellular protective membranes: epidermis, other epithelia.

(d) Muscular sheets: tunicae musculares. These consist usually of smooth, rarely of striated, muscle fibers, supported and held together by interstitial connective tissue, which also carries vessels and nerves. They occur in the walls of most hollow organs, e.g., the digestive, urinary, and reproductive tracts, and the arteries and veins. The muscle fibers lie parallel in layers. Most muscular tunics are composed of longitudinal and circular layers. Oblique layers are found in some organs; rarely the entire tunic consists of irregularly interwoven fibers.

(e) Nervous membranes: tunicae nervosae. These are composed of nervous elements and a special supporting tissue, e.g., the retina and the olfactory epithelium.

(f) Connective tissue membranes. (These have been described on pp. 39–43.) They may consist of loose, regular, or irregular dense connective tissue with elastic fibers and often muscle fibers or bundles. Occasionally they also contain adipose tissue.

2. Composite Membranes

(a) **The serous membranes,** tunicae serosae, line the walls of the closed body cavities (thoracic and abdominal) and invest the organs contained in them. Their structure varies with the mechanical stress to which they are subjected. Generally, they are made up of an epithelial covering layer, a thin lamina propria consisting of collagenous and elastic tissue, and a loose stratum subserosum. The epithelium covering the free surface is of the simple squamous type and is called mesothelium (see p. 23 and Fig. 31). The nonglandular, thin *lamina propria* is often separated from the epithelium by a limiting layer of elastic tissue. It commonly consists of connective tissue with flat interwoven collagenous bundles and a delicate elastic net, which becomes denser in the deeper layers. It contains vessels, nerves, and, in some parts, smooth muscle fibers. Close-meshed nets of lymph capillaries occur immediately under the epithelium, and larger lymphatics are found in the subserous layer. The *subserosa,* when present, exhibits a loose structure and sometimes contains large quantities of adipose tissue. Its function is to attach the serosa to the underlying tissues. The surface of the serous membranes is lubricated by serous fluid, which contains lymphocytes, macrophages, and mesothelial cells.

The detailed description of the serosa sometimes gives the false impression that it is a fixed, independent structure, whereas it is actually dependent upon the existence of a body cavity. It arises as the lining of the coelom in the embryo, and it is obliterated by transformation of the mesothelium to connective tissue wherever two serous surfaces adhere and eliminate the cavity. This occurs in certain developmental adhesions and in postnatal inflammations.

(b) **The synovial membranes,** tunicae synoviales, line the joint cavities, tendon sheaths, and bursae. They are covered by an incomplete layer of flattened fibroblasts resting on collagenous connective tissue. Villous processes and folds are often present, and the entire surface is lubricated by a thin layer of fluid containing mucin and various types of free cells. (See *tendon sheaths,* p. 43.)

(c) **The mucous membranes,** tunicae mucosae, line cavities and tubes which communicate with the outside through the natural body openings, where they are continuous with the skin. They are elastic, extensible, and contain vessels and nervous tissue. The following layers are recognized: (1) the *epithelial layer* (lamina epithelialis, stratum epitheliale; Figs. 123–125,a), (2) the connective tissue of the mucosa, *lamina propria mucosae* (stratum proprium, tunica propria; Figs. 123; 124,b;

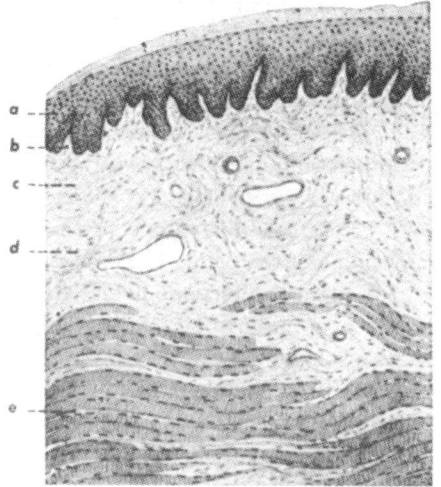 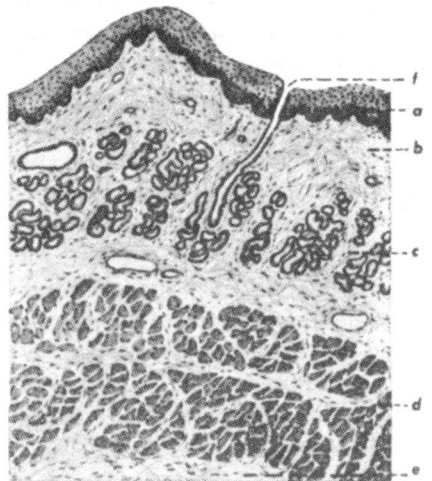

Figure 123 (left). Section through a cutaneous mucous membrane without glands (dental pad of ox). *a,* squamous epithelium with stratum corneum; *b,* papillary body; *c,* lamina propria blending into *d,* submucosa, which shows sections of blood vessels; *e,* striated muscle in longitudinal section.

Figure 124 (right). Section through a cutaneous mucous membrane with glands in the submucosa (canine esophagus). *a,* squamous epithelium; *b,* lamina propria; *c,* lamina submucosa with glands; *d,* tunica muscularis; *e,* loose connective tissue; *f,* opening of the excretory duct of a gland.

125,*e*), (3) the *lamina muscularis mucosae* (stratum musculare mucosae; Fig. 125,*g*), which is essentially restricted to the digestive tract, and (4) the *lamina submucosa* (stratum submucosum).

The lamina epithelialis and lamina propria are frequently separated by a basement membrane. When glands are encountered in the propria, we often distinguish a lamina glandularis (Fig. 125,*e*) from the remaining, nonglandular lamina subglandularis (*f*).

The muscularis mucosae is a thin muscular sheet intervening between the lamina submucosa and the lamina propria (Fig. 125,*g*). Commonly it sends muscle fibers into the latter (*i*). Smooth muscle fibers may also occur in mucous membranes which lack a lamina muscularis mucosae. The muscularis mucosae should not be confused with the tunica muscularis (Fig. 124,*d*), which is much thicker and lies subjacent to the entire mucous membrane.

The surface of a mucous membrane may be smooth or exhibit elevations or depressions, e.g., papillae (Fig. 183), villi, folds, furrows (Fig. 125,*l*), and pits (Fig. 125,*b*). Lymph nodules are frequently seen in mucous membranes. These may be single or aggregated.

A loose connective tissue membrane, the lamina submucosa (Fig. 124,*c*), binds the mucous membranes to adjacent tissues. It conveys the vascular and nervous trunks to the mucosa and contains any ganglia that may be present. It also makes the mucosa movable upon the underlying tissue and permits the formation of folds.

It is composed of loose connective tissue with elastic fibers and often contains fat and sometimes glands and lymph nodules.

The mucous membranes may be classified as (1) cutaneous mucous membranes, (2) glandular mucous membranes, and (3) transitional mucous membranes.

(1) The *cutaneous mucous membranes* (Figs. 123, 124) resemble the skin in structure. Their lamina epithelialis consists of stratified squamous epithelium, whose superficial layers may in some cases form a *stratum corneum* (Fig. 123). The tough lamina propria is made up of fibrillar, densely woven, feltlike connective tissue. Its most superficial layer, the *pars papillaris* (papillary body; Fig. 123,b,c) forms microscopic conical or cylindrical projections, the microscopic papillae. Often it gives rise to macroscopic papillae, which also have a microscopic papillary body covered by epithelium (Fig. 183). Folds, ridges, and leaflike processes of the mucous membrane may be formed as modifications of the macroscopic papillae. When the muscularis mucosae is absent, the lamina propria blends into the submucosa without any sharp demarcation. As a rule, glands are lacking in the lamina propria. The latter is often penetrated, however, by the excretory ducts of the submucous glands (Fig. 124,c) and those that lie entirely outside the mucous membrane. Muscle fibers are always present in these mucous membranes, and sometimes a continuous muscularis mucosae is found under the propria. The cutaneous

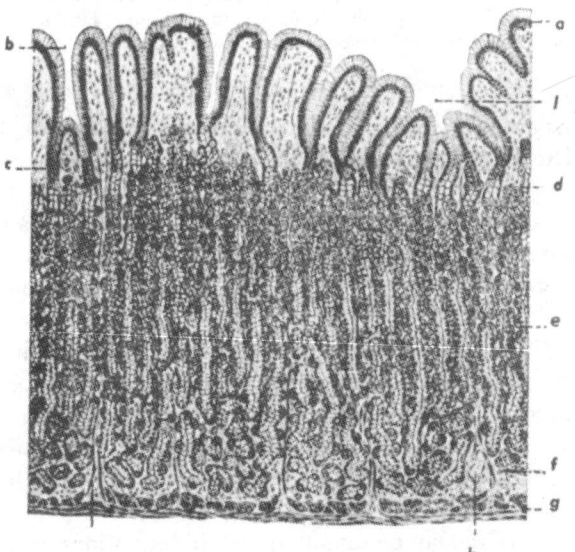
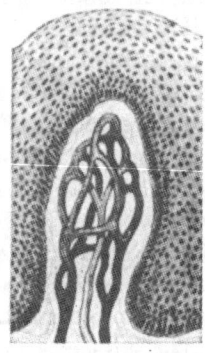

Figure 125 (left). Section through a glandular mucous membrane (canine stomach). *a*, simple columnar epithelium; *b*, gastric pits; *c* and *d*, excretory ducts of tubular glands; *e*, body of a gland in the stratum glandulare of the lamina propria; *f*, stratum subglandulare; *g*, muscularis mucosae; *i*, interglandular muscle bundles derived from the muscularis mucosae; *k*, blood vessels; *l*, gastric furrow.

Figure 126 (right). Microscopic papilla from a papillary body of the oral cavity, showing a capillary loop. Stratified squamous epithelium overlies the papilla.

mucous membranes occur in the oral cavity, pharynx, esophagus, pars oesophagea of the equine stomach, forestomach of ruminants, and vestibulum vaginae.

(2) The *glandular mucous membranes* (Fig. 125) have a columnar surface epithelium which is sometimes ciliated and often secretes mucin. The lamina propria contains glands (lamina glandularis) and consists of reticular or similarly constituted connective tissue. The surface of the glandular mucosae often bears slender projections called villi. There may also be crest- or ridgelike elevations, temporary and permanent folds and furrows (Fig. 125,*l*), pitlike depressions, follicles, tubercles, etc.

The mucous membranes contain blood and lymph vessels, nerves, and ganglia. The vascular and nervous trunks lie in the submucosa. Their ramifications and capillary beds extend up to the deep surface of the epithelium, forming subepithelial capillary nets (Fig. 126). The glands are surrounded by periglandular capillary nets.

(3) *Transitional mucous membranes* are those which have a transitional epithelium and whose propria forms no papillary body but may contain glands. A submucosa may be present.

(d) **The skin** differs from cutaneous mucous membranes in that it contains hair and tubular and sebaceous glands.

VIII

The Circulatory System

THE circulatory system consists of the blood vascular system and the lymphatic system. The former is made up of the heart, arteries, veins, and capillaries. All these hollow organs have one histological characteristic in common, a thin, delicate cellular lining membrane, the endothelium. This membrane forms the walls of the capillaries and the innermost layer of the arteries, veins, heart, and lymphatics. Its function is to provide a frictionless surface for the flow of blood and lymph and to prevent intravascular clotting. The endothelial cells of the capillaries are elongated and flat (Fig. 127,c). With the increase in caliber in the arteries (b) and veins (a), the cells become wider and finally polygonal, in many cases even square. Around the endothelium of arteries, veins, and lymphatics are deposited concentric layers of muscular and connective tissue, which vary with the type, size, and function of the vessels. Three layers are commonly recognized: the tunica intima (or interna), media, and adventitia (or externa).

A. BLOOD VESSELS

The functions of the blood vessels are manifold. They serve as conduits for the blood; they regulate the blood supply to the various parts of the body; and they mediate the nutrient exchange between blood and tissues. All vessels, particularly the larger ones, take part in fulfilling the first function. The regulatory and nutritive activity falls to the smaller arteries and capillaries. The type of work is reflected in the structure of the wall. The large arteries must be tough and elastic, because they are called upon to withstand strong pulsating pressure exerted upon their walls. Therefore we find here a prevalence of supportive elements, especially elastic tissue, which is capable of absorbing the force of the pulse. The remaining arteries are usually rich in muscle fibers; the contractility of their walls makes possible the regulation of the distribution of blood throughout the body. The thin walls of the capillaries facilitate the exchange of metabolites between blood and tissues. The veins have only a small amount of pressure to withstand; they carry a large volume of blood at low velocity. Therefore they have a larger lumen and thin yielding walls, which show greater variations in their make-up than those of the arteries. The heart, which furnishes the main propelling force for the circulation, has undergone a high degree of differentiation from the original simple tubular form.

1. Capillaries

The capillaries[1] (Figs. 54*; 127,c,d; 128) are extremely delicate tubules of about the same diameter as an erythrocyte. Their walls are formed by endothelial cells, held together by a soft intercellular cement. These endothelial cells are flat, fusiform, and often curved like a trough. They have scalloped or serrated edges and

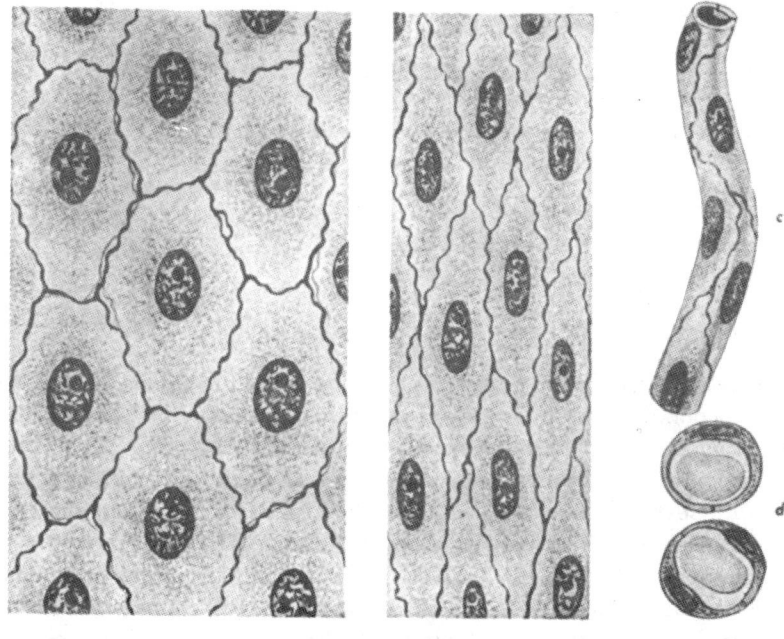

Figure 127. Endothelial lining of blood vessels. a, vein; b, artery; c, capillary; d, cross sections of capillaries containing red blood corpuscles.

elongated, flattened nuclei. The capillaries are surrounded by a connective tissue sheath, in which reticular fibers may be demonstrated by the silver staining method. Often they are also enveloped by pericytes, whose numerous processes encompass the entire tube (Fig. 129). It is doubtful that these cells are responsible for capillary contraction as asserted by their discoverer, Rouget, who considered them to be branched muscle cells. Modern investigators have defined capillaries as vessels that do not have muscle fibers in their walls.[2] The pericytes are probably histiocytes; they are phagocytic and leave the capillary wall in response to stimuli.

[1] L. *capillus* hair: vessels with hair-sized lumina.
[2] E. R. Clark, and E. L. Clark, Microscopic Observations on the Extra-endothelial Cells of Living Mammalian Blood Vessels, *Am. J. Anatomy 66* (1940): 1–49.
* Fig. 54 is on p. 51.

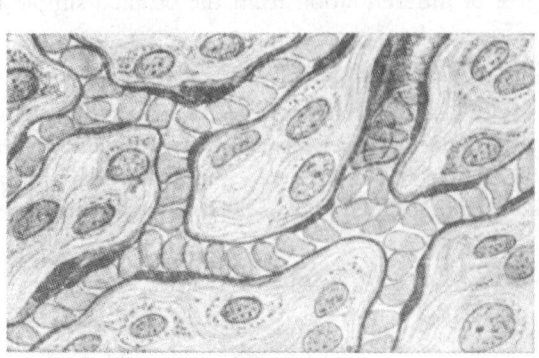

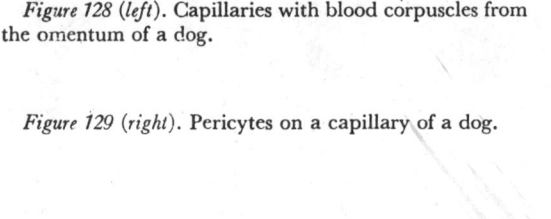

Figure 128 (left). Capillaries with blood corpuscles from the omentum of a dog.

Figure 129 (right). Pericytes on a capillary of a dog.

In the liver, spleen, bone marrow, and certain endocrine glands, the thin-walled vessels that connect the arteries and veins are called *sinusoids*. They have an irregular lumen which is wider than that of a capillary. Their lining cells differ from ordinary endothelium in many particulars. The cell boundaries cannot be demonstrated with silver nitrate, nor can the cells be isolated. Many of the cells are phagocytic and project irregularly into the lumen. They are members of the reticulo-endothelial system. In the spleen the lining cells are apparently separated by spaces through which the blood cells pass.

It is also impossible to demonstrate the outlines of the endothelial cells in the capillaries of the renal glomeruli, the chorioid, and the intestinal villi, and, generally, in young, newly formed capillaries.

The capillaries form nets or loops, whose meshes are wider or narrower according to the metabolic activity of the vascularized tissue. Changes in the diameter of the capillaries are under nervous control. Many believe that the contractility of the capillary endothelium itself is an important factor in regulating capillary flow, but most of the direct evidence for this comes from amphibia. Studies of mammalian capillaries indicate that the changes in diameter are accomplished mainly by regulation of the flow of blood to or from the capillaries[3] (p. 113). Often the capillaries are separated from the parenchyma by delicate connective tissue. The capillary wall is permeable to gases (e.g., oxygen) and dissolved substances. Leukocytes are able to migrate through the soft intercellular cement of the capillary wall or even the endothelial cytoplasm. Capillaries are absent from cartilage and most epithelia.

---

[3] *Ibid.*

2. Arteries

When viewed in cross section, the arteries present a small circular lumen. Their walls contain a triple framework of collagenous, elastic, and muscular constituents. These elements are interconnected and interwoven and show tendencies toward a lamellar arrangement. The arterial wall is characterized by its great thickness. In the histological preparation the arterial lumen usually contains no blood.

The intima of the smallest arteries (Fig. 130) is made up of an endothelial tube and the inner elastic membrane (tunica elastica interna, *b*). The latter becomes in larger arteries a fenestrated membrane with conspicuous corrugations resulting from contractions of the circular smooth muscle fibers. In the precapillary vessels or *arterioles*, the tunica elastica interna slowly fades out. The tunica media (*c*) is made up of circular layers of smooth muscle varying from one layer in the smallest to several in the larger arteries. Peripheral to this we find the adventitia (*d*), composed of longitudinal collagenous and elastic fibers, which blend into the surrounding tissue without any sharp lines of demarcation, as is the case with the adventitia of all vessels.

In the medium-sized or *muscular arteries* (Figs. 131, *left;* 132) we find an additional layer intervening between endothelium and internal elastic membrane. This is a thin stratum of collagenous, elastic, and muscular fibers which varies in composi-

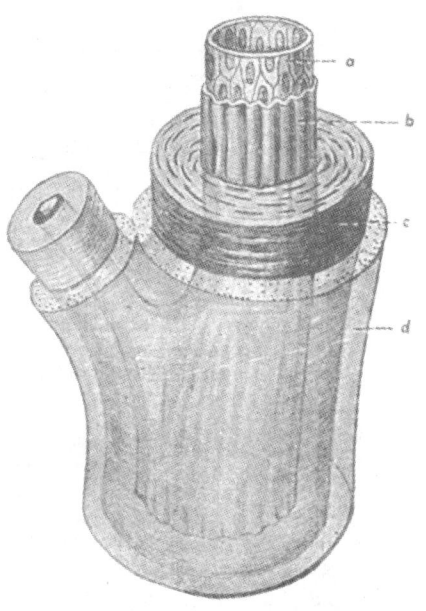

Figure 130. Three-dimensional reconstruction of a muscular artery. *a*, endothelial tube; *b*, tunica elastica interna; *c*, tunica media with circular muscle fibers; *d*, adventitia.

tion with species, age, body region, and kind of vessel. The intima cells which occur in it are able to store vital dyes, have a fusiform or star-shaped appearance, and resemble in nature the reticular connective tissue cells. In older animals the intima and especially its subendothelial collagenous tissue become more conspicuous. The layer adjoining the tunica elastica interna is the media (Figs. 131,*c;* 132,*b*). It consists of a collagenous framework with elastic fiber nets and smooth muscle tracts, most of which are circular. There are very few longitudinal or spiral fibers. The adventitia contains many longitudinally directed elastic fiber nets, which are concentrated near the media and constitute the elastic membrane of the adventitia or tunica elastica externa.

The largest arteries, the *elastic arteries* (Fig. 131, *right*) such as the aorta and the iliac, femoral, subclavian, and vertebral arteries are lined by an endothelium whose cells are more nearly polygonal. The intima is heavier (except in small

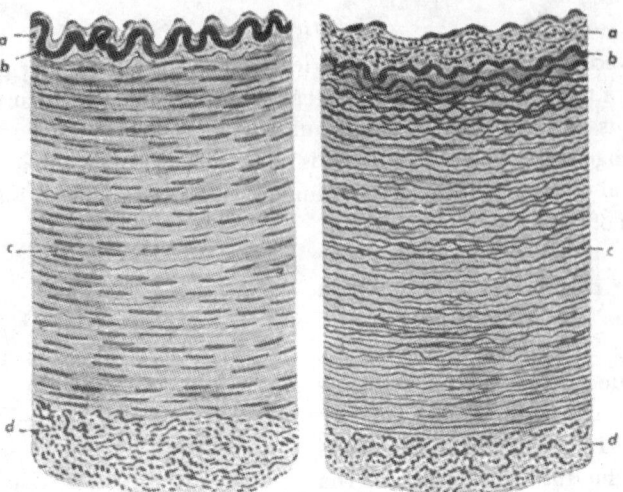

Figure 131. Left: section through the wall of a muscular artery (common digital of horse). Right: an elastic artery (common carotid of horse). a, intima; b, tunica elastica interna; c, media; d, adventitia. The elastic tissue is shown in black.

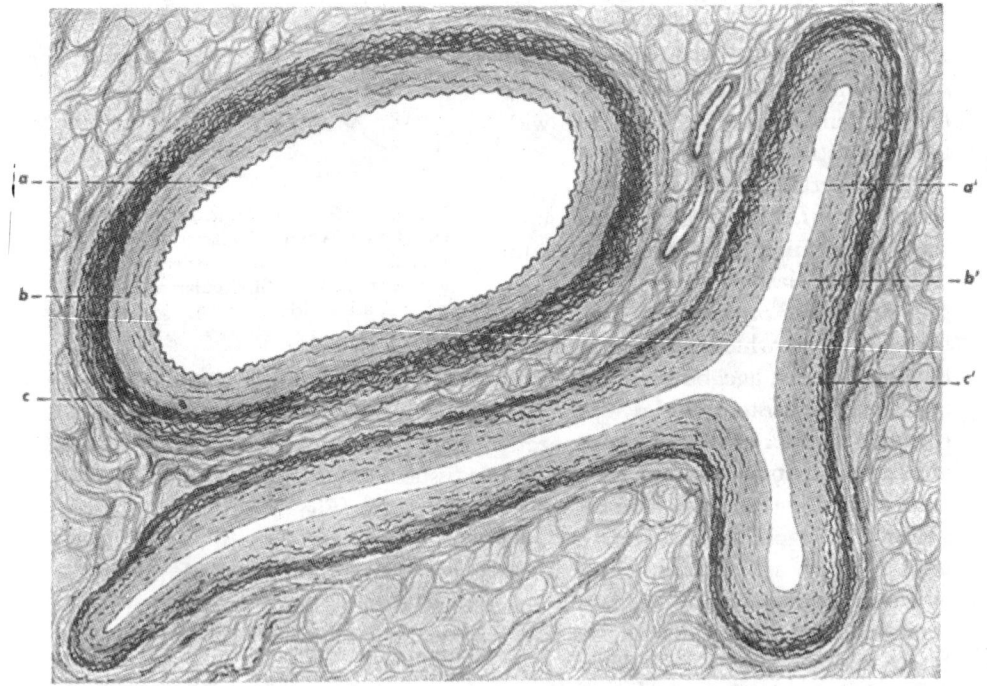

Figure 132. Cross section through the femoral artery and vein of a dog; elastic tissue stained black with resorcin-fuchsin (35 X). a, intima with tunica elastica interna; b, media; c, adventitia of the artery; a', intima; b', media; c', adventitia of the vein.

domestic animals), and its elastic fibers become denser as they approach the media. An elastica interna is not distinguishable from the many elastic layers in the thick media, which shows a preponderance of elastic as compared to muscular elements. The elastic fibers form a series of concentric fenestrated membranes or nets enclosing between them layers of muscle fibers oriented circularly, obliquely, or longitudinally (as at the origin of the aorta). Obliquely directed elastic fibers and membranes cross the smooth muscle layers to connect the elastic laminae. The rather thin adventitia lacks an external elastic membrane, and elastic fibers in general are scarce or absent. Longitudinal smooth muscle fibers or fat, however, may be encountered here.

A homogeneous basophilic (chromotropic) substance occurs between the fibrous and cellular elements of the arterial walls. It resembles mucin in staining reaction and increases with advancing age, especially in the central portions of the elastic arteries. It contains collagenous fibers.

In the transition from elastic to muscular arteries, the decrease in elastic fibers in the media is quite abrupt in the horse but more gradual in the other domestic mammals. It does not always occur at the same relative distance from the heart. The same artery in different species, or even in different individuals of one species, may vary from the elastic to the muscular type. The decrease in elastic fibers in the media is generally accompanied by a comparable increase of such elements in the adventitia, so that strongly muscular arteries are characterized by an abundance of elastic fibers in the adventitia. The arteries of the ox possess an unusually heavy adventitia. Wherever arteries are directly apposed to bone or are protected against the stress of traction or pressure (e.g., in the intracranial cerebral arteries) or supported by neighboring muscles, the wall undergoes a thinning process at the expense of the elastic elements. This thinning may be rather marked (e.g., in the aorta of the horse as it passes through the aortic hiatus of the diaphragm.)

3. Veins

The veins are vessels that conduct blood toward the heart, and this definition is applied without regard for the degree of oxygenation of the blood contained. They usually have a wider lumen and thinner walls than the corresponding arteries (Fig. 132). They exhibit greater variations in structure and have a more collagenous character due to the decrease in muscular and elastic elements. Because of the flaccidity of their walls, the veins—in contrast to the arteries—are either filled with blood in sections or, more commonly, collapsed. Their layers are not so sharply defined as those of the arteries. In the course of the veins toward the heart, the usual three-layered structure is first attained in the veins of the extremities, which are subjected to greater demands and, like the large venous trunks, have a more resistant wall. The smallest veins as well as the veins of bone, meninges, retina, liver, and spleen lack a tunica media.

The endothelial cells of the intima are nearly polygonal (Fig. 127,a). The few elastic fibers present run longitudinally. An elastica interna is usually absent and is replaced by nets of elastic fibers. In the larger veins (especially those of the pelvis) longitudinal smooth muscle fibers are encountered, which are sometimes united into bundles and which may cause the formation of longitudinal ridges encroaching upon the lumen of the vessel.

The media is thinner than that of the accompanying arteries. The muscle fibers are often oriented longitudinally (in contrast to those of the arteries), but sometimes also circularly or spirally. In some veins the muscle elements predominate (as in the extremities); in others, the connective tissue framework. Veins of less

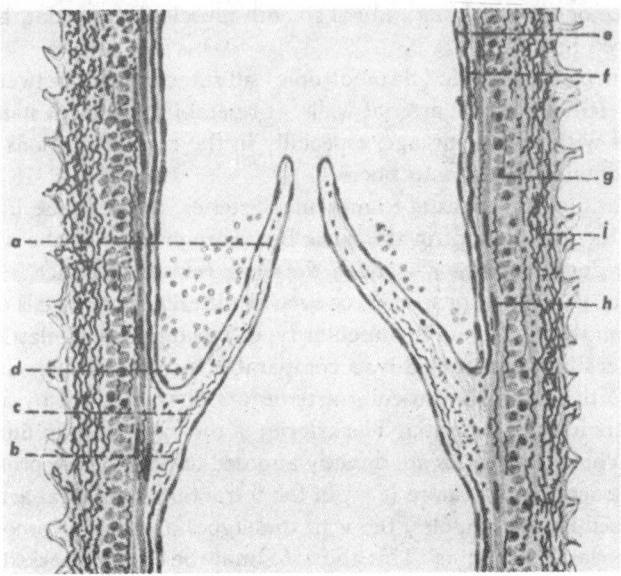

Figure 133. Longitudinal section through a cutaneous vein of a dog (70×). *a*, valve leaflet; *b*, valve base; *c*, elastic fibers in the inner wall of the valve; *d*, valve sinus; *e*, endothelium; *f*, tunica elastica interna; *g*, media; *h*, longitudinal muscle fibers; *i*, adventitia.

than 100 μ in diameter lack muscle fibers. The larger portal veins are more muscular, the smaller ones more elastic.

The adventitia is generally the thickest of the three layers. Often it is thicker than that of the corresponding arteries. It is relatively rich in longitudinal elastic fibers and nets of fibers. It is a loose connective tissue membrane, which often (e.g., in the visceral veins) contains whole bundles of longitudinally directed muscle fibers. These are altogether absent in the adventitia of small veins. Near the heart the walls of the terminal portion of the large veins contain more or less extensive tracts of cardiac muscle fibers. These occur in the adventitial layer closest to the media.

The valves with which most veins are equipped (Fig. 133,*a*) open toward the heart so as to prevent a backflow of blood. They are paired semilunar folds of intima, consisting of a thin layer of connective tissue with a subendothelial layer of elastic fibers on the side toward the lumen. Occasionally they may contain smooth muscle fibers as well. The wall of the vein is often thinned in the area of the valves. Valves are absent in veins of less than 1 to 1.5 mm. in diameter and in those of the central nervous system, lung, kidney, uterus, bone, and other organs.

For a description of the cavernous blood spaces, see *corpora cavernosa* (p. 275).

VASA VASORUM. Blood and lymph vessels are found in the walls of the larger arteries and veins. The arteries enter by way of the adventitia and form a capillary net there and in the media. Lymphatics usually occur in the adventitia, but they may also be found in the aorta immediately under the endothelium.

NERVES. The wall of the blood vessels contains unmyelinated and myelinated nerves, which form nets upon emerging from their myelin sheaths. From these nets delicate fibers arise, part of which end on the smooth muscle fibers of the media; others form sensory receptors in the adventitia similar to those in the epi- and endocardium. The sensory fibrils are probably always derived from myelinated nerve fibers. The nerve endings in the carotid sinus and aortic arch are concerned with the reflex regulation of blood pressure. Pacinian corpuscles are constantly present in the adventitia of the abdominal aorta. The capillaries also have been found to be innervated by extremely delicate unmyelinated fibers. Nerve cells have been seen in the adventitia of the large vessels of the body cavities.

Structures Regulating Circulation. Arteries and veins exhibit special structural features as well as direct anastomoses which serve to regulate peripheral circulation and control the distribution of blood.

The arteries are the main sites of constricting and occlusive mechanisms. In addition to sphincter-like smooth muscle rings in the media we also find in the intima longitudinal bundles of smooth muscle cells which form long ridges projecting into the lumen of the vessel. They occur mainly in those organs whose blood requirements are subject to great fluctuation (p. 275). These muscular pads are capable of constricting or even occluding the lumen. In contraction they become thicker and are brought closer together by the simultaneous contraction of the circular fibers. The umbilical arteries have a similar mechanism which prevents the newborn from bleeding to death when the umbilical cord is severed.

Another kind of occlusive mechanism is illustrated by certain polygonal epithelioid cells. They are characterized by a homogeneous, hyaline cytoplasm and a vesicular nucleus. They occur in the small arteries and arterioles—in the media and also inside and outside its muscle fibers. They are derived from the same kind of cells as the smooth muscle fibers and are therefore designated *epithelioid musculature* (Fig. 134). They occur either singly or in groups and are said to cause a reduction in the diameter of the lumen by swelling.

The veins of many organs are equipped with occlusive mechanisms. These take the shape of sphincter-like muscle rings, muscular spirals, or longitudinal muscular ridges in the intima which project into the lumen. The veins bearing such structures are as a rule small, and their occlusion not only throttles the venous drainage but causes engorgement of the corresponding capillary bed. The resulting increase in capillary pressure and the diminished rate of flow facilitate the transfer of fluids to the surrounding tissue. This arrangement is advantageous in such organs as the kidney and salivary glands. Constricting mechanisms in veins are especially frequent in connection with arteriovenous anastomoses.

In many parts of the body arteries pass directly into veins. By means of these shunts, the *arteriovenous anastomoses*, a part of the capillary bed can be by-passed. The anastomotic vessels are important in regulating the flow of blood into the capillary system. The structure and arrangement of the anastomoses vary from organ to organ. A very simple situation obtains in the submucosa of the stomach,

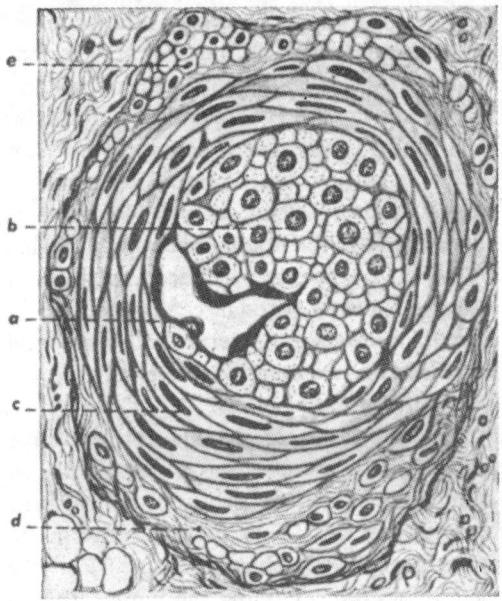

Figure 134. Cross section through an anastomotic vessel of the glomerulus caudalis of a baboon (460×). *a*, endothelium; *b*, epithelioid musculature of the intima; *c*, circular muscle layer of the media; *d*, adventitia with epithelioid cells (*e*).

for example. Here small branches of comparatively large arteries abruptly assume the characteristics of veins. In such cases the origin of the anastomosis is guarded by a ring or roll of smooth muscle cells. In other arteriovenous anastomoses (e.g., in salivary glands, intestine, and kidney) the efferent veins possess constricting mechanisms in the form of strong muscle rings alternating with sacculations.

Another kind of arteriovenous anastomosis has vessels of greater length. These are characterized by their faculty of complete occlusion, accounted for by the presence of longitudinally directed smooth muscle tracts or epithelioid cells. The more tortuous the anastomoses, the more numerous are the epithelioid cells, which may occasionally make up the entire vascular wall. A continuous elastica interna is absent. Arteriovenous anastomoses with epithelioid cells are especially rich in nerves. The efferent veins lack a constricting mechanism.

In the distal part of the tail of long-tailed mammals occur small groups of such anastomotic vessels, held together by muscular connective tissue. They are called *glomeruli caudales* (Fig. 134). They are always present in large numbers and resemble in structure the glomus coccygeum (coccygeal gland) in man.

Although the significance of the glomeruli caudales is obscure, there are structures of similar morphology which have been extensively investigated by physiological methods. These are the aortic and carotid bodies. The carotid body (glomus caroticum) is located near the division of the common carotid artery (on the first part of the occipital in the dog). The aortic bodies (glomera aortica) are near the origins of the subclavian arteries and between the aorta and pulmonary artery. The epithelioid "glomus cells" are richly supplied with nerve endings. The carotid body has been shown to be a chemoreceptor sensitive to anoxia or to an increase in hydrogen ion or carbon dioxide concentration. It initiates compensatory circulatory and respiratory reflexes. It is probable that the aortic bodies have the same function.[4] These structures were heretofore erroneously included in the paraganglia, or chromaffin system.

B. HEART

The wall of the heart, like that of the vessels, consists of three concentric laminae: the endocardium, the myocardium, and the epicardium.

(1) The Endocardium (Fig. 135,*a*). This membrane bears an internal layer of endothelial cells resting on delicate connective tissue. Under this is a thick stratum consisting mostly of flat nets of elastic fibers which become more numerous toward the myocardium. They are especially prominent in the atria. The densely woven endocardium is followed by a loose subendocardium that blends with the perimysium of the heart muscle. The subendocardium contains isolated strands of cardiac muscle and Purkinje fibers (p. 116 and Figs. 103,*a;* 135,*b*).

(2) The Epicardium. The visceral layer of pericardium forms the epicardium, which is a tough serous membrane of varying thickness. It contains numerous elastic fibers, which are laid down densely in laminae, especially in the deeper portions. On its free, pericardial surface it is covered by simple epithelium consisting of squamous to low columnar cells. It is closely attached to the myocardium and also covers vessels, nerves, and adipose tissue. The fat is distributed in a definite manner and is especially abundant in the grooves of the heart. The heart is encircled in the coronary groove by a wreath of nerve cells and fibers. Dense aggregates of ganglion cells are present in the subepicardium, especially at the point of entrance of the vena cava cranialis.

(3) The Myocardium. The myocardium (Fig. 135,*c*) consists of cardiac muscle fibers in a connective tissue framework which is continuous with both the epicardium and endocardium. It contains elastic fibers, vessels, nerves, and terminal Purkinje fibers. The cardiac muscle fibers are connected in a narrow-meshed syncytium. The bundles have a complex course.

The impulse for the heartbeat arises at the *sinoatrial node*, which is located in the

---

[4] C. F. Schmidt and J. H. Comroe, Functions of the Carotid and Aortic Bodies, *Physiol. Rev.* 20 (1940): 115.

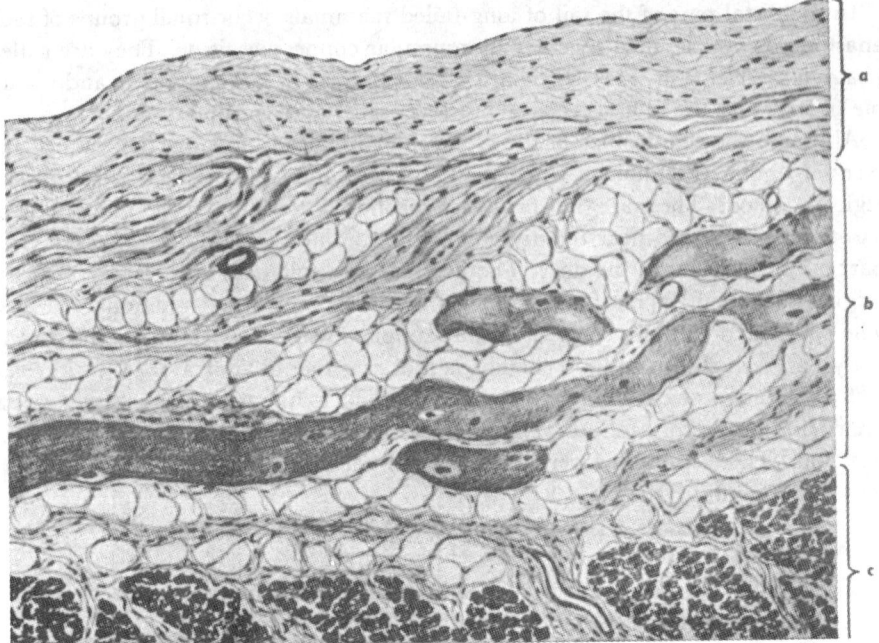

Figure 135. Cross section through cardiac muscle of a horse showing the endocardium. *a*, endocardium; *b*, subendocardium showing Purkinje fibers in longitudinal section; *c*, cross section of cardiac muscle fibers. (Note the large caliber of the Purkinje fibers as compared to the ordinary cardiac muscle fibers.) (After Ackerknecht.)

ventral wall of the cranial vena cava at the point of entrance into the right atrium. The sinoatrial node is rich in connective tissue and elastic fibers and consists of a highly irregular fabric of very narrow Purkinje fibers surrounded by nets of nerves. The transition of Purkinje fibers to ordinary cardiac muscle fibers is gradual and accompanied by an increase in width and distinctness of the striations. Nerve cells have been found in the sinoatrial node of man and most domestic mammals.

The musculature of the atria is separated from that of the ventricles by the tendinous annuli fibrosi. The impulse for the heartbeat is conducted across this barrier by the *atrioventricular bundle of His*. The bundle originates at the *atrioventricular node* in the atrial septum near the orifice of the coronary sinus. The node contains an irregular network of narrow Purkinje fibers and in all animals except the horse also contains nerve cells. There is some disagreement as to whether the atrioventricular node receives impulses from ordinary cardiac fibers of the atrium or via dispersed Purkinje fibers from the sinoatrial node. The result is the same. The atrioventricular bundle, composed of Purkinje fibers three or four times the diameter of ordinary cardiac fibers (135,*b*), divides into branches which descend on both sides of the ventricular septum and spread out in the ventricles. They gradually lose their subendocardial position and specialized structure and pass into the regular fibers of the myocardium. The bundle of His is surrounded by a connective tissue sheath enclosing many blood vessels, nerve cells, and nonmyelinated nerve fibers, which envelop the muscle fiber tracts.

The moderator bands (mm. transversi cordis) extend from the septum to the ventricular wall. Some are muscular and others are tendinous. The larger ones contain Purkinje fibers.

The four *fibrous rings* (annuli fibrosi) around the ostia at the base of the heart are the regions of attachment of the valves. The aortic and pulmonic rings are made up of densely woven connective tissue which is poor in elastic fibers. The aortic ring contains islands of hyaline cartilage, fibrocartilage, or, in the ox, bone.

The *heart valves* have an endocardial layer of varying thickness on either side of a stratum proprium. In the case of the semilunar valves this middle layer is covered on the arterial side by a rather heavy sheet of predominantly collagenous fibers, which is the continuation of the arterial intima. The ventricular surface is covered by a much thinner extension of the endocardium, which is rich in elastic fibers. The stratum proprium is connective tissue containing chondroid cell complexes (in the pig, dog, and cat) and basally some blood vessels. The nodules found in the middle of the free border consist of loose connective tissue with embedded chondrocytes. The stratum proprium of the atrioventricular valves is made up of connective tissue rich in elastic fibers, into which the chordae tendineae are inserted. The atrioventricular valves also contain blood vessels and, near their base, longitudinal and transverse bundles of cardiac muscle fibers.

The numerous blood vessels of the heart are located in the perimysium and fol-

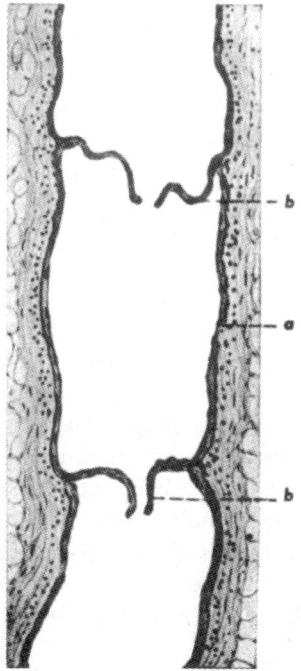

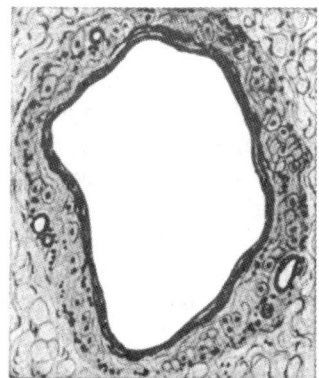

Figure 136 (left). Longitudinal section through a nonmuscular lymph vessel of a sheep (70×). *a*, wall; *b*, valves.

Figure 137 (right). Muscular lymph vessel of an ox (90×).

low its branchings. They form capillary nets, which are oblong in the myocardium and polygonal in the epi- and endocardium. The lymphatics form interconnected nets in all three layers. The nerves of the heart are many and contain predominantly, though not entirely, nonmyelinated fibers. Multipolar autonomic ganglion cells are present, especially at the atrioventricular junction. The sensory fibers form numerous nets in the epi- and endocardium. Unmyelinated motor fibers with single, somewhat thickened endings lie on the surface of the muscle fibers or may even enter them. (See section on nerve endings, p. 333.)

C. LYMPHATICS

The lymphatics are accessory to the blood-vascular system. They arise in the region of the tissue spaces and in the villi of the intestine (as lacteals). Their function is to collect the tissue fluid which has escaped the blood capillaries, to filter it through the lymph nodes inserted in their course, and to return it to the blood stream. The lymphatics conduct their fluid centripetally like the veins, which they parallel and into which they empty. Their structure is similar to that of the veins, though more delicate.

The lymph capillaries begin, according to the now prevalent view, as blind terminal twigs. They form nets with wider and more irregular meshes than the blood capillaries. Like the blood capillaries, they consist only of an endothelial tube, but their diameter is greater and they frequently show irregular dilatations.

The lymphatics in a stricter sense, i.e., those connecting the capillaries with the lymphatic trunks, are composed of an endothelial tube and a connective tissue sheath, which may also contain muscle fibers (Figs. 136, 137). They show great variation in structure, not only among the species but also from one body region to the other.

The lymphatic trunks, including the thoracic duct (Fig. 138), have a three-layered wall which is much thinner in relation to their caliber than that of the blood vessels. The layers exhibit much local variation in regard to demarcation, development, and composition. The intima, which lacks the elastica interna of blood vessels, consists of a lining endothelium, loose connective tissue, and nets of delicate longitudinal elastic fibers. The media is made up of predominantly circular smooth muscle fibers, elastic elements, and connective tissue. The thickness of the musculature is subject to local irregularities. The adventitia is composed of connective tissue bundles, and a few variously oriented smooth muscle bundles. It becomes looser peripherally.

The lymph vessels and trunks possess delicate valves (Fig. 136,b) of the same structure as those of the veins. The constrictions at the valves cause the lymph vessels to assume a string-of-pearls appearance. The larger lymphatics are supplied with vasa vasorum and nerves much like the corresponding blood vessels.

Associated with the lymphatic system are several kinds of spaces without a proper endothelial lining. The tissue spaces of the connective tissues are unlined intercommunicating spaces filled with tissue fluid (Fig. 122,g). In osseous tissue, this system is represented by the canaliculi, while the matrix of cartilaginous tissue appears to be uniformly permeated by tissue juice.

The perivascular spaces of spinal and cerebral vessels also play a part in metabolism. They communicate with the subarachnoid spaces.

At present, some authorities favor the viewpoint that the serous cavities (the pleural, peritoneal, and pericardial cavities) are not parts of the lymphatic system. This view finds support in the fact that the mesothelium is neither structurally nor

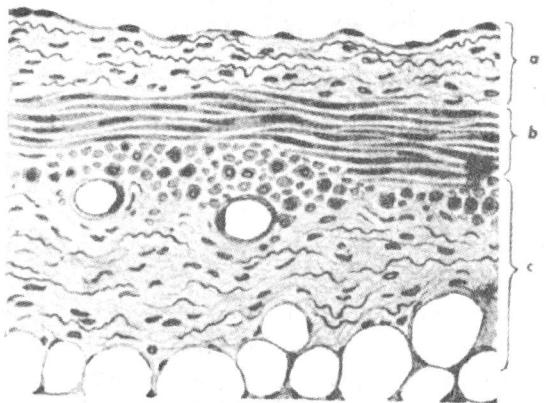

Figure 138. Cross section through the thoracic duct of a horse. *a*, intima with endothelium and elastic fibers; *b*, media with circular smooth muscle fibers; *c*, adventitia with longitudinal muscle fibers and vasa vasorum.

embryologically related to the lymphatic endothelium. On the other hand the serous fluid is quite similar to lymph in composition, and experiments with intravital dyes have demonstrated that serous cavities and lymphatics intercommunicate.

The subdural and subarachnoid spaces of the brain, the chambers of the eye, and the peri- and endolymphatic spaces of the inner ear communicate at least in part with lymph vessels.

The lymph sinuses of the lymph nodes are described on p. 124.

IX

Blood-forming Organs

THE hemopoietic system includes the lymph nodules and tonsils which occur, in and under the mucosae, as well as the lymph nodes, the spleen, and the bone marrow. While the latter produces the myeloid elements (erythrocytes and granulocytes), the others give rise to the lymphocytes. The activity of the closely related organs to be described is not restricted to blood formation. They are also concerned with blood destruction, in which the reticulo-endothelial system (p. 37) plays an important role. This system is well represented·in the hemopoietic organs by the widely distributed reticular tissue and in the lymph sinuses and blood sinusoids by the phagocytic cells.

A. LYMPHATIC ORGANS

All these structures contain reticular tissue (p. 36), the meshes of which are filled with lymphocytes. In addition to the formed lymphatic structures (the nodules, tonsils, nodes, and spleen) there are many diffuse lymphocytic infiltrations in the body. They occur in many mucous membranes of the digestive, respiratory, and genital systems and in the conjunctiva.

1. Subepithelial Lymph Nodules

Grossly, the subepithelial lymphatic tissue gives a granular or flattened nodular appearance to the mucosa of the digestive, respiratory, and urogenital tracts. It is characterized by the absence of afferent lymphatics and by its relationship to the surface epithelium. The nodules occur singly, aggregated, or in special structures, the tonsils.

Of all the domestic animals, swine have, in their digestive tracts, the most abundant subepithelial lymphatic tissue. It is particularly massive in the cardial gland zone of the stomach.

When examined under low magnification, lymphatic tissue appears to consist only of fine granules (Fig. 139). These are the nuclei of the lymphocytes, which hide the reticular framework. The latter is seen only after artificial removal of part of the lymphocytes.

a. Solitary Lymph Nodules

Solitary lymph nodules (Figs. 139, 250) are spheroid or ovoid masses of lymphatic tissue, often well defined by a capsule. They are more numerous in youth. They can develop postnatally or retrogress. Located centrally or eccentrically in the nodule is usually a lighter area, the *germinal center*, which does not differ materially from those of other lymphatic structures. The germinal center appears lighter because it is composed of hemocytoblasts and large lymphocytes. These cells have more cytoplasm than the small lymphocytes in the peripheral zone, and their nuclei do not stain so densely. Many of the cells of the germinal center show mitotic figures, indicating active proliferation. When this activity ceases, the germinal center is obliterated by small lymphocytes.

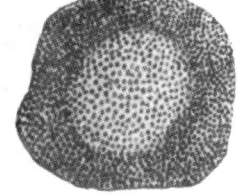

Figure 139. Solitary lymph nodule with germinal center.

Another type of light central area in a lymph nodule is the *reaction center*. This contains macrophages and cellular debris, and is regarded as a response to an irritant. The reaction center does not contain mitotic lymphocytes.

Blood vessels surround the nodule and capillaries penetrate it. The lymph nodules are not intercalated in the lymph stream, but they are closely surrounded by a network of lymph capillaries, by means of which cells and fluids are probably borne away.

b. Aggregated Lymph Nodules

Aggregated lymph nodules (Fig. 251) occur mainly in Peyer's patches in the intestinal tract. The patches are constant structures, which arise early in embryonic life. They are larger in the young.

c. The Tonsils

The tonsils (Fig. 140) are lymphatic organs that form, with solitary nodules and diffuse lymphatic tissue, a "pharyngeal ring" around the passage from mouth to pharynx. There is also an incomplete ring around the choanae. We find the lingual and palatine tonsils in the fauces, the pharyngeal tonsil on the caudal wall of the pharynx, and the tubal tonsils in the pharyngeal end of the Eustachian tube (in ruminants and swine). There are two types of tonsils: those with crypts and those without.

A *tonsillar crypt* is a blind, sometimes branched evagination of the surface epithelium surrounded by lymphatic tissue (Fig. 140,*B*,*e*). A single crypt together with its lymphatic tissue is called a *tonsillar follicle* (Fig. 141). A collection of follicles constitutes a tonsil of the first type. The tonsils with crypts, or follicular tonsils, include the palatine tonsils of man, horse, ruminant, and swine; the lingual tonsil of man, horse, and ox; the tubal tonsils of swine; and the tonsillae paraepiglotticae of sheep, goat, and swine.

The tonsils without crypts are formed of a simple lamina of lymphatic tissue. The increase of mucosal surface area, characteristic of tonsils, is achieved here by a bulging outward or a forming of folds (Fig. 140,*A*). In this class belong the pala-

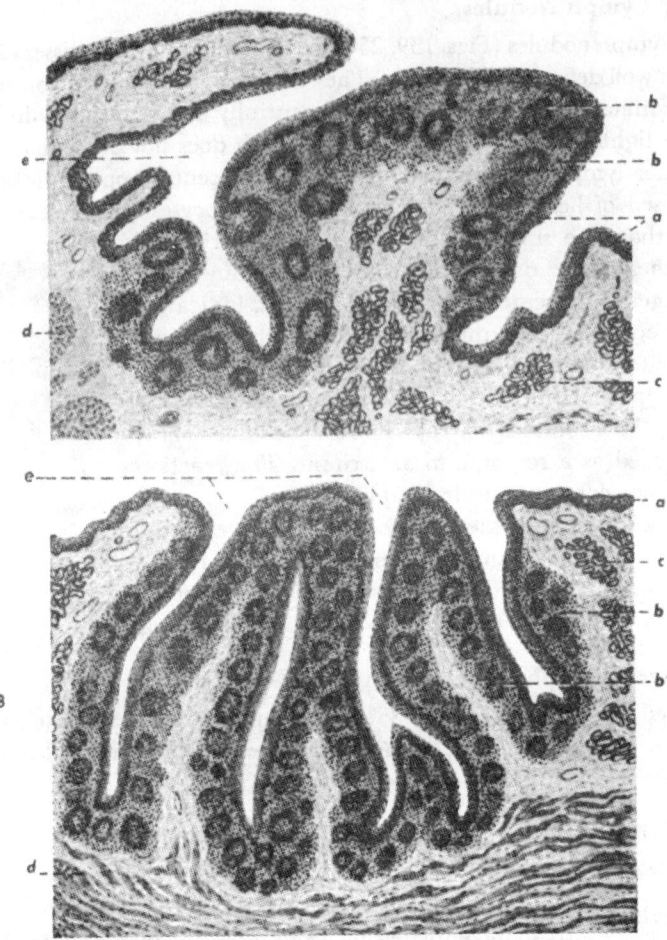

Figure 140. Section through the palatine tonsil of the dog (above) and the sheep (below). *a*, stratified squamous epithelium; *b*, lymphatic tissue with *b'*, nodules; *c*, mucous glands; *d*, striated musculature; *e*, tonsillar sinus (above) and crypts (below).

tine tonsils of carnivora, the pharyngeal tonsil of all domestic animals, and the tubal tonsil of ruminants.

The palatine tonsil of the ox is not visible on the surface. The crypts and associated mucous glands open into a common tonsillar sinus, which has a short passage to the surface. The prominent palatine tonsil of the horse has slitlike crypts, some of which are common openings for several follicles. The horse also has a tonsilla palatina impar at the origin of the soft palate. In swine, the palatine tonsils are not in the lateral walls of the fauces but on the soft palate. The smooth palatine tonsil of the dog is partially concealed by a fold of mucosa which forms a cavity, the tonsillar sinus, around the tonsil (Fig. 140,*A*,*e*). Note that some of the tonsillar tissue is in the wall of the sinus.

The tonsils lie in the propria mucosae, occasionally extending deep into the submucosa, where they are incapsulated by a condensation of connective tissue. The collagenous fibers near the lymphatic tissue pass over into its reticulum.

The tonsillar tissue is separated from the oral or pharyngeal cavity by the surface epithelium. In the follicular tonsils, the surface epithelium lines the crypts. The epithelium is often infiltrated with lymphocytes to such an extent that the cells and even the boundaries of the epithelium cannot be distinguished in sections. In such places the epithelial cells are sometimes loosened and the clefts between them

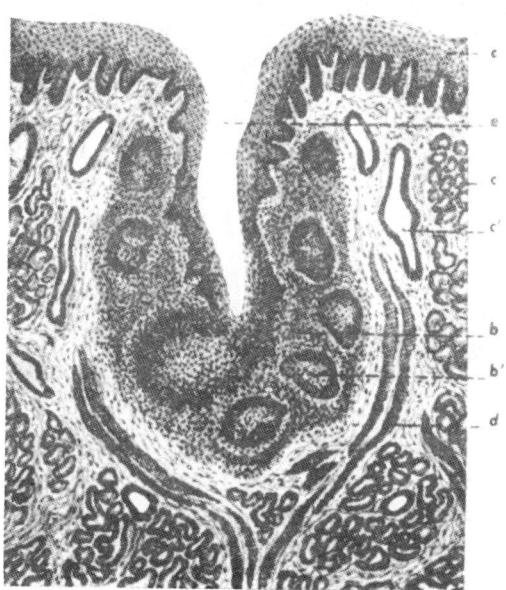

Figure 141. Section of a tonsillar follicle from the root of the bovine tongue. *a*, stratified squamous epithelium; *b*, lymphatic nodule; *b'*, germinal center; *c*, mucous glands; *c'* their excretory ducts; *d*, striated muscle in longitudinal section; *e*, crypt.

packed with lymphocytes. We assume that the lymphocytes are motile and capable of migrating through the epithelium.

In the lymphatic tissue are nodules with germinal (or reaction) centers (*b'*). The crypts often contain free nuclei, epithelial cells, granulocytes, lymphocytes, and masses of detritus.

In the vicinity of the tonsils are *tonsillar glands* (*c*) which are mucous as a rule, but mixed in carnivora. The ducts do not open into the crypts but on the mucosal surface.

In general the tonsils are larger in young animals.

The tonsils have no afferent lymphatics. The nets of lymph vessels around the lymphatic tissue arise under the epithelium and communicate with well-developed lymphatics in the connective tissue framework and vicinity.

2. Lymph Nodes

In addition to differences in structure, the lymph nodes differ from the lymphatic organs discussed above in having both afferent and efferent vessels. They are inserted in the course of the lymphatics so that the lymph must flow through them.

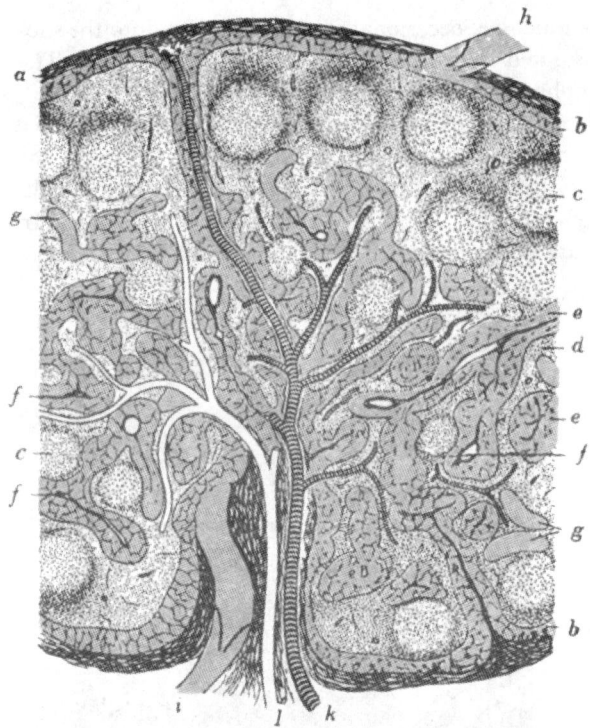

Figure 142. Diagram of a lymph node. The entire lymph sinus system is yellow. *a*, capsule; *b*, marginal sinus; *c*, nodule; *d*, medullary cord; *e*, intermediate sinus; *f*, trabecula; *f'* trabecula with vessel; *g*, sinus without reticulum; *h*, afferent, and *i*, efferent, lymphatics; *k*, artery; *l*, vein. (After Heudorfer.)

The lymph nodes (Figs. 142, 143) are surrounded by a connective tissue capsule containing elastic and smooth muscle fibers. Septa detached from the capsule extend a short distance toward the interior, forming shallow compartments, and are continued by trabeculae (Fig. 143,*b*). The trabeculae are best developed in the central portion. They anastomose and continue into the stroma of the hilus (Fig. 143,*f*). The framework divides the node into communicating compartments filled with reticular tissue (Fig. 144,*f*). Collagenous fibers of the framework penetrate far into the reticular tissue. The latter is filled with lymphocytes, except for the spaces next to the capsule and trabeculae, which comprise the lymph sinuses.

In the lymph nodes of most mammals and man, we can distinguish a cortex and a medulla. The cortex surrounds the medulla everywhere except at the hilus. The cortex consists of massive lymphatic tissue with nodules and germinal centers, while in the medulla the lymphatic tissue is arranged in anastomosing cords which may also contain germinal centers (Figs. 143,*d*; 142).

Between the framework (capsule and trabeculae) and the lymphatic tissue lie the *lymph sinuses*. These are spaces of varying width, traversed by reticular cells and fibers that attach the lymphatic tissue to the framework (Fig. 144,*c*). The lymph flows through these irregular passages from the afferent lymphatics, which penetrate the capsule, to the efferent lymphatics, which leave at the hilus. The efferent vessels are fewer and larger than the afferents. There is no structural dif-

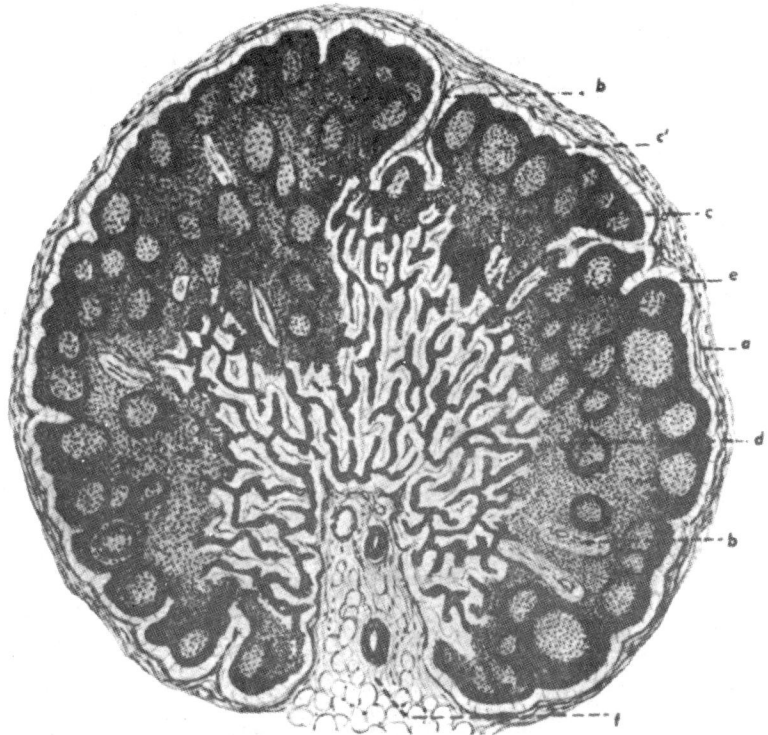

Figure 143. Section of a bovine mesenteric lymph node (13×). *a*, capsule; *b*, trabecula; *c*, cortical substance with germinal centers (*c'*); *d*, medulla; *e*, marginal sinus; *f*, hilus with vessels and fat.

ference between them. The lymph sinuses are not lined by ordinary endothelium but by flattened macrophages and reticular cells. These do not form a continuous wall. The lining cells are part of the reticulo-endothelial system. The first and most important site of phagocytosis of foreign material is in the sinuses of the lymph nodes. The lymphocytes, which are formed primarily in the germinal centers of the cortical nodules, are carried into the sinuses and the efferent vessels by the lymph that permeates the node. They also wander directly into the blood stream through the thin walls of the veins.

The cells in the meshes of the reticular tissue are predominantly lymphocytes, but there are also granulocytes (especially eosinophils), plasma cells, cell debris, free erythrocytes, and free macrophages. The latter often contain phagocytosed erythrocytes and leukocytes. Plasma cells (Fig. 56) are apparently differentiated from lymphocytes. They have a small, round, eccentrically placed nucleus with coarse chromatin particles. The cytoplasm is strongly basophilic. In addition to the formation and destruction of blood elements, the lymph nodes serve as a regional filtration system which retains soot particles, pigments, bacteria, and other particulate matter. Under the influence of irritants the lymph nodes can enlarge by growth of the cortical nodules and the budding of new nodules.

From accidental causes erythrocytes may appear temporarily outside the blood stream in such numbers as to give a red color to part or all of a lymph node. Such red nodes should not be confused with hemal nodes (p. 128). The erythrocytes enter the sinuses from the afferent lymphatics, and probably also by migration through the thin walls of the veins in the lymphatic tissue. They are disposed of by phagocytosis or carried on through the vasa efferentia. Many lymph nodes (renal lymph

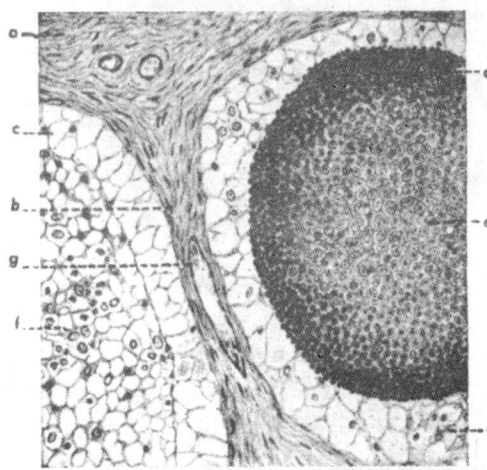

Figure 144. From a lymph node of the horse. *a*, capsule; *b*, trabecula; *c*, lymph sinus around cortical nodule; *d*, small lymphocytes; *e*, germinal center; *f*, reticulum of a nodule with the lymphocytes brushed out; *g*, blood vessel in a trabecula.

nodes of sheep and goats) contain blood almost invariably. Perhaps their blood and lymph vessels are connected.

The blood vessels usually enter at the hilus when one is present (Figs. 142, 146). The larger arteries run in the trabeculae and give off branches to the capsule. Small branches course through the medullary cords, branching as they go, and enter the cortical nodules, where they form capillary nets. When germinal centers develop, they displace the capillaries to the periphery of the nodule. From the resulting denser peripheral network, vascular loops pass into the germinal center. The endothelium of the veins varies greatly in thickness. The veins do not run in the same medullary cords as the arteries. The nerves are probably vasomotor; they accompany the blood vessels.

Species Differences. The preceding description does not apply to the lymph nodes of swine. In this animal the lymphatic tissue that contains germinal centers and corresponds to the cortex of the node in other species occupies a more central position. The peripheral zone is filled with a tissue that is comparable to that of the medulla of other species, although it has a somewhat different structure (Fig. 145,*d*). The afferent vessels penetrate the capsule at one or, rarely, several points (Fig. 146, *bottom*). They pass in thick trabeculae directly to the interior of the node and empty into the sinuses surrounding the trabeculae. The vasa efferentia

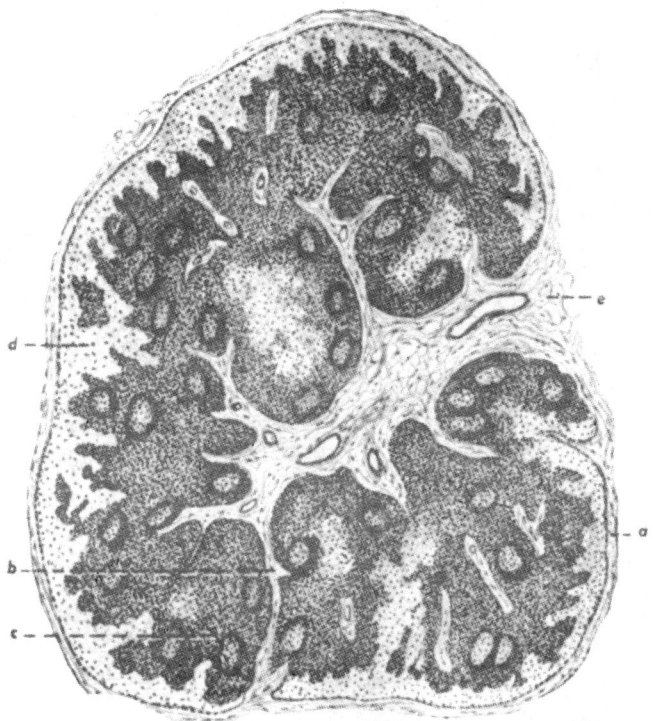

Figure 145. Section of a cervical lymph node of a pig. *a*, capsule; *b*, trabecula; *c*, tissue which corresponds to the cortex of the lymph nodes of other animals; *d*, tissue which corresponds to the medulla of other animals; *e*, hilus.

are formed by the confluence of sinuses that pass through the peripheral tissue. They leave the node at several points on the surface. It is worthy of note that the same type of nodular lymphatic tissue always lies closer to the afferent vessels, whether in swine or in other species.

The relative amount of cortical and medullary substance fluctuates greatly, especially as the development of these substances is influenced by different physiological conditions. They may be equally well developed, it may appear that only one or the other is present, or it may be difficult to say whether the parenchyma is cortical or medullary in structure. All of these conditions appear in the horse. Fusion of individual cortical nodules is common (Fig. 143). The largest germinal centers occur in the ox, the most numerous in swine.

Involution of the lymph nodes with age is manifested in a decrease in numbers of lymphocytes, a reduction in the number, size, and definition of germinal centers, and a greater development of reticular and elastic fibers. There is also an adipose transformation of the parenchyma, which may become reduced to vestiges. In fat animals (e.g., swine) the parenchyma may contain fat cells at an early age. An accidental involution occurs in starvation and wasting diseases and as a

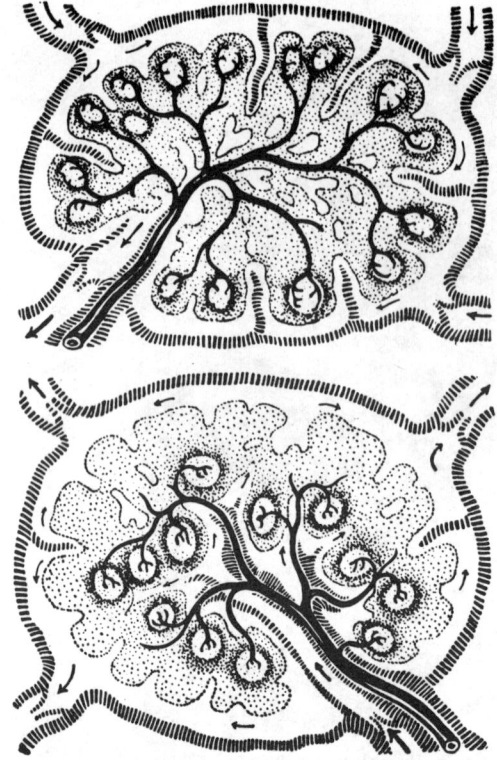

Figure 146. Diagram of canine lymph node (above) and porcine lymph node (below). Capsule and trabeculae are striped; lymph passages are white; lymphatic tissue is dotted, with cortical (above) or central (below) nodules; arteries are black. Capillaries, veins, and reticulum are omitted. (After Baum-Grau.)

result of roentgen radiation. After removal of the cause, the original structure is restored.

Among the birds, only waterfowl (e.g., ducks and geese) have true lymph nodes. These occur in the cervical and lumbar regions. Perhaps they are only modified portions of the walls of the lymphatics. They develop by the proliferation of cord-like, branched mesenchymal growths from the wall of the lymph vessel into the lumen. The lumen is thus divided into numerous lymph spaces. Only a central sinus passing through the entire node is left clear. The mesenchymal cords change to reticular connective tissue and become filled with lymphocytes. Nodules develop in the central ends of the cords, narrowing the central sinus. The sinus spaces are not traversed by reticulum. Capsule and trabeculae are missing. Blood vessels enter from all sides and ramify in the passages. Lymph nodes are lacking in the chicken. Lymphatic tissue is widely distributed in the avian body, especially in the digestive tract. Lymphatic tissue is also abundant in the walls of the branches of the portal vein in the liver (Fig. 270), in the serous membranes, and in the vicinity of the cutaneous arteries.

Hemal nodes (Fig. 147) occur only in the ruminants. They are independent of the lymphatic system, but may occur in the regions where lymph nodes are found (especially in the retroperitoneal fat). They have no lymph vessels. The parenchyma

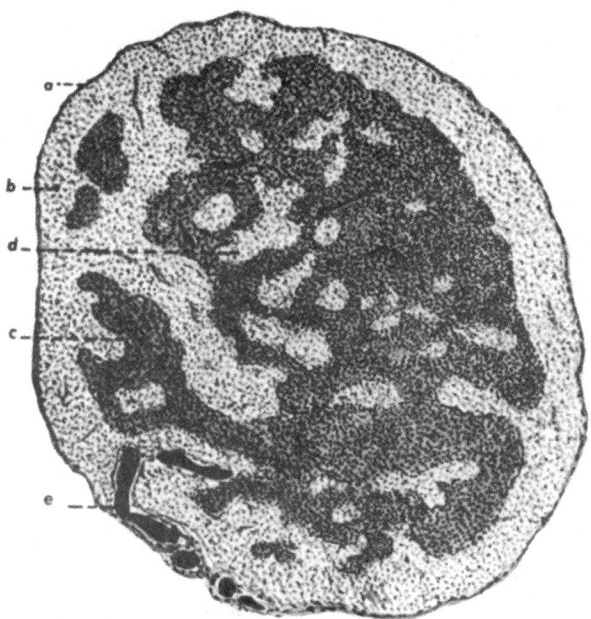

Figure 147. Section of a hemal node of a sheep (60×). All of the sinuses are distended with erythrocytes. *a*, capsule; *b*, marginal sinus; *c*, lymphatic tissue; *d*, intermediate sinus; *e*, blood vessels injected with black mass.

is a uniform mass of lymphatic tissue in which large numbers of erythrocytes are congregated. Macrophages with phagocytosed erythrocytes and pigment are also present. The wide sinuses (*b,d*) give the impression of being swollen with blood. The framework is not well developed. Hemal nodes have many structural similarities to the spleen, especially in the vascular walls, and are probably similar in function.

3. Spleen

The spleen is closely related to the blood-forming organs and can be classified with them until its position in the organism is better understood. In addition to blood formation, it is also active in blood destruction, hemoglobin and iron metabolism, and, by virtue of its reticulo-endothelial components, in blood filtration. The spleen also serves as a blood storage organ, which takes up large numbers of blood corpuscles, withholds them from the circulation, and releases them again.

The framework of the spleen consists of a capsule and trabeculae (Fig. 148). The connective tissue capsule is rich in elastic fibers and smooth musculature, which lies in the deeper zones. In the horse and ox, the muscle fibers are arranged in layers; in other domestic animals they are interwoven. The serosa is intimately attached to the capsule, except in horses and ruminants, where it is looser. Thick muscular trabeculae containing blood vessels radiate to the capsule, branching

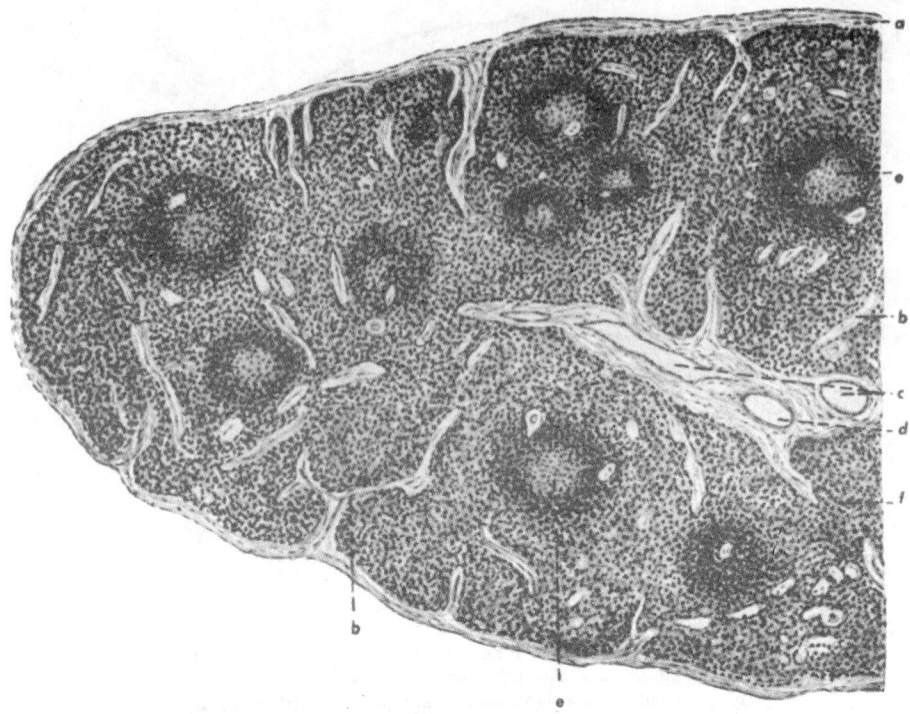

Figure 148. From the spleen of a cat (30×). *a*, capsule; *b*, trabecula; *c,d*, vessels in a trabecula; *e*, splenic corpuscle (white pulp); *f*, red pulp.

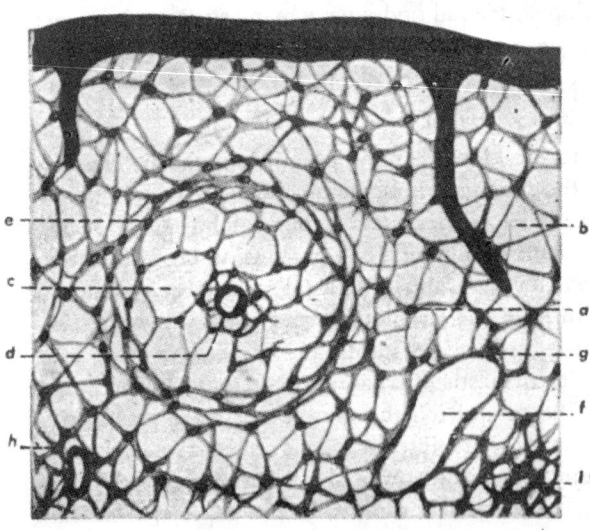

Figure 149. Diagram of the distribution of the reticular tissue in the splenic parenchyma. The reticular fibers are not represented. *a*, cellular reticulum of the red pulp; *b*, its meshes; *c*, wide-meshed reticulum of the white pulp with *d*, a central artery; *e*, condensed reticulum on the boundary between red and white pulp; *f*, sinusoid; *g*, connection of the reticulum with lining cell; *h*, condensation of the reticulum on an artery after its emergence from the white pulp; *i*, thicker syncytial condensation on a sheathed artery.

and anastomosing to form a complicated, netlike framework. Many fine trabeculae do not join the others but fuse with the branching veins, strengthening their delicate walls. There is also a trabecular system that is independent of the blood vessels.

The splenic parenchyma is a mixture of red pulp and white pulp. The red pulp is a soft, dark, reddish-brown substance that fills the communicating spaces in the framework. Within the red pulp are the whitish, splenic (Malpighian) corpuscles. These are spherical or ellipsoid, about the size of a pinhead, and visible with the naked eye as the white pulp.

A cellular *reticulum* (Fig. 149) extends in all directions throughout the red and white pulp. It is reinforced by fibers which are mostly intracellular and are clearly demonstrated only by special methods. This network adapts itself by expansion or

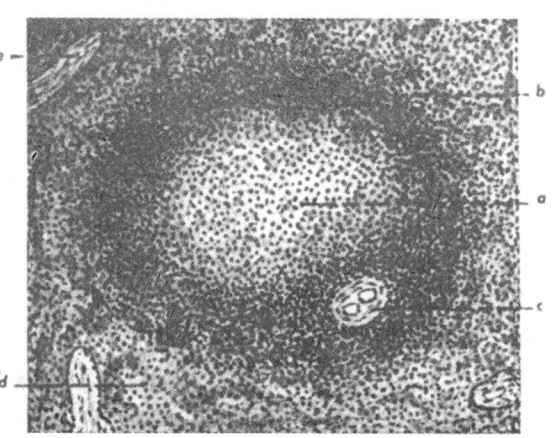

Figure 150. Splenic corpuscle from the spleen of a cat (125×). *a*, germinal center; *b*, small lymphocytes; *c*, artery of the white pulp at a bifurcation; *d*, red pulp; *e*, trabecula.

collapse to the changing functional conditions of the spleen. The cells and fibers of the reticular tissue connect the small vessels of the pulp to the framework. In so doing they support the vessels and take part in the structure of their walls. The meshes of the reticulum are narrower in the red pulp than in the splenic corpuscles. The border between white and red pulp is marked by a close-meshed zone containing elastic fibers. Where the reticulum is attached to certain portions of the arteries, it becomes denser (*h*), and this condensation is so marked on the sheathed arteries (*i;* see also below) that the network is replaced by a syncytial layer. The reticulum of the red pulp is especially strong in the cat and swine.

The *white pulp* (Figs. 148,*e;* 150; 152,*a*) arises by transformation of the adventitia of the arteries to lymphatic tissue shortly after they pass from the trabeculae into the parenchyma. This lymphatic sheath accompanies the arteries and their branches, expanding at intervals to form nodules—the splenic corpuscles. The artery may pass through the center of the nodule or, more commonly, through one side. Therefore, each splenic corpuscle contains a small artery of variable position, falsely called the central artery (Figs. 150,*c;* 152,*g*). The artery is not visible in every corpuscle in a section because some sections are cut parallel to the artery, not through it. Like the cortical nodules of the lymph nodes, the splenic corpuscles sometimes show a lighter central area, the germinal center, which is often missing in the spleens of aged animals.

The development and extent of the white pulp fluctuate among individuals and are dependent upon conditions of age, nutrition, etc. The corpuscles are especially large in the ox. In the cat the white pulp appears as nodules; in the dog, as nodules and cords.

The spaces between the white pulp and the trabeculae are filled by the *red pulp* (Fig. 148,*f*). This contains, in addition to the arterial branches that emerge from the white pulp, the venous sinuses or sinusoids. The reticulum spreads out be-

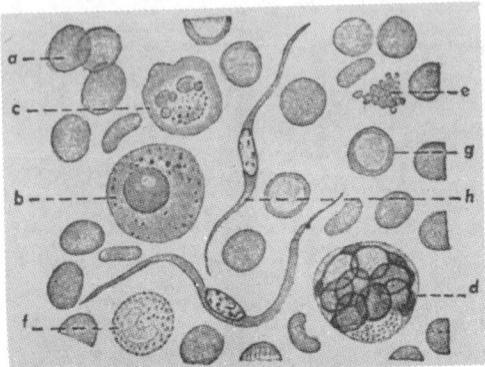

Figure 151. From a teased preparation of the spleen of the dog (fresh, 700×). *a*, erythrocytes; *b*, phagocyte; *c*, phagocyte with pigment; *d*, phagocyte with erythrocytes; *e*, free pigment; *f*, granulocyte; *g*, lymphocyte; *h*, lining cell of a sinusoid.

tween the vessels, containing in its meshes cells of various kinds (Fig. 151). The elements of the circulating blood are always present. In addition to lymphocytes, the red pulp harbors granulocytes. Eosinophils are unusually numerous in the horse. Basophils are rare in all species. Granulocytes may develop postnatally from myelocytes in the spleen of ruminants and carnivora. Erythroblasts are present in young animals. The most numerous blood elements are the erythrocytes, many of which do not re-enter the circulation but undergo degeneration. The destruction of red cells is particularly well demonstrated in the horse and swine. The remains are engulfed by the abundant large macrophages, which may also contain brown pigment, lipids, and degenerate white blood cells. The lining cells of the sinusoids and the fixed macrophages of the reticulum are also important in the phagocytosis and digestion of cellular detritus and foreign substances. Hemosiderin, an iron-containing pigment of yellowish-brown color derived from hemoglobin, is present in granules or clumps; it may be either intracellular or free in the meshes of the reticulum (*c,e*). Heavy deposits of pigment are found in adult horses (in 5 percent of old animals), swine, and ruminants. Locally produced, iron-free, wear-and-tear pigments are also present. Lobulated giant cells (megakaryocytes) have been identified, especially in the red pulp of carnivora and swine. In ruminants and swine, smooth muscle fibers occur in the red pulp. They are connected with the trabeculae.

There are apparently two quantitatively different types of mammalian spleens.

The "storage" spleen of the horse, dog, and cat is relatively large, rich in trabeculae and muscle, and poor in white pulp. The abundant red pulp serves as storage space for blood elements, and the muscular framework acts to empty the spleen. The contrasting type is the "defense" spleen, which is small and has few trabeculae and muscle fibers but abundant lymphatic tissue. The red pulp, the storage space of the spleen, is poorly developed in the rabbit, only moderately so in man. The ruminant and swine belong to an intermediate group.

Blood Vessels. The arrangement of the blood vessels is essential to an understanding of the structure of the spleen. The number of splenic arteries entering at the hilus varies with the species. Their larger branches ramify with the trabeculae,

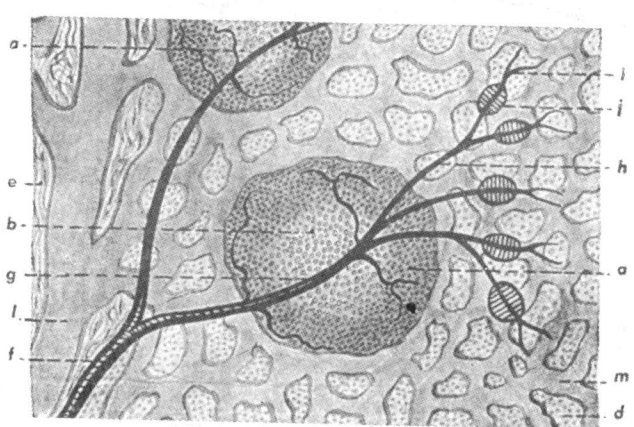

Figure 152. Blood vessels of the spleen, diagrammatic. *a*, splenic corpuscle; *b*, germinal center; *d*, red pulp; *e*, trabecula; *f*, artery; *l*, vein; *g*, central artery; *h*, artery of a penicillus; *i*, sheathed artery; *k*, arterial capillary; *m*, sinusoid.

and after reduction to a diameter of 0.1 to 0.2 mm. they pass out into the pulp (Fig. 152,*f*). After a course that is usually short, the arteries pass through the splenic corpuscles, which receive tufts of anastomosing capillaries. The vascularization of the corpuscles fluctuates with their constant growth and retrogression. Upon emerging from the white pulp, the arteries break up into fine branches like the bristles of a brush (the penicillus, Fig. 152,*h*). These soon become *sheathed arteries* as their muscular connective tissue coat is replaced by a spindle-shaped condensation of the reticulum consisting of rounded cells and argyrophil fibers. The sheath cells lie next to the endothelium and are considered to be an especially active part of the reticulo-endothelial system. The sheaths are extensible and may also serve to support the delicate vascular wall under the stress of volume changes in the spleen. A passive valvular action on the capillary branches has been described.[1] The sheaths vary in form among the species.

The sheathed arteries are continued as the somewhat wider *arterial capillaries*. These are endothelial tubes supported by the surrounding reticulum with its lattice fibers. Occasionally in man and dog the arterial capillaries open directly into the sinusoids (closed circulation). However, the present understanding is that most

[1] David W. MacKenzie, A. O. Whipple, and M. P. Wintersteiner, Studies on the Microscopic Anatomy and Physiology of Living Transilluminated Mammalian Spleens, *Am. J. Anatomy* 68 (1941): 397–456.

arterial capillaries are not complete tubes conducting to the sinusoids but that they open into the meshes of the red pulp. This is called an open circulation.[2] At their termination, the arterial capillaries dilate to form an ampulla, and the endothelial cells become so dissociated as to be indistinguishable from reticulum cells. The blood elements pass through the red pulp, either rapidly in direct channels or slowly in the meshes of the reticulum. They enter the sinusoids at their origins or through apertures in the walls and are borne away by the venous drainage.

The *sinusoids* (the venous sinuses, Fig. 152,*m*) vary in structure among the species. Their lining cells play an important role in the reticulo-endothelial system.

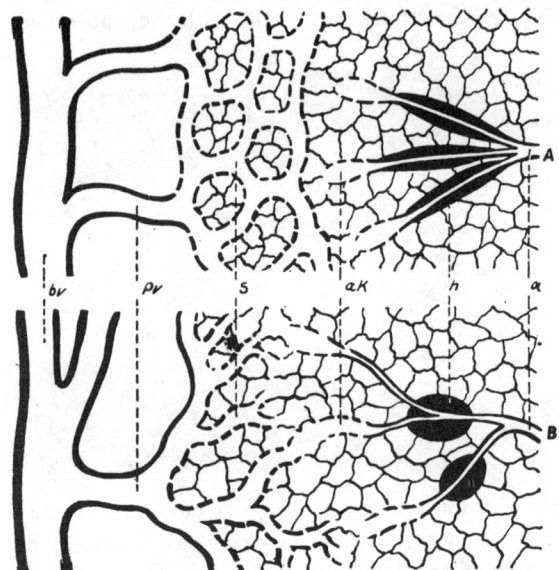

Figure 153. Diagram of the course of the arteries after leaving the white pulp in the spleen of man and dog (*A*), and in the spleen of ruminant, horse, swine, and cat (*B*). *a*, artery dividing to form a penicillus; *h*, sheathed artery; *ak*, arterial capillaries; *s*, sinusoids; *pv*, pulp veins; *bv*, trabecular veins. (After Hartmann.)

In man they form an irregular network which extends through the greater part of the red pulp. They are thin-walled vessels of variable diameter, formed by longitudinal ribbon-like cells (littoral cells, Fig. 151,*h*) which are separated by narrow slits. Some authors claim that they are actually connected by an invisible membrane. The littoral cells anastomose, and their nuclei bulge into the lumen. They are held together by circular fibers (Fig. 154) that are continuous with those of the reticulum. The wall of the sinus is regarded as a condensation and regular arrangement of the reticular tissue to form a latticework. The inner, longitudinal strips of the lattice are formed by the reticular cells, elongated and differentiated into fixed macrophages, while the outer circular elements are reticular fibers. The blood elements can pass through the spaces in the wall from the meshes of the red pulp into the sinusoids and vice versa. The sinusoids are connected with the trabecular veins by numerous short pulp veins (Fig. 153,*pv*).

The sinusoids in domestic animals are not so well developed as they are in man. The condition in the dog most closely resembles that of man. A prominent network

[2] *Ibid.* See also David Gall, A Simple Technique for the Microscopy of Living Tissues in situ with Some Observations on the Splenic Circulation, *Ann. Trop. Med. and Paras.* 42 (1948): 54–66.

of sinusoids is lined by cells which are connected by transverse bridges. Thus the sinusoid is surrounded by a cytoplasmic lattice, in which the lattice of reticular fibers is embedded. In the horse, ruminant, swine, and cat (Fig. 153,*B*), the sinusoids are subordinate to the rest of the red pulp. They begin as individual roots in the reticulum and form no network but converge in large trunks. Their tubular lumen is at first only a channel in the reticulum, but the meshes of the wall become narrower as the sinusoids grow larger, until the completely enclosed pulp veins are reached.

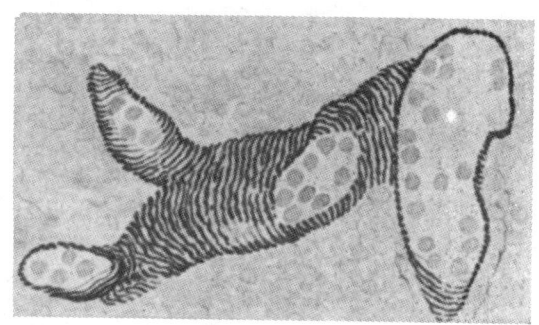

Figure 154. Sinusoid with circular fibers from the spleen of the dog; stained with orcein (450×).

The trabecular veins run with the arteries (Fig. 152,*l*) to the hilus. In the horse and ox there are many connections between the pulp veins and the subserous venous plexus.

The lymph vessels occur in the serosa and in the capsule. There are few in the trabeculae and none in the parenchyma.

The nerves are mostly unmyelinated (Figs. 114, 363) and supply the musculature of the vessels and trabeculae. The myelinated fibers are apparently sensory.

B. RED BONE MARROW

The color of red bone marrow is due to its great vascularity and to the numerous hemoglobin-containing blood corpuscles. It occurs mainly in the short and flat bones and in the epiphyses of long bones of adults. In the young it occurs in all bones. It consists of delicate reticular tissue (Fig. 155,*d*) which has dye-storing and phagocytic properties and is free of elastic fibers. The reticulum condenses on the walls of the marrow cavity to form a connective tissue membrane, the endosteum.

The meshes of the reticulum are filled with erythrocytes and granulocytes and their precursors (p. 92).[3] In addition to the mature erythrocytes and granulocytes, the following types are present:

1. Hemocytoblasts (myeloblasts) are relatively large cells with a spherical nucleus and basophilic, nongranular cytoplasm. They are descended from reticular cells, probably give rise to most of the elements of the bone marrow, and are more numerous in young animals than older ones.

---

[3] M. Lois Calhoun, Technic for Obtaining Bone Marrow from the Horse and Cow, *Vet. Student* (Iowa) *8* (1946): 143; Frank Bloom and L. M. Meyer, The Morphology of the Bone Marrow Cells in Normal Dogs, *Cornell Vet. 34* (1944): 13–18.

2. Erythroblasts (Fig. 156,*f**) are numerous and usually lie in groups. The cytoplasm varies in staining properties with the hemoglobin content (polychromasia). The more mature (i.e., rich in hemoglobin) the cytoplasm, the more eosinophilic it becomes. The nucleus is round, dark, and often seen in mitosis. With the loss of the nucleus, these cells become the erythrocytes, which pass between the lining cells of the sinusoids and enter the circulation.

3. Myelocytes (Fig. 156,*c**) are large cells with round or ovoid nuclei. Mitoses are abundant. With advancing maturity the nucleus becomes indented and the cell is called a metamyelocyte. Myelocytes contain specific granules, which increase with maturity. The neutrophil myelocytes predominate over the eosinophil and basophil. The different types develop into the corresponding granulocytes, which migrate into the sinusoids.

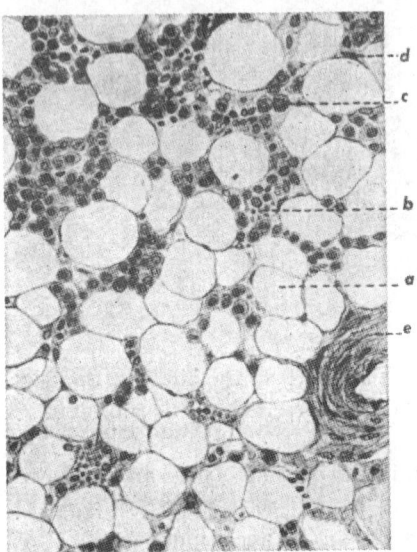

Figure 155. From the red bone marrow of a goat. *a*, fat cell; *b*, erythrocytes; *c*, myelocyte; *d*, nucleus of a reticular cell; *e*, part of an arterial wall.

4. Lymphocytes are rare in the vicinity of the vessels, but are found in the lymph nodules that occur in the bone marrow (in man and the cat).

5. Plasma cells (p. 39) are rare.

6. Megakaryocytes (Fig. 156,*a**) occur in variable numbers. They are finely granular giant cells characterized by a large polymorphous nucleus.

7. Monocytes are very rare.

8. Fat cells (Fig. 155,*b*) develop from reticular cells.

9. Osteoclasts (Fig. 84,*a**) lie in the marrow near the bone (or cartilage). Osteoblasts belong to the osseous tissue.

BLOOD VESSELS. The arteries of the marrow are derived from the nutrient artery of the bone and the numerous small arteries that enter the marrow via Volkmann's canals. The capillaries empty into sinusoids, which unite to form the veins. The thin, perhaps perforate, walls of the sinusoids are composed of flattened reticular cells and a latticework of reticular fibers. The lining cells and those in the reticulum belong to the reticulo-endothelial system. Lymph vessels seem to be absent.

A physiological reduction of the red bone marrow begins in adult animals with the diaphyses. The red marrow is replaced by yellow or fatty marrow, which is composed mainly of fat cells and has nothing to do with blood formation. After a substantial loss of blood, the yellow marrow can change into red marrow again. In emaciated animals the fat in the cells partially disappears and is replaced by a mucous fluid. This gelatinous bone marrow also occurs in old horses in good condition. In birds the bone marrow, which is rich in fat and heterophil leukocytes, is displaced to a large extent by air (in the pneumatic bones, e.g., the humerus).

* Fig. 84 is on p. 89 and Fig. 156 on p. 93.

X

Organs of Internal Secretion, the Endocrine Glands

THE endocrine glands differ as widely in origin, structure, and location as in the nature of their secretions. They are especially rich in wide, thin-walled blood vessels. Unlike the secretions of exocrine glands (p. 29), their products are not conveyed to the outside, i.e., the skin or a mucous surface, by way of an excretory duct. Instead they are secreted directly from the glandular cells or follicles into the lymph or blood stream. The endocrine glands are the sources of important specific substances, called *hormones*,[1] which are carried in the blood to organs whose activity they stimulate or depress. Thus they exert an important governing influence on the entire organism. Whenever these chemical agents are absent or deficient, grave disturbances in function occur, which may be alleviated by the administration of an extract or the substance of the organ in question. Hormones are also used therapeutically to produce certain physiological effects (e.g., adrenalin or pitressin is used to raise blood pressure, and oxytocin to cause uterine contractions, etc.). In addition to the purely endocrine glands there are others which show both exocrine and endocrine activity (e.g., the pancreas, testis, and ovary). Finally, there are structures not classed as endocrine glands (the liver, placenta, epithelium of the small intestine, reticulo-endothelial cells, and others) that produce an internal secretion. The glands to be discussed here are characterized by their functional unity; they are closely interrelated.

A. THYROID GLAND

The embryonic thyroid gland consists of tortuous, branching epithelial cords and tubes. Originally it possesses a duct which opens on the root of the tongue. This thyroglossal duct, however, is reduced to vestiges in the embryonic period. The glandular substance is divided prenatally into numerous compartments by invading connective tissue. The thyroid gland (Figs. 157*, 158, 159) at the time of birth is a ductless alveolar gland. It is surrounded by a connective tissue capsule (Fig.

---

[1] Gr. *hormaein* to excite, to rouse. * Fig. 157 is on p. 94.

159,*a*), which gives off septa of varying thicknesses to the interior. These divide the organ into flat or round interconnected lobules. The lobules consist of vesicles of varying sizes—the *thyroid follicles* (Figs. 157,*c,d**; 159,*b*). In young animals the follicles often retain their embryonic continuity and are usually smaller than in adults. Between the follicles there is delicate, fat-free connective tissue, which contains many blood and lymph capillaries. It also contains in young animals varying quantities of primitive cells which may give rise to more follicles. The follicles are completely closed and are surrounded by a network of delicate reticular fibers.

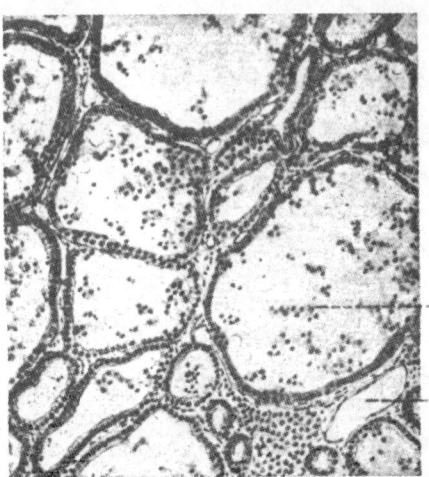

Figure 158. Section through the thyroid gland of a three-year-old ox. *a*, dislodged epithelial cells in the colloid; *b*, blood vessel.

They are usually spherical or ovoid in shape, but some are tubular or sacculated. The cells lining the follicles have a large round nucleus. They are closely apposed to the interfollicular connective tissue or capillaries. Their shape is cuboidal or low columnar, and they are joined to each other by terminal bars. Functional changes are manifested in the size of the cells and the relative abundance of intracellular inclusions. As a rule, all the cells of one follicle are in the same functional state, but there are differences in this respect among the follicles.

The follicles contain *colloid*, a viscous fluid rich in iodine secreted by the cells. In the colloid there are free epithelial cells, which occur in such numbers in the adult ox as to suggest a holocrine secretion (Fig. 158). They are replaced by mitosis. The colloid may appear homogeneous or finely granular; it is usually acidophilic, but some follicles show varying degrees of basophilia. The vacuoles in the colloid are probably a fixation artefact (Fig. 157,*f**).

The thyroid gland stores its secretions in the closed follicles in the form of colloid or thyroglobulin, the storage form of the hormone. When the impetus for the mobilization of the colloid is given by the thyrotrophic hormone of the hypophysis, the thyroglobulin is hydrolyzed to thyroxine, the absorbable form. As such it is reabsorbed by the follicle cells and thrown into the blood stream from their basal surface. During resorption and basal secretion the epithelium becomes taller.

The thyroid gland undergoes certain changes with advancing age. These include flattening of the epithelium, an increase of fat and pigment granules in the cells, and thickening of the colloid. Pregnancy and the time of year influence the structure of the thyroid gland; there appears to be an increase in the cell size and the

---

* Fig. 157 is on p. 94.

size of the gland in the winter. Differences among breeds and localities have also been recognized.

The blood vessels are numerous (Figs. 157*; 158,*b*). The arteries, some of which are equipped with occlusive mechanisms, give rise to very dense capillary nets, which surround the follicles in basket fashion. From them arise numerous veins. The lymph vessels originate as perifollicular capillary nets. They continue in the supporting framework and communicate with a lymphatic net in the capsule. Ganglia are often present along with the nerves, which supply vasomotor and secretory fibers to the vessels and the basal surface of the gland cells.

The thyroid gland is a very important organ. Its hormone, thyroxine, which contains iodine, governs the rate of metabolism. It also influences the nervous system, growth (especially of bone), and the mental and physical development of the organism. The gland is controlled by the hypophysis. There are important interrelations between the thyroid gland, on the one hand, and the adrenals, the sex glands, mammary glands, and thymus on the other. Their exact nature is not clear in all cases.

Often we encounter accessory thyroid glands. These have the same structure and function as the regular thyroid gland and are especially common in poultry.

They must not be confused with the parathyroid glands. The ultimobranchial bodies are derived from the last (fifth) pharyngeal pouch. There is some disagreement to their fate, and they vary with the species. In animals in which they remain distinct from the thyroid, they are cellular aggregates or cystlike structures lined with simple ciliated columnar epithelium. They never contain colloid and may persist in the tissue of the thyroid gland or its vicinity for varying lengths of time; they stay longest in cattle.

B. PARATHYROID GLANDS

The parathyroids are separate organs in spite of their close developmental and anatomical relationship to the thyroid and thymus. They possess a thin con-

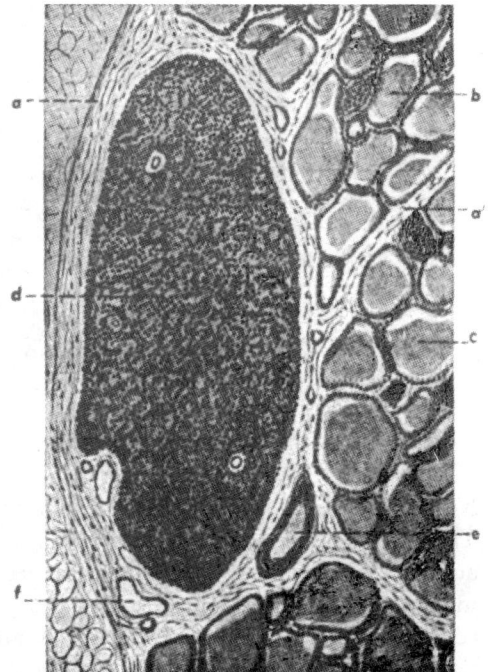

Figure 159. Thyroid and parathyroid glands of a dog (35×). *a*, common capsule; *a'*, interstitial connective tissue; *b*, thyroid follicle; *c*, colloid; *d*, parathyroid gland; *e*, artery; *f*, vein.

* Fig. 157 is on p. 94.

nective tissue capsule, which is often absent when the glands are deeply embedded in the thyroid substance (Fig. 159,d). The interstitial connective tissue may be heavy, as in the dog and ox, or delicate, as in sheep, goats and young animals in general. It may contain abundant adipose tissue in older individuals. It surrounds the glandular parenchyma, which is richly supplied by sinusoidal capillaries. The parenchymal cells are polygonal, finely granular, and show little affinity for stains. A condensed layer of ectoplasm outlines them sharply. They form cords, islets, or clusters between strands of connective tissue. Larger cell aggregates are also seen.

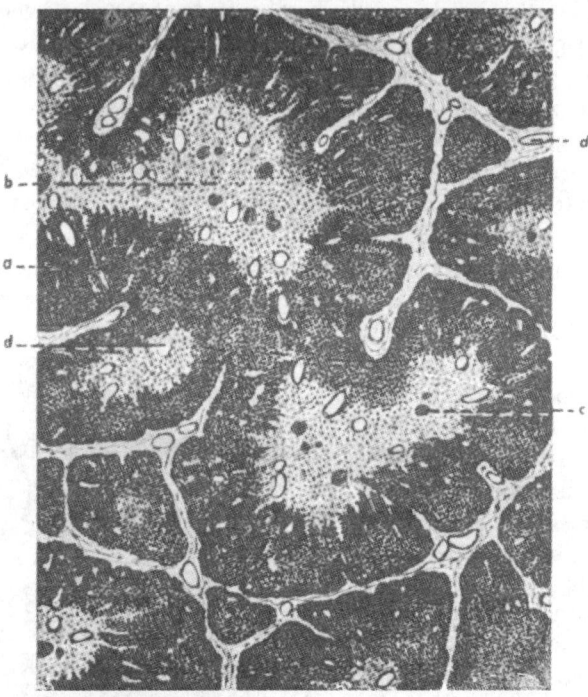

Figure 160. Section from the thymus of a twelve-week-old cat showing a nearly complete lobule. *a,* cortex; *b,* medulla; *c,* Hassall's body; *d,* blood vessel in the interstitial connective tissue.

No arrangement characteristic for any particular species or age has been described The variation in stainability of the cells apparently reflects the state of secretory activity. (The markedly oxyphilic cells seen in man have not been reported in domestic animals other than the ox).[2] Glycogen, fat, and granules are present in the cells, especially in older animals. All cells are surrounded by a reticular connective tissue framework. Near the periphery of the organ one occasionally finds vesicles lined with epithelium and filled with a homogeneous substance. These may originate by the accumulation of secretions in the parenchyma.

[2] Michael Levine, Oxyphil Cells in the Parathyroid Glands of the Cow and Steer, *Anat. Rec. 39* (1928): 293–297.

The parathyroid glands are richly vascularized. Their sinusoids have a wide lumen, sometimes resembling cavernous spaces (e.g., in sheep). Larger lymphatics are absent. Nerves supplying vessels and parenchyma are numerous. In the dog Pacinian corpuscles are also found.

The function of the parathyroid glands consists of the secretion of a hormone (parathormone), which regulates calcium and phosphorus metabolism. Removal of the glands results in lowered blood calcium and fatal parathyroid tetany.

C. THYMUS

The thymus does not have the structure of a typical endocrine gland. It is composed of pyramidal or polygonal lobules, which are joined to each other by loose connective tissue. The lobules (Fig. 160) average 5 to 13 mm. in size. In stained sections they are seen to consist of a dark cortex and a lighter medulla. Often the medullary substance is continuous through several lobules. The superficial portion of the lobule is often notched and subdivided into smaller compartments, separated by connective tissue. These subdivisions have a diameter of about 1 mm. and consist mostly of cortical substance. More centrally they blend with the undivided medulla. Cortex and medulla look very much like lymphatic tissue. Embryologically, however, the thymus is not related to the lymph nodes, since the derivation of its reticulum is not mesenchymal but entodermal. It develops by transformation of a purely epithelial primordium which grows caudad from the third and fourth pharyngeal pouches. The meshes of the cortical reticulum contain large numbers of small lymphocytes (thymocytes, Fig. 161,*b*). The reticular cells are easily recognized by their large pale nuclei. Eosinophils and plasma cells are also present. The lymphocytes migrate from the neighboring mesenchymal tissue into the thymus primordium, pushing the epithelial cells apart. The epithelial cells are thus transformed into stellate cells, connected by their processes to form a reticulum. The intimate mingling of epithelium and mesenchyme is peculiar to the thymus.

The medullary substance (Fig. 160,*b*) of the lobules differs from the cortical substance in that the reticular cells have more cytoplasm, the thymocytes are fewer and show no mitotic figures, and Hassall's bodies are present (Fig. 161,*a*). The latter are spheroid structures of varying size and consist of concentric layers of flat epithelial cells. The innermost cells are often transformed into hyaline masses.

Hassall's corpuscles are transitory structures. They originate by hypertrophy of

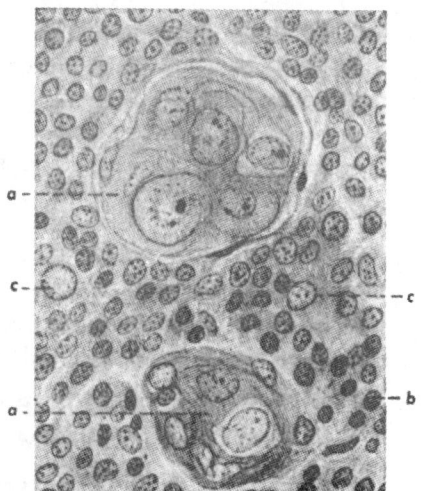

Figure 161. Section from the medulla of the thymus of a dog (600×). *a*, Hassall's body; *b*, lymphocytes; *c*, nuclei of entodermal reticular cells.

isolated medullary reticular cells, followed by the apposition of more reticular cells. During the growth of the corpuscle the center undergoes degenerative changes, i.e., karyolysis, hyaline degeneration, fatty changes, calcification, and invasion of leukocytes. Hassall's corpuscles are the most characteristic feature of the thymus gland and are common to all species. Their number may be an index of thymus activity. In man about 1,350,000 such corpuscles are present at the time of puberty. Only half of these remain by the twentieth year.

The medullary substance also contains at times epithelial cells with abundant cytoplasm and large nuclei. These may occur singly or in groups. Multinucleated giant cells also occur here. Occasionally cysts are encountered in the medulla. They contain clumps of material and are lined with epithelium, which may be ciliated. They are most often seen in old horses.

The blood vessels (Fig. 160,d) of the thymus are ensheathed in lymphatic tissue, which takes an active part in the production of lymphocytes. The arteries lie in the medulla near the cortex and supply capillary nets, which become especially dense toward the surface of the cortex. These are drained by veins which course around the lobules on their surface. The lymphatics encircle the medulla and are continued as netlike lymph channels, which lie in the periphery of the lobules and are drained by interlobular vessels. The nerve fibers present are mainly vasomotor. Only a few have free endings in the medulla.

Age involution of the thymus gland apparently begins with the change of feed at weaning time and becomes pronounced at puberty. It takes effect mainly in the cervical portions; remnants of the thoracic portion persist in cattle and dogs up to old age. The parenchyma is reduced, partly by emigration of lymphocytes and partly by reticular cell phagocytosis of lymphocytes, and is gradually replaced by fatty tissue. In addition to age involution we also recognize *accidental involution* due to exhaustion, malnutrition, cachectic diseases, x-ray treatments, and other factors. In this case, the reticular cells enlarge, and the cortical thymocytes decrease rapidly in number, starting at the periphery.

The function of the thymus gland is unknown. Because its period of largest size coincides with that of the development and growth of the organism, and because the period of its most rapid decline begins with puberty, great efforts have been made to demonstrate a thymic hormone with growth-promoting properties or with power to retard sexual development pending the completion of the maturation process. The results have been inconclusive. The thymus does, however, produce lymphocytes and, to some extent, also plasma cells and myelocytes.

D. ADRENAL (SUPRARENAL) GLANDS AND CHROMAFFIN TISSUE

The adrenal glands consist of two developmentally, morphologically, and physiologically distinct parts: the cortex, derived from the coelomic mesoderm, and the medulla, derived from the same ectodermal tissue as the sympathetic ganglion cells. The two portions develop at first independently and later combine to form one organ.

The connective tissue capsule (Fig. 162,*g*) contains elastic and smooth muscle fibers, occasionally also pigment, and detaches many thin, well-vascularized processes, which penetrate to the corticomedullary junction.

The meshes of the cortical framework contain cell cords. In the peripheral part of the cortex, the *zona fasciculata*, they are radially arranged in solid cell columns (Figs. 162,*b;* 164). In the inner part of the cortex, the cords lose their regularity and form a network, the *zona reticularis* (Fig. 162,*c*). In horses, swine, and carnivores the cell cords become wider peripherally as their polygonal cells change to long columnar cells, which are laid down transversely. Near the capsule these wide cell cords are connected by arches, forming the *zona arcuata* (Figs. 162,*a;* 163). In ruminants, which lack the zona arcuata, the round cell strands often turn parallel to the surface immediately under the capsule. The arrangement simulates in section the round cell masses of the human zona glomerulosa. The cortical cells contain nuclei that are poor in chromatin. The cords appear in sections to be one to four cells wide. The cytoplasm contains many lipoid droplets, which are mixtures of fatty acids, phospholipids, and cholesterol compounds. They are especially abundant in the outer zona fasciculata. Granules of ascorbic acid (vitamin C) may be demonstrated histochemically. There is a high degree of correlation between the activity of the cortex and the amount of lipoid material and ascorbic acid. A brownish-yellow pigment occurs intracellularly in the zona reticularis. Lipids as well as pigment increase with age. The cortical cell cords are separated only by a delicate reticular connective tissue from the capillaries, which are especially large (sinusoids) in the zona reticularis.

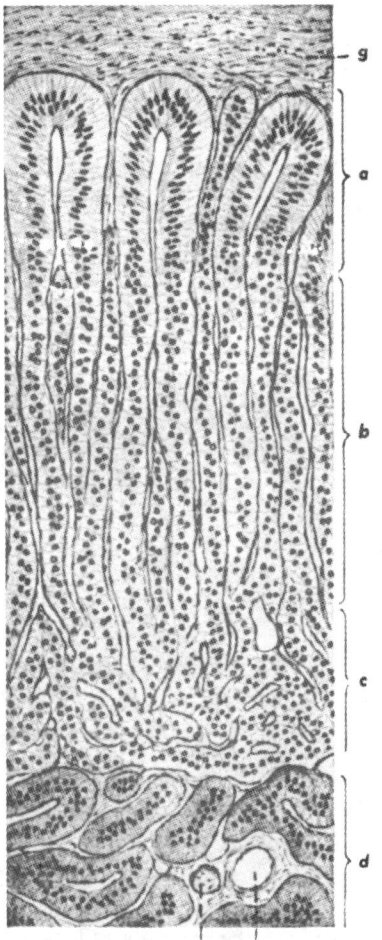

Figure 162. Cross section of the adrenal gland of the horse; potassium dichromate preparation (60×). *a*, zona arcuata; *b*, zona fasciculata; *c*, zona reticularis; *d*, medulla (chromaffin tissue); *e*, nerve fiber in cross section; *f*, blood vessel; *g*, capsule.

The medulla (Figs. 162,*d;* 165) contains sympathetic ganglion cells, which are especially abundant in ruminants, and the chromaffin medullary cells, which stain yellow or brown when fixed with chromic acid. They also stain green with ferric chloride and are readily stained with basic dyes. They shrink easily on fixation. The chromaffin cells are polygonal (columnar in swine and sheep). Their abundant cytoplasm lacks lipoid inclusions, but shows a fine chromaffin granulation which varies with the adrenalin content of the gland. The cells form anastomosing strands or clusters separated by sinusoids. The large, pale nuclei are located in the central portion of the cell cords. The fine netlike connective tissue framework contains elastic fibers.

In both cortex and medulla mitoses are normally present indicating continuous destruction and replacement of cells. In the cortex this replacement process occurs mainly in the peripheral layers. It is not unusual to find medullary substance in the area of the cortex and vice versa. Accessory cortical tissue is occasionally encountered nearby, retroperitoneally, and in the vicinity of the internal genital organs.

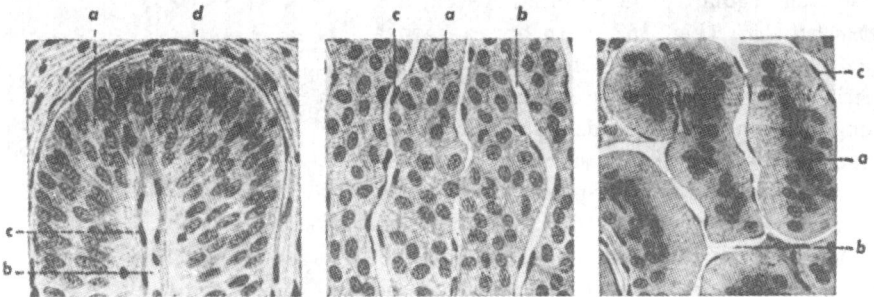

Figure 163 (left). Zona arcuata of the equine adrenal gland (350×). *a*, cortical cells; *b*, capillary; *c*, its endothelium; *d*, capsule.

Figure 164 (center). Zona fasciculata of the equine adrenal gland (350×). *a*, cells; *b*, capillaries; *c*, their endothelium.

Figure 165 (right). Cell cords from the adrenal medulla of a horse (350×). *a*, medullary cells; *b*, sinusoids; *c*, lining cells.

In addition to arteries that penetrate the cortex without branching until they reach the medulla, there are also arteries that branch in the capsule and supply the cortical capillary nets. These become sinusoidal in the zona reticularis and continue into the medulla. The medullary veins (except those in ruminants) contain in their walls longitudinal strands of muscle, which probably regulate the rate of drainage. They converge to form a single central vein for the whole gland. Sinusoids and capillaries are in close contact with the parenchymatous cells. The lining cells of the sinusoids are part of the reticulo-endothelial system. Lymphatics have been found in association with the larger blood vessels.

The numerous nerves are of sympathetic origin. Most of them go to the medulla (Fig. 162,*c*), where they form such dense nets that each cell is surrounded by nerve fibers. Sympathetic ganglion cells are present in the medulla.

Extirpation of the adrenal glands causes progressive weakness, a pronounced drop in blood pressure, and death. The survival period varies with species and age. The cortex is the vital portion of the gland. It secretes a number of steroid hormones, not all of which have been identified chemically. Nor has any one of the recognized substances been identified with a particular function of the cortex. The cortical hormones are concerned with water and electrolyte metabolism, carbohydrate metabolism, and protection against shock. The cortex also yields an androgenic hormone like that of the testis. Cortical tumors cause sexual precocity and virilism in females. Conversely, the structure of the cortex is influenced by estrus, pregnancy, and castration. The medulla secretes adrenalin, which is a specific stimulant to sympathetic nerves and thus acts on all regions of the body that receive sympathetic innervation. It is valued therapeutically as a vasoconstrictor and cardiac accelerator, producing a rise in blood pressure. It also raises the blood sugar level.

The Paraganglia. Chromaffin tissue in the animal body is not restricted to the adrenal medulla. Chromaffin cells of the same derivation and possibly the same function occur singly or sometimes in macroscopically visible nodules in ganglia or nerve fibers throughout the area of distribution of the sympathetic nerves. They are also found in a series of separate spheroid or fusiform bodies, the paraganglia. These bodies contain chromaffin cells embedded in richly vascularized and innervated connective tissue. Smaller paraganglia are especially frequent in the thoracic and cervical portions of the sympathetic system, in the vicinity of the large abdominal vessels, on the surface of the adrenal glands, at the renal hilus, in the broad ligament of the uterus, and elsewhere. The paired organ of Zuckerkandl at the point of origin of the caudal mesenteric artery is a larger paraganglion. The paraganglia are much larger in young animals. All these structures are included in the chromaffin system, the foremost representative of which is the adrenal medulla.

E. HYPOPHYSIS CEREBRI (PITUITARY GLAND)

The hypophysis (Fig. 166) consists of two parts differing in origin, structure, and function. One, the pars nervosa, is derived from an outpouching of the floor of the diencephalon, while the other originates as a dorsal evagination of the stomodeum and is called the pars buccalis. In the embryo the buccal part, or Rathke's pouch, lies close to the pars nervosa and fuses with it, later becoming separated from the primitive oral cavity by constriction of its stalk. The wall of Rathke's pouch that fuses with the pars nervosa undergoes little further growth. It is called the pars intermedia. Lateral proliferations of the pars buccalis surround the infundibulum (a) to form the pars tuberalis, which extends to the tuber cinereum of the brain. The rest of the wall of Rathke's pouch forms the pars distalis or anterior lobe. In man and horse this lobe is closely applied to the pars intermedia, but in other animals a vestigial hypophyseal cavity (c) persists. The pars nervosa is intimately fused with the pars intermedia to form the posterior lobe and represents the thickened solid end of the infundibulum. The lumen of the infundibulum (b) may extend down into the pars nervosa, as in carnivores, swine, and to some extent in horses, or it may end before reaching the hypophysis (as in ruminants). The pars nervosa of ruminants and swine lies caudodorsally in a depression in the buccal part. In solipeds and carnivores it is enclosed by the latter on all sides.

The nomenclature of the hypophysis has been complicated by overlapping terms derived from gross anatomy, histology, and embryology. The following scheme is offered by way of clarification:[3]

---

[3] Maximow and Bloom, p. 302.

Embryology	Adult Histology	Gross Anatomy Physiology Pharmacology
	Pars tuberalis —	Pars tuberalis
Pars buccalis	Pars distalis —	Anterior lobe
	Pars intermedia	Posterior lobe
Pars nervosa —	Pars nervosa	

The terms anterior lobe and posterior lobe, while not strictly applicable to solipeds and carnivores, are well established in the literature of endocrinology.

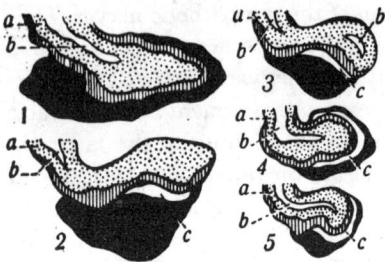

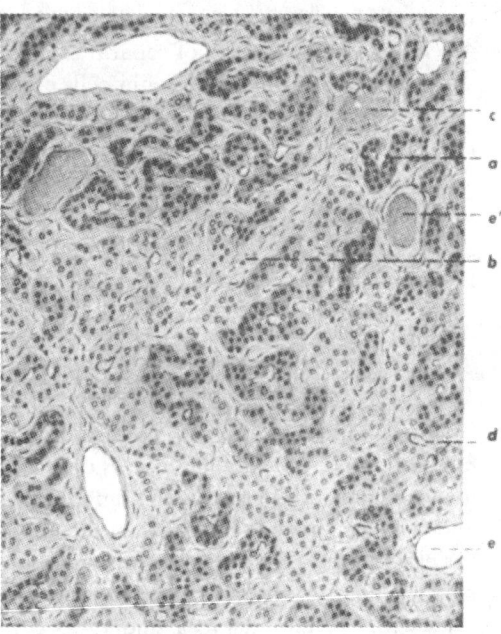

Fig. 166. Median section through the hypophysis of domestic animals, schematic. 1, horse; 2, ox; 3, pig; 4, dog; 5, cat. Black = pars distalis; shaded = pars intermedia and tuberalis; stippled = pars nervosa. a, infundibulum with adjacent pars tuberalis; b, infundibular cavity; c, hypophyseal cavity.

Figure 167 (right). Section through the pars distalis of a goat. a, cell cords; b, interstitial connective tissue; c, colloidal material in b; d, capillary; e, blood vessel; e', colloid.

The *pars distalis* (Fig. 167) contains a meshwork of highly vascular connective tissue. In it we find the parenchyma, composed of tortuous and often branching cell cords of varying length and width, which are surrounded by a reticular fiber sheath. Three main types of cells are present. The more numerous *chief* or *chromophobic* cells (Fig. 168,a*) are characterized by a pale-staining, nongranular cytoplasm. The remaining cells are larger and contain easily stained granules in their cytoplasm. The *acidophil* or *alpha* cells take a red stain (b) and the *basophil* or *beta* cells take a blue stain (c) with hematoxylin-eosin. They are separate cell types and do not represent different stages of secretion. Their close apposition to the thin-walled, sinusoidal blood vessels facilitates secretion into the blood stream. The number and distribution of the cells named seems to depend on the prevailing physiological state, but the beta cells are usually the rarest. The granular cells often

* Fig. 168 is on p. 149.

contain fat. Between them there are occasionally deposits of colloidal material which are more common in older animals. The hypophyseal cavity (residual lumen, interglandular cleft) is lined by cuboidal or columnar epithelium, which may be ciliated and contains goblet cells. The cavity is filled with a colloidal mass which often contains blood, cells, and fat.

The *pars intermedia* (Fig. 166) consists of a connective tissue framework occupied by basophilic cells, which often form dense masses. Glandlike follicles also occur. They are lined with epithelium and contain a colloidal substance. Islands of well-differentiated tissue of the pars distalis type occur regularly in the intermediate lobe—of the ox, for example.

The *pars tuberalis* contains many sinusoidal blood vessels and cellular tubes with stratified epithelial lining and colloidal masses in their lumina. It may be responsible for the production of the diabetogenic principle of "anterior pituitary" extract.

The vascular connective tissue framework of the *pars nervosa* houses neuroglia-like cells with interwoven processes. Certain of these cellular elements, the pituicytes, show fine granules and droplets indicative of secretory activity. The pars nervosa contains intra- and extracellular pigment, which increases in amount with age. Basophilic cells and spheroid hyaline corpuscles may also be present. In addition to this there is a netlike plexus of nerve fibers, which arise in the centers of the diencephalon and reach the pars nervosa via the infundibulum. True nerve cell bodies are lacking. The infundibular cavity and canal are lined by ependyma.

The arteries originate from the internal carotid and the circle of Willis. The pars distalis and pars tuberalis are especially well vascularized. The veins drain into the cavernous sinus. The pars intermedia and the pars nervosa receive few blood vessels. The vasomotor nerves originate at the carotid plexus. It is uncertain whether secretory nerves are present in the pars distalis.

During pregnancy the pars distalis undergoes marked enlargement; there is a multiplication of cells intermediate between chromophobe and acidophil. These "pregnancy cells" are not as distinct in animals as in man and vary among the species. Castration also results in an enlargement of the pituitary. This, however, is due to an increase in the number of basophil cells. Ascorbic acid is demonstrable in the pars distalis and possibly plays a part in the secretory process. In man and occasionally also in animals (e.g., horses and cats) there occurs, at the original opening of the craniopharyngeal canal a pharyngeal hypophysis whose structure resembles that of the pars distalis.

The anterior lobe of the hypophysis is a vital organ. Six of its hormones have been isolated: (1) the growth-producing hormone, (2) the thyrotrophic hormone, (3) the adrenocorticotrophic hormone, (4) the follicle-stimulating hormone, which causes the development of ovarian follicles and spermatozoa, (5) the luteinizing hormone, which causes ovulation and formation of the corpus luteum and stimulates the interstitial cells of the testis, and (6) prolactin, which initiates milk secretion and maintains the corpus luteum. Other effects of anterior pituitary extracts are ketogenic, insulin-antagonizing, diabetogenic, parathyrotrophic, pancreatrophic, and mammogenic.

The posterior lobe is not essential to life. Posterior pituitary extract is divided into two substances of considerable therapeutic importance. Pitressin raises blood pressure by vasoconstriction and also has an antidiuretic effect. Oxytocin stimulates contraction of the uterine musculature and causes expulsion of the milk in the mammary gland. The hypothalamic autonomic centers and the pars nervosa are closely interrelated.

F. EPIPHYSIS CEREBRI (PINEAL BODY)

The connective tissue capsule of the epiphysis sends off processes (Fig. 169,*b*) toward the interior. These vary in development with the species and age. They form a network, incomplete centrally, whose meshes are occupied by glia cells. The epithelioid pineal cells are located either singly or in groups in the feltwork formed by the fibers of the glia cells. The large, light nuclei and the cytoplasm often contain droplet-like homogeneous inclusions. The cells are characterized by long, slender processes, which have club-shaped endings terminating in the connective tissue septa. Nerve fibers enter through the epiphyseal stalk (*e*) and permeate every part of the organ. Nerve cells are absent. Brownish-black pigment is often present intra- or extracellularly, especially in old animals. Calcareous concretions (brain sand), amyloid bodies, and, in the ox, a few smooth and striated muscle fibers are also encountered. The pineal body is not especially rich in blood vessels.

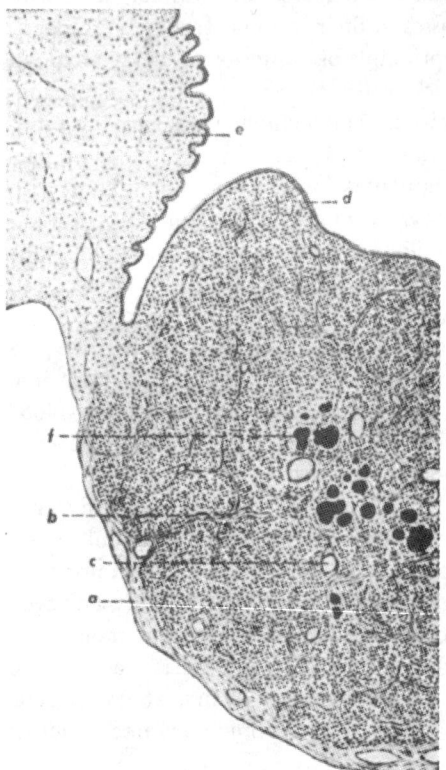

Figure 169. Horizontal section through one half of the epiphysis of a goat. *a,* capsule; *b,* trabecula; *c,* vessels; *d,* ependyma; *e,* epiphyseal stalk; *f,* mineral concretions.

The structure of the epiphysis of young animals (e.g., in the ox) differs from that of the adult. Perhaps its function is altered at puberty. Changes developing with age include an increase in connective tissue, glia, mineral deposition, and cyst formation.

The exact function of the pineal body is as yet undetermined. The pineal cells are credited with an internal secretion, but the hormone has not been isolated. Its probable action is inhibition of genital development. The cessation of pineal activity is said to produce mental and physical precocity.

The endocrine components of the pancreas, sex glands, intestine, etc. will be taken up in the chapters dealing with these organs.

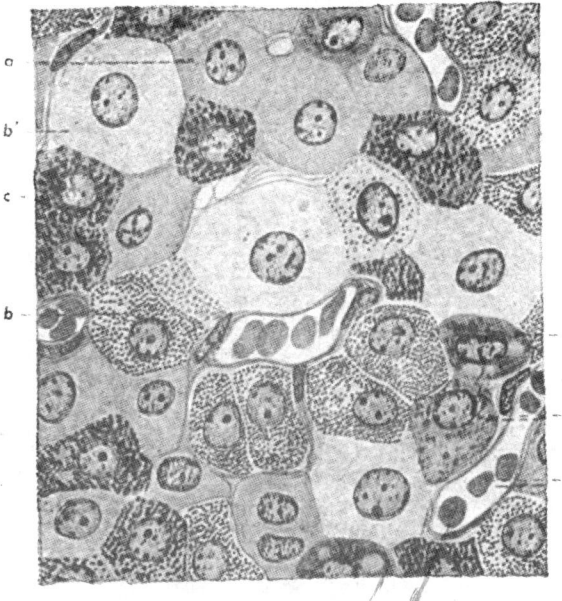

Figure 168. Cell group from the pars distalis of the hypophysis (900×). *a,* chromophobe; *b,* acidophil; *b',* acidophil depleted of granules; *c,* basophil; *d,* degenerating cell; *e,* sinusoid.

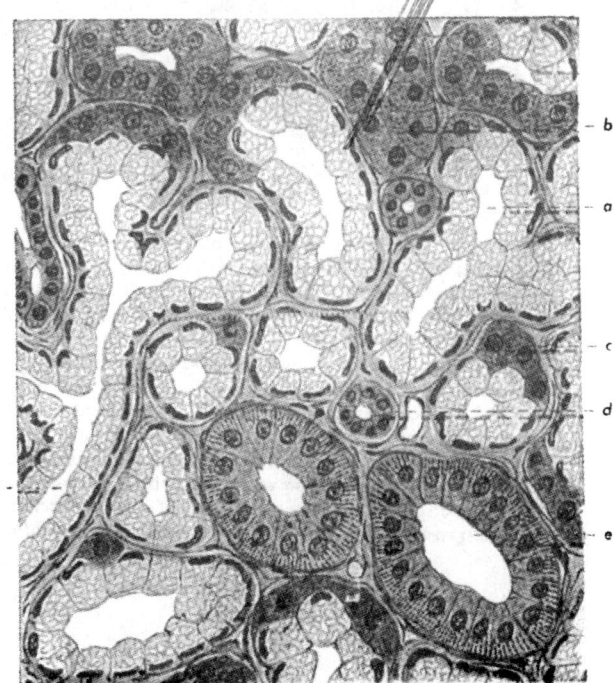

Figure 176A. Section of a mixed gland (mandibular gland of the ox); hemalumeosin. *a,* mucous, and *b,* serous, end-pieces; *c,* serous demilune; *d,* intercalated duct; *e,* striated tubule; *f,* mucous tubule.

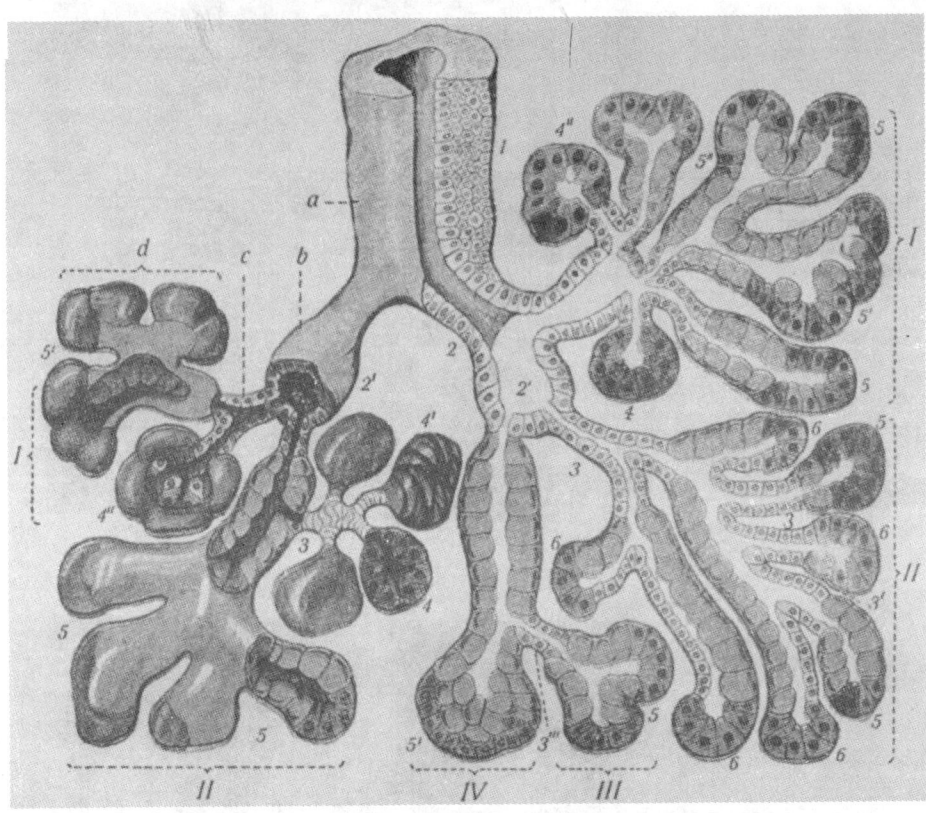

Figure 177. Scheme of the mandibular gland of domestic mammals. *I*, horse and small ruminants; *II*, ox; *III*, ox and pig; *IV*, carnivores. *a*, excretory duct; *b*, striated tubule; *c*, intercalated duct; *d*, secretory end-pieces. The parts of the gland are represented in three dimensions on the left and in section on the right. *1*, excretory duct; *2*, striated tubules with dilatations (*2'*); *3*, intercalated ducts; *3'* mucous transformation; *4*, simple serous acini with a canal-like lumen and secretory capillaries; *4'*, three-dimensional representation of basket cells. In section, these appear as black, elongated triangles apposed to the basement membrane; *4''*, compound serous end-pieces. They contain "separating" cells derived from the intercalated ducts. Red cells contain serous granules only; pink cells contain amphitropic granules. *5*, mixed end-pieces composed of mucous cells and serous end complexes, which show various shapes and may be simple or divided (*5'*); *6*, mucous transformation of cells of intercalated ducts; *3'''*, absence of mucous transformation of intercalated ducts at points of bifurcation. (After Ziegler)

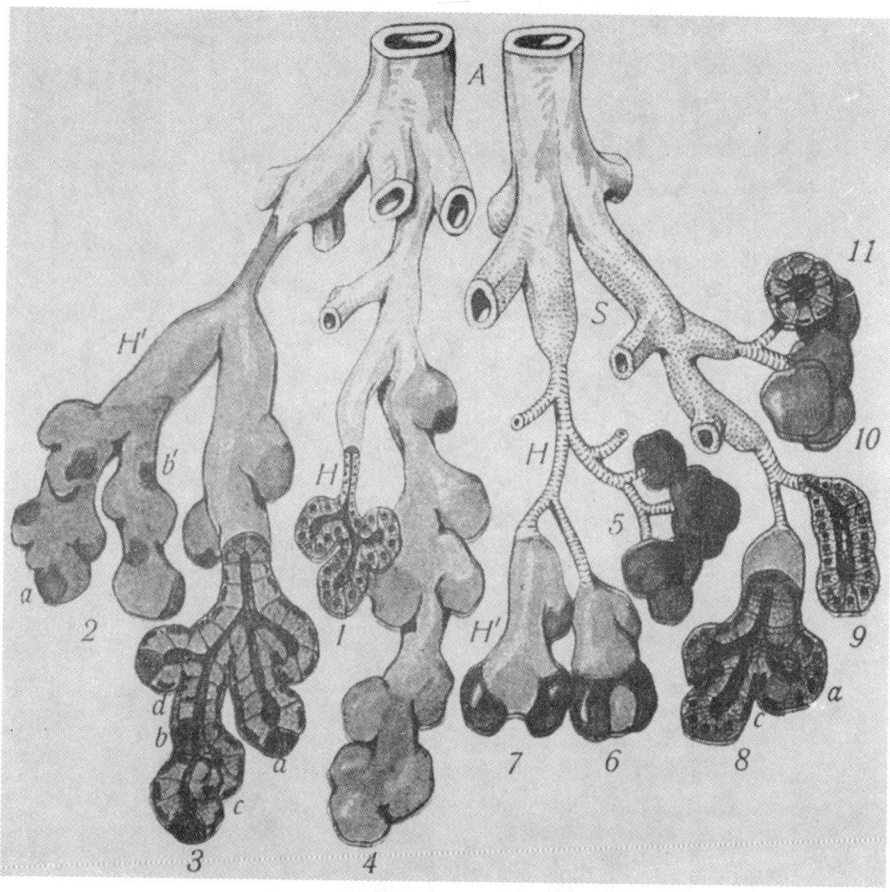

Figure 178. Structural scheme of the sublingual glands. *1–4*, glandulae sublinguales minores; *5–11*, glandulae sublinguales majores. *A*, excretory duct; *H*, intercalated duct; *H'*, mucous transformation of intercalated duct, opened in *3; S*, striated tubule. Red = cells in the serous phase. Gray = mucin-containing cells. Blue = mucous cells, of intercalated duct origin in *3* and *8*. At *3,d* and *11*, note the secretory capillaries, which do not occur in ordinary mucous end-pieces. (After Ziegler.)

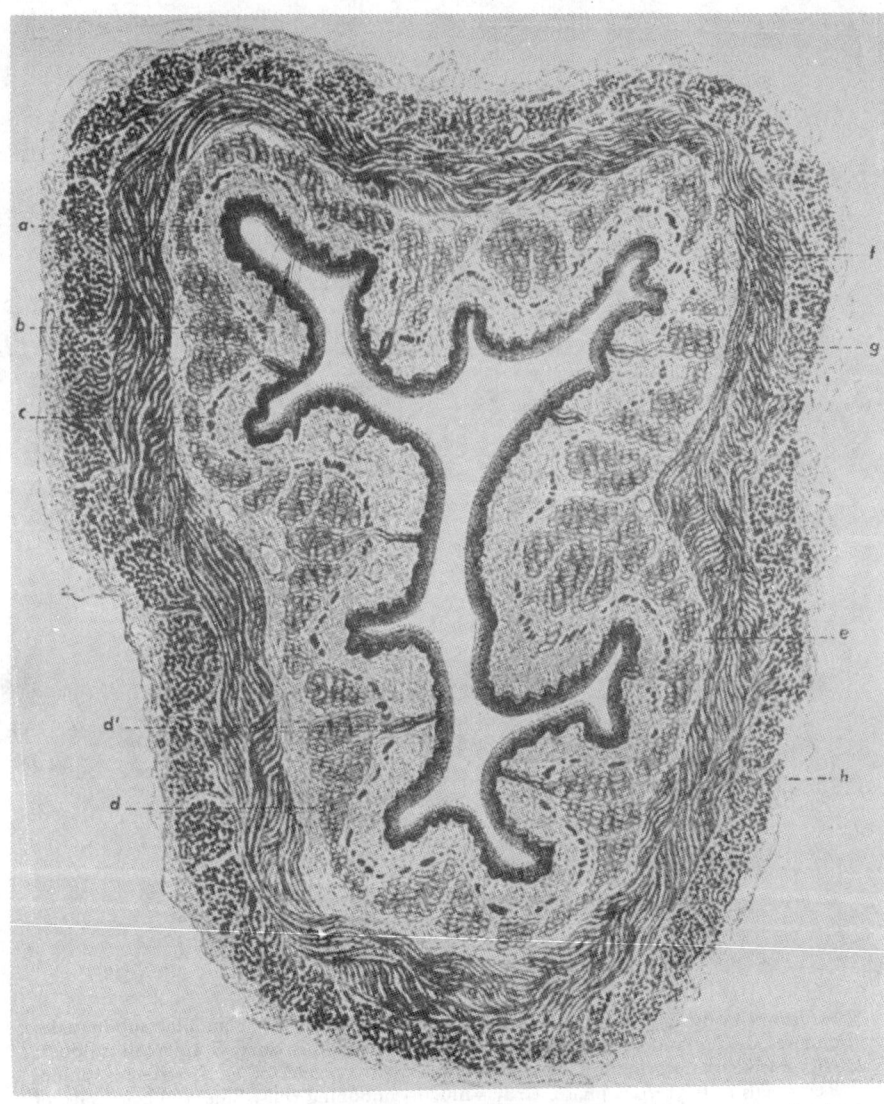

Figure 208. Cross section through the esophagus of the dog (11 ×); stained with hemalum-eosin. *a*, stratified squamous epithelium; *b*, lamina propria; *c*, muscularis mucosae; *d*, mucous glands in the submucosa; *d'*, excretory duct of a mucous gland; *e*, lymphatic; *f*, inner, *g*, outer layer of the muscularis; *h*, adventitia.

XI

The Digestive System

THE function of the digestive system is to reduce the nutrients present in the food to simpler absorbable and assimilable constituents. These can then be utilized either to meet the energy requirements of the organism or to build up its tissues and organs.

The digestive tube is lined by a continuous mucous membrane which begins at the mouth and ends at the anus. It contains—except for some sections—glands in its wall. In addition to these, there are also separate glands, which retain their embryonic connection with the mucosa by means of their excretory ducts. These are the salivary glands, pancreas, and liver. The following layers of mucosa are recognized (Figs. 123–125):

1. The lamina epithelialis, which is made up of stratified squamous epithelium from the mouth to the glandular stomach, and of simple columnar epithelium from there to the anus.

2. The lamina propria.

3. The lamina muscularis mucosae, which, however, is absent in the oral cavity, pharynx, rumen, and portions of the esophagus.

4. The lamina submucosa, which is lacking in a few portions of the wall of the mouth.

The next layer peripheral to the mucosa is the muscular coat (tunica muscularis) consisting usually of an inner circular and an outer longitudinal sheet. This is covered by a serous or fibrous layer (tunica serosa or fibrosa). This description does not hold for the oral region.

A. SALIVARY GLANDS

The salivary glands may be classified on the basis of their secretions and the epithelium of their end-pieces as serous, mucous, and mixed glands.

The saliva they furnish has chemical and mechanical functions. The mechanical action is connected mainly with the mucous secretion, which aids in the formation of a bolus and serves as a lubricant in the act of swallowing. The chemical action is accomplished by the thin watery secretion of the serous cells, which serves to adjust the pH, to dilute or dissolve the food, to make it possible to taste the food, and, when an enzyme is present, to hydrolyze the higher carbohydrates.

The glandular end-pieces are surrounded by a basement membrane (Fig. 45; see also p. 22), on the inner surface of which is a layer of flat, star-shaped myoepithelial cells (Figs. 170,*e;* 173,*a*). These are joined to each other by their cytoplasmic processes to form a basket-like shell around the secretory cells. Therefore they are also called basket cells (Fig. 177,*4'**).

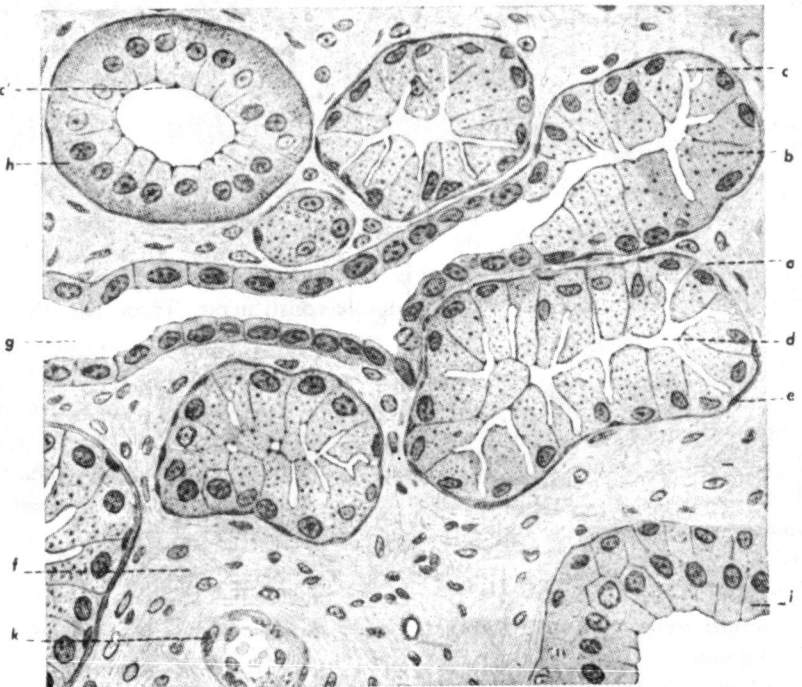

Figure 170. Serous gland from the planum nasolabiale of the ox. *a*, basement membrane; *b*, secretory cells; *c*, secretory capillaries; *c'*, terminal bars; *d*, lumen of a secretory end-piece; *e*, basket cells; *f*, interglandular connective tissue; *g*, intercalated duct; *h*, striated tubule; *i*, part of the wall of an excretory duct; *k*, blood vessel.

The small glands of the oral cavity are branched tubuloalveolar glands embedded in the submucosal connective tissue (Fig. 193,*b*). They occur either singly or in groups, so dense in places that they have the appearance of one large, continuous gland complex. The larger salivary glands, however, are true compound tubuloalveolar glands, consisting of large and small lobules (Fig. 171). They have grown away from the oral cavity, with which they remain connected by means of one or several excretory ducts. (Regarding the interlobular tissue of glands, see p. 99.)

---

* Fig. 177 is on p. 150.

(a) **Serous glands** have end-pieces (Figs. 170; 171,*b;* 172,*d*) with a narrow, canal-like lumen (wider in sheep and goats), from which secretory capillaries (Figs. 44; 170,*c;* 173,*c;* 174,*b*) extend between the pyramidal or polygonal gland cells. The spherical nucleus lies in the proximal half of the cell but not against the wall. The serous cells show inclusions of dark, strongly refractive secretory granules, which vary in number, arrangement, and staining properties (Fig. 173).

The appearance of the cells varies with their functional status. They may be

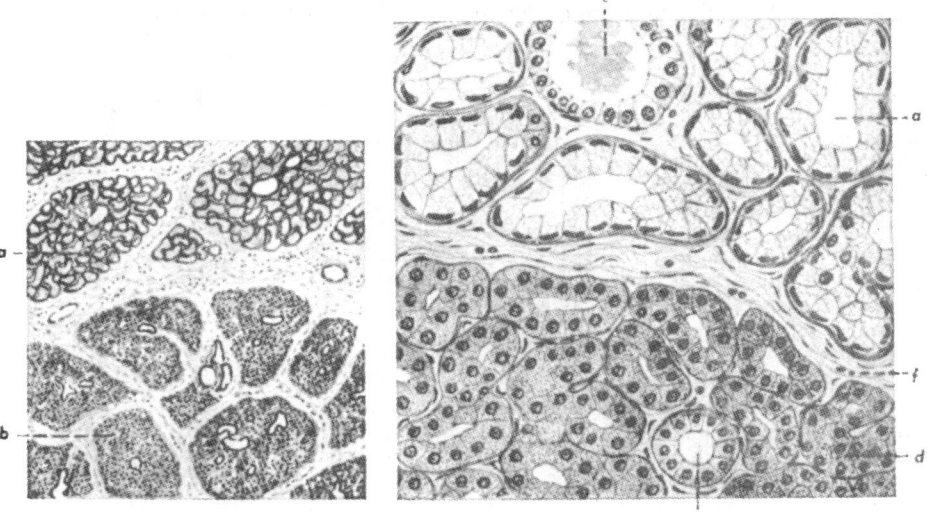

Figure 171 (left). Mucous and serous glands occurring side by side (buccal gland of the goat). *a*, mucous gland; *b*, serous gland.

Figure 172 (right). Mucous and serous gland occurring side by side (buccal gland of the goat). Higher magnification than that of Fig. 171. *a*, sections through mucous end-pieces; *c*, interlobular excretory duct; *d*, sections through serous end-pieces; *e*, excretory duct; *f*, connective tissue.

large and nearly filled with coarse secretory granules, or smaller with only a few secretory granules near the free surface. The granules are the precursors of the secretion. They may or may not be liquefied before extrusion. The parotid gland, which, in the ruminant, secretes continuously and furnishes a very thin, watery fluid, exhibits three phases of activity in neighboring zones. These phases are storage, secretion, and exhaustion. In the secretory stage the cells become lower and the lumen becomes larger. In the stage of exhaustion the cells fill up with acidophil protein substances, which in the storage phase are transformed into secretory granules. The interstitial and perivascular connective tissue contains an abundance of mast cells.

(b) **The mucous glands** have tubular end-pieces (Figs. 171,*a;* 172,*a;* 175,*b*) most of which have a wide lumen. Secretory capillaries are absent. The mucous cells, when examined in the fresh state, are less refractive than the cells of the serous glands and turn turbid on treatment with acetic acid. With hematoxylin-eosin, the secretion of the mucous cells stains blue, while the cytoplasm of the serous cells, and especially their secretory granules, stain red (Fig. 176A*). When full of secretion, mucous cells are often markedly distended and occupied, except for a narrow strip of basal cytoplasm, by light, coarse secretory granules or droplets (Fig. 42). The granules are demonstrable only by special methods; they may be stained with mucin stains (e.g., mucicarmine). They become confluent by most of the common fixation methods and natural postmortem changes. The cell then appears transparent, reticulated, and more or less light-colored in accordance with its functional state (Fig. 175,b). The pressure of the contents of the mucous cell flattens the nu-

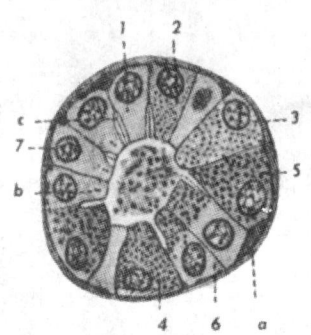

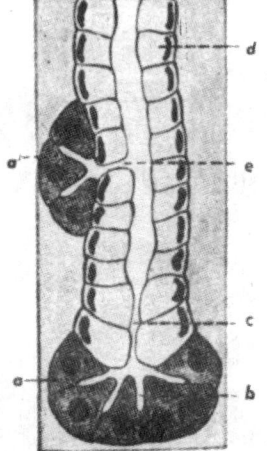

Figure 173. Schematic representation of the functional stages of a serous gland. *1–4,* consecutive stages in the filling of the cell with secretory granules; *5–7,* stages in emptying the cell. *a,* basement membrane with basket cells; *b,* diplosome; *c,* intercellular secretory capillaries.

Figure 174 (right). Schematic representation of secretory capillaries (*b*) in serous demilunes (*a,a'*). *c,e,* clefts connecting the secretory capillaries with the lumen of the end-piece; *d,* mucous cell of the end-piece.

cleus against the basal wall where it lies surrounded by a small amount of finely granular cytoplasm. When the droplets of mucin are extruded, they swell in water and form mucus. The depleted cell is smaller, the cytoplasm is finely granular, and the nucleus is more nearly spherical. At this stage the cells resemble empty serous cells. They may be differentiated from the latter by the presence of a few mucigenous granules in their distal portions and by their lack of intercellular secretory capillaries.

(c) **The mixed glands** either have separate serous and mucous end-pieces (Fig. 175), or the same end-piece may contain both mucous and serous cells singly or in groups. In the second case the end-piece is usually elongated (Figs. 174, 176, 176A*).

The mixed salivary gland of the second type has been found in man and domestic animals to arise by mucous transformation of the branched intercalated ducts of the serous acini. As this transformation progresses, the acini lose their spherical shape at their junctions with the former ducts. Finally they are merely caplike structures at the end of the mucous tubes. The shorter the intercalated duct, the longer the mucous portion (Fig. 177*). Such a mixed gland contains, in addition to purely serous end-pieces, mixed end-pieces in which the two kinds of

---

* Fig. 176A is on p. 149 and Fig. 177 on p. 150.

cells are arranged in a single layer around the lumen (less common) or the end of the mucous tubule is capped by an outer group of serous cells. These parietal complexes are crescent-shaped in section and are therefore known as *serous demilunes* (Figs. 176; 176A,*c**; 177*; 178,*a**). Branches of the lumen extend between the mucous cells to the secretory capillaries of the demilunes (Fig. 174,*c*).

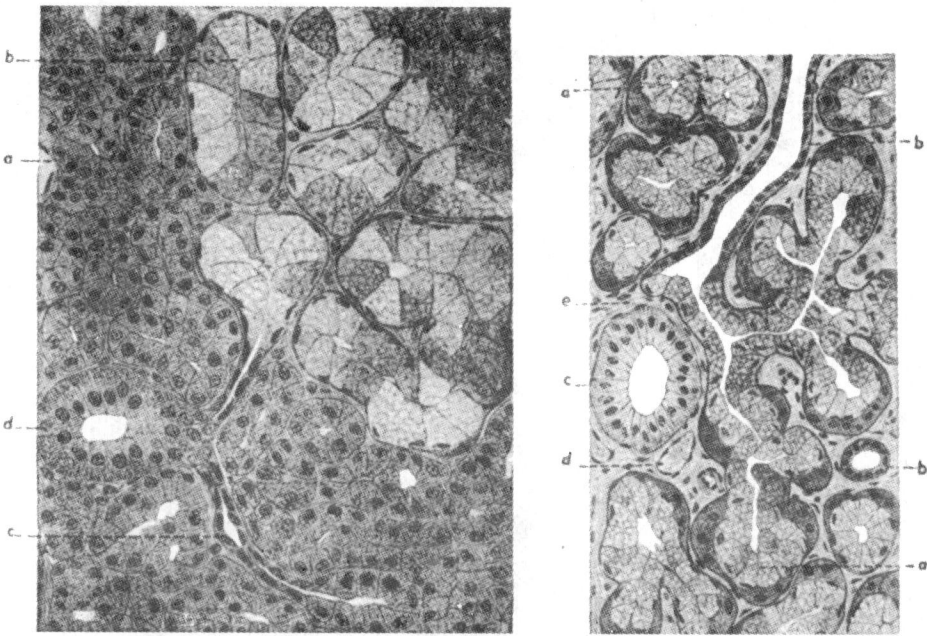

Figure 175 (left). Portion of a mixed gland (parotid of a pup). *a*, serous end-pieces; *b*, mucous end-pieces; *c*, intercalated duct; *d*, striated tubule.

Figure 176 (right). Portion of a mixed gland (marginal lingual, in a horse). *a*, sections through mixed end-pieces with serous demilunes; *b*, intercalated ducts; *c*, striated tubule; *d*, blood vessel; *e*, interglandular connective tissue.

In addition to the true demilunes there are also groups of nonsecreting mucous cells, called pseudolunulae or Stöhr's crescents. These lack secretory capillaries.

Fig. 177* shows the variation in arrangement of serous and mucous cells of the mandibular gland in different species.[1] Fig. 178* illustrates the structure of the sublingual glands. Many of the cells combine serous and mucous characteristics and give an "amphitropic" staining reaction. They have secretory capillaries. According to their functional status, they may have the appearance of serous (*1,5,6*) or mucous (*4,10,11*) cells.[2]

---

[1] Hermann Ziegler, Beiträge zum Bau der Unterkieferdrüse der Hauswiederkäuer, *Zeitschr. f. Anat. 82* (1927): 73–121.

[2] Hermann Ziegler, Zur Morphologie gemischter Hauptstücke in sublingualen Speicheldrüsen von Haustieren, *Zeitschr. f. mikrosk.-anat. Forsch. 39* (1936): 100–104.

* Fig. 176A is on p. 149, Fig. 177 on p. 150, and Fig.178 on p. 151.

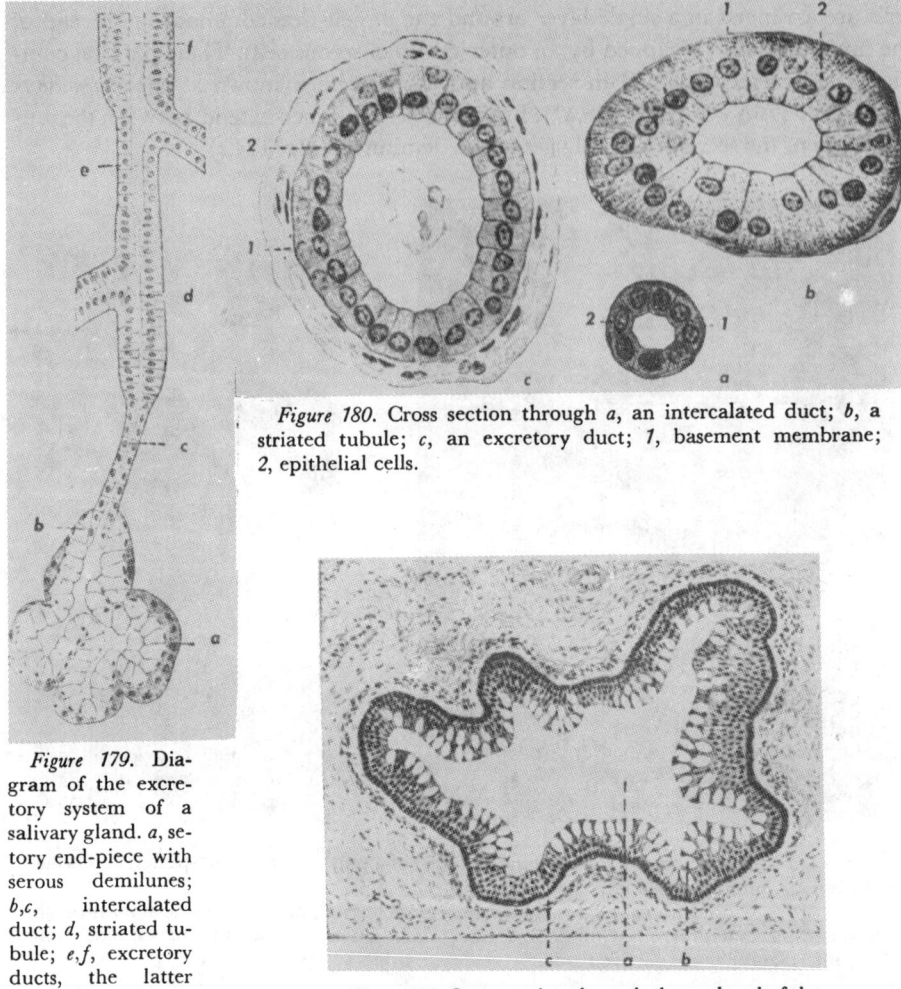

Figure 180. Cross section through a, an intercalated duct; b, a striated tubule; c, an excretory duct; 1, basement membrane; 2, epithelial cells.

Figure 179. Diagram of the excretory system of a salivary gland. a, setory end-piece with serous demilunes; b,c, intercalated duct; d, striated tubule; e,f, excretory ducts, the latter with two-layered columnar epithelium.

Figure 181. Cross section through the oral end of the ductus mandibularis (a), showing goblet cells (b) in the epithelium and the connective tissue sheath (c).

(d) **The excretory ducts** of the small glands of the oral cavity are immediately continuous with the secretory end-pieces. In the larger salivary glands, the end-pieces pass first into narrow tubules lined by simple, low cuboidal (rarely squamous), epithelium. These are called *intercalated ducts* (Fig. 179,c). While still within the lobule they join to form wider tubes, called *striated tubules* or salivary ducts (Figs. 170,h; 179,d), whose thin basement membrane bears a simple columnar epithelium composed of high, strongly eosinophilic cells. These cells show basal striations presumably caused by parallel rows of mitochondria. The striations are taken as evidence of secretory activity, and the tubules have been credited with the secretion of calcium salts. In purely mucous glands, striated tubules are usually not present. In the parotid gland of the ruminant a considerable number of mast cells are found around the salivary ducts and within their actively secreting two-layered epithelium. The mast cells increase with age. The larger striated tubules are partly inter-lobular and show sinus-like enlargements that serve to store secretions.

The ducts continue as interlobular excretory ducts (Figs. 177,*1**; 179,*e;* 180,*c*). At the beginning these have a simple columnar epithelium, the cells of which lack striations but may show evidence of apocrine secretion. The larger excretory ducts have two-layered columnar epithelium (Figs. 170,*i;* 179,*f*). The terminal portions are lined by stratified high columnar epithelium (Figs. 177,*1**; 181), which in some glands contains a few goblet cells. Near the opening the epithelium changes to the stratified squamous type. The collagenous tunica propria (Fig. 180) of the inter-lobular (excretory) ducts contains elastic and smooth muscle fibers, but that of the striated tubules is thinner; it sometimes also contains smooth muscle fibers. The tunica propria of the intralobular tubules and intercalated ducts consists either of basket cells and a basement membrane or of a very thin lamina of collagenous fibers with flattened nuclei.

Table 2. Character of the Salivary Glands

Serous Glands	Mucous Glands	Mixed Glands
Parotid (contains mucous end-pieces in young carnivores and lambs)	Labial glands of sheep, goats, and carnivores	Mandibular gland
	Lingual glands, except those listed elsewhere	Sublingual gland
Ventral buccal gland of cattle and its ventral portion in sheep and goats		Marginal glands of the tongue of the horse
	Middle and dorsal buccal glands of cattle	Glandula frenularis of sheep and goat
Ebner's glands under the cir-cumvallate and foliate pa-pillae	Ventral buccal gland of car-nivores, and its dorsal por-tion in sheep and goats	Glands of the root of the tongue in horse and ox
		Buccal glands of horses and swine
		All glands not mentioned un-der mucous or serous glands

There is no agreement regarding the homology of the salivary glands of birds. The small angularis oris gland is considered the homologue of the parotid. The glands lying between the rami of the mandible are assumed to correspond to the mammalian mandibular gland, and those on the side of the tongue to the sublin-gual gland. All the oral glands of the chicken are of the mucous type.

VESSELS AND NERVES. The arteries, which may be equipped with epithelioid mus-cle cells, especially along the excretory duct system, pass into extensive capillary nets. The parenchymatous capillaries surround the salivary ducts and secretory end-pieces. The lymphatics run with the ducts in the interlobular connective tis-sue. Lymph nodules are found in some salivary glands. The nerves, along whose course nerve cells occur singly or in groups, end either on blood vessels or in the form of delicate nets around the basement membrane, where they form epilemmal fibers. The finest among these penetrate the basement membrane and end between the secretory cells (hypolemmal fibers).

---

* Fig. 177 is on p 150.

Saliva is a colorless, stringy fluid, mostly water, which contains, in addition to desquamated epithelial cells, the so-called salivary corpuscles. These are swollen leukocytes from the lymph nodules and tonsils.

B. ORAL CAVITY

The oral cavity and associated organs function in the prehension of food and its immediate processing, i.e., mastication, insalivation, and bolus formation. The cavity is lined with a cutaneous mucous membrane (p. 104), characterized by stratified squamous epithelium and a relatively high papillary body. Wherever the epithelium is exposed to severe wear, it is thickened and, except in man and dog, covered by a heavy stratum corneum. This applies to the dental pad of ruminants (Fig. 123) the dorsum of the tongue, the hard palate, the oral surface of the soft palate, and the labial and buccal mucosa of ruminants. The lamina propria, which forms the papillary body, is fine-fibered superficially but coarser elsewhere. It is densely woven and generally does not contain glands of its own, but transmits the ducts of the submucosal and large compound glands. In certain parts macroscopic papillae are found, each of which has a papillary body (Fig. 183). The tunica propria passes, usually without demarcation, into the submucosa, which in turn lies on striated muscle. The latter is absent in the region of the hard palate. The submucosa consists of loose fibroelastic tissue and is sometimes rich in adipose cells. Occasionally it is absent, in which case it is replaced by muscle and intermuscular connective tissue. In many places the submucosa and intermuscular tissue of the walls of the mouth contain glands. These are absent on the tip and the larger portion of the body of the tongue, the hard palate, and the gums. Lymphatic nodules and follicles are also present.

VESSELS AND NERVES. The blood vessels form a deep submucous, and also a more superficial, close-meshed network, which lies in the tunica propria and supplies the subepithelial net of capillaries. These penetrate into the papillae (Fig. 126). The lymphatics form narrow nets in the lamina propria and wide ones in the submucosa. Lymph nodules are especially abundant in the mucosa of the soft palate (Fig. 184,g) and the base of the tongue, but diffuse lymphatic tissue may appear instead. Certain parts of the oral mucosa are exceedingly rich in nerves (e.g., the tongue and lips). Terminal twigs of sensory nerves enter the epithelium and end either freely between the epithelial cells or in the form of specialized nerve endings, such as taste buds and tactile bodies. Autonomic nerve fibers supply blood vessels and glands.

1. Lips

The middle layer of the lips (Fig. 182,B) is made up of muscle, tendon, connective tissue, and glands. Externally it is covered by the skin and subcutis (A) and internally by the oral mucosa and submucosa (C). The skin gradually blends into the mucosa at the labial margin (D). Here the hair and skin glands become smaller and rarer and finally disappear, while the papillae of the papillary body become larger and more numerous. A loose subcutis is poorly developed or absent since the connective tissue of the corium is directly continuous with the intermuscular tissue. The submucosa contains aggregates of labial glands (5; see also p. 159),

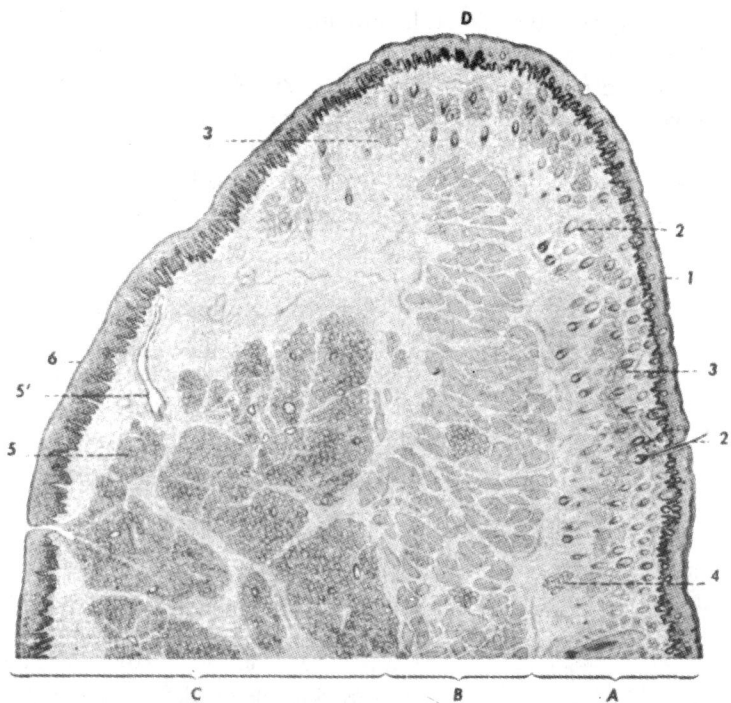

Figure 182. Sagittal section through the lip of a donkey. *A*, skin and subcutis; *B*, middle layer; *C*, oral mucosa and submucosa; *D*, labial margin;
1, stratum corneum of the epidermis; *2*, hairs in sagittal and oblique sections; *3*, sebaceous gland; *4*, tubular skin gland; *5*, labial gland with *5′*, its
excretory duct; *6*, stratum corneum of the squamous epithelium of the
mucosa. The middle layer (*B*) shows mainly striated muscle bundles in
cross section but also groups of glands in the intermuscular connective
tissue.

which may extend into the lamina propria. The labial mucosa of ruminants forms
macroscopic papillae (Fig. 183). The epithelial cover (Fig. 183,*b*) which coats the
papillary body or connective tissue core possesses a distinct stratum corneum (*c*).
Arteriovenous anastomoses, whose walls contain epithelioid cells, occur in the lips
of all domestic animals and are especially well developed and numerous in cattle
and pigs. The labial integument (Fig. 182,*A*) contains many special nerve endings and, in some species, tactile hairs. The skin of the upper lip forms part of the
smooth, moist *planum nasolabiale* of the ox and the *planum rostrale* of swine. These
structures bear only a few tactile hairs and are supplied with large serous glands
(Fig. 170). The glands also occur in the hairless *planum nasale* of the sheep and goat,
but not in the dog.

2. Cheeks

The cheeks consist of the skin, a muscular and glandular middle layer, and a
generally nonglandular mucosa, which, in dogs and ruminants, may be pigmented.
The buccal mucosa of ruminants bears macroscopic papillae (Fig. 183), which
play an important mechanical role in the prehension and mastication of food. Out-

side the mucosa, extending from the submucosa through the muscles into the sub-cutis, we find the buccal glands.

In solipeds and pigs the *buccal glands* are mixed glands with serous demilunes. In cattle the ventral buccal gland is serous. In sheep and goats the ventral half of the ventral gland is serous. The middle and dorsal buccal glands are mucous. In car-nivores the dorsal buccal gland is the zygomatic (or orbital) gland, which contains serous demilunes. The ventral one is a mucous gland.

3. Hard Palate

The ridges of the hard palate are formed by thickenings of the firm, tough mucosa. The sub-mucosa contains layers of venous plexuses, the cavernous tissue of the hard palate. The caudal portion contains groups of mucous glands, which are sparse in the horse and absent in the pig.

4. Soft Palate

The soft palate (Fig. 184) has a middle layer of muscle and connective tissue, which is covered on its oral surface by a cutaneous mucous. mem-brane (*a*) and on the aboral surface by a mucosa bearing pseudostratified ciliated epithelium (*a'*). The cutaneous mucous membrane of the oral surface is reflected around the free edge of the palate and onto a narrow distal zone on the respiratory surface. Only then does it change into pseudostratified ciliated epithelium. An ex-tensive layer of mucous glands underlies the oral portion of the palatine mucosa (*c*). On the respir-atory surface, where the mucosa has no papillary body, there are glands in the lamina propria and in the submucosa (*c'*).

Diffuse lymphatic tissue and lymph nodules also occur on both surfaces of the soft palate. In the horse and pig, tonsillar follicles are present. In the pig, the many closely aggregated follicles form a paired compact mass, which represents the palatine tonsil of other animals and man.

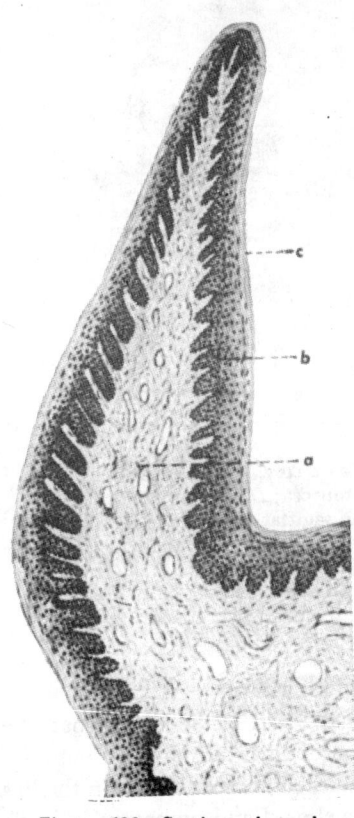

Figure 183. Section through a macroscopic papilla from the oral cavity of the ox. *a*, connective tissue core; *b*, squamous epithelium; *c*, its stratum corneum.

The mucosa of the sublingual floor of the mouth lacks glands. Only the horse and goat have, near the sublingual caruncle, a small group of mucous glands and some lymphatic tissue (glandula and tonsilla paracaruncularis, respectively). Be-hind the middle incisors occur a number of paired epithelial cords or tubes.

The plica pterygomandibularis and the rostral pillar of the soft palate (arcus

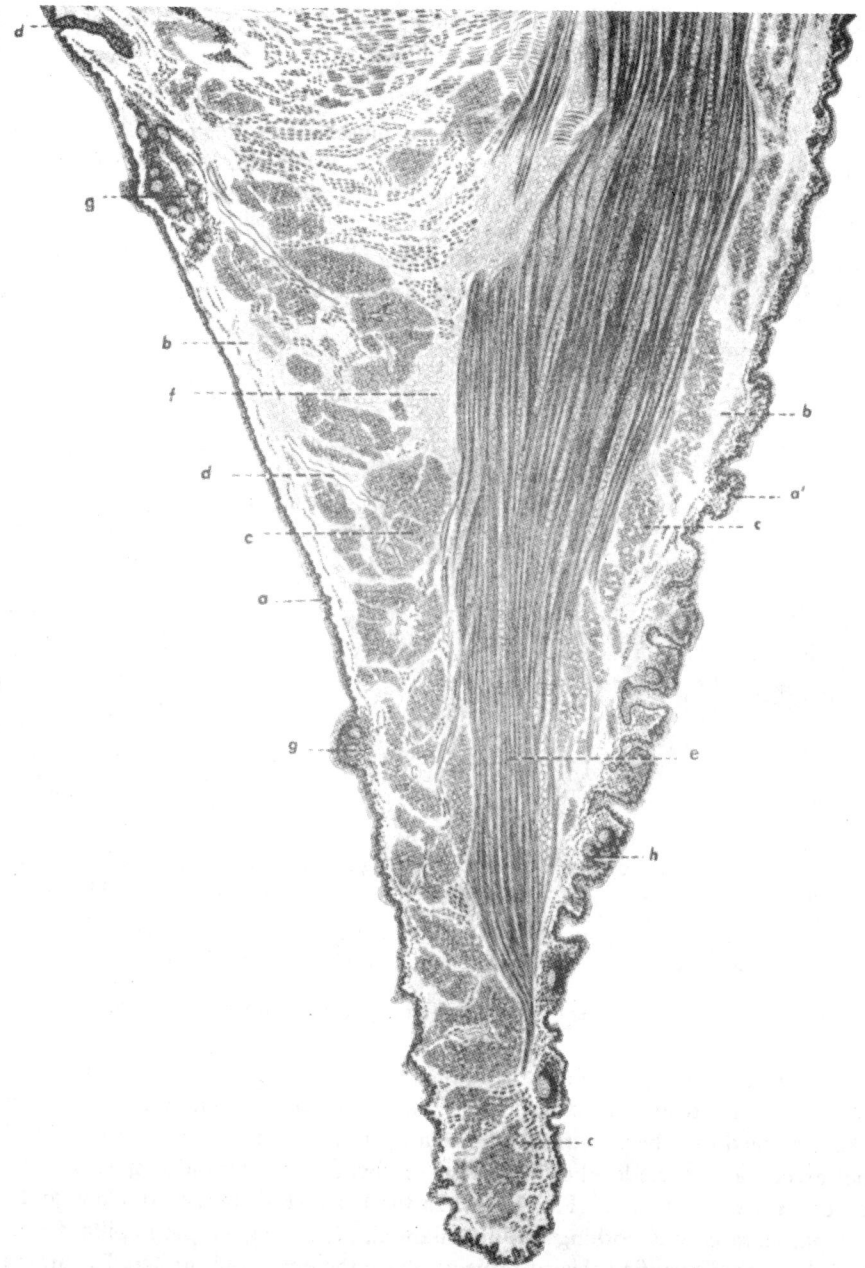

Figure 184. Sagittal section through the soft palate of a pig. *a*, squamous epithelium of the oral aspect; *a'*, ciliated columnar epithelium of the pharyngeal aspect; *b*, lamina propria; *c*, glands; *d*, excretory ducts of glands; *e*, striated muscle of the middle layer in longitudinal section; *f*, adipose tissue; *g*, macroscopic papillae containing lymph nodules; *h*, lymph nodules of the pharyngeal mucosa.

palatoglossus) contain tubuloalveolar mucous glands. The rostral pillar of the horse and dog also contains lymph nodules and follicles.

5. Tongue

This organ consists essentially of striated muscle and intermuscular connective tissue, which is rich in fat cells. The connective tissue attaches the rather tough mucous membrane to the muscular mass. The lingual mucosa is rich in nerves and special nerve endings. It forms both a microscopic papillary body and macroscopic papillae. In certain places glands and lymph nodules are present. The epithelium of the tongue is thickest and has the heaviest stratum corneum on the dorsal surface.

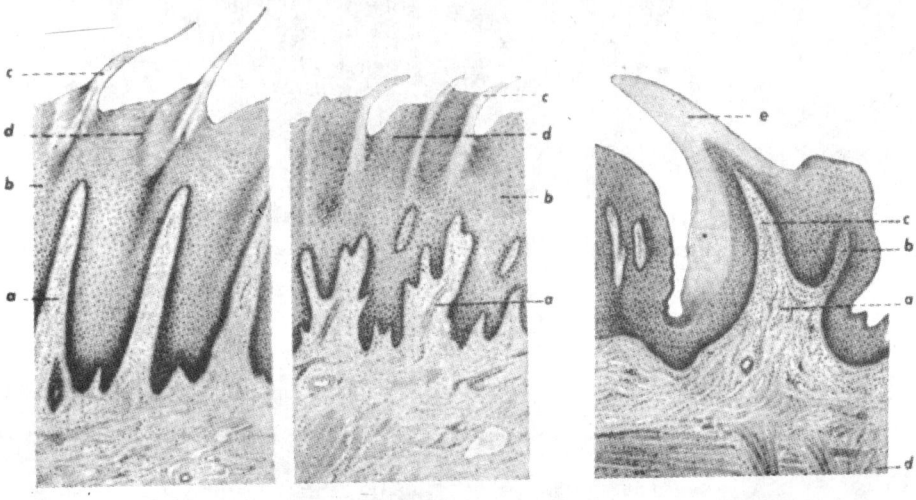

A   B

Figure 185 (left). Longitudinal section (30×) through the tip of the tongue of a horse (*A*) and a goat (*B*). *a*, connective tissue core; *b*, epithelium; *c*, papilla filiformis (cornified thread); *d*, interpapillary epithelium.

Figure 186 (right). Longitudinal section through a filiform papilla of a cat (30×). *a*, connective tissue core with *b*, small, and *c*, large, mucosal papilla; *d*, striated muscle; *e*, horny spine.

The tongue bears various papillae, which are named for their characteristic gross morphology:

(a) The *filiform papillae* (Figs. 185, 186) have a mechanical function and consist of a connective tissue core derived from the lamina propria and an epithelial cover characterized by a heavy stratum corneum. In most species the papillary core does not extend above the level of the glossal epithelium; the visible projection is made up entirely of epithelium (Fig. 185,*c*). In the horse (Fig. 185,*A*), donkey, and pig, the papillary core is nothing but an enlarged, elongated, simple papilla, from the top of which a cornified thread projects above the epithelial surface. In ruminants (Fig. 185,*B*) the connective tissue core gives rise to several small secondary papillae, whereas the epithelial coat is raised into a single cornified cone. In carnivores (Fig. 186) the connective tissue core extends above the surface epithelium and bears papillae of unequal sizes. The caudalmost of these is especially large (it is most distinct in the cat) and bears a thick caudally directed horny tooth (Fig.

186,*e*). This primary papilla is braced by a rostral supporting papilla. Large conical papillae, whose core projects beyond the surface of the tongue, occur in all domestic mammals except the horse and donkey.

(b) The *fungiform papillae* (Fig. 187), whose connective tissue core (*d*) is rich in
nerves and characterized by a papillary body, have a relatively soft epithelium
containing taste buds (*e*). Taste buds are very sparse in the fungiform papillae of
cattle and horses. They are more numerous in sheep and swine, very abundant in
carnivores, and especially so in the goat. In this animal they may occupy nearly
the entire free surface of the papilla. The taste buds of the cat and the dog are conspicuous for their size.

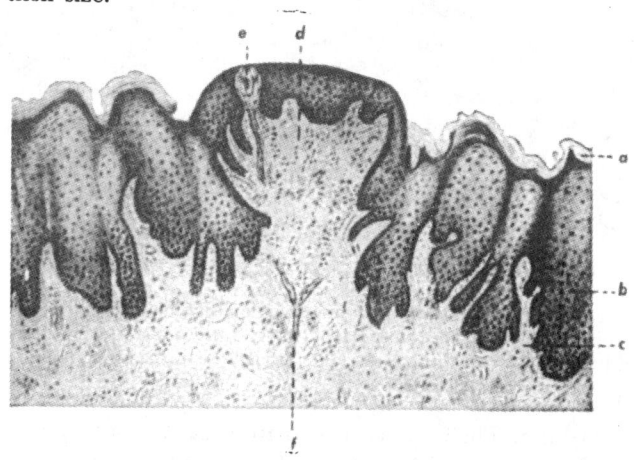

Figure 187. Section through a fungiform papilla and surrounding tissue of a sheep (30×). *a*, stratum corneum; *b*, stratum profundum of the epithelum; *c*, papillary body; *d*, connective tissue
core of the fungiform papilla; *e*, taste bud with nerves; *f*, nerve.

(c) The *circumvallate papillae* (Fig. 188) are surrounded by a cleft (*b*) lined with
epithelium. They project above the lingual epithelium only slightly or not at al!.
Their connective tissue core bears microscopic papillae and is rich in nerves and
lymphocytes. The epithelial surface facing the moat is not invaded by connective
tissue papillae, but contains many taste buds (*d*). Deep to the papillae lie groups of
serous (Ebner's) glands (*e*), whose excretory ducts (*f*) open into the moat at various
levels.

The circumvallate papillae bear the most taste buds in swine and dogs and the
fewest in cats. In the horse, ruminants, and swine taste buds are distributed over
the entire papillary wall of the moat, while in carnivores the gustatory field is restricted to the bottom of the moat and is therefore very small. Taste buds are usually absent in the surface epithelium of the papilla as well as in the peripheral wall
of the moat. In addition to the serous glands, mucous glands also occur under the
papilla in the horse. These, however, secrete onto the lingual mucosa.

(d) The *foliate papillae* (Fig. 189) consist of a series of parallel connective tissue
leaves, rich in nerves and bearing secondary papillae that project into the covering

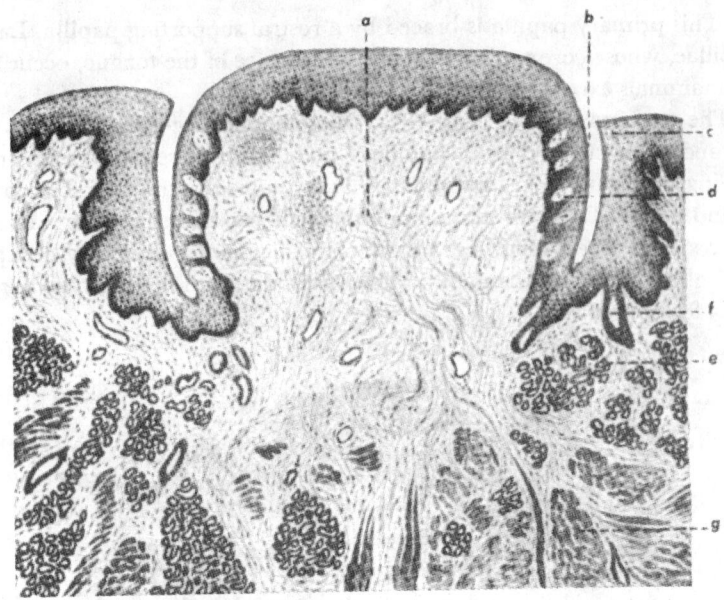

Figure 188. Section through a circumvallate papilla of the sheep (30×).
a, connective tissue core; *b*, moat; *c*, wall; *d*, taste buds in the squamous
epithelium; *e*, serous (Ebner's) glands; *f*, excretory duct of a gland; *g*, striated muscle in cross section.

squamous epithelium. They are separated from each other by gustatory furrows
(*b*). The epithelium covering the sides of the leaves bears taste buds. Deep to the
papillae lie serous glands whose ducts empty into the gustatory furrows. They are
especially abundant in the horse and dog, which have mucous glands also. Foliate
papillae are absent in ruminants, and rudimentary and without taste buds in cats.

Taste Buds

These are found in the epithelium of the fungiform, foliate, and circumvallate
papillae of the tongue; they are also found widely separated in the soft palate, the
epiglottis, and the free edge of the vocal folds. They are ellipsoid bodies embedded
in an upright position in the epithelium of the mucous membrane. The surface
epithelium over the tip of the bud is pierced by the taste pore (Fig. 191,*d*).

The taste bud is made up of supporting cells and neuroepithelial cells. Its outer
layer is formed by the peripheral supporting cells (Figs. 190; 191,*b*). These are
curved narrow cells with an ellipsoid nucleus, which surround the central cells
like barrel staves. They taper distally to a fine point, while their proximal end is
blunt or indented. In the interior of the bud we encounter the central supporting
cells, which are shorter and straighter than the peripheral ones and rounded off
on the distal end. In some species the taste buds also contain basal supporting
cells. These lie deep to the other supporting cells and are connected to them by
means of processes. Among the supporting cells lie about six neuroepithelial cells
(Figs. 190; 191,*a*). These are slender cells, thickened slightly in the region of the

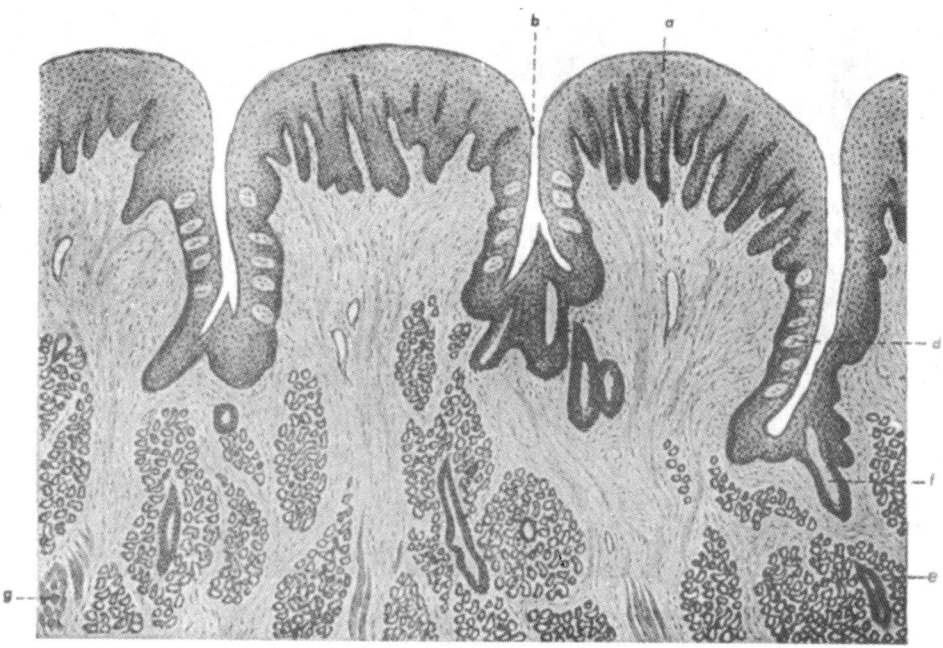

Figure 189. Section through a foliate papilla of the horse (30×). *a*, connective tissue core; *b*, gustatory furrow; *d*, taste buds in the squamous epithelium; *e*, serous glands; *f*, excretory duct of a gland; *g*, striated muscle in cross section.

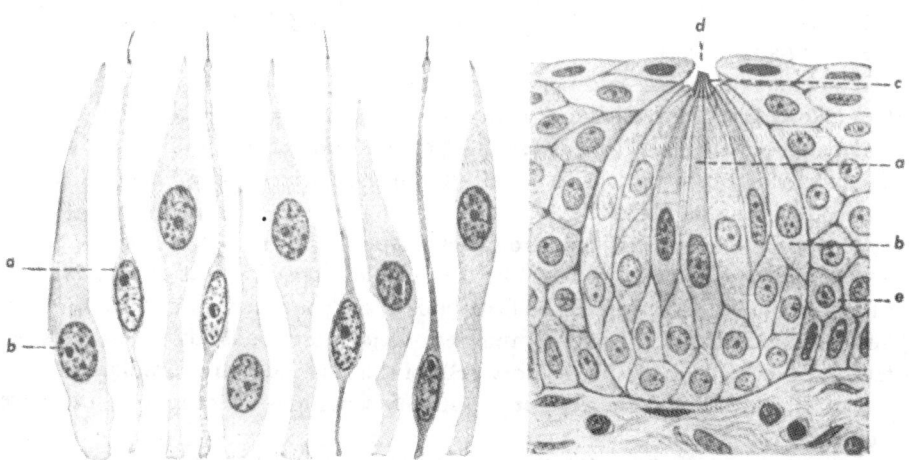

Figure 190 (left). Cells from a taste bud (600×). *a*, taste cells; *b*, supporting cells.
Figure 191 (right). Taste bud from a foliate papilla of the rabbit (420×). *a*, taste cell; *b*, supporting cell; *c*, taste hair; *d*, taste pore; *e*, surrounding epithelium. (After Sobotta.)

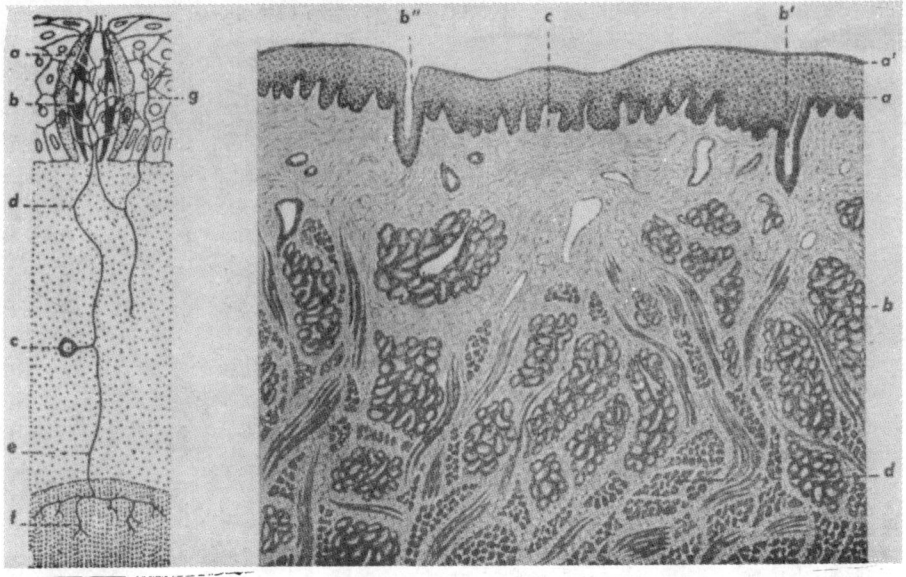

Figure 192 (left). Diagram of a taste organ. *a*, supporting cell; *b*, taste cell; *c*, nerve cell: *d*, nerve fiber conducting toward the cell body, showing intragemmal distribution of nerve endings; *e*, nerve fiber conducting away from the cell; *f*, its ending in the medulla oblongata; *g*, intergemmal distribution of nerve endings.

Figure 193 (right). Section from the root of the tongue of the horse. *a*, stratum profundum, *a'*, stratum corneum of the squamous epithelium; *b*, mucous glands with *b'*, their excretory duct, and *b''*, their opening on the surface; *c*, papillary body; *d*, striated muscle.

nucleus, and resemble the central supporting cells. They are characterized by a hairlike cuticular rod (Fig. 191,*c*) on their distal extremity. Because the supporting cells become shorter toward the center of the bud, a slight pit is formed, into which the taste hairs project.

Numerous nonmyelinated nerve fibers ascend from the secondary nerve plexus (see below) into the epithelium, where they ramify extensively and end as inter- and perigemmal[3] fibers (Fig. 192,*g*). A smaller number enter the bud and send delicate branches to its cells, especially the neuroepithelial ones. These fibers are called intragemmal fibers.

The taste organs of the horse are melon-shaped, while those of the sheep and ox are close-set ovoid buds, which, like the spindle-shaped buds of swine, extend a little into the tunica propria. The taste buds of the goat are very small and irregularly ellipsoid. The dog possesses minute spherical taste buds; those of the cat are few and poorly defined. The sensory cells of the taste buds are stimulated by dissolved substances, and the resulting gustatory sensations affect reflexly the secretion of digestive juices.

The *lingual glands* (Fig. 193,*b*) are situated partly in the submucosa, partly in the intermuscular tissue, and are especially abundant on the root, on the margins,

---

[3] L. *gemma* bud, i.e., taste bud.

and near the gustatory organs of the tongue. Those of the gustatory region are the serous glands of Ebner previously mentioned. The remaining glands are all mucous except the mixed glands of the margin of the tongue in the horse, the glands of the root of the tongue in the horse and the ox, and the glandula frenularis (of Nuhn) in the sheep and the goat.

As special structures of the tongue should be mentioned the lingual fibrous cord of solipeds, the dorsal prominence of the ruminant tongue, and the lyssa of carnivores.

The lingual fibrous cord of equines is a middorsal structure, located under the lamina propria between the muscles. It consists of exceedingly dense fibroelastic tissue interspersed with fibrous and hyaline cartilage, fat, and some striated muscle fibers. Lingual muscles are inserted on it.

The dorsal prominence of the ruminant tongue presents a well-defined area of thickening of the mucosa. It is spongy in the center, and its squamous epithelium bears a heavy stratum corneum and peculiar macroscopic lenticular papillae. Mucous glands are present in some parts.

The lyssa[4] of carnivores is made up of a collagenous sheath enveloping adipose tissue. In the dog there are also striated muscle fibers in the middle portion, in addition to blood vessels and nerves, and the caudal part contains islands of cartilage and chondroid supporting tissue. A similar cord of fat occurs in the septum linguae of the pig. This, however, is not a homologue of the lyssa of carnivores.

VESSELS AND NERVES. The blood vessels of the tongue are arranged like those of other cutaneous mucous membranes and striated muscle. In the dog the blood vessels contain mechanisms that make possible a considerable and rapid enlargement of the tongue in the heat-regulatory process of panting. In many places the blood vessels show a tortuous course and the veins are located in tissue spaces that permit venous engorgement. The lymphatics of the mucosa of the tongue form a deep, submucous, wide-meshed net and a fined subepithelial superficial one, which extends up into the papillae. Lymphatic tissue is restricted almost entirely to the region of the root of the tongue. It occurs as diffuse lymphatic tissue, lymph nodules, and lingual follicles. The latter are found mainly in solipeds, swine, and cattle. When the follicles are numerous, they are regarded collectively as a lingual tonsil. There is an extraordinary abundance of nerves in the tongue. They form at first a coarse plexus of myelinated fibers. This is the primary plexus and contains ganglia. From it nonmyelinated fibers emerge and form a subepithelial secondary plexus, from which the nonmyelinated fibers enter the epithelium and terminate either freely between the epithelial cells or in tactile bodies or taste buds. In the tunica propria some terminal bulbs of Krause occur (see p. 330).

For a description of the tonsils—lingual, palatine, pharyngeal, and tubal—and the lymphatic ring of the pharynx, see p. 121.

6. Gums

The gums (gingivae) have a basis of tough connective tissue with abundant elas-

---

[4] L. *lyssa* rabies. This structure was thought to be a worm that caused rabies.

tic fibers (Fig. 194,*f*). They are nonglandular and lack true lymph nodules. The propria forms a papillary body and is firmly fused with the periosteum throughout most of its extent. The squamous epithelium possesses a thick stratum corneum in the region of the dental pad of ruminants (Fig. 123). The striated muscle underlying the dental pad is presumably derived from the lip musculature.

7. Teeth

The gross parts of a tooth are the *root*, which is sunk in the alveolus; the projecting *crown;* and the intermediate *neck*, which is surrounded by the gum. In some

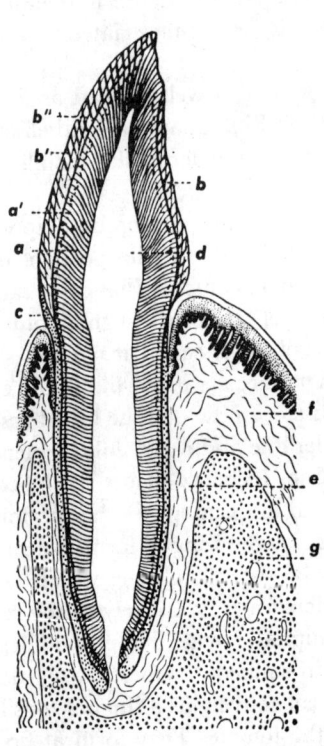

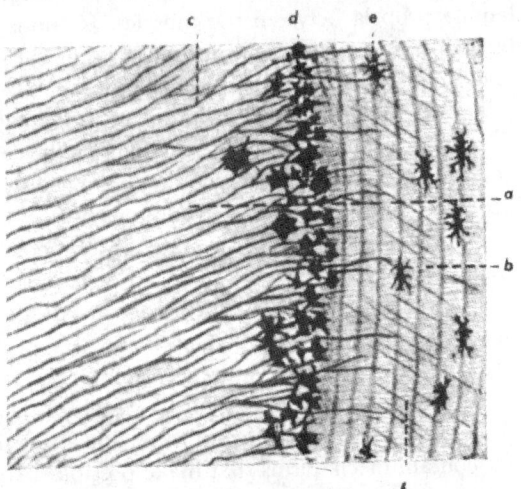

Figure 194 (left). Sagittal section through a bovine incisor in situ. *a*, dentin with dentinal tubules; *a'*, interglobular spaces; *b,b',b''*, enamel; *c*, cementum; *d*, pulp cavity; *e*, periodontal membrane; *f*, gingiva; *g*, mandible with alveolus.

Figure 195 (right). Dentinocemental junction from a longitudinal section through the root of a molar tooth of a pig. *a*, dentin; *b*, cementum; *c*, dentinal tubules; *d*, small interglobular spaces of the granular layer of Tomes; *e*, lacunae of the cementum; *f*, Sharpey's fibers.

domestic animals there is no constriction at the neck, and the enamel-covered *body* of the tooth extends far down into the alveolus. Histologically we have to consider the three hard substances: dentin, enamel, and cementum, as well as the soft dental pulp and the periodontal membrane.

(a) The dentin (Figs. 194,*a;* 195,*a;* 198–201,*a*), the main substance of the tooth, is a peculiar tissue in which the cells, called *odontoblasts*, remain on the inner surface lining the pulp cavity and send long processes out through the calcified substance. The latter resembles the intercellular substance of bone. It contains collagenous fibrils which run generally parallel to the surface—in the crown, parallel to the occlusal surface. When decalcified, dentin resembles cartilage. It is perforated by fine canaliculi, the *dentinal tubules* (Fig. 195,*c*). The elongated odonto-blasts (Fig. 202) form a single layer of cells around the pulp and each sends a proc-ess (Tomes's fiber) into the dentin. These densely packed fibers run through the radial dentinal tubules to the surface of the dentin and undergo extensive division and ramification on the way. The dentinal tubules have special, highly resistant walls (Neumann's sheaths), which can be isolated. They begin as free openings on the internal wall of the dentin and continue to the surface, tapering along their course. They and the fibers they contain branch repeatedly, first close to their ori-gin and again in the more peripheral layers of dentin. They show S-shaped curves, waves, and spiral turns. Most of the branches of the dentinal tubules end blindly. Loop-shaped anastomoses occur also in the more superficial layers. In rare cases

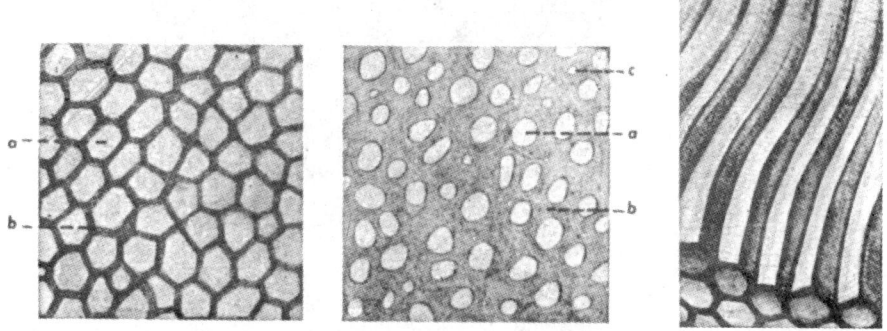

Figure 196 (left and center). Cross sections through enamel prisms. *Left:* near the surface. *Right:* near the dentin. *a*, enamel prisms; *b*, cementing substance; *c*, dentinal tubules in cross section.

Figure 197 (right). Enamel prisms in longitudinal and transverse section.

dentinal tubules extend into the enamel or cement substance (Figs. 195 near *e;* 196,*c*).

In the superficial layers of the dentin there are small uncalcified areas called the interglobular spaces. The globules referred to are the spherical mineral deposits that enlarge and finally coalesce in the calcification of the dentin. The interglobu-lar spaces are more numerous in the root, where they form Tomes's granular layer (Fig. 195,*d*) just under the cementum. In the crown they are less numerous and deeper in the dentin. Here they form the lines of Owen (Fig. 194,*a'*). The inter-globular spaces are actually filled with organic intertubular substance, and the dentinal tubules continue uninterruptedly through them.

The dentin contains some unmyelinated nerve fibers from the pulp.

(b) **The enamel,** which covers the crown, (Fig. 194,*b*) is free from cellular ele-ments. The hardest substance in the body, it consists almost entirely of inorganic material. In addition to a small amount of cementing substance, it contains long, slender, hexagonal, calcified rods called enamel prisms (Figs. 196, 197). Each prism exhibits cross striations. The prism bundles run in spirals and waves to the outer enamel surface. The variation in the curves of the bundles gives the false

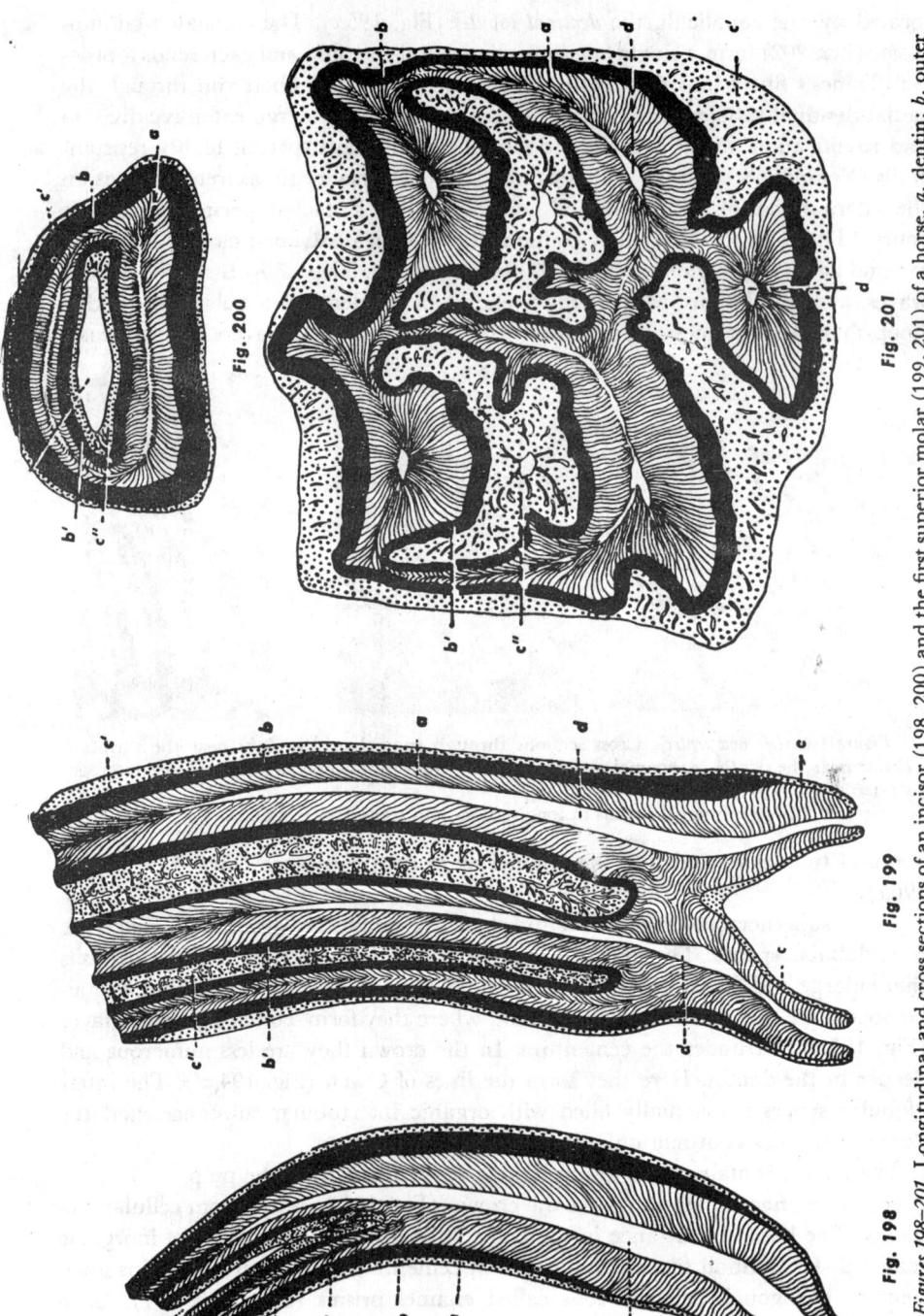

Fig. 200

Fig. 201

Fig. 199

Fig. 198

Figures 198–201. Longitudinal and cross sections of an incisor (198, 200) and the first superior molar (199, 201) of a horse. *a,* dentin; *b,* outer enamel of the crown; *b',* invaginated enamel lining the infundibulum; *c,* cementum of the root; *c',* outer cementum of the crown; *c'',* cementum deposit in the infundibulum; *d,* pulp cavity; *e,* infundibulum or cup.

impression that they cross. Here and there elongated spaces filled with cementing material occur between the prisms. A structureless, brittle, tightly adherent, and highly resistant cuticle covers the free surface of the enamel.

In the brachydont[5] teeth of carnivora, swine, and man, the enamel is restricted to the crown, which it covers like a hood. In the hypsodont[6] teeth of the horse, the enamel not only covers the crown but extends far down on the root and is also invaginated into the infundibula. On the sides of the cheek teeth it forms folds and deep grooves (Figs. 198–201,b). The incisors of the ruminant are brachydont. The ruminant cheek teeth are hypsodont but not so long as those of the horse. The occlusal surface of the teeth of herbivores is entirely covered by enamel at the time of eruption, but, as the tooth wears, the dentin is exposed between the peripheral enamel (b) and the infundibular enamel (b'). This results in an efficient grinding surface marked by prominent enamel ridges.

(c) **The cementum** (Figs. 194,c; 195,b) is slightly modified bone. It consists of lamellae that run nearly parallel to the surface, and it contains isolated lacunae (Fig. 195,e) which house the cells and give off anastomotic canaliculi. There are also collagenous Sharpey's fibers (f), but few vascular canals. Where the cementum is thinnest, lacunae are absent. The fibrillar bundles of the intercellular substance are perpendicular to the surface. The cementum envelops every root and occasionally overlaps the enamel in the region of the neck (Fig. 194). In the teeth of herbivores (except the incisors and three lower premolars of ruminants) the cementum also invests the entire crown and more or less fills the grooves and infundibula (Figs. 198–201,c). The infundibulum or cup of the equine incisor is therefore an invagination of enamel and cementum down into the dentin (Figs. 198; 200,e).

(d) **The dental pulp,** which occupies the pulp cavity (Figs. 194; 198; 199,d), consists of soft connective tissue containing numerous blood vessels and nerves, but no elastic fibers. Structurally it resembles embryonic connective tissue. The ground substance of this connective tissue contains interlacing collagenous fibrils (but no bundles), between which are located many anastomosing cells. The most superficial of these form a layer of contiguous odontoblasts (Figs. 202; 206,f). These are characterized by basal nuclei and a granular cytoplasm. They are columnar in shape and give off a long process, the fiber of Tomes, into the dentinal tubules. Basal and lateral processes are also present.

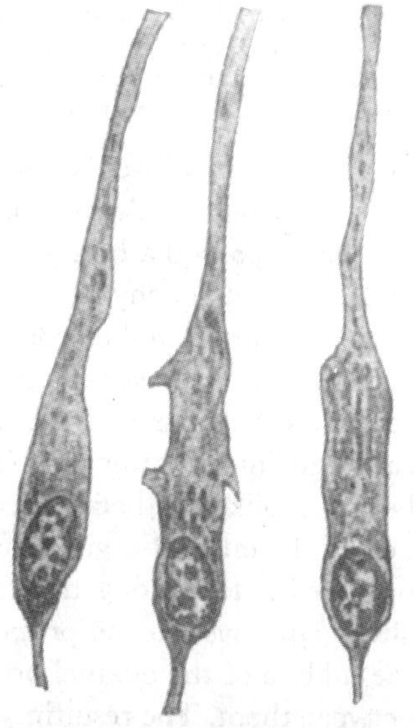

Figure 202. Isolated odontoblasts from a bovine fetus. Note the long dentinal fibers (of Tomes) and the torn lateral and basal pulp processes.

---

[5] Gr. *brachys* short, i.e., the enamel-covered portion or body of the tooth is short.

[6] Gr. *hypsi* high, i.e., the enamel-covered portion of the tooth is long and prismatic.

These have free endings in the pulp (pulp processes) or unite with similar processes from neighboring cells (commissural processes). In old teeth the pulp cavity is gradually reduced by the growth of the dentin.

(e) The periodontal membrane or alveolar periosteum (Figs. 74; 194,*e*) fills the space between the alveolar wall and the root of the tooth. It consists of tough connective tissue, which lacks elastic fibers. Its collagenous bundles are continued into the alveolar wall and the dental cementum as Sharpey's fibers (Fig. 195,*f*), thus providing extraordinarily firm anchorage.

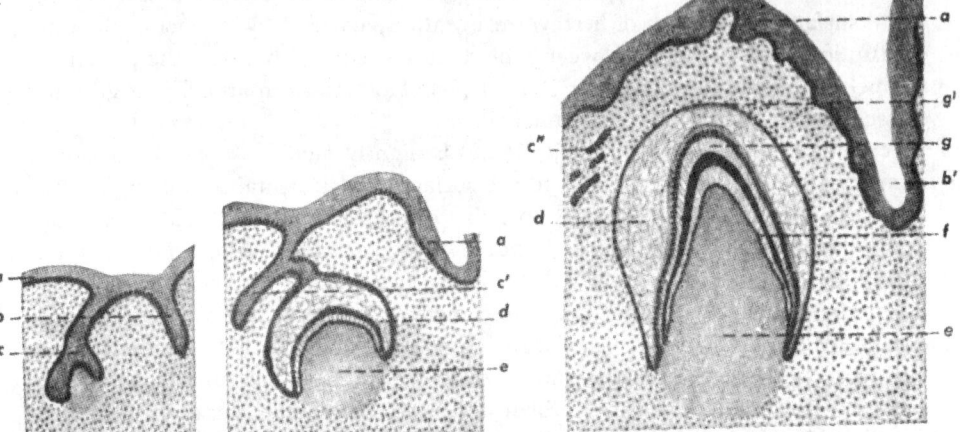

Figures 203–205 (left to right). Development of the teeth. *a*, oral epithelium; *b*, labial lamina separating the lip from the jaw; *b'*, labial furrow; *c*, dental lamina with early enamel organ; *c'*, part of dental lamina that gives rise to permanent teeth; *c''*, its vestiges; *d*, enamel organ; *e*, dental papilla; *f*, dentin; *g*, inner, and *g'*, outer, enamel epithelium.

Development of the Teeth

On the edges of the prospective jaws the oral epithelium undergoes a thickening and develops into a horseshoe-shaped ridge, the *dental lamina*, which grows into the underlying mesenchyme. On its labial surface clubbed thickenings (Fig. 203,*c*) are formed, whose number corresponds to that of the deciduous teeth. These are the primordia of the *enamel organs*, and they are met by an equal number of highly cellular elevations of the connective tissue the *dental papillae* (Fig. 204,*e*). These cause an invagination of the epithelial outgrowths so that each papilla comes to bear a caplike epithelial cover, the enamel organ (Figs. 204; 205,*d*). The connection of the enamel organ with the dental lamina becomes more and more slender but persists for a long time as a narrow isthmus. The dental lamina degenerates after giving rise to the primordia of the permanent teeth. Meanwhile the cells in the middle of the enamel organ become stellate in shape, and a fluid accumulates between them. The resulting tissue resembles mucous connective tissue and is called stellate reticulum or enamel pulp (Figs. 205,*d;* 206,*e*). It splits the remainder of the enamel organ into the external (Fig. 205,*g'*) and internal (*g*) enamel epithelium. The former is flat and later contributes to the enamel cuticle. The cells of the internal enamel epithelium lie in apposition to the odontoblast layer of the dental

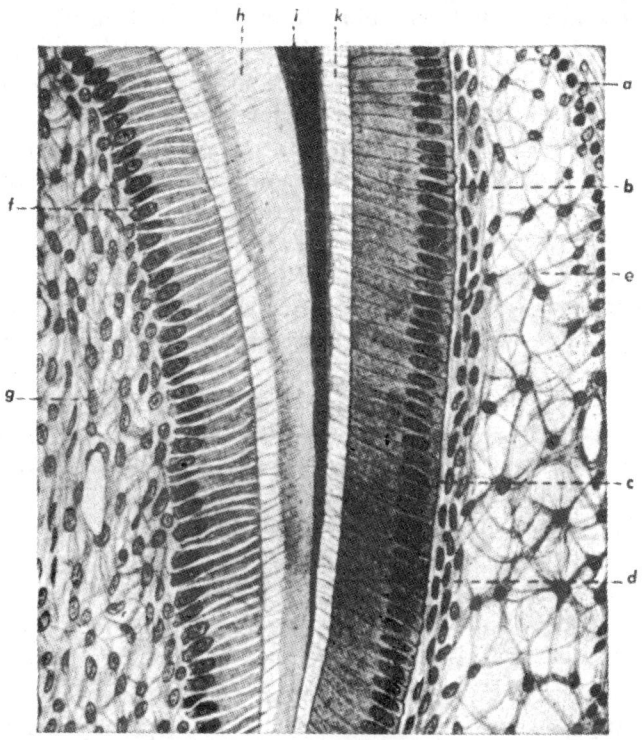

Figure 206. Section through the proximal margin of a
tooth from a newborn pup (300×). *a*, outer, *b*, inner, enamel
epithelium; *c*, its basement membrane, and *d*, cuticle;
e, enamel pulp; *f*, odontoblasts; *g*, dental papilla; *h*, dentin;
i, enamel; *k*, enamel prisms (rods). (After Bonnet.)

papilla. They are high columnar cells (Fig. 206,*b*) with a cuticular border (*d*) facing the papilla. At the line of reflection near the base of the papilla they pass into
the external enamel epithelium (Fig. 205). The connective tissue surrounding each
tooth primordium condenses to form a two-layered sheath, the *dental sac*.

The formation of the hard tooth substances begins with the deposition of uncalcified dentin (Fig. 206,*h*). This is done by the odontoblasts, which leave cytoplasmic strands, the dentinal fibers of Tomes, embedded in the dentin as they re-
cede. Shortly after the start of dentin calcification the deposition of enamel begins.
The dentinal ends of the cells of the internal enamel epithelium, called *ganoblasts*,
produce long cuticular processes which become calcified and cemented together to
form the enamel prisms. The preliminary calcification proceeds from the dentin outward. Later the enamel matures, i.e., the organic matter is almost completely replaced by minerals. Maturation proceeds from the apex of the crown to the neck.
Thus the formation of the crown of the tooth is completed. The root formation
does not begin until shortly before the eruption of the tooth when, starting at the
line of reflection of the enamel organ, the inner and outer enamel epithelia begin to

grow down around the papilla, forming the *epithelial sheath* of Hertwig. Under its cover the papilla lays down the root dentin, whereupon the epithelial sheath begins to degenerate. The cementum is formed on the dentin by the inner layer of the dental sac, whose mesenchymal cells develop into osteoblasts and penetrate the epithelial sheath. If the tooth remains in the cementum-producing dental sac until its eruption, then the entire tooth is coated with cement. If, however, the tooth breaks through the dental sac prior to the beginning of cementum deposition, the crown remains free. Cementum-free crowns are the rule in the brachydont teeth of man, swine, and carnivores, but the teeth of Equidae and most of the cheek teeth of ruminants are completely covered by a coating of cement. Just before the eruption of a tooth the enamel organ forms the enamel cuticle and degenerates. The remaining dental papilla becomes the pulp of the tooth. The periodontal membrane is derived from the dental sac. In the multicuspid teeth (of Carnivora and Omnivora) the dental papilla consists of several parts. At the tip of each cusp a cap of enamel and dentin is formed. Later these coalesce and make up one single crown. In the ridged teeth of herbivores the enamel organ sends deep folds and invaginations into the large papilla, resulting in enamel folds and infundibula in the finished tooth. In compound teeth the epithelial sheath of Hertwig forms as many compartments as the tooth will have roots.

The formation of a distinct root results from the fact that the pulp cavity, which at first was wide open at its basal end, is quickly reduced by the growth of the dentin to a root canal containing only a strand of connective tissue with vessels and nerves. Following the constriction and division of the pulp, the activity of its osteoblasts is restricted to the formation and growth of the root branches, while the longitudinal growth of the body of the tooth ceases. This description applies to the brachydont condition found in man and carnivores. In hypsodont teeth (tusks of the boar, incisors of rodents, teeth of the horse, and cheek teeth of ruminants) the enamel-covered body of the tooth shows a high degree of longitudinal development. This is made possible by the fact that root formation and constriction of the pulp cavity are delayed. The longitudinal growth is continued at the basal edge of the tooth around the open pulp cavity. The tusks of the boar grow throughout life. The cheek teeth of Equidae show a true longitudinal growth only until the fourth to sixth year. At this time the basal part of the pulp is split and constricted as the root branches are formed, and growth of the body of the tooth ceases. Bovine teeth have a shorter growth period than equine teeth.

The deciduous teeth originate as described. The permanent teeth arise later on by the formation of tooth primordia at the free edge of the dental lamina. The process is identical with that leading to the formation of the deciduous teeth. The primordia of the molars arise from a caudal extension of the dental lamina.

OROPHARYNX OF BIRDS. Because of the absence of a soft palate, the cranial portion of the digestive tract of birds is made up of a single oropharynx, with which the nasal cavity communicates by a median cleft in the roof of the mouth. It is lined by cutaneous mucous membrane. The squamous epithelium, which lies on a papillary body, shows regions of cornification on the dorsum of the tongue and the roof of the mouth down to the entrance to the larynx. The propria contains an abundance of mucous glands throughout. These occur either as simple glands, which have their own excretory ducts, or as larger glandular masses (e.g., around the tongue). The mucosa is exceedingly rich in diffuse or nodular aggregates of lymphocytes. These often surround the excretory ducts of the glands or accumulate around the secretory end-pieces. They are especially abundant around the entrance into the esophagus.

The tongue of gallinaceous birds is elongated and pointed. It contains the entoglossal bone, which joins the basihyoid caudally and ends in a cartilaginous point rostrally. The cornified layer of the dorsum is continued over the point of the tongue and on its lower surface. Macroscopic, caudally directed, cornified papillae occur in a transverse row on the root of the tongue and in several rows across the roof of the mouth. The last of these, the palatine row, marks the border between the mouth and the pharynx.

The oropharyngeal mucosa and the yellow skin around the base of the beak contain special nerve endings called Grandry's corpuscles and Herbst's corpuscles (p. 328). Structures resembling taste buds have been described on the root of the tongue and elsewhere.

The mammalian pharynx is described under the respiratory system, p. 234.

C. ESOPHAGUS

The wall of the esophagus consists of a cutaneous mucous membrane and a muscular tunic, which, in the cervical region, is covered by a loose fibrous adventitia. In the thoracic region the latter is replaced by a serous membrane.

The base of the longitudinally folded mucosa is a tunica propria made up of closely woven collagenous fibers with some elastic fiber nets interspersed. Its well-developed papillary body is overlain by superficially cornified, stratified squamous epithelium (Figs. 207,b; 208,a*). The muscularis mucosae is made up of longitudinal fibers. It is complete in man, but in solipeds, ruminants, and the cat it consists at first only of isolated bundles. Only in the caudal half does a more or less continuous sheet appear. In the dog and pig it is lacking entirely in the initial portion. In the caudal half, muscle bundles make their appearance but form a continuous layer only in the vicinity of the stomach. In some domestic animals and man the loose submucosa contains numerous mucous glands (Figs. 124; 208,d*), whose excretory ducts (d') traverse the tunica propria. The loose structure of the submucosa permits the formation of the mucosal folds, which in turn allow for great distention of the esophagus.

In the dog the glands form a continuous stratum that extends to the vicinity of the stomach. In the pig the glandular layer begins to fade out at about the middle of the esophagus. Caudal to this point, glands are few and small, but occur singly as far as the cardia. In the horse, ruminants, and the cat, glands are present at the pharyngoesophageal junction only. The esophageal mucosa of man and the pig con-

---

* Fig. 208 is on p. 152.

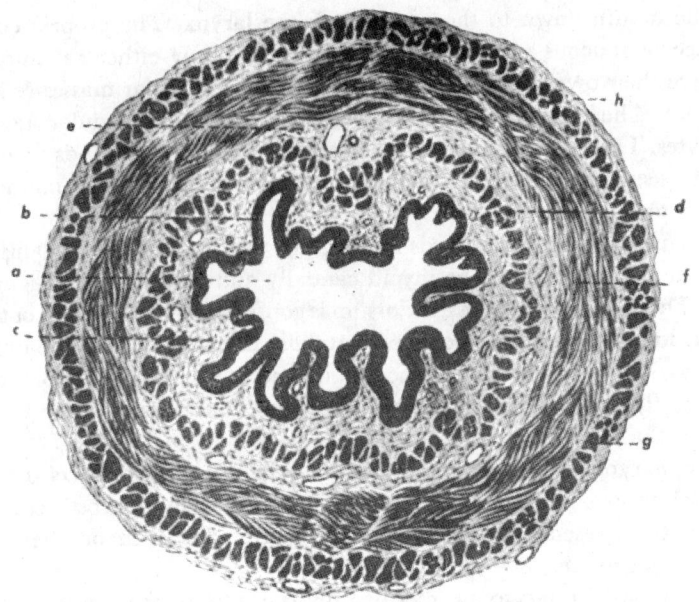

Figure 207. Cross section through the esophagus of the cat. *a*, lumen; *b*, squamous epithelium; *c*, tunica propria; *d*, muscularis mucosae; *e*, submucosa; *f*, internal layer of circular muscle; *g*, external layer of longitudinal muscle; *h*, serosa.

tains lymph nodules also. These are especially numerous in the pig, where they lie adjacent to the glands.

The tunica muscularis (Figs. 124,*d;* 207,*f,g;* 208,*f,g**) is made up of striated muscle with some smooth muscle at the caudal end. It is formed of two main layers whose fibers at first cross each other obliquely, then take a spiral course. Gradually an inner circular and an outer longitudinal layer become distinct. The outer ·longitudinal layer increases in thickness caudally in the horse only. The inner circular layer becomes thicker toward the stomach in all animals, especially in the horse. In addition to these continuous main layers there are also incomplete accessory layers.

The transition from striated to smooth musculature occurs in the pig just cranial to the cardia. In the horse and cat it takes place at the beginning of the caudal third to fifth of the esophagus. In ruminants and dogs the entire tunica muscularis is composed of striated muscle, which in ruminants is continued on the outside of the esophageal groove and the rumen (p. 184).

The entire esophageal wall is rich in elastic tissue. It increases in quantity wherever there is a thickening of the wall or a constriction of the lumen.

VESSELS AND NERVES. The vascular trunks run longitudinally in the submucosa. Their branches ramify and form capillary nets in all layers, especially in the subepithelial. The secretory end-pieces of the glands are surrounded by capillaries.

* Fig. 208 is on p. 152.

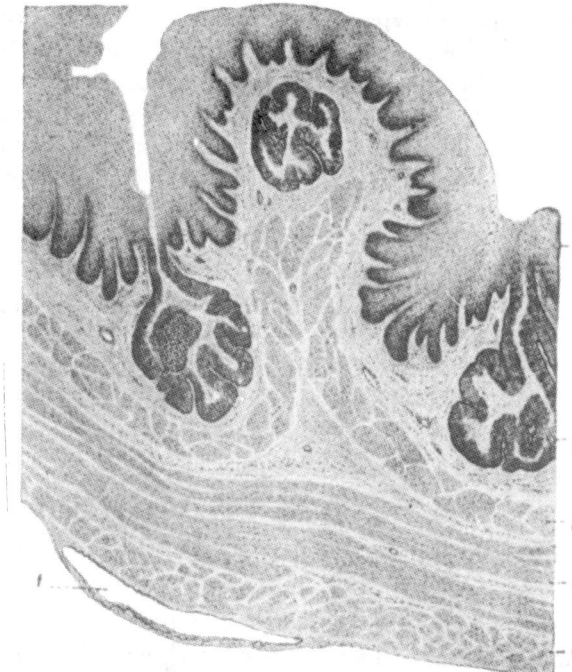

Figure 209. Cross section through the esophageal wall of the chicken, caudal to the opening into the crop (40×). *a,* stratified squamous epithelium; *b,* propria with mucous glands; *c,* muscularis mucosae; *d,* circular muscle layer; *e,* longitudinal muscle layer; *f,* air sac in the adventitia.

Large venous plexuses are present at the cranial end of the esophagus. The large lymphatics of the submucosa are equipped with valves (Fig. 208,*e**). The nerve trunks are also found in the submucosa. Their branches penetrate all layers. In the epithelium they end intercellularly in the usual manner. Nerve cells occur in the plexuses located in the submucosa and between the main layers of muscle.

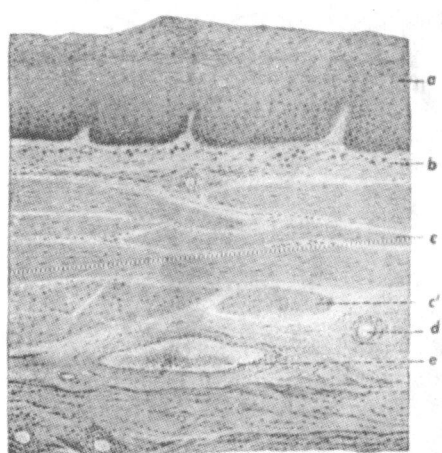

Figure 210. Section through the wall of the crop of the chicken (75×). *a,* stratified squamous epithelium with cornified and partly desquamated cells; *b,* lamina propria with papillary body and lymphocytes; *c,c',* muscle layers; *d,* artery; *e,* vein.

ESOPHAGUS OF BIRDS. The entrance to the esophagus is marked by a dorsal and a ventral transverse row of papillae. The stratified squamous epithelium is thrown into folds and overlies a papillary body (Fig. 209,*a*). The tunica propria contains numerous saclike mucous glands, each of which has a collecting sinus (*b*). The secretory end-pieces are lined by a layer of columnar cells with basal nuclei. Lymphocytic aggregates are present in the vicinity and may bulge into the interior of the gland or displace the gland

* Fig. 208 is on p. 152.

cells. These aggregates become more numerous near the stomach, forming the so-called esophageal tonsil. The musculature consists of an inner longitudinal layer, which follows the folds and must be considered the muscularis mucosae (*c*). This is followed by a layer of circular muscle (*d*); peripheral to this in the chicken is another thin layer of longitudinal muscle (*e*). The outer coat is formed by loose connective tissue. The crop (Fig. 210) is a dilatation of the esophagus and resembles the latter in structure. The folds of mucosa are not as high as those in the esophagus. The epithelium is thick and superficially cornified. The propria is rich in lymphatic tissue. Glands are present only occasionally in the chicken and pigeon crop. They are regularly present in geese and ducks. The musculature of the wall is arranged in the same strata (*c,c′*) as that of the esophagus proper. Before and during brooding time "crop milk" is produced in the pigeon crop, which consists of two symmetrical sacs. The milk originates by a fatty transformation of the superficial cells of the proliferated epithelium and serves as nourishment for the young.

D. STOMACH

The wall of the stomach consists of a mucosa with its submucosa, and muscular and serous tunics. The true gastric mucosa is characterized by the presence of gastric glands. Only the stomachs of man and carnivores are lined by gastric mucosa exclusively. In solipeds and swine the esophageal portion or forestomach bears a cutaneous mucosa (Fig. 211,*III,IV*). Ruminants have a stomach consisting of

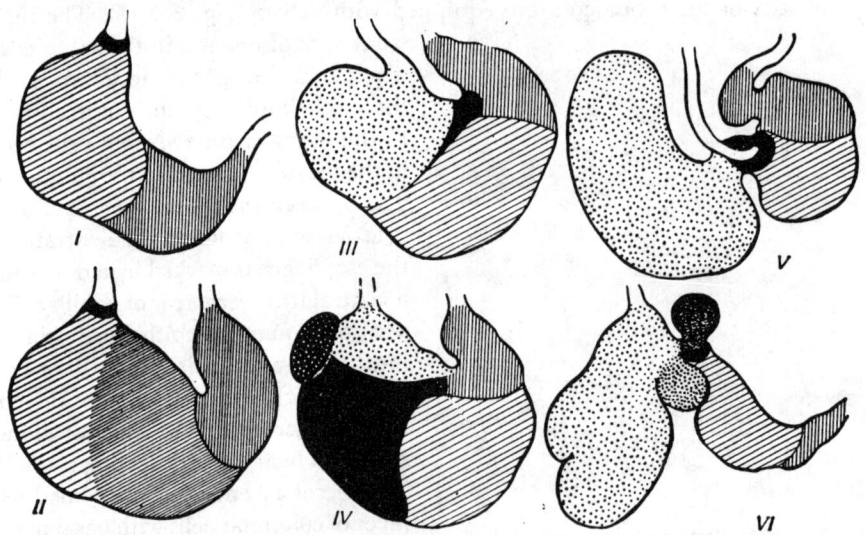

Figure 211. Diagrammatic representation of the stomach. *I*, man; *II*, dog; *III*, horse; *IV*, pig; *V*, hamster; *VI*, ruminant. Black = area of cardial glands; white stippling = diverticulum ventriculi; diagonal shading = fundic gland area (in *II*: dark and light zones); vertical shading = pyloric gland area; black stippling = forestomach (in *VI*: light stippling = rumen; denser stippling = reticulum; very dense stippling = omasum).

four compartments: three nonglandular diverticula comprising the forestomach and a true glandular stomach.

1. The Forestomach of the Ruminant

The wall of the forestomach consists of a nonglandular cutaneous mucous membrane, a two-layered muscular tunic, and a serosa. There is an abundance of elastic tissue in the wall especially in the region of the esophageal groove and the omasal laminae.

VESSELS AND NERVES. The larger blood vessels run in the submucosa, while in the propria the smaller branches form a subepithelial capillary net, which extends into the papillary body (Fig. 126). The tunica muscularis has the usual long-meshed capillary nets (Fig. 91). The larger lymphatics are found in the submucosa. They arise in part in the propria, where we often find rather large lymph vessels, especially in the omasal leaves and the walls of the cells of the reticulum. There is also a subserous net. Between the longitudinal and circular muscle layers and in

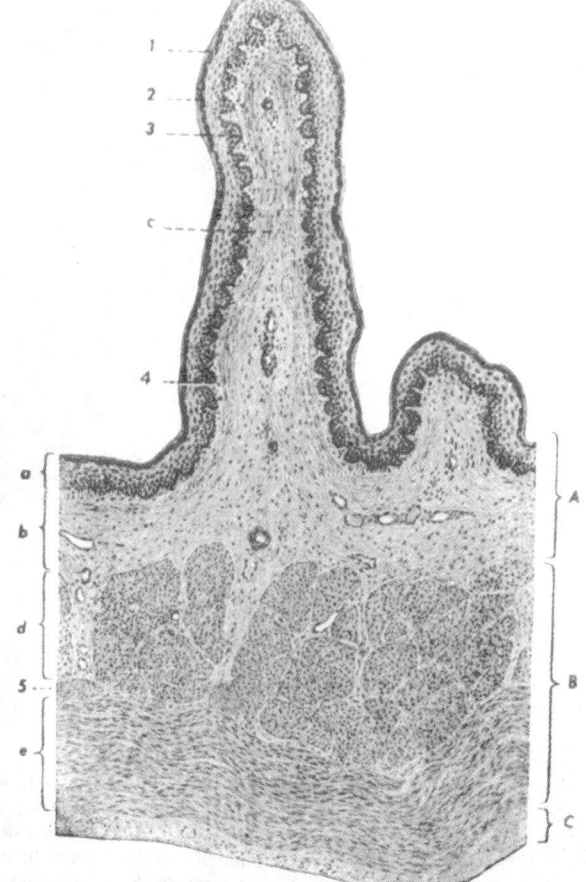

Figure 212. Section through the bovine rumen, the plane of section having passed through large and small papillae. *A,* mucosa; *B,* muscularis; *C,* serosa; *a,* squamous epithelium; *b,* lamina propria blending gradually into the submucosa; *c,* condensed connective tissue; *d,* inner, *e,* outer muscle layer; *1,* stratum corneum; *2,* stratum granulosum; *3,* germinal layer of the squamous epithelium; *4,* papillary body; *5,* ganglion.

the submucosa, the nerves form plexuses containing many ganglia (Fig. 212,*5*), especially in the wall of the reticulum. The intermuscular nerve plexus is also dense in the omasum. The autonomic nervous system controls the complex motor mechanism of the ruminant forestomach.

(a) Rumen (Paunch)

The mucosa (Fig. 212,*A*) forms large tongue-shaped or conical papillae, which may reach a length of 1 cm. in cattle and which are provided with a papillary body (*4*). The mucosa contains neither glands nor lymph nodules. The squamous epithelium (*a*) varies in thickness and is covered by a stratum corneum (*1*). The stratum granulosum and stratum lucidum (see *skin*, p. 335) are more or less continuous. The cells of the stratum lucidum often swell to become nucleated vesicles with a cornified wall and nonstainable cytoplasm. This "primary swelling" occurs mostly in areas where the stratum corneum exerts little pressure on the underlying cells. Here the swollen cells join the stratum corneum as vesicular horn cells with.

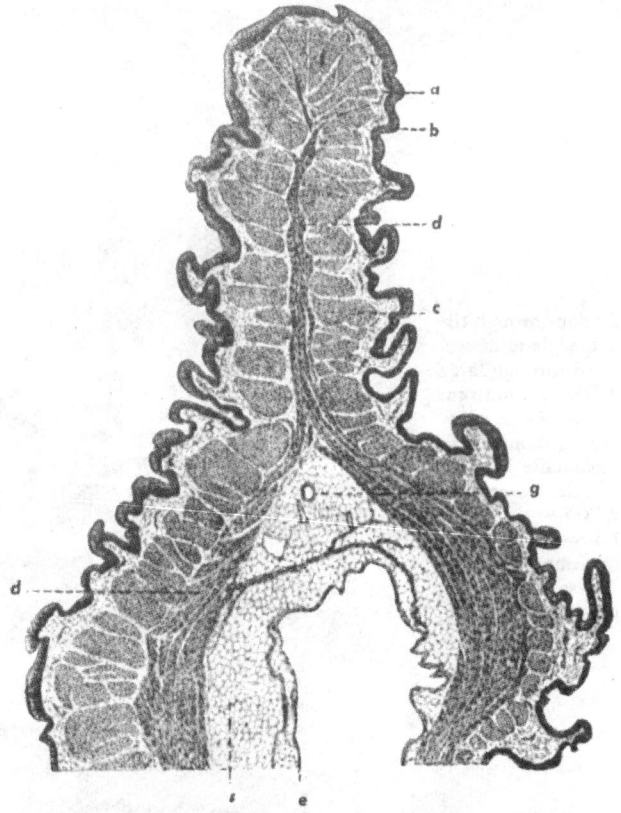

Figure 213. Cross section through a ruminal pillar of the sheep. *a*, lamina propria; *b*, squamous epithelium; *c*, muscle derived from the internal muscle layer of the ruminal wall; *d*, intermediate muscle lamella, derived from the outer muscle layer of the ruminal wall; *e*, serosa; *f*, fat; *g*, blood vessel.

little reduction in volume. In places where the stratum corneum is under tension, as on the tops of the papillae, the cells undergo the usual flattening in the process of cornification. A "secondary swelling" caused by the fluids of the forestomach occurs in the superficial cells of the stratum corneum in places where desquamation is retarded by lack of friction. Similar phenomena are to be observed in the reticulum and omasum. The propria consists of a dense feltwork of fine collagenous and many elastic fibers. The submucosa (b) is loose and thin and blends into the propria without any sharp line of demarcation. It condenses somewhat near the muscular tunic. The muscularis mucosae is absent. However, a denser, more deeply staining sheet of connective tissue, which extends into the papillae, may be mistaken for it (c).

The tunica muscularis (Fig. 212,B) is composed of two layers. In the outer layer the fibers are directed essentially craniocaudally, but in many places they take a more oblique or even a dorsoventral course. At the grooves of the rumen, some fibers of the outer coat bridge the groove and others dip into it to become the central layer of the corresponding *pillar* on the inside (Fig. 213,d). The fibers of the inner muscular layer have a generally circular arrangement. Where they enter the grooves, they take up a course parallel to the groove and form the bulk of the corresponding pillar (Fig. 213,c). The ruminal pillars contain an abundance of elastic fibers. Near the cardia, bundles of striated muscle from the esophagus spread out on the ruminal wall.

The serosa (Fig. 213,e) bridges the ruminal grooves, where the loose subserosa is especially thick and contains fat, nerves, and the large vessels.

The rumen harbors great numbers of microorganisms. The bacterial fermentation of cellulose and other carbohydrates carried on here is an important factor in ruminant digestion. Bacteria also synthesize amino acids and proteins in the rumen and play an important part in the synthesis of the B-complex of vitamins. Protozoa are regularly found adhering to the ruminal mucosa in histological sections. Their part in ruminal digestion is not as clearly established as that of the bacteria, but it is considered to be of lesser significance. The ruminal movements further the chemical and microbiological processes by churning the contents, and the papillae aid in comminution of the solid constituents.

b. Reticulum (Honeycomb)

The mucosa forms characteristic permanent folds, whose sides are covered with closely adjacent vertical ridges while their free edge bears conical papillae with cornified tips. The detailed structure of the mucosa resembles greatly that of the rumen. In every large fold of the reticulum we find a band of smooth muscle fibers (Fig. 214,g) which run in the same direction as the fold itself and are continuous with the muscularis mucosae of the esophagus. The reticular folds begin at the cardia. Wherever the reticular folds intersect (Fig. 215), the muscle bundles pass from one fold into the other, forming a continuous network. A muscularis mucosae is otherwise absent.

The muscular tunic, which is somewhat thickened at the apex of the reticulum, consists of two layers whose fibers follow an oblique course and cross at right angles.

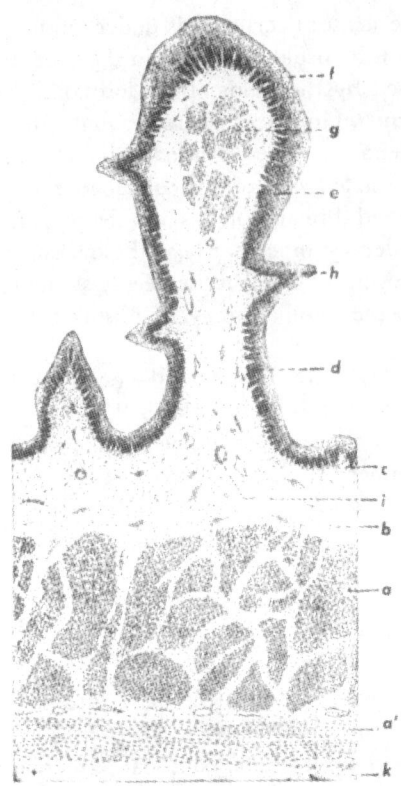

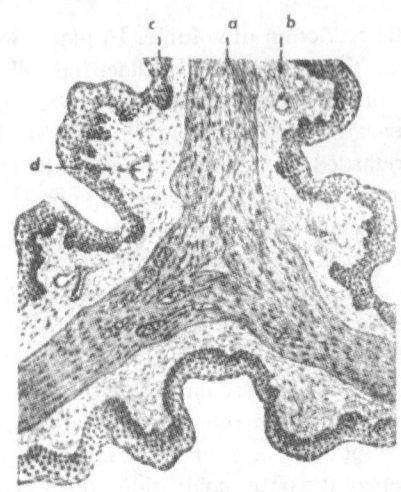

Figure 214 (left). Cross section through a reticular fold and the wall of the reticulum of the sheep. *a,* inner circular, *a',* outer longitudinal muscle layer; *b,* submucosa; *c,* lamina propria; *d,* papillary body; *e,* squamous epithelium; *f,* its stratum corneum; *g,* muscle cord of the fold; *h,* macroscopic papilla; *i,* vessels; *k,* serosa.

Figure 215 (right). Point of intersection of three reticular folds, cut near the free edge. *a,* muscle cord; *b,* lamina propria mucosae; *c,* squamous epithelium; *d,* vessels.

Both are continuous with the musculature of the esophagus and esophageal groove. The internal layer (Figs. 216,*i;* 217,*e*) runs into the muscle of the lips of the esophageal groove, while the external sheet makes up the transverse muscle of the floor of the groove (Figs. 216,*f;* 217,*h*).

The digestive processes in the reticulum are the same as those in the rumen.

The *esophageal* (or reticular) *groove* has a structure similar to that of the rest of the reticulum. Its wall is exceptionally rich in elastic tissue. Its cutaneous mucous membrane contains no glands except in sheep. The muscularis mucosae (Fig. 217,*c*) is incomplete. It is most conspicuous in the lips of the groove and forms a complete layer near the omasum, with whose muscularis mucosae it is continuous. It is also continuous with the muscular bands of the reticular folds. On the floor of the groove is a thick sheet of transverse muscle fibers (*h*), which in turn is followed by a thin longitudinal layer containing both smooth fibers (*i*) and bundles of striated muscle (*k*). The latter are continuations of the esophageal musculature. They predominate over the smooth muscle at the cardia but fade out toward the end of the groove. The thick longitudinal (smooth) muscle of the lips of the groove (Figs. 216; 217,*e*) is derived from the inner muscular layer of the esophagus. It forms a loop over the cardia corresponding to the cardial loop of animals with sim-

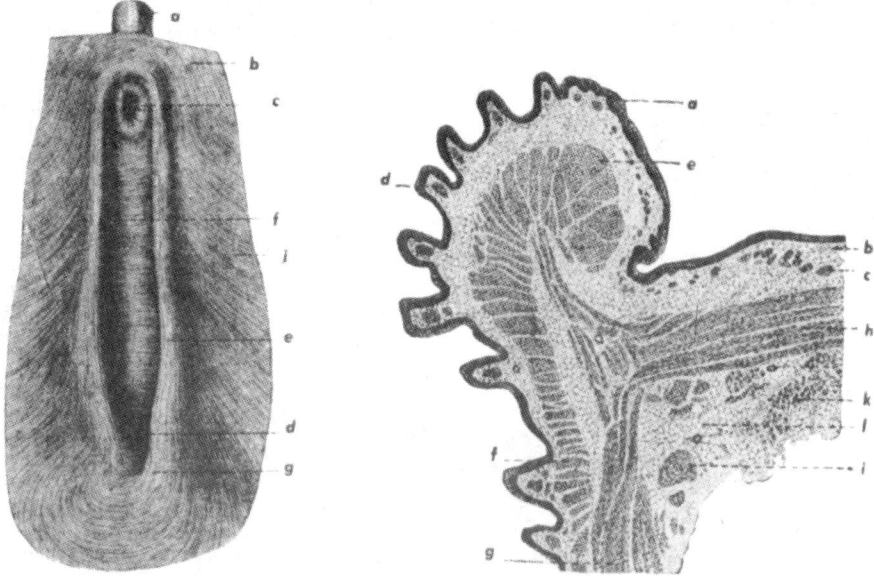

Figure 216 (left). Musculature of the esophageal groove of the ox, as seen from the inside. *a*, esophagus; *b*, reticular musculature and apex of the cardial loop; *c*, cardia; *d*, reticulo-omasal orifice; *e*, crura of the muscle loop and longitudinal muscles of the lips of the groove; *f*, transverse muscle layer of the floor of the groove; *g*, fusion of the muscles of the two lips of the groove, encircling the reticulo-omasal orifice; *i*, inner circular muscle layer of the reticulum.

Figure 217 (right). Cross section through one lip and part of the floor of the esophageal groove of the sheep. *a*, squamous epithelium; *b*, lamina propria; *c*, muscularis mucosae; *d*, bundles derived from *c*, in the folds of the esophageal groove (beginnings of the reticular folds); *e*, cross section of the longitudinal musculature of the lips, which passes into the inner muscle layer of the reticulum (*f*); *g*, outer muscle layer of the reticulum, which passes into *h*, the transverse muscle layer of the floor of the groove; *i*, smooth, and *k*, striated, longitudinal muscle tracts of the floor of the groove; *l*, adipose tissue.

ple stomachs.[7] At the ventral end of the esophageal groove the muscle fibers pass into the sphincter of the reticulo-omasal orifice. At the sides of the groove the fibers spread out into the inner layer of the reticulum. Most of the transverse muscle on the floor of the groove passes over to the wall of the reticulum, but a thin sheet curves around into the lips and is inserted on the longitudinal muscle (Fig. 217).

In the young, especially the suckling, animal the esophageal groove contracts reflexly to form a tube, which conducts the milk to the abomasum by the shortest route. In older animals water and food enter the rumen directly.

c. Omasum (Manyplies)

The cutaneous mucous membrane contains dense capillary nets immediately under the epithelium. It has neither glands nor lymph nodules but possesses a distinct muscularis mucosae (Fig. 218*B,c*) and forms the characteristic omasal laminae, which are studded with macroscopic papillae. The papillae are so directed that the movement of the laminae works the solid food from the reticulo-omasal

[7] S. Sisson and J. D. Grossman, *The Anatomy of the Domestic Animals*, Figs. 358a, 421.

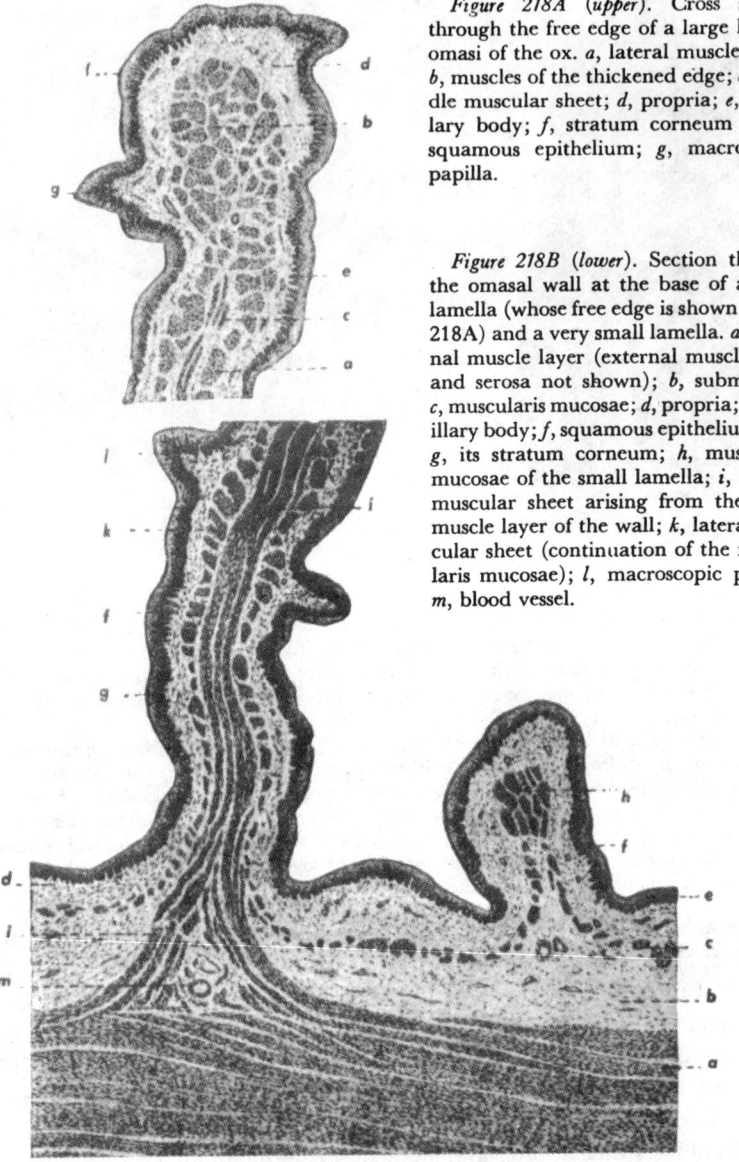

Figure 218A (upper). Cross section through the free edge of a large lamina omasi of the ox. *a*, lateral muscle sheet; *b*, muscles of the thickened edge; *c*, middle muscular sheet; *d*, propria; *e*, papillary body; *f*, stratum corneum of the squamous epithelium; *g*, macroscopic papilla.

Figure 218B (lower). Section through the omasal wall at the base of a large lamella (whose free edge is shown in Fig. 218A) and a very small lamella. *a*, internal muscle layer (external muscle layer and serosa not shown); *b*, submucosa; *c*, muscularis mucosae; *d*, propria; *e*, papillary body; *f*, squamous epithelium with *g*, its stratum corneum; *h*, muscularis mucosae of the small lamella; *i*, middle muscular sheet arising from the inner muscle layer of the wall; *k*, lateral muscular sheet (continuation of the muscularis mucosae); *l*, macroscopic papilla; *m*, blood vessel.

orifice up into the interlaminar spaces and out at the abomasal end. The laminae are folds which include the entire mucosa with the muscularis mucosae and the submucosa. The larger laminae contain in addition a layer of the tunica muscularis, the fibers of which extend toward the free edge and fuse with the marginal thickening of the muscularis mucosae (Figs. 218*A,c;* 218*B,i*). Thus a cross section of a larger omasal leaf shows three muscle layers: the intermediate layer and, separated from it by a thin stratum of submucosa on either side, the two layers of muscularis mucosae (Figs. 218*A*,*a*; 218*B*,*k*), whose fibers are directed toward the abomasum at right angles to those of the middle layer. The muscularis mucosae occasionally sends fibers into the papillae of the omasal laminae. The larger papillae usually contain a peculiar tissue that stains blue in hemalum-eosin preparations and resembles mucous connective tissue. It contains large cells with distinct membranes and shrunken cytoplasm. Droplets in the cells give a mucoid reaction.

The tunica muscularis is composed of an outer thin longitudinal layer and an inner thicker circular layer (218*B*,*a*) whose innermost stratum is continued into the larger omasal leaves as their intermediate muscle sheet (*i*).

The vela terminalia (valvulae terminales, Fig. 219) are folds of mucous membrane containing a muscularis mucosae (*d*). In the ox the omasal surface is covered by cutaneous mucous membrane. In the sheep and goat the vela are folds of the abomasal mucosa. Between the two mucosal surfaces there is loose connective tis-

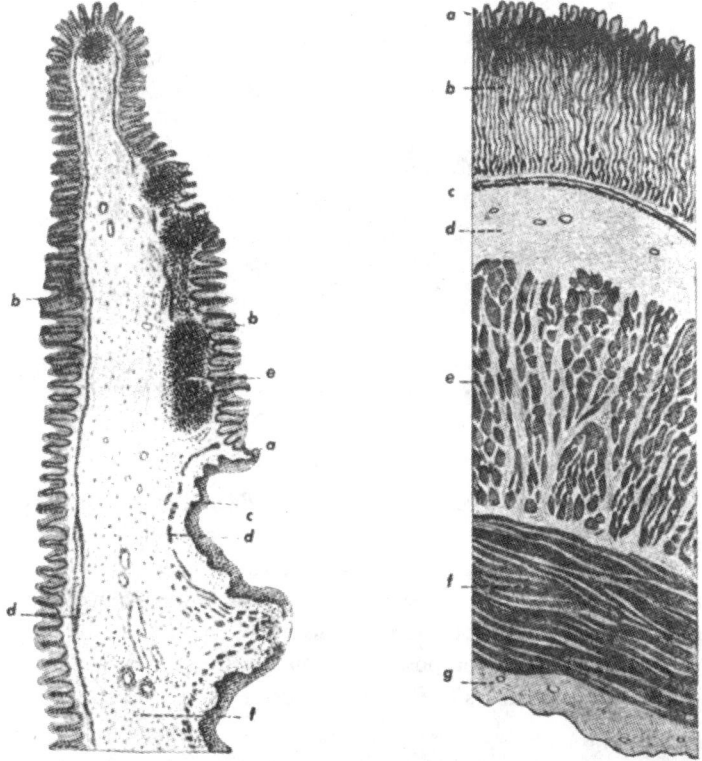

Figure 219 (left). Cross section through the velum terminale of the goat. *a*, mucocutaneous junction; *b*, gastric glands; *c*, squamous epithelium; *d*, muscularis mucosae; *e*, lymphatic tissue; *f*, submucosa.

Figure 220 (right). Section through the stomach wall of the dog ($\times$5$\times$). *a*, gastric pits with gastric epithelium; *b*, lamina propria (glandular layer); *c*, muscularis mucosae; *d*, submucosa; *e*, inner circular, *f*, outer longitudinal muscle layer of the tunica muscularis; *g*, serosa.

sue and fat. At the junction of glandular and cutaneous mucosa, lymph nodules (*e*) are always present.

The floor of the omasum is covered by a thin, folded mucous membrane, which in goats often contains mucous or mixed glands. The thick musculature is made up of a thin external longitudinal layer and a very heavy inner transverse sheet. The latter thickens toward the abomasum and forms the omasal pillar. The lips of the omasal groove show a strong muscularis mucosae composed of longitudinal fibers.

The function of the omasum is apparently comminution. The ingesta between the laminae are squeezed almost dry, and the particles are finer at the abomasal end than at the reticular end. Fluids pass directly from the reticulum to the abomasum through the omasal groove.

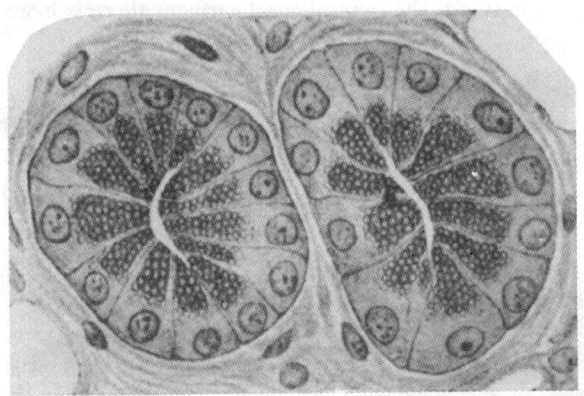

Figure 221. Cross section through two gastric pits from the cardial gland region of the pig. The mucigenous granules are well fixed.

2. THE GLANDULAR STOMACH

The stomach has several functions which are reflected in its structure. It secretes the gastric juice for enzymatic digestion. It acts mechanically in mixing and breaking down the food and moving it into the intestine. It also serves as a storehouse and filling mechanism for the intestine. Finally it is important as a bacteriostatic organ inhibiting the growth of microorganisms taken in with the food. The wall of the stomach (Fig. 220) is composed of a mucosa (*a–d*), a tunica muscularis consisting of smooth muscle fibers (*e,f*), and a serosa (*g*).

a. Tunica Mucosa

The mucosa of the stomach consists of the surface epithelium (*1*), the glandular lamina propria (*2*), a muscularis mucosae (*3*), and a loose submucosa (*4*).

(1) **The Surface Epithelium.** This begins abruptly at the jagged border of the thick stratified squamous epithelium of the esophageal mucosa. It consists of a single layer of high (20–30 μ) columnar cells with terminal bars. The ellipsoid nucleus lies in the basal half of the cell (Fig. 223*). The cytoplasm of a fresh cell shows

* Fig. 223 is on p. 201.

a finely granular basal zone containing the nucleus, and a distal zone in which the centrioles and mucigenous granules are found (Fig. 221). If the cell is not fixed soon after death, the granules change into a confluent mucous mass which protrudes from the cell. The epithelial cells of ruminants have a striated border, which is obliterated during the secretion of mucus. The surface epithelium is continued into depressions in the gastric mucosa, which serve to increase the amount of secreting surface area. These depressions are the *gastric pits* or *foveolae* (Figs. 221–222; 223*; 224,*b*). Toward the bottom of the pits the cells become shorter and wider, and often show mitoses, by means of which worn-out cells are replaced. Their nuclei are spherical and located in the basal half. Leukocytes (Fig. 223,*h**) are often present between the epithelial cells.

(2) **The Lamina Propria.** The lamina propria (or glandularis) contains the

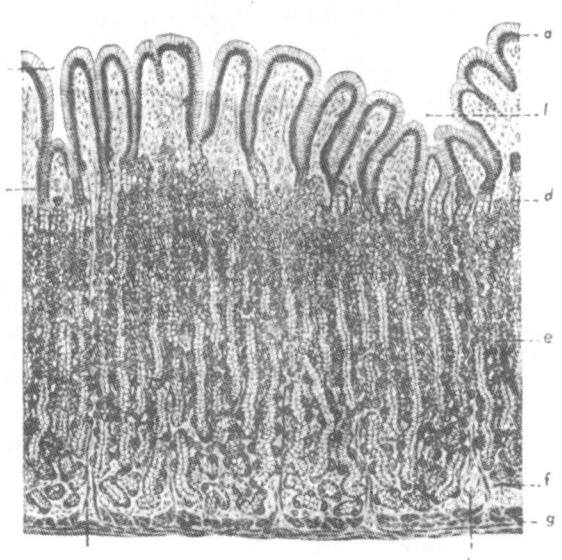

Figure 222. Section through the fundic gland region of the dog. *a*, columnar epithelium of the surface of the stomach; *b*, gastric pits; *c,d*, necks of the glands; *e*, body of a gland; *f*, stratum subglandulare; *g*, muscularis mucosae giving off interglandular muscle bundles (*i*); *k*, vessel; *l*, gastric furrow.

gastric glands, supported by a delicate, sparse, connective tissue framework. The latter is predominantly reticular connective tissue (Figs. 224; 225,*c**; 230,*e*) in which we find, in addition to fine elastic fibers, smooth muscle fibers and bundles (Fig. 229,*b'*) derived from the muscularis mucosae. The reticular connective tissue condenses into a reticular membrane on the epithelium, the muscle cells, and the capillaries.

Around the glands the supportive framework forms a thin fibrillar glandular sheath. There is less connective tissue between the glands than between the gastric pits. In certain areas (but not in the cardial gland zone) the glands are divided into groups (Figs. 227, 235) by heavier strands of supporting tissue. The connective tissue between the pits and below the glands is rich in leukocytes including eosinophils and plasma cells, especially in the pig.

---

* Figs. 223 and 225 are on p. 201.

The plicae villosae of the pyloric mucosa are nonglandular projections between the pits, while the gastric furrows (Figs. 222,*l*; 227,*a*) are depressions in the tunica propria.

The gastric glands are simple tubular glands and are usually branched. Several of them open into one gastric pit. The pits open into the furrows or on the raised areas between the furrows. The glands vary from 1 to 1.5 mm. in length. They are of three types: fundic, pyloric, and cardial glands.

(a) **The fundic glands** were so named because they were first discovered in the fundus. Actually they are not restricted to this region of the stomach. They are less branched and less contorted than the other glands and have a neck distinct from the glandular body.

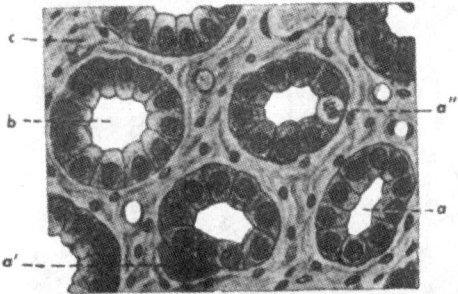

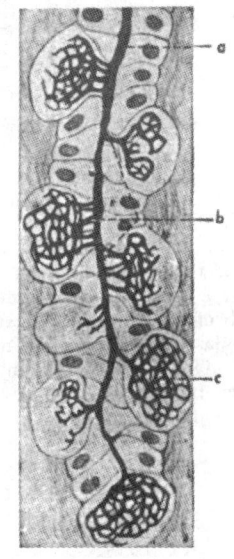

Figure 224. Cross section through the necks of fundic glands and the bottoms of gastric pits in a dog's stomach. *a*, section through the neck of a gland showing transitional cells; *a'*, parietal cell; *a''*, mitotic figure; *b*, section through a gastric pit; *c*, interglandular tissue.

Figure 226 (right). Secretory canaliculi of fundic glands. *a*, glandular lumen; *b*, intercellular drainage channels of the secretory canaliculi; *c*, network of the intracellular secretory canaliculi in the parietal cells.

The upper part of the neck (Fig. 223,*c**) is lined by cuboidal cells connected by a series of transitional forms with the foveolar epithelium. In the lower part of the neck are the *mucous neck cells* which give a special mucin reaction and have a flat basal nucleus (*d*). There are also parietal cells in the neck (see below).

The body of the gland (Figs. 223,*e,f**; 225*) contains two kinds of cells: chief and parietal. The *chief cells* (Figs. 223,*c,f**; 225,*a**) are cuboidal-to-columnar or wedge-shaped and contain rather coarse secretory granules. In hemalum-eosin preparations the cytoplasm of the chief cells remains nearly unstained. Their nuclei are spheroid and are located near the basal end.

The secretory phases of the chief cells are easily discernible. The cells are large and turbid in the fasting animal and become smaller during digestion. Their coarse granules diminish in number during digestion, but there is a relative increase in the finely granular cytoplasm. The chief cells furnish the proteolytic enzyme pepsin as well as rennin.

* Figs. 223 and 225 are on p. 201.

The *parietal cells* (Figs. 223,*g**; 225,*b**) are larger than the chief cells. Their outer portion is rounded and the inner portion is pyramidal. Their finely granular cytoplasm gives them a frosted-glass appearance when fresh and makes them look lighter than the chief cells. They contain no secretory granules. The central nucleus is occasionally double. The parietal cells stain deeply with acid dyes (e.g., eosin).

The parietal cells may lie outside the chief cells, or they may be wedged between them, or, especially in the neck, they may border directly on the lumen. They con-

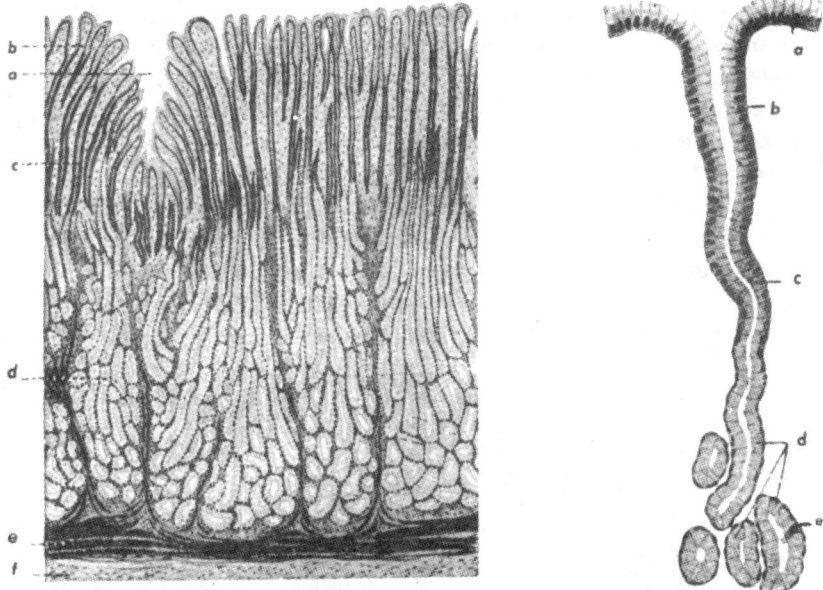

Figure 227 (left). Section through the pyloric mucosa near the duodenum of a pig. *a,* gastric furrow; *b,* gastric pit (foveola); *c,* excretory duct; *d,* body of gland (densely packed and very tortuous); *e,* muscularis mucosae; *f,* submucosa.

Figure 228 (right). Pyloric gland of the pig. *a,* surface epithelium; *b,* epithelium of the gastric pit; *c,* excretory duct; *d,* body of the gland; *e,* Stöhr's cell.

tain a network of intracellular secretory canaliculi (Fig. 226,*c*), which in exceptional cases communicates directly with the lumen but is usually connected with the latter by a small canal which runs between the chief cells (*b*). The parietal cells are most numerous in the upper part of the body and in the neck of the gland (Fig. 222), where they often occur in groups. They are rarer in the gland fundus (Fig. 225*).

The parietal cells produce the precursors of hydrochloric acid, which activates pepsin and rennin, aids directly in the digestion of proteins, acts as an antiseptic and bactericide, and may, to a slight degree hydrolyze sucrose.

(b) The pyloric glands (Figs. 227–229) open into much deeper pits and are also more branched than the fundic glands. Their branches are often very tortuous and sometimes wound up in a ball. In the deepest portion of the gastric pits there

* Figs. 223 and 225 are on p. 201.

is a gradual transition to glandular epithelium (Fig. 228,c,d). The relative length of the gastric pit and the body of the gland varies with the species and the region of the stomach. The cells of the glandular epithelium are cuboidal or pyramidal (Figs. 228,d; 229,a). They resemble the mucous neck cells of fundic glands. They contain a few dark granules but chiefly much larger, light, mucigenous granules. The deeply staining nucleus is basal and often strongly flattened.

Between the cells of the pyloric glands the narrow eosinophilic Stöhr's cells are quite commonly found (Figs. 228,e; 229,c). True secretory canaliculi are probably absent in the pyloric glands. The foveolae are deep in solipeds and ruminants, but shallow and scarcely discernible in carnivores. As to the secretory phases of the pyloric glands, it is known that prior to secretion the cells are large and light, while afterwards they are small and turbid. The cells that are full of secretion have a flat basal nucleus, whereas the empty cells have a round nucleus. In addition to small amounts of proteases, the pyloric glands secrete mainly mucus.

(c) The cardial glands (Figs. 230–232) are highly branched and often coiled into a ball. The portion of the foveola corresponding to the excretory duct usually enters deeply into the lamina propria, while the body of the gland is commonly short. The epithelial cells of the pits resemble those of the surface epithelium but are more cuboidal (Figs. 230; 231,c). They produce mucus. The body of the gland

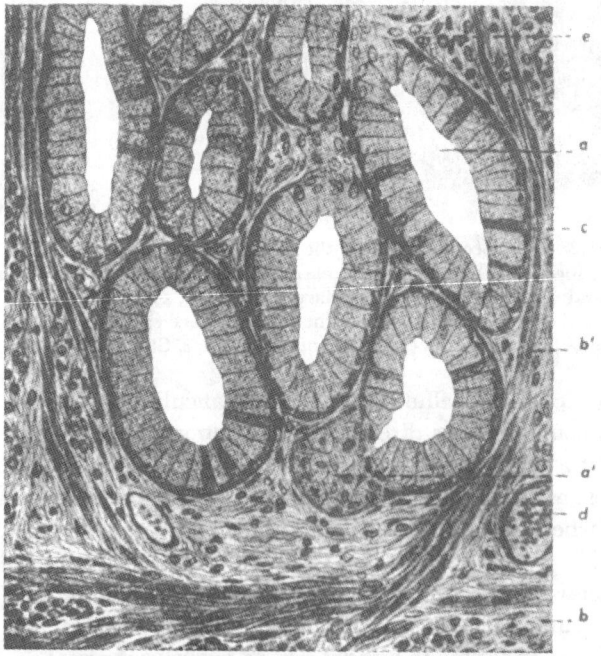

Figure 229. Section through the deepest part of the pyloric mucosa of the pig. a, section through the fundus of a gland; a', oblique section through a glandular tube; b, muscularis mucosae; b', ascending muscle bundles of the muscularis mucosae; c, Stöhr's cells; d, blood vessel; e, interglandular tissue.

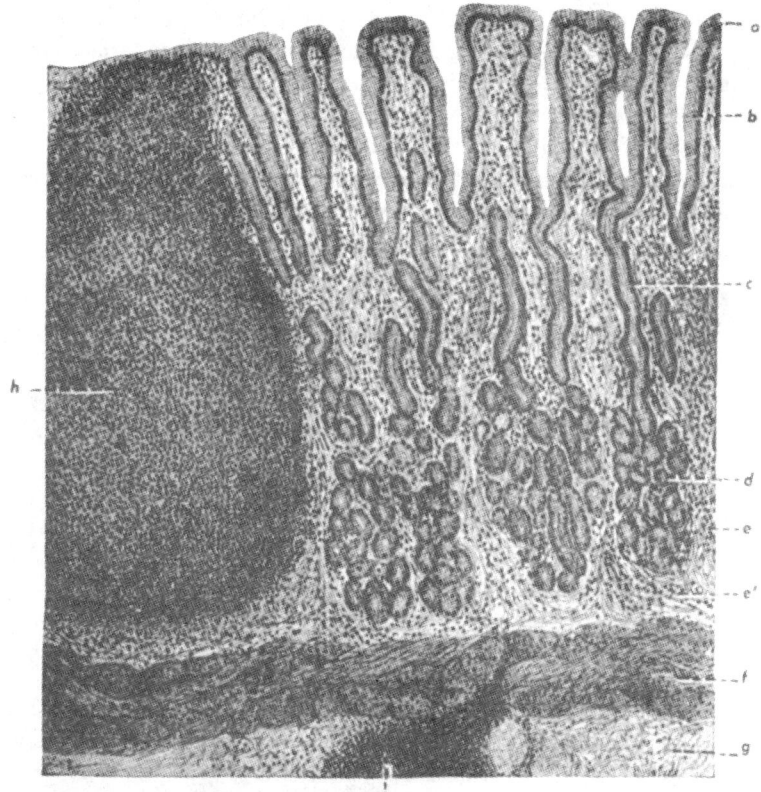

Figure 230. Section through the mucosa of the cardial gland area of the pig. *a*, surface epithelium of the stomach; *b*, epithelium of the gastric pits; *c*, excretory duct; *d*, body of the gland; *e*, interglandular tissue; *e'*, subglandular tissue; *f*, muscularis mucosae; *g*, submucosa; *h*, lymph nodule in the propria, and *i*, in the submucosa (only partly shown).

has a relatively wide lumen and is lined by pyramidal or cuboidal cells with a basally located nucleus (Figs. 231,*d;* 232,*a*). The cells contain granules in their distal portion. They stain similarly to the fundic parietal cells and do not react with mucin stains (Bensley[8] to the contrary). As with fundic and pyloric glands, transitional cells are found between the epithelial cells of the pits and those of the glands. The functional stages of the cardial gland cells resemble those of the serous salivary glands to a considerable degree.

In those areas where the zones of the three kinds of glands border on each other, we find a mixture of glands. We also find transitional glands, i.e., pyloric and cardial glands with parietal cells. These also occur in the region adjacent to the esophageal mucosa.

(3) **Muscularis Mucosae.** Under the propria lies the muscularis mucosae (Fig.

8 R. R. Bensley, The Cardiac Glands of Mammals, *Am. J. Anatomy* 2 (1902): 105–156.

230,*f*; 233,*a*). The muscle fibers may be irregularly interwoven or stratified. Fiber bundles extend into the propria (Fig. 233,*f*) to the vicinity of the surface epithelium.

The muscularis mucosae probably plays a part in the emptying of the glands. It influences the periodically changing topography of the mucosa and, by constriction or dilatation of the veins, the flow of blood in the mucosal capillaries.

In carnivores a lamina subglandularis intervenes between the muscularis mucosae and the blind ends of the glands. This becomes stratified in two layers in older

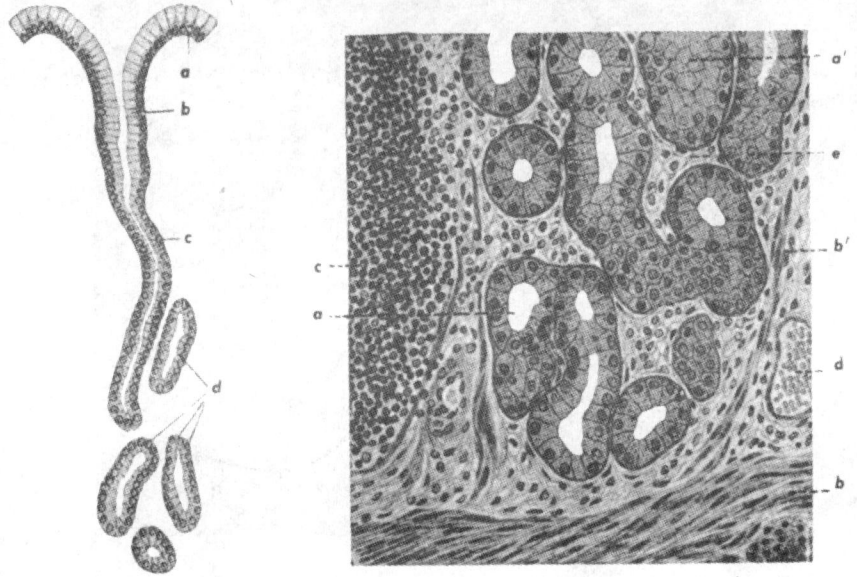

Figure 231 (left). Cardial gland of the pig. *a*, surface epithelium; *b*, epithelium of the gastric pit; *c*, epithelium of the excretory duct; *d*, epithelium of bodies of glands in cross section.

Figure 232 (right). Section through the fundus of cardial glands in the pig. *a*, cross section through the fundus of a gland; *a′*, tangentially cut glandular tube; *b*, muscularis mucosae; *b′*, ascending muscle bundles of the muscularis mucosae; *c*, portion of a lymph nodule; *d*, blood vessel; *e*, interglandular tissue.

individuals. Its inner layer, stratum granulosum (Fig. 233,*c*), which borders directly on the glands, is rich in cells, but the outer stratum compactum (*b*), which lies adjacent to the muscularis mucosae, is composed of an elastic network and a dense, almost hyaline, homogeneous collagenous substance. This layer is highly resistant and probably protects the gastric wall against perforations by bone splinters.

(4) Submucosa. The submucosa (Figs. 220,*d*; 234*A*,*5*) is composed of loose connective tissue and many elastic fiber nets. It permits movement of the mucosa on the underlying tunica muscularis. It often contains numerous adipose cells as well as the larger vessels, nerves, and ganglia.

Besides glands, the gastric mucosa contains lymph nodules (Figs. 230,*h,i*; 232,*c*; 235,*h*) either singly or in groups. These nodules are especially abundant in the pig. The region of the cardial glands and the transitional areas between the gland zones

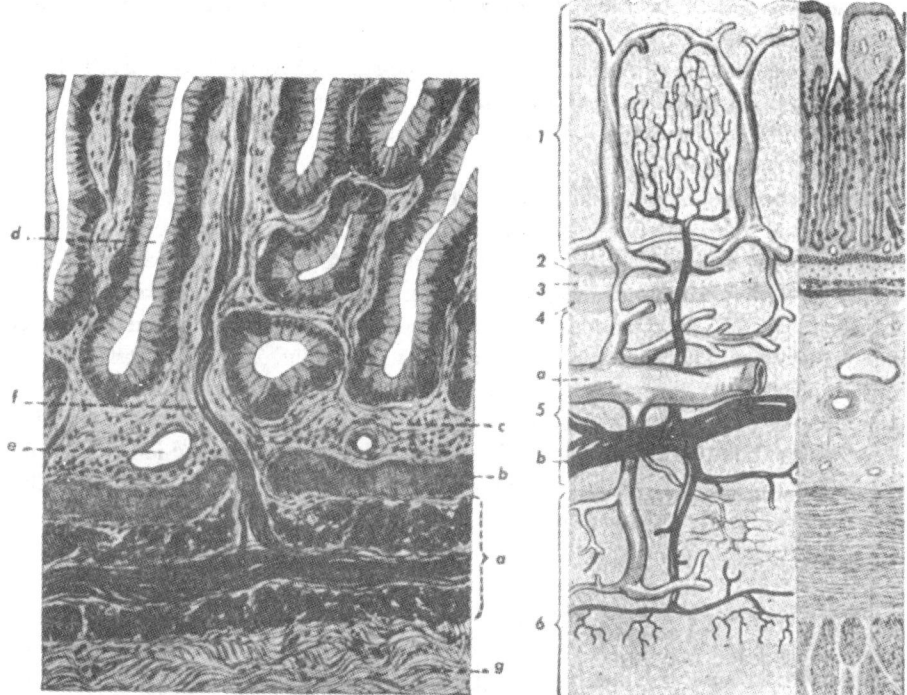

Figure 233. Section from the stomach of the cat. *a*, three-layered muscularis mucosae; *b*, stratum compactum; *c*, subglandular and periglandular tissue; *d*, section through glands; *e*, blood vessel; *f*, interglandular muscle strands derived from the muscularis mucosae; *g*, submucosa.

Figure 234A. Schematic section through the stomach wall, with and without vessels. *1*, lamina propria; *2*, stratum granulosum; *3*, stratum compactum; *4*, muscularis mucosae; *5*, submucosa; *6*, two-layered tunica muscularis; *a*, vein; *b*, artery.

are especially well provided with such lymphatic structures. The lymph nodules are usually located in the propria and, more rarely, in the submucosa. In the vicinity of the nodules the surrounding tissues as well as the surface and glandular epithelium are infiltrated with leukocytes and thereby obscured. Gastric pits and glands are displaced from their normal position. Lymph craters, lined with surface epithelium, occur in the stomach of the pig. Under the epithelium is a cluster of 20 to 30 lymph nodules, which extends down into the submucosa and is surrounded by a connective tissue capsule.

b. Tunica Muscularis

The muscular tunic of the stomach (Figs. 220,*e*,*f*; 249,*d*,*e**) is made up of an incomplete *outer longitudinal layer* and an *outer oblique layer* occurring near the cardia. In addition there is an *inner circular layer*, which is reinforced in the pyloric part of the stomach, the scene of stronger contractions and true mixing of the ingesta. The sphincter pylori is part of this layer, as is the muscular core of the torus pyloricus

* Fig. 249 is on p. 202.

of swine. On the left, an *inner oblique layer* forms the sphincter cardiae and the cardial muscle loop.

VESSELS AND NERVES. The blood vessels of the stomach (Figs. 234A, 234B) form a submucosal net which gives off twigs into both the mucosa and the muscularis. In the latter they form capillary nets with oblong meshes (Fig. 91), which receive additional blood from the subserous net and from the arteries going to the submucosa. From the submucosal net, branches are given off toward the lumen at fairly regular intervals. These penetrate through the muscularis mucosae, which they supply by collateral branches, and form in the lamina propria a capillary meshwork, which surrounds each of the glands, including their openings. The venules that originate from the capillary areas form submucous and subserous venous plexuses, which give rise to the efferent veins (Fig. 234A,*a*). Arteriovenous anastomoses (p. 114) are present in the submucosa of the stomach. The lymphatics form a plexus in the propria. This plexus drains the periglandular and perivascular tissue spaces. The lymphatic trunks lie in the submucosa, from which they open into an intermuscular network of lymphatics. The nerves are derived from the vagus and sympathetic and form plexuses with many ganglia in the submucosa and intermuscular connective tissue. A similar situation is found in the intestine (p. 213).

SPECIES DIFFERENCES. The esophageal region or forestomach of the horse has a cutaneous, nonglandular mucosa (Fig. 211,*III*). This mucosa possesses a papillary body and is covered by a superficially cornified stratified squamous epithelium, which, at the margo plicatus, changes abruptly to the columnar epithelium of the glandular stomach. Aboral to the margo plicatus is a narrow, rather light-colored

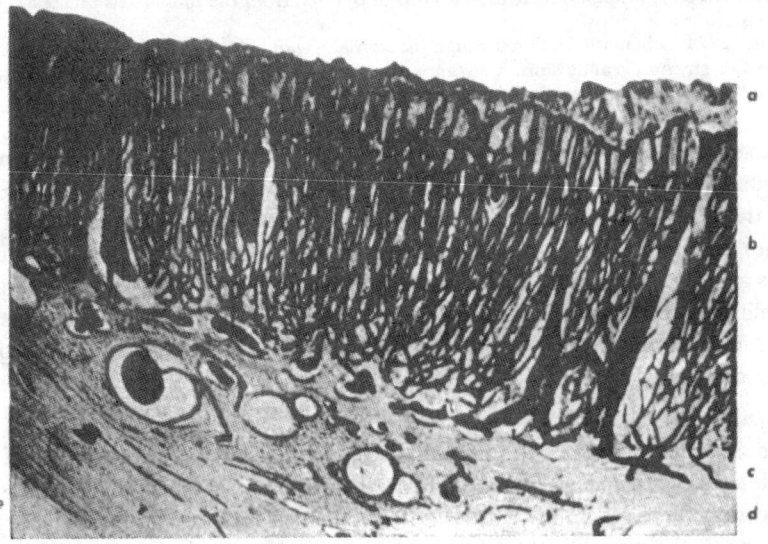

Figure 234B. Section through the stomach wall of the cat with blood vessels injected (40×). *a*, region of the gastric pits; *b*, gastric gland zone; *c*, muscularis mucosae; *d*, submucosa; *e*, muscularis (a portion of the circular layer).

zone which contains pyloric glands, scattered cardial glands, and lymphatic aggregates. At the greater curvature and on both stomach surfaces the cardial zone passes into the much thicker fundic gland mucosa. The transitional area between the two zones is very narrow and is marked by an admixture of fundic glands and by the appearance of parietal cells on the pyloric and cardial glands. The red-brown fundic gland zone is separated by a broad intermediate zone from the yellow-gray, thin pyloric mucosa. The latter occupies the pyloric region and the lesser curvature, where it meets the esophageal region and blends into the cardial transitional zone.

In the abomasum of the ruminant (Fig. 211,*VI*) we recognize a fundic and a pyloric gland region and an unimportant cranial transitional zone, which contains cardial, fundic, and pyloric glands. The thin mucosa of the extensive fundic gland zone is thrown into high, permanent folds and contains relatively short fundic glands. The pyloric mucosa is thicker, has no folds, and contains densely crowded pyloric glands.

In the stomach of swine (Fig. 211,*IV*) we distinguish a small esophageal part or forestomach, a very large cardial gland area, subdivided into two sections, and the fundic and pyloric regions. The esophageal part has a nonglandular, tough, cutaneous mucous membrane bearing stratified squamous epithelium. The cardial gland area includes the diverticulum ventriculi, which is especially rich in lymph nodules. The thin mucous membrane of the cardial zone contains many lymph nodules and the cardial glands (p. 192). The fundic mucous membrane is about twice as thick and contains long fundic glands. The fundic glands in the middle of

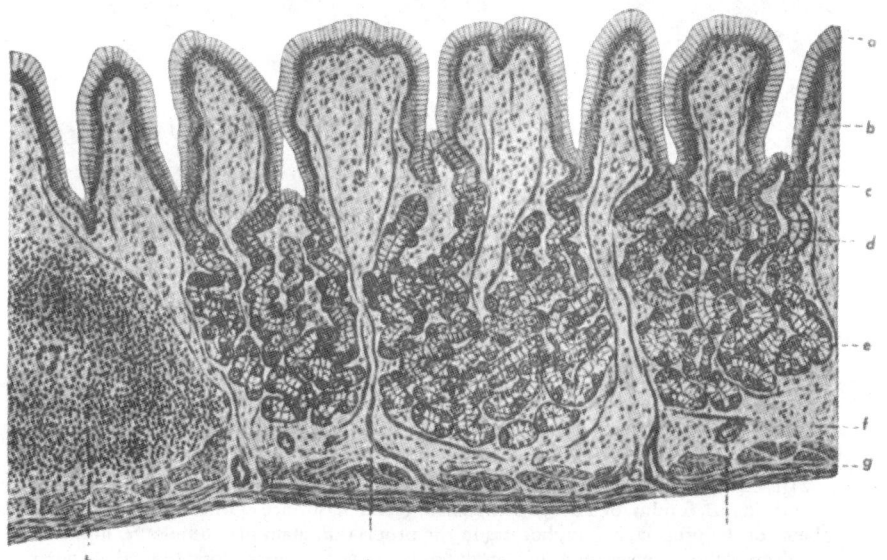

Figure 235. Section through the mucosa of the light zone in the fundic gland area of the dog. *a*, surface epithelium; *b*, gastric pits; *c,d*, neck of a gland; *e*, body of a gland; *f*, stratum subglandulare; *g*, muscularis mucosae; *h*, portion of a lymph nodule; *i*, ascending muscle bundles, derived from *g; k*, vessel.

the region are peculiar in that the parietal cells on the upper portion of the long glandular body are located in special recesses of the propria outside the glandular tube. The pyloric mucosa is somewhat thinner than the fundic and contains the pyloric glands, which are shorter, more tortuous, and more branched than the fundic glands and show a clublike enlargement at their blind end. Lymph craters are found here and in the transitional zones, and isolated parietal cells occur in pyloric and cardial glands.

The stomach of carnivores (Fig. 211,*II*) is divided into a fundic gland region and a pyloric gland region. Adjoining the cardia there is a narrow transitional zone containing cardial glands with and without parietal cells, true fundic glands, and pyloric glands with and without parietal cells. The thicker and darker fundic gland mucosa is subdivided into a small lighter-colored zone with a thinner mucous membrane and a larger aboral dark zone with a thick mucous membrane. In the former (Fig. 235) the gastric pits are deep. The glands appear in groups, are short and tortuous, and do not reach the muscularis mucosae. They contain fewer parietal cells than do the true fundic glands. A stratum compactum is absent. The darker subdivision (Fig. 222) contains true fundic glands and shallower pits than

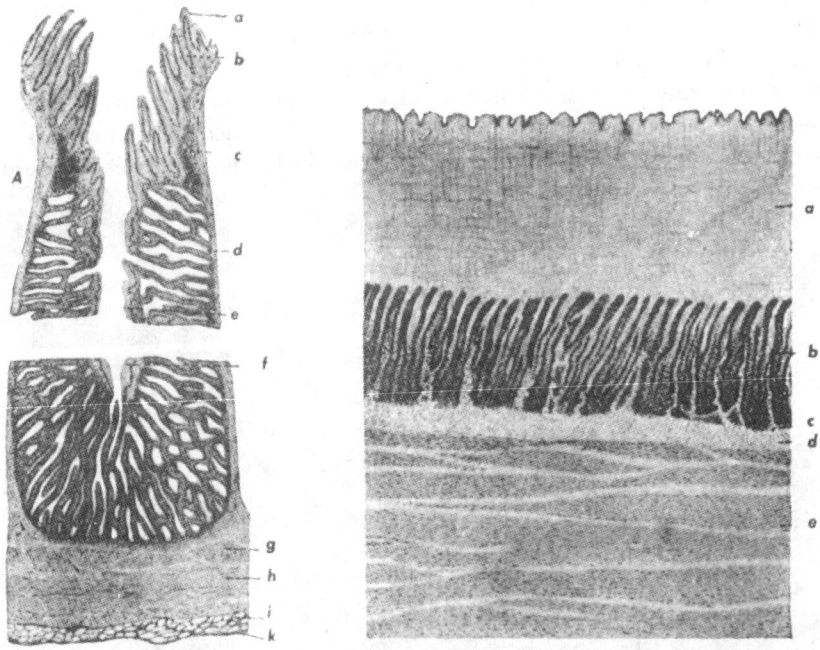

Figure 236 (left). Section through the wall of the proventriculus of the chicken (40×). *A,* opening, *B,* fundus, of a deep (compound) gland. *a,* surface epithelium; *b,* superficial glands of the propria; *c,* lymphocytes in the propria; *d,* glandular tubules; *e,* lumen of the deep gland; *f,* epithelium of the glandular lumen; *g,* inner longitudinal, *h,* outer circular, muscularis layer; *i,* subserosa with its longitudinal muscle layer; *k,* serosa.

Figure 237 (right). Cross section through the gizzard of the chicken (60×). *a,* horny layer; *b,* glandular layer; *c,* subglandular layer of the lamina propria; *d,* submucosa; *e,* muscularis.

either of the adjacent zones. The thinner, lighter pyloric mucosa has deep gastric pits and pyloric glands.

In poultry the stomach consists of the small, spindle-shaped proventriculus (glandular stomach) and the voluminous gizzard (ventriculus or muscular stomach). The two parts are connected by a necklike constriction. The mucous membrane of the glandular stomach (Fig. 236) exhibits longitudinal folds and is covered by a mucigenous, simple, high columnar epithelium (a), which is sharply marked off from the stratified squamous epithelium of the esophagus. As the epithelium dips into the small superficial glands of the propria (b), it becomes more cuboidal and loses its mucin reaction. In addition, the mucosa contains the deep compound glands of the propria, which are 2 mm. long (A,B). At the openings, which project like papillae, the mucosal epithelium dips into the comparatively wide lumen of the collecting sinuses (e). From these radiate branched secretory tubules lined by simple cuboidal epithelium. The glands are separated from each other by thin, highly vascular connective tissue septa, which show large aggregates of lymphocytes. The tunica muscularis consists of an inner thin longitudinal layer (g), an outer circular layer (h), and a very thin, partially absent subserous longitudinal sheet (i). The passage connecting proventriculus and gizzard contains no deep glands in its wall.

The lens-shaped gizzard (Fig. 237) presents a body with dorsal and ventral portions and the cranial and caudal blind sacs. The thick wall is composed of bundles of smooth muscle (e) which arch around the borders from one lateral aponeurosis to the other. Central to the muscle layer we find the connective tissue submucosa (d) and next the glandular layer, consisting of straight tubules lined by mostly cuboidal epithelium. The secretion of these glands is given off toward the lumen, solidifies, and forms over the inner surface a hard, keratinoid plate 1 mm. in thickness, which has a striated appearance in section and a rough grinding surface.

E. THE INTESTINAL TRACT

In the intestinal tract, which is at the same time an absorptive and an excretory organ, the most important processes of enzymatic digestion occur. These are brought about by the bile and the pancreatic and intestinal juices. The intestinal movements aid digestion by mixing and propelling the ingesta.

The intestinal wall consists of a mucosa, a muscularis, and a serosa.

1. Tunica Mucosa

The mucosa contains glands and lymph nodules and may be subdivided into the following layers:

a. The lamina epithelialis.

b. The lamina propria, which forms the lamina glandularis (Fig. 238,b) and in the small intestine also forms the nonglandular villi in the stratum villosum (Fig. 238,a).

c. The lamina muscularis mucosae (Figs. 238,e; 249,b'*).

---

* Fig. 249 is on p. 202.

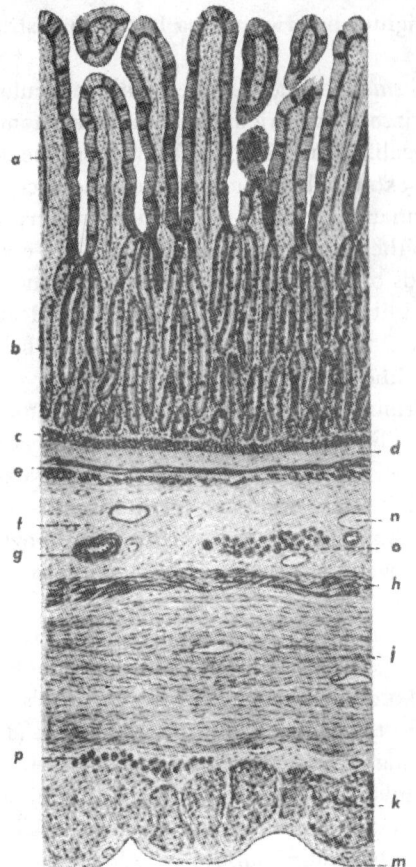

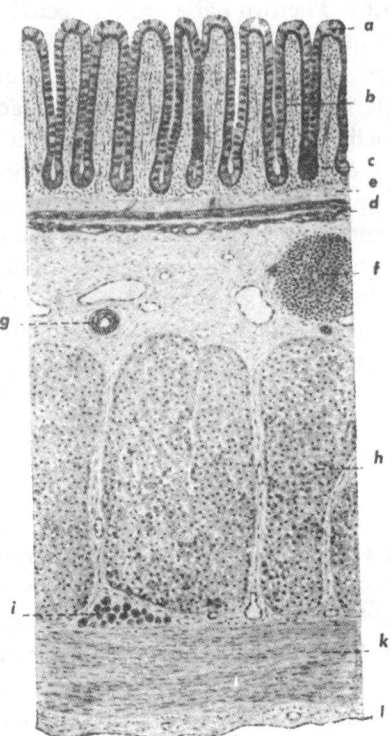

Figure 238 (*left*). Cross section through the small intestine of the dog (52×). *a*, villi; *b*, glands of Lieberkühn; *c*, stratum granulosum; *d*, stratum compactum; *e*, muscularis mucosae; *f*, submucosa; *g*, blood vessels; *h*, oblique, *i*, circular, *k*, longitudinal, layers of tunica muscularis; *m*, serosa; *n*, lymphatic; *o*, ganglion of Meissner's, *p*, of Auerbach's, plexus. The goblet cells of the surface epithelium are shown in black.

Figure 239 (*right*). Longitudinal section through the wall of the colon of a dog. *a*, surface epithelium; *b*, goblet cells; *c*, propria with glands of Lieberkühn; *d*, muscularis mucosae; *e*, stratum compactum; *f*, portion of a submucosal lymph nodule; *g*, artery; *h*, circular, *k*, longitudinal, layer of the muscularis; *i*, ganglion of the myenteric (Auerbach's) plexus; *l*, serosa.

d. The loose, large-meshed submucosa (Figs. 238,*f;* 249,*c′**), which contains the duodenal glands.

a. Lamina Epithelialis

The surface epithelium is simple and consists of columnar and goblet cells. Its *columnar cells* (Figs. 240; 244,*a*) are narrow and high and reach their greatest height on the villi. Their free surface bears a shiny cuticular border (Figs. 240,*a;* 241,*b;* 244,*a′*), which frequently appears to be striated. It is perforated by fine pores, into

---

* Fig. 249 is on p. 202.

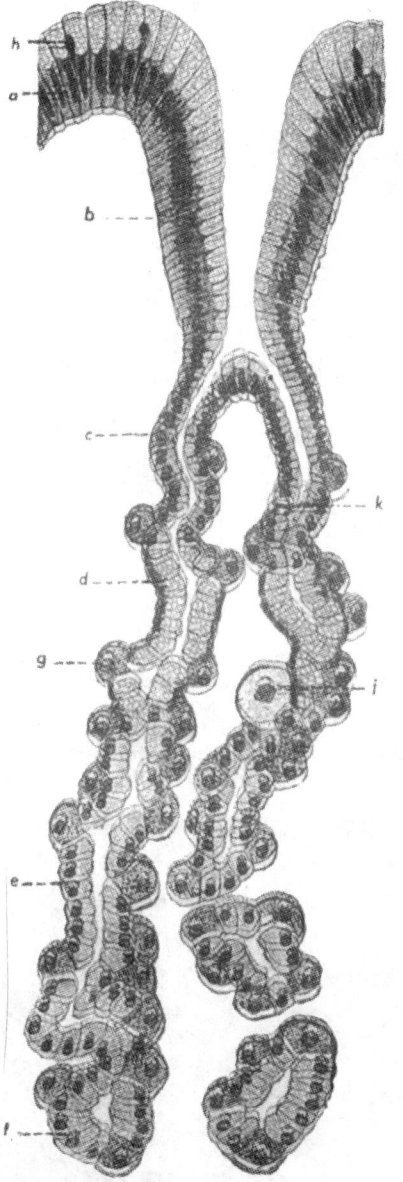

Figure 223. Fundic gland of the dog; stained with hemalum-eosin. *a*, gastric surface epithelium; *b*, epithelium of a gastric pit; *c*, epithelium of the neck of a gland near its opening; *d*, mucous neck cells near the body of the gland; *e,f*, chief (zymogenic) cells from the middle and fundus of the gland; *g*, parietal cells; *h*, leukocyte; *i*, large parietal cell; *k*, mitotic figure.

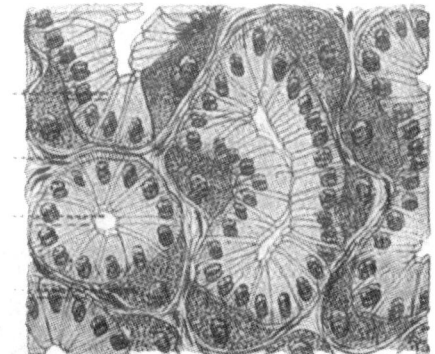

Figure 225. Cross section through the deepest portion of the fundic glands of the pig; stained with hemalum-eosin. *a*, chief cells; *b*, parietal cells; *c*, interglandular connective tissue; *d*, glandular lumen.

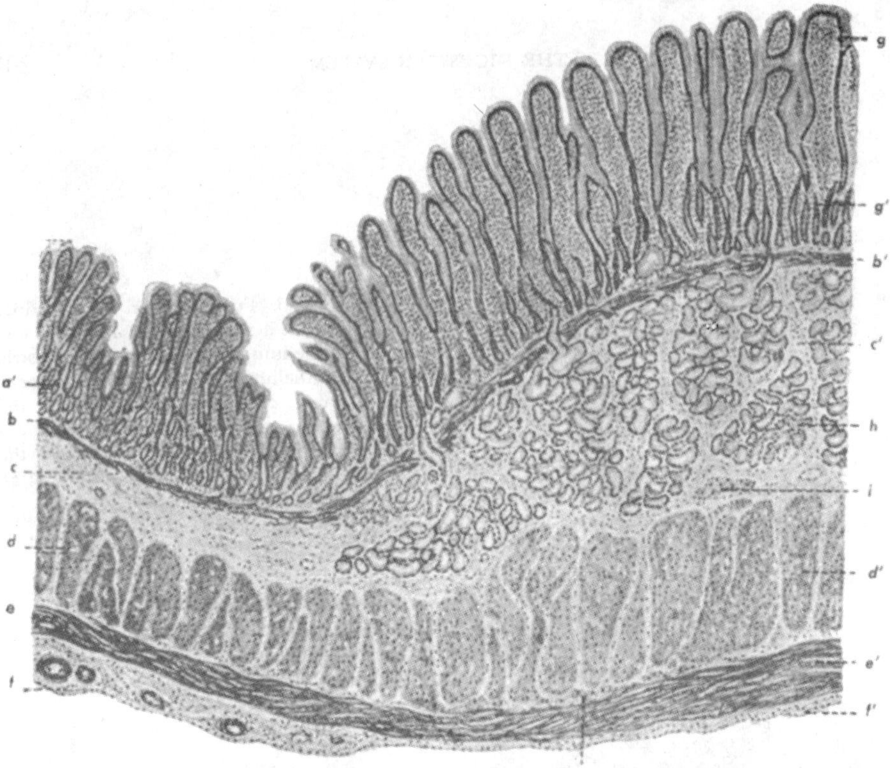

Figure 249. Longitudinal section through the gastrointestinal junction; stained with hemalum-eosin. *a*, surface epithelium of the stomach; *a'*, pyloric glands; *b*, muscularis mucosae of the stomach; *b'*, muscularis mucosae of the intestine; *c*, gastric, *c'*, intestinal, submucosa; *d*, circular layer of the gastric, *d'*, of the intestinal, tunica muscularis; *e*, longitudinal layer of the gastric, *e'*, of the intestinal, tunica muscularis; *f*, gastric, *f'*, intestinal serosa; *g*, surface epithelium of the small intestine; *g'*, glands of Lieberkühn; *h*, duodenal (Brunner's) glands; *i*, ganglion of Meissner's, *i'*, of Auerbach's, plexus. Note the transition from the stomach to the duodenum which is especially pronounced in the glands and the submucosa.

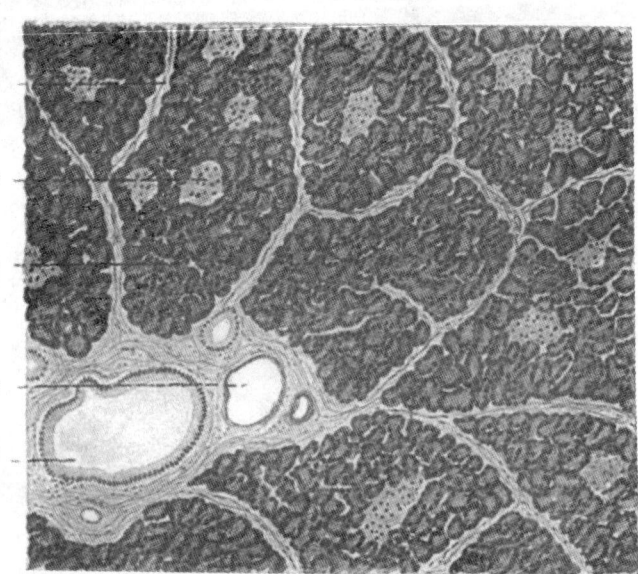

Figure 258. Section of the pancreas of the dog, at a low magnification; stained with hemalumeosin. *a*, islet of Langerhans; *b*, pancreatic lobule; *c*, interlobular connective tissue; *d*, excretory duct; *e*, blood vessel.

which rodlike, contractile cytoplasmic processes project. The cuticular border is demonstrable in the glandular epithelium in the upper part of the glands only. In the large intestine the border becomes lower and less distinctly striated. Intercellular clefts are present, which are filled with tissue fluid and sealed distally by a network of terminal bars. The cytoplasm of columnar cells exhibits several zones differing in their granule content. It is surrounded by a layer of ectoplasm and contains an abundance of fat droplets during fat absorption. The centrioles lie immediately below the cuticle, and the ellipsoid nucleus occupies a basal position.

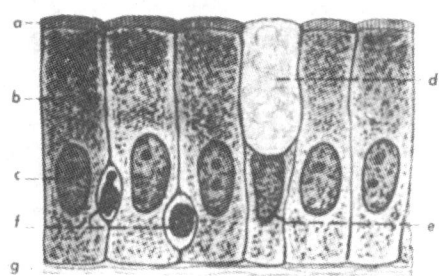

Figure 240. Surface epithelium from an intestinal villus of the donkey. *a*, cuticular border; *b*, cytoplasm; *c*, nucleus; *d*, goblet cell; *e*, its nucleus; *f*, nuclei of leukocytes; *g*, basement membrane.

The *goblet cells* (Figs. 240,*d;* 241,*c;* 242,*a''*) usually occur singly between the columnar cells. They contain varying amounts of mucin. Their nucleus is basally located, but their diplosome is embedded in the mucous masses of the distal cell half. Between the epithelial cells leukocytes are often encountered (Figs. 240,*f;* 241,*d*). These are wandering cells, which often penetrate into the lumen of the bowel, where they perish.

The columnar cells actively participate in the absorptive processes. Through its striated free surface, the epithelium takes up absorbable material from the intestinal contents and passes it on to the blood or lymph by way of the basal portion of its cells. The fatty acids and glycerol resulting from fat hydrolysis in the intestine are resynthesized within the epithelial cell to yield once more neutral fat, in which state it leaves the cells and enters the lacteals. The mucus secreted by the goblet cells protects the intestinal surface against mechanical irritation and noxious effects of the enzymes. In the large intestine it also acts as a lubricant aiding the movement of the thickened intestinal contents.

b. Lamina Propria

The lamina propria has a supporting framework of reticular tissue with elastic fibers and smooth muscle bundles. This contains various kinds of leukocytes (often eosinophils, plasma cells, lymphocytes), glands, and lymph nodules. The villi are projections of the tunica propria covered by surface epithelium.

The Intestinal Villi (Figs. 238,*a;* 241–243; 247,*a;* 249). These structures serve to increase the intestinal surface area available for absorption. They are roughly conical projections measuring on the average 0.5–1 mm. in length and 0.2 mm. in width. In the center of each villus occurs a tubular lymph space, lined by en-

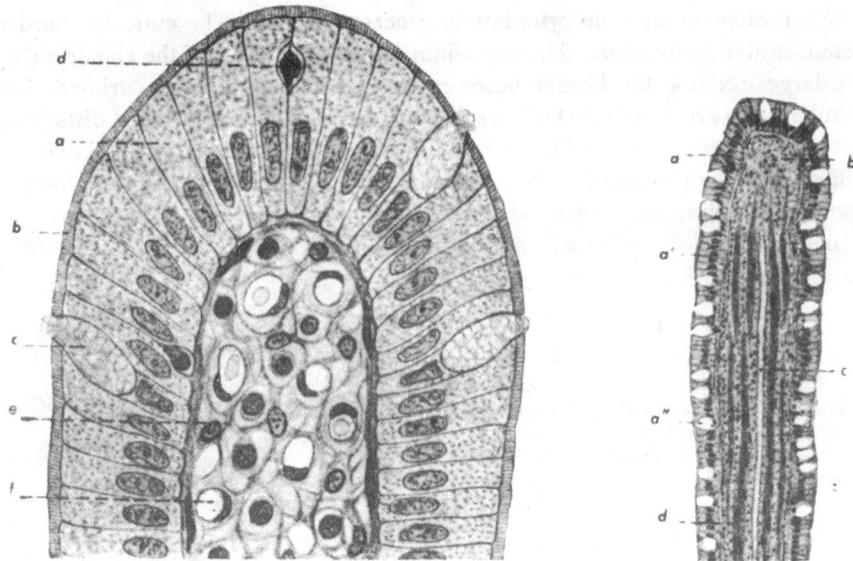

Figure 241 (left). Longitudinal section through the tip of an intestinal villus of the horse. *a,* columnar cell of the surface epithelium; *b,* cuticular border; *c,* goblet cells; *d,* leukocytes; *e,* reticular connective tissue of the villus; *f,* blood capillary.

Figure 242 (right). Longitudinal section through an intestinal villus of the cat. *a,* columnar cell of the surface epithelium; *a′,* its cuticular border; *a″,* goblet cell; *b,* connective tissue of the villus; *c,* central lacteal; *d,* smooth muscle bundles.

dothelium and known as a lacteal (Figs. 242; 243,*c*). Only in thicker villi, e.g., in sheep, do two or more lacteals occur. The reticular spongy stroma of the villi contains leukocytes, fat droplets, capillaries, nerves, and bundles of smooth muscle fibers (Figs. 242; 243,*d*). These originate in the muscularis mucosae and rise between the glands (Fig. 245,*i*) into the villi, where their number is increased. The bundles of longitudinal fibers extend to the tip of the villus, becoming thinner and sparser along the way. Often they appear in a central layer close to the lacteal and in another, peripheral layer. Toward the surface of the villus the stroma condenses into a limiting layer (Fig. 241) which is covered by flattened cells and contains blood vessels and smooth muscle fibers. Delicate, frequently perforated collagenous or elastic membranes extend transversely across the stroma of the villi. A net of fine elastic fibers is also present. This is densest around the lacteal.

The carnivores (Fig. 242) possess the longest and most slender villi; the ruminants (Figs. 247, 251) have the shortest and thickest ones. Shape, size, and number of villi vary in the different sections of the small intestine. Contraction of the smooth muscle fibers causes a shortening of the villi with the formation of circular folds of the epithelium. This widens the lacteals and presses their contents into the efferent lymphatics. The transverse elastic fibers and membranes, which are stretched in the process, cause the villi to return to their former shape and size. The contraction incident to fixation causes a withdrawal of the stroma from the epithelial cover in histological preparations.

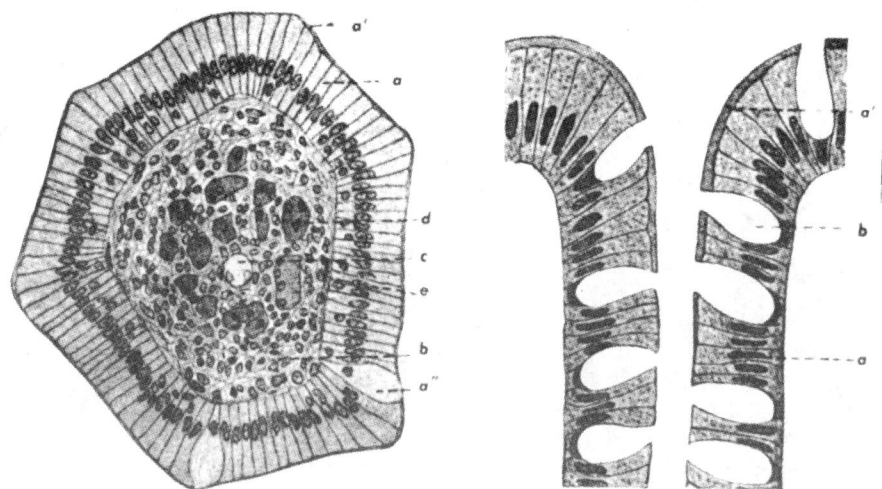

Figure 243 (left). Cross section through an intestinal villus of the horse. *a*, surface epithelium; *a'*, its cuticular border; *a''*, goblet cell; *b*, connective tissue of the villus; *c*, central lacteal; *d*, smooth muscle bundles in cross section; *e*, basement membrane.

Figure 244 (right). Beginning of a gland of Lieberkühn in the colon of a dog. *a*, columnar cell of the glandular epithelium; *a'*, cuticular border; *b*, goblet cell.

The Intestinal Glands (Glands of Lieberkühn, Figs. 238,*b;* 239,*c;* 244; 246; 247,*b;* 249,*g'**). The glands are tightly packed, usually simple tubules, which resemble the fingers of a glove. They are found in the propria from the pylorus to the anus. The glands are surrounded by a reticular sheath and consist of glandular epithelium with a thin basement membrane. The epithelium is made up of the same elements as the surface epithelium, with which it is continuous. The columnar cells of the glands, however, are lower (Fig. 244,*a*), and their cuticular border becomes less and less distinct in the deeper portions of the gland until it finally disappears altogether. Goblet cells (Figs. 244,*b;* 245,*c*), which may arise at any time by transformation of ordinary columnar cells, are more abundant here than in the surface epithelium. Their goblets, however, are smaller. Goblet cells are most plentiful in the glands of the large intestine (Fig. 239,*b*). Here the goblet cells may even be in the majority or occur alone, but as a rule they alternate with columnar cells. These may often be so narrow that they are overlooked on casual examination. Usually only ruminants show goblet cells in the blind ends of the glands of the small intestine. These cells occur in the glands of the large intestine of all species, but are smaller. Mitotic figures are regularly encountered in the glandular epithelium. The cells produced here are pushed up to replace worn-out surface cells. Wandering cells also occur in the glandular epithelium. They are especially numerous near the lymph nodules.

In the small intestine and cecum the gland fundus contains the specialized, markedly granular *cells of Paneth* (Fig. 246,*c*), which are absent in carnivores and swine. The glands of Lieberkühn open on the surface epithelium between the villi.

---

* Fig. 249 is on p. 202.

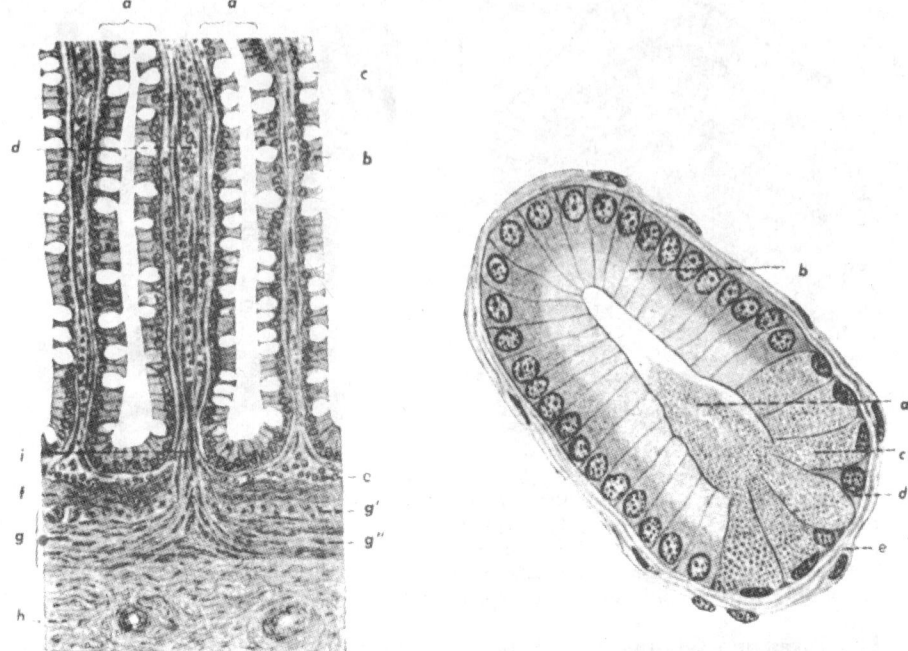

Figure 245 (left). Glands of Lieberkühn from the small intestine of the dog: villi not shown. a, glands; b, columnar, c, goblet, cell of the glandular epithelium; d, interglandular tissue; e, stratum granulosum; f, stratum compactum; g, muscularis mucosae; g', circular, g", longitudinal layers of g; h, submucosa; i, muscle bundle entering the glandular layer from g.

Figure 246 (right). Fundus of a gland of Lieberkühn from the small intestine of the horse (oblique section). a, lumen with secretory granules; b, columnar cell of the glandular epithelium; c, cell of Paneth filled with granules; d, compressed columnar cell; e, basement membrane.

Between the glands of Lieberkühn in the duodenum we also encounter excretory ducts of the submucosal glands as they pass through the propria.

Enterochromaffin or *argentaffin* cells occur in all domestic animals along the entire gastrointestinal tract, especially in the epithelium of the glands of Lieberkühn, but also in the surface epithelium and between the duodenal gland cells. They occur singly or, more rarely, in groups. They are characterized by a peculiar, fine granulation in the basal portion of the cell. Their significance is not clear. They have also been found in the epithelium of the bile and pancreatic ducts, as well as in the glands of the gall bladder of the ox.

Generally the glands of the large intestine are farther apart than those of the small intestine, but they are longer and straighter (except in goats, in which all the intestinal glands are tortuous) and have a wider lumen.

The glands of Lieberkühn of the small intestine furnish mucus and several enzymes which attack peptides, fats, and carbohydrates. They also produce enterokinase, which activates the trypsinogen of the pancreatic juice. Which of the gland cells produce the enzymes has not been satisfactorily determined. In the large intestine much mucus and little if any enzyme is secreted. Bacterial fermentation and putrefaction predominate here.

Between the blind endings of the glands of Lieberkühn and the muscularis mucosae of horses and carnivores lies the thin lamina subglandularis. In carnivores this layer is subdivided into a stratum granulosum (Figs. 238,c; 245,e), which contains many leukocytes, and a nearly homogeneous stratum compactum bordering on the muscularis mucosae (Figs. 238,d; 245,f). The horse has only a stratum granulosum, which is relatively poor in cellular elements.

c. Muscularis Mucosae

The muscularis mucosae (Figs. 245,g; 247,c; 249,b'*; 251,c) consists of bundles of smooth muscle fibers, which are often arranged in two sheets perpendicular to one another. They also interweave. In the area of the duodenal glands the muscularis mucosae is discontinuous and even absent in parts because it splits into separate strands, which dip into the glandular layer. It may also be interrupted in spots by the nodules of Peyer's patches (Fig. 251).

d. Submucosa

The submucosa (Figs. 247,d; 249,c'*) consists of loose fibrillar connective tissue and elastic fiber nets. It contains fat cells, lymph nodules, autonomic ganglia (Figs. 238,o; 239,i), nerves, and vessels. Its thickness varies with the intestinal region and

* Fig. 249 is on p. 202.

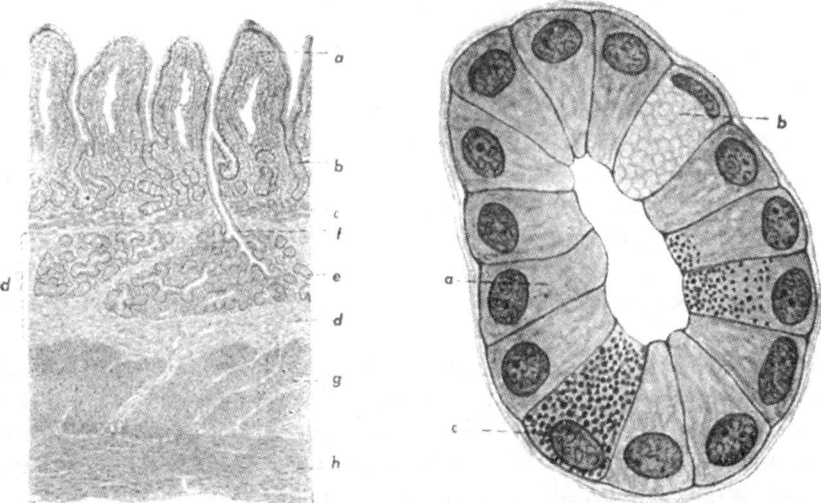

Figure 247 (left). Longitudinal section through the wall of the duodenal gland zone of the ox. *a,* villi showing central lacteals; *b,* glands of Lieberkühn; *c,* muscularis mucosae; *d,* submucosa; *e,* lobule of a duodenal gland; *f,* its excretory duct; *g,* circular, *h,* longitudinal, layer of the tunica muscularis.

Figure 248 (right). Cross section through the body of a duodenal gland of the horse (750×). *a,* serous cell; *b,* mucous cell; *c,* cell of Paneth.

the individual. It is heaviest in the duodenal gland zone of solipeds and thinnest in ruminants.

The Duodenal Glands (Brunner's Glands; Figs. 247,*e;* 248; 249,*h**). These are branched tubuloalveolar glands. Their lobules are usually located in the submucosa but may project into the lamina propria or even lie entirely within it. Their lighter staining reaction makes it easy to differentiate them from the glands of Lieberkühn. The secretory portion is lined with low columnar cells (Fig. 248,*a*), which, in carnivora, resemble the cells of the pyloric glands and very likely are related to them. The cells rest on a basement membrane and have basally located

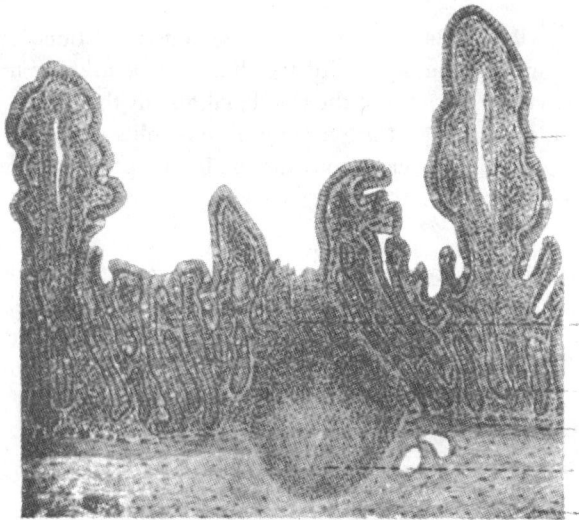

Figure 250. Section through a solitary lymph nodule in the mucosa of the small intestine of the pig. *a*, villus; *b*, gland of Lieberkühn; *c*, muscularis mucosae; *d*, submucosa; *e*, lymph nodule with *f*, its germinal center.

spheroid or flattened nuclei. Around the lobules and between the end-pieces we find muscle fibers or muscle bundles, which are derived from the muscularis mucosae. The unbranched excretory duct of the duodenal glands (Fig. 247,*f*) is lined with columnar cells resembling those of the surface epithelium. Isolated goblet cells occur between the columnar cells. The duct passes through the glandular layer of the propria and ends between the villi on the surface, or occasionally in a gland of Lieberkühn.

The duodenal gland zone begins at the pylorus. Its length is subject to individual variation: carnivores—1.5 to 2 cm., man—10 to 15 cm., goat—20 to 25 cm., sheep —60 to 70 cm.; pig—3 to 5 meters, ox—4 to 5 meters, soliped—5 to 6 meters. In the pig and the horse, lobules occur which are purely serous or have both serous and mucous cells side by side. Paneth cells (in the horse, Fig. 248,*c*), goblet cells (in the horse, ox, and sheep), narrow, dark cells (Stöhr's cells), and degenerating cells have been found in the glandular epithelium. In the lumen and interstitial tissue stratified coagula are frequently encountered (horse, pig). The mucous secretion of the duodenal glands contains an amylase and enterokinase. Secretory capillaries are absent.

* Fig. 249 is on p. 202.

Lymph Nodules. In the intestine these occur as isolated solitary nodules (Figs. 239,*f;* 250,*e,f*) or in larger groups in the form of Peyer's patches (Fig. 251,*e*). In addition to these, diffuse lymphatic aggregates are present in many sections of the intestine.

The usually spheroid, pyriform, or ovoid solitary nodules are located, at the beginning of their development, entirely in the lamina propria. Later they are found at varying depths. Small nodules confined to the propria are relatively rare. Most of the nodules are more deeply located, with a large, well-circumscribed portion in the submucosa and a smaller, poorly defined part in the propria (Fig. 250).

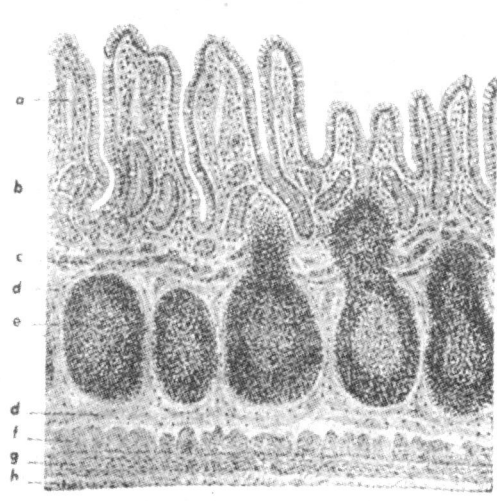

Figure 251. Longitudinal section through the jejunal wall of the goat at the site of a Peyer's patch. *a,* villus; *b,* gland of Lieberkühn; *c,* muscularis mucosae; *d,* submucosa; *e,* lymph nodule; *f,* circular, *g,* longitudinal, muscle layers; *h,* serosa.

There are also lymph nodules that lie entirely within the submucosa. Often a false impression of a submucosal position is created by sections that strike only the thick submucosal part of a nodule. Their number, size, and shape vary greatly with the species, intestinal region, individual, age, constitution, and other factors. Their size ranges from microscopic to more than 2 mm. in diameter. The intestine of swine is especially rich in lymphatic organs.

Peyer's patches are aggregates of lymph nodules (Fig. 251). They are plaquelike elevations or depressions in the mucosa, usually on the side opposite the attachment of the mesentery, and commonly lie in the propria and submucosa. The single nodules in the patch often coalesce so that only the germinal centers give a clue to the location of the component nodules. In young growing animals the solitary nodules and patches are larger and more numerous than in adults. The number of nodules in a patch may vary widely. Patches occur which consist of but a few (2–5) nodules. On the other hand, such masses of nodules may be present that the resulting plaques measure several meters (up to 3.5 in swine). Wherever obstructive mechanisms are present in the intestine, as in the ileocecal region, causing a relative stasis of the contents, lymphatic structures, usually plaques, are present in large quantities. In the large intestine the solitary nodules are more frequent than in the small intestine, but the patches are fewer.

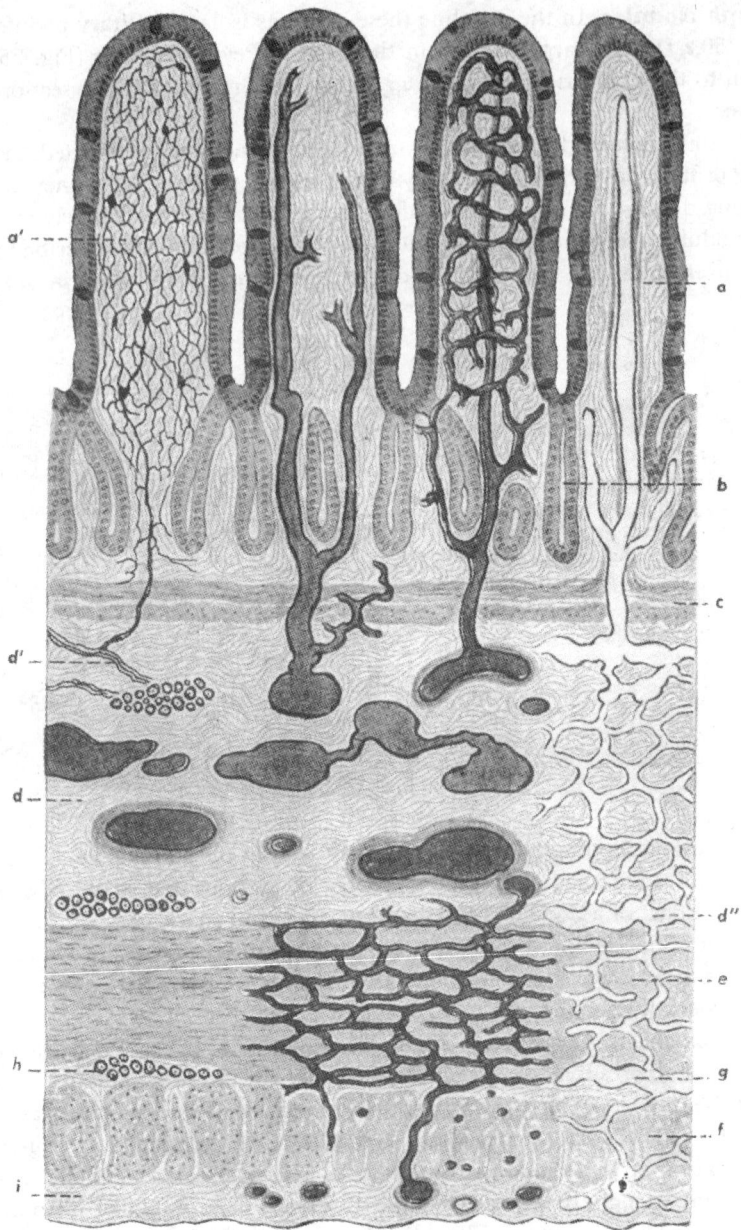

Figure 252. Cross section through the small intestine showing blood vessels, lymphatics, and nerves. Arteries and blood capillaries shown in red, veins in blue, lymphatics in white, nerves black. *a*, villus with lacteal and smooth muscle fibers; *a'*, villus with nerve plexus; *b*, gland of Lieberkühn; *c*, two-layered muscularis mucosae; *d*, submucosa; *d'*, submucosal (Meissner's) plexus; *d''*, lymphatic network; *e*, circular, *f*, longitudinal, muscle layer; *g*, lymphatic network in the intermuscularis; *h*, myenteric (Auerbach's) plexus with nerve cells in the intermuscularis; *i*, serosa.

In the vicinity of lymph nodules the intestinal wall often presents a changed appearance (Figs. 250, 251). The muscularis mucosae is interrupted, split, or displaced, and the glands of Lieberkühn and Brunner are pushed aside by the nodules. The glandular and surface epithelium contains many leukocytes near the lymph nodules and sometimes has an eroded appearance. In the region of the nodules the propria, too, is always rich in leukocytes. Wherever the nodules are deeply embedded, the villi of the intestine are unchanged; where the nodules are superficial, the villi are shorter than usual or lacking entirely. They are often so rich in leukocytes that they look like projections of lymphatic mucous membrane. On the site of a group of nodules the mucosa may also show a crater-shaped depression which lacks glands and villi.

Similar conditions prevail in birds. In all species of birds the lymphatic structures increase in number toward the vent. The lymphatic tissue reaches the highest degree of development in the ceca, where it is often arranged around crypts and exhibits a tonsil-like character.

2. Tunica Muscularis

The muscular tunic of the intestine (Figs. 238,*h,i,k;* 239,*h,k;* 247,*g,h;* 249,*d',e'**) consists of an outer thinner longitudinal layer and an inner circular layer. The two layers are connected by the intermuscular connective tissue. The longitudinal layer of the large intestine of man, horse, and pig forms taeniae (see p. 213) between which there is only a thin layer of longitudinal muscle fibers. The small intestine of carnivores has, in addition to the usual two layers, an innermost thin layer of oblique fibers, which immediately adjoins the submucosa (Fig. 238,*h*).

The intestinal wall is relatively rich in elastic tissue. It contains numerous fine-to-medium-thick elastic fibers, which in some portions form continuous nets throughout the entire thickness of the intestinal wall. In the muscularis there is an accumulation of elastic tissue in the intermuscular stratum. The intestinal wall of the carnivores is richest in elastic tissue, which makes up a continuous dense network below the blind ends of the glands of Lieberkühn. This elastic layer is thin in the horse, ox, and pig and hardly demonstrable in the goat and sheep.

THE BLOOD VESSELS OF THE INTESTINAL WALL (Fig. 252). The arteries enter the intestinal wall from the mesentery, perforate the longitudinal muscle layer, and give off branches into the stratum intermusculare, forming a plexus from which the muscular tunic is supplied. The trunks of the arteries penetrate through the circular muscle layer and into the submucosa, where they divide into many anastomosing branches and make up the submucous arterial plexus. This gives off short arteries to the glands of the mucosa and, in the small intestine, to the long arteries of the villi. The former penetrate the muscularis mucosae and form abundant periglandular capillary nets. The latter divide into several branches in the propria. Each branch as a rule ascends directly to the tip of a villus, where it gives rise to a capillary net, which, in turn, is drained by the veins of the villus. In the glandular layer the veins of the villi (Fig. 252) and the veins arising from the periglandular

---

* Fig. 249 is on p. 202.

capillary nets combine to form venous trunks, which form a submucous plexus. This plexus gives rise to larger venous trunks, which run with the arteries through the muscularis and enter the mesentery.

The small intestine also has a shunting mechanism in its circulatory system. In man and rodents the tips of the villi contain an arteriovenous connecting loop. The arteries of the villi do not branch until they reach the tips of the villi, where the divide into a nutrient branch to the capillary net and a thicker second branch, which passes immediately into the vein (Fig. 253). Except during the actual process of digestion the arterial branch to the capillary net is blocked off, causing the blood to be shunted into the vein. During digestion and absorption the entire

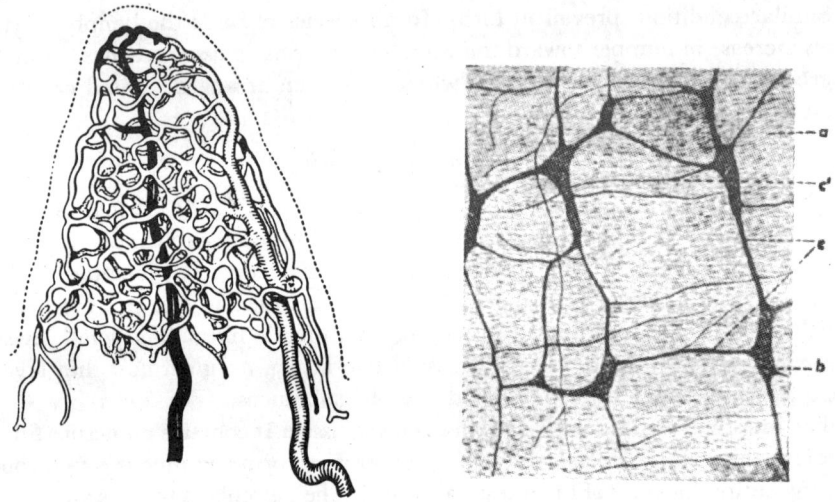

Figure 253 (left). Tongue-shaped papilla from the jejunum of the rat, showing injected blood vessels (190✕). Black = artery; shaded = vein; white = capillaries on the surface toward the observer; stippled = away from the observer. (After Spanner.)

Figure 254 (right). Myenteric plexus. *a*, muscle; *b*, nerve cells; *c*, nerve fibers; *c′*, delicate rami of *c*.

capillary system is also filled with blood. The villi of horses, carnivores, and pigs lack arteriovenous loops. Instead they have arteriovenous anastomoses in the submucosa, which make possible a partial by-passing of the capillary circuit while digestion is not taking place. The anastomoses precede the villous circulation. They are composed of arteries equipped with occlusive mechanisms (p. 113), which enter special venous plexuses. The venous plexuses give rise to submucosal veins that are equipped with sphincters and intervening nonmuscular, highly dilatable sections. When the sphincters contract, these sections serve as blood reservoirs. The blood and lymph vessels of the large intestine are quite similar to those of the stomach.

LYMPHATICS OF THE INTESTINAL WALL (Figs. 238,*n*; 252). Every intestinal villus contains a wide, blindly ending lymphatic, called a lacteal (*a*). At the base of the villi the lacteals divide into branches, which unite into a plexus situated below the villi. From this plexus originates a network, which surrounds the glands of the propria. Nets of lymph capillaries also surround each lymph nodule. Lymph capillaries arising in the propria penetrate the muscularis mucosae and empty into the submucous net of lymphatics, which are equipped with valves (d''). Some of the lymphatics of the muscularis empty into this net. Most of them, however, drain into an intermuscular (g) and a subserous net. All these nets are interconnected by transverse branches and give rise to the trunks that pass into the mesentery.

NERVES. The nerves of the intestine (Fig. 252) are mostly unmyelinated and form three plexuses, in which we find groups of multipolar nerve cells. The coarser myenteric plexus of Auerbach (Figs. 252,h; 254) lies in the stratum intermusculare between the two muscle layers (Figs. 238,p; 239,i) and gives off axons ending on the muscle fibers. It is connected by numerous branches with the finer submucosal plexus of Meissner (Fig. 252,d'). The latter furnishes the fibers that supply the mucosa. They, too, form a plexus with which ganglia are associated. These nerve fibers are derived from parasympathetic nerves (the vagus and pelvic nerve) and sympathetic nerves. The stomach is quite similarly innervated (see p. 196).

REGIONAL DIFFERENCES. The small intestine is characterized by the presence of villi, which are lacking in the large intestine. Duodenum, jejunum, and ileum do not show constant differential features that apply to all species of domestic animals. Generally speaking, the occurrence of duodenal glands is confined to the first portion of the small intestine (pars duodenalis), but their area of distribution does not coincide with that of the anatomical duodenum (see p. 208). The ileum of the horse is distinguished by a particularly heavy muscularis. In other species the thickness of the muscularis also increases in the ileum, except in cattle, where it decreases.

The large intestine lacks villi (Fig. 239). Its mucosa is thicker; its glands of Lieberkühn are longer and straighter (they are tortuous in goats only) and very rich in goblet cells. The large intestine of man, solipeds, and swine possesses flat bands of longitudinal muscle, the taeniae. In the cecum and large colon of the horse the taeniae are so rich in elastic fibers and so poor in muscular elements that they may be considered elastic bands. The taeniae of swine are also rich in elastic tissue.

The rectum lacks taeniae. Its surface epithelium does not show a well-developed cuticular border. The rectal glands contain an abundance of goblet cells. The muscular tunic is heavier than that of the colon, especially in the horse and ox. In the terminal portion of the rectum the serosa is replaced by a loose collagenous adventitia. The rectal wall is exceedingly rich in elastic tissue.

In ruminants the termination of the rectum exhibits a zona columnaris consisting of 5–8 permanent longitudinal folds of mucosa (rectal columns) and the intervening sinuses. The mucosa in this region contains patches of lymph nodules.

INTESTINAL TRACT OF BIRDS (Fig. 255). The intestine begins with the long U-shaped duodenal loop, which encloses the pancreas. Next follow the loops of small intestine suspended by a long mesentery. The beginning of the large intestine is marked by the openings of the two ceca. The short colon soon widens into the cloaca, into which the urinary and genital tracts also open. The cloaca opens at

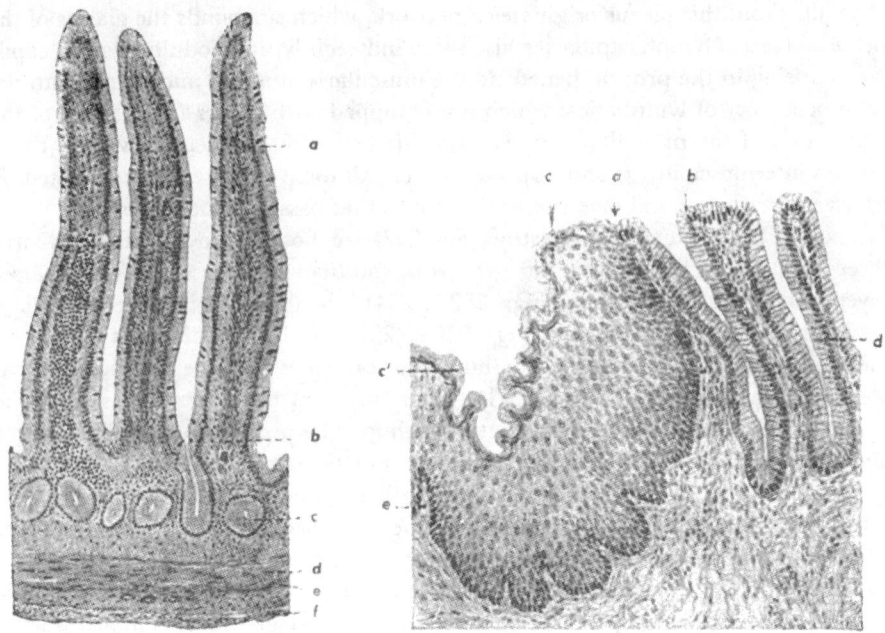

Figure 255 (left). Cross section through the small intestine of the chicken (55×). *a,* epithelium of the villi with cuticular border and interspersed goblet cells; *b,* propria with lymphocytes; *c,* glands of Lieberkühn; *d,* inner circular, *e,* outer longitudinal, layer of the tunica muscularis; *f,* serosa.

Figure 256 (right). Section through the mucosa of the anorectal junction of a calf. *a,* change of epithelium (linea anorectalis); *b,* columnar epithelium of the rectal mucosa; *c,* stratified squamous epithelium of the anal mucosa showing *c',* the stratum corneum; *d,* glands of Lieberkühn of the rectum; *e,* papillary body of the anal mucosa.

the vent. The entire intestinal mucosa is characterized by the presence of regularly arranged villi, which are very long in the duodenum (1.5 mm.) but gradually become shorter and thicker. The structural relationships resemble those of the mammalian intestine to a high degree. The simple columnar epithelium (*a*) bears a cuticular border, contains goblet cells, and covers the stroma of the villi, which contain in addition to the usual elements a central lacteal surrounded by bundles of smooth muscle. The propria (*b*) has the characteristics of diffuse lymphatic tissue. It often contains eosinophils. The epithelium of the short glands of Lieberkühn (*c*) is remarkable for the many mitotic figures present. The muscularis mucosae consists of longitudinal fibers and is bordered by a generally poorly developed submucosa. The tunica muscularis (*d,e*) is composed of an inner thicker circular layer and an outer longitudinal layer. Duodenal glands are absent. The ceca (in the chicken 15–25 cm.; in the pigeon 5–6 mm.) arise from the intestine by a narrow tubular segment, which is equipped with a sphincter. Masses of lymphocytes are present in the mucosa. The villi become shorter as they approach the blind end and finally disappear altogether. Large tonsillar follicles containing germinal centers are present in the lamina propria. They cause a bulging of the mucosa. At the

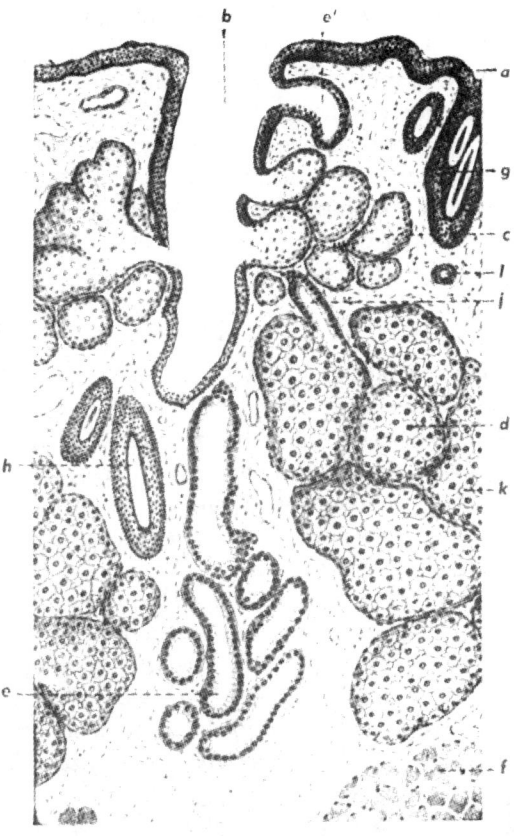

Figure 257. Group of glands of the circumanal region of the dog (70×). *a*, epidermis; *b*, distended hair follicle acting as collecting sinus for secretions; *c*, holocrine sebaceous glands; *d*, circumanal gland; *e*, tubular gland; *e'*, its opening; *f*, striated muscle; *g*, hair follicles with hairs; *h*, oblique section of a hair; *i*, excretory duct of *d* (disputed, see text); *k*, intercellular spaces (artefacts?); *l*, artery.

apex of the bulge is the opening of the crypt, which may be lined by columnar epithelium. At the cloacal end of the intestine the villi become low and broad, the glands grow longer, and the goblet cells more numerous.

The Anal Mucosa (Fig. 256). The cutaneous mucous membrane has a papillary body (*e*) and stratified squamous epithelium (*c*). At the anorectal line it passes abruptly into the rectal mucosa (*a*). In swine and carnivores it forms a zona columnaris ani, which contains both diffuse and nodular lymphatic tissue. Venous erectile tissue is also present. In the dog and pig only, we find the tubuloalveolar *anal glands*, which in swine furnish a mucous secretion, in dogs a fatty one. They open outside the columnar zone in the zona intermedia. The anal mucosa is otherwise free of glands except for the terminal section, the zona cutanea, which is characterized by a cornified epithelium, hairs, and sebaceous and tubular glands.

In the dog the *circumanal glands* (Fig. 257,*d*) occur here. These have recéntly been reinvestigated by Parks[9] and found to consist of an upper sebaceous portion with a patent duct to a hair follicle, and a deeper, nonsebaceous portion. The non-

---

[9] Harold F. Parks, *Morphological and Cytochemical Observations on the Circumanal Glands of Dogs*, Ph.D. thesis, Cornell University, Ithaca, N.Y., 1950.

sebaceous lobules are solid masses of large polygonal cells with pale nuclei. They contain proteinaceous cytoplasmic granules. These were formerly interpreted as secretory granules, and it was claimed that a serous secretion was discharged through intercellular canaliculi 1–2 μ in diameter into patent excretory ducts. Parks, who was unable to demonstrate secretory canaliculi between the cells and who found that the ducts to this portion of the gland were solid, not patent, concludes that the nonsebaceous cells exhibit no evidence of secretory activity.

Lateral and ventral to the anus of carnivores are the anal sacs with their anal sac glands (see Chapter XVII).

F. THE PANCREAS

The pancreas (Figs. 258*, 259, 260*) is a compound tubuloacinous gland. The framework, vessels, nerves, lobule formation, and basement membrane of the secretory end-pieces all show the same relationships as the corresponding portions of the salivary glands. The pancreas differs from the salivary glands in the peculiarity of its glandular epithelium, the absence of striated tubules and basket cells, and the presence of the islets of Langerhans. In dogs and cats the interstitial tissue contains Pacinian corpuscles.

The conical or pyramid-shaped secretory cells (Figs. 259,a; 260,c*) are arranged in a single layer. They resemble serous cells but are distinguished by the presence of two zones. The inner zone is coarsely granular, while the somewhat shiny outer (basal) zone appears almost homogeneous or may present faint radial striations. The spheroid nucleus lies in the outer zone, but in such a manner that a portion of it projects into the inner zone. A centriole is found near the nucleus. During secretion an eosinophilic spheroid or crescent-shaped structure is often present close to the nucleus. Its significance is not clear.

The two zones of the secretory cells have different staining properties (Fig. 259), and their relative extent varies with the functional status of the cell. In the fasting animal the strongly refractive and acidophilic zymogen granules of the inner zone are numerous and the inner zone is large. In the digesting animal the granules, which are the precursors of the digestive enzymes, are extruded, making the cell smaller and its outer zone wider.

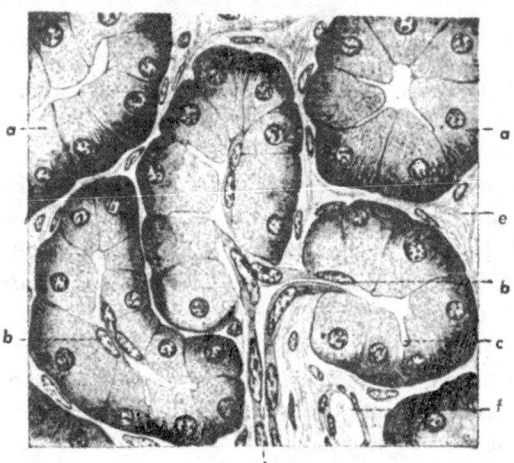

Figure 259. Section from the pancreas of the ox, at a high magnification; stained with hemalum-eosin. *a,* secretory cells; *b,* centroacinar cells; *c,* secretory capillary; *d,* intercalated duct; *e,* interalveolar tissue; *f,* blood vessel.

* Fig. 258 is on p. 202 and Fig. 260 on p. 220.

The lumen of the end-piece is narrow and sends secretory capillaries between the gland cells (Fig. 259,c). The glandular end-pieces are continued by long intercalated ducts lined by flat or cuboidal epithelium (d). Their initial portions often appear inside the lumen of the end-pieces as centroacinar cells (b), which are applied to the inside of the secretory cells but permit the secretory capillaries to pass to the lumen. The intralobular intercalated ducts pass immediately into interlobular ducts (Fig. 258,d*), which are lined by simple columnar epithelium. The cells of this epithelium become higher as the ducts grow larger and are acidophilic like the striated tubules of the salivary glands. Basal striations, however, are absent. The lamina propria of the interlobular ducts of the ox contains smooth muscle fibers.

The exocrine secretion of the pancreas contains an abundance of enzymes, which effect the digestion of proteins, fats, and carbohydrates.

The pancreas of all mammals contains small (0.04–0.2 mm.) partially encapsulated cell aggregates: the *islets of Langerhans* (Figs. 258,a*; 260,b*). These are networks of cellular cords whose meshes are filled by sinusoidal capillaries. There is no connection with the excretory ducts. Fine secretory granules are occasionally visible in the cytoplasm of the cells. The latter have so little affinity for the usual stains that the islets appear as lighter spots in stained sections. Special staining methods, however, have shown at least three and possibly four types of cells to be present in the islets. Which of these types are separate cells and which are merely different metabolic stages of the same cell are problems that have not been satisfactorily solved. The size and number of the islets are subject to great variation. On the average there is an islet to every 1–3 sq. mm. The total number of islets in man is estimated at 0.75 to 1.5 million. The total volume of the islet tissue would amount to 1 cc. The islets of Langerhans are endocrine organs and furnish one hormone governing sugar metabolism—insulin—and one concerned with lipid metabolism—lipocaic.

The pancreas has one or two excretory ducts that run part of their course outside the gland and enter the duodenum (extrapancreatic ducts). Because the human nomenclature is not applicable to the dog, ox, or pig, it seems advisable to use the term *Wirsung's duct* for the one that terminates close to the bile duct and to refer to the other as the *duct of Santorini* (the accessory duct in man). The epithelium lining the ducts is columnar and contains goblet cells. The larger interlobular and extrapancreatic ducts have mucous glands and smooth muscle cells in their walls. The latter increase in the extrapancreatic ducts, especially where they pass through the wall of the duodenum, and assume a sphincterlike character at the orifice. The muscular elements form a substantial tunic in cattle, carnivores, and solipeds but are less abundant in sheep and goats. They are absent from the duct system of swine and from the duct of Santorini in horses and dogs, except for a terminal sphincter.

The vessels and nerves are like those of the salivary glands (see p. 159).

THE PANCREAS OF THE FOWL. The structure is tubuloacinous. Because of the even

* Fig. 258 is on p. 202 and Fig. 260 on p. 220,

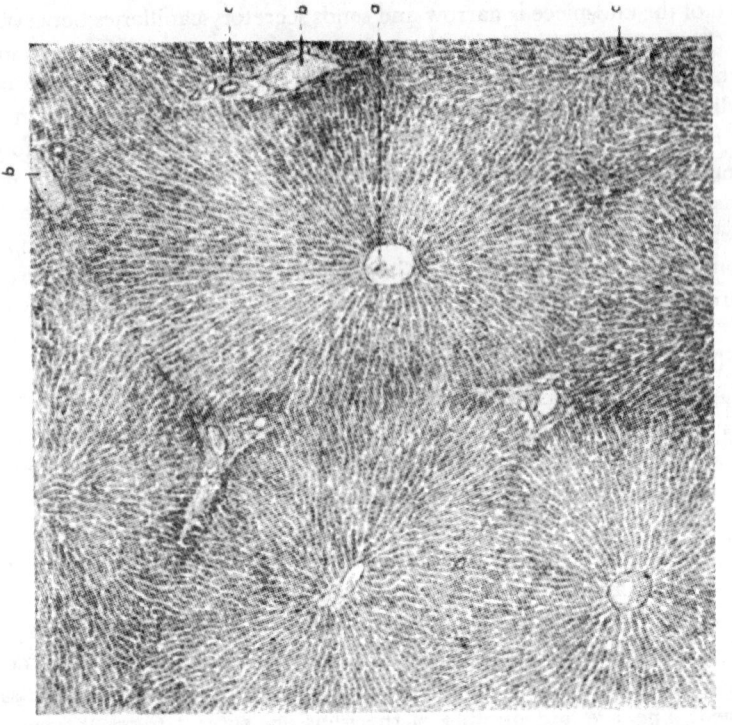

Figure 262. Section from the liver of the horse. *a*, central vein; *b*, branch of portal vein; *c*, bile ducts.

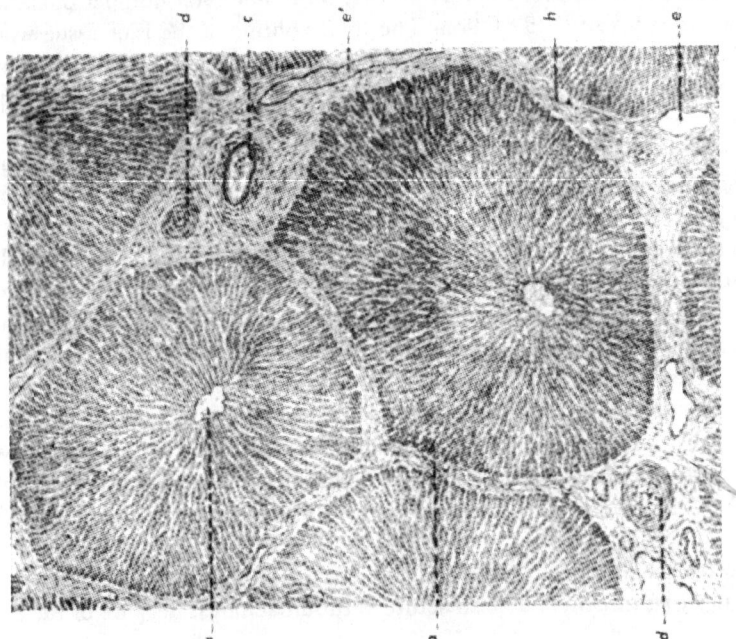

Figure 263. Section from the liver of a pig. *a*, central vein; *b,h*, interlobular connective tissue; *c*, bile duct; *d*, branch of hepatic artery; *e,e'*, branches of portal vein.

distribution of connective tissue, there is no pronounced lobulation. The perivascular connective tissue occasionally contains lymph nodules. The pancreas of the chicken is rich in islets.

G. THE LIVER

The liver is an important metabolic organ of many functions, most of which are concerned with the blood. Only a brief listing of its fields of activity can be attempted here. The liver maintains the glucose level of the blood by drawing upon its stores of glycogen and by producing glucose from fats and proteins. Fats are stored and undergo extensive metabolic changes in the liver. The end products of protein catabolism are converted to urea and discharged into the blood for excretion by the kidney. The liver synthesizes the proteins of the blood plasma. It converts carotene to vitamin A and stores it, as well as part of the B-complex. The erythrocyte-maturing factor is produced in the liver. The liver has a detoxicating action on substances absorbed from the intestine. Its reticulo-endothelial components are important in this protective function and play a part in blood destruction. Bile, the exocrine secretion of the liver, is a viscous fluid that contains desquamated columnar cells, granular masses of bile pigment, mucin, bile acids or salts, and lipids, including cholesterol. The bile salts play an important role in digestion, especially of fats. The bile pigments are waste products of hemoglobin metabolism.

On the surface or in sections of pig livers (Fig. 261), there are roundish-polygonal fields of about 1–1.5 sq. mm. in area, which are the gross manifestation of the lobular structure of the liver. In other domestic mammals and man these lobules are not sharply defined structures, but their boundaries are indicated by the regular intervals between the vessels (Fig. 262). The liver lobules make up the parenchyma of the liver, of which they are the smallest functional units. Each lobule includes a central vein (see p. 221) and the surrounding parenchyma, whose sinusoids are all drained by the central vein. The lobules are irregularly polyhedral prisms, 1.5–2.5 mm. in length, and are often curved. They are smaller in young, growing animals than in adults. Often, especially near the periphery of the liver, the lobules are joined at the points of exit of the central veins, forming lobule complexes (Fig. 269).

The liver is covered by a thin coat of peritoneum, the capsula serosa, below which there is another, usually very thin, loose connective tissue layer, the capsula fibrosa (Glisson's capsule). The latter condenses in the region of the hilus (porta hepatis) into a heavier connective tissue mass, which sheathes the vessels, nerves, and ducts, and invades the organ as the interstitial tissue, finally surrounding the lobules as interlobular tissue. The quantity of interlobular tissue varies with species and determines the distinctness of the lobules. The interstitial tissue of the liver is also directly continuous with the fibrous capsule over the whole surface. The interlobular connective tissue is connected with the intralobular reticular fiber framework (Fig. 263), which forms a supporting envelope around the sinusoids and condenses into a sheath around the central vein.

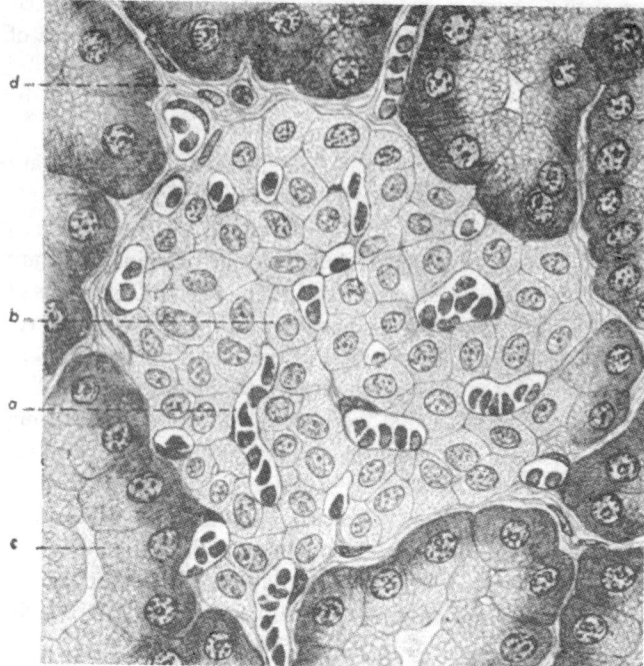

Figure 260. Section through an islet of Langerhans in the pancreas of the ox (400×). *a*, capillary; *b*, cell cord; *c*, exocrine secretory end-piece; *d*, interlobular connective tissue.

Figure 265. Liver section from a rat that has been injected with lithium carmine (600×). *a*, hepatic cell; *b*, hepatic sinusoids; *c,c'*, reticulo-endothelial (Kupffer) cell with stored dye particles; *c''*, resting Kupffer cell.

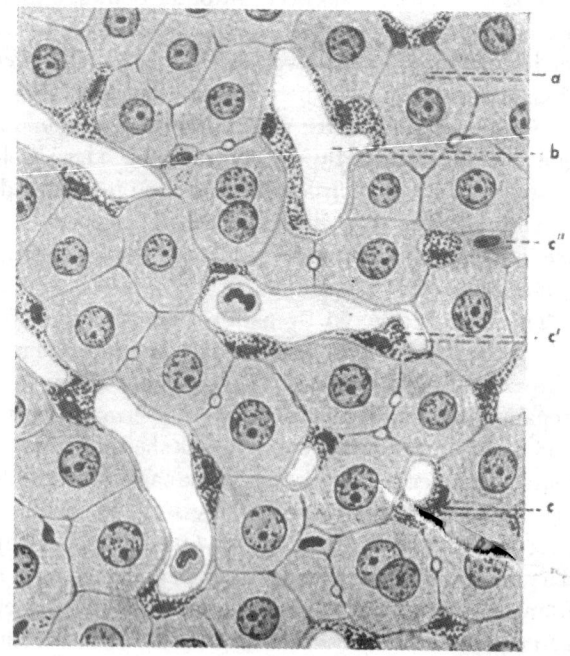

Between the lobules we find, in addition to nerves, the vasa interlobularia (Figs. 261,*c,d,e;* 262,*b,c*) or *portal triad* consisting of branches of the portal vein, the hepatic artery, and the bile ducts. They course around the lobules and along their edges. The *central vein,* the V. intralobularis (Figs. 261,*a;* 262,*a*), lies in the center of each lobule. Between the afferent interlobular vessels and the efferent, intra-lobular central vein the lobule is permeated by a dense venous plexus consisting of sinusoids (Figs. 266*, 268), in whose meshes the liver cells lie. Here is where the actual work of the liver is carried on. The liver cells receive material from the neighboring sinusoids and empty their own products into them.

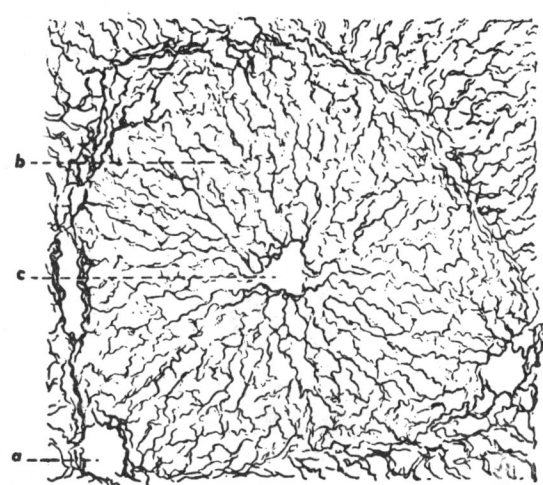

Figure 263. Reticular fibers in a liver lobule of a calf; silver impregnation. *a,* interlobular vessels; *b,* reticular fiber net; *c,* central vein.

Hepatic Cells. The arrangement of the liver cells is usually described as cordlike (Figs. 261, 262), but recent studies by Elias on man, horse, cat, dog, and rabbit,[10] as well as certain widely published older illustrations (Fig. 266*), indicate that the cells are arranged in plates (laminae). These are generally one cell thick, curved, perforated, and connected by many anastomoses. They radiate from the central vein in the same manner as the sinusoids, which fill all the interlaminar spaces and anastomose through the holes in the laminae.

The liver cells (Fig. 264) lack a basement membrane. This circumstance facilitates the exchange of materials with the blood. The cells are irregularly polyhedral and 20–25 μ in diameter. Those of young, growing animals are smaller by 2–7 μ than those of adults. The surface of the cell is condensed into a relatively firm layer of ectoplasm. The cell contains a spheroid nucleus of highly variable size and little chromatin. Two or more nuclei may be present. Mitoses have been seen in the liver of the rat.[11] Yellow and brownish pigment is characteristic for the cytoplasm of hepatic cells. Fat droplets, glycogen flakes or granules, and mitochondria in the

---

[10] Hans Elias, A Re-examination of the Structure of the Mammalian Liver, *Am. J. Anatomy 84* (1949): 311–328, and *85* (1950): 379–456.

[11] H. W. Beams and R. L. King, The Origin of Binucleate and Large Mononucleate Cells in the Liver of the Rat, *Anat. Rec. 83* (1942): 281–297.   * Fig. 266 is on p. 225.

form of granules or threads may be present. The appearance of the liver cells varies greatly according to their functional status. In the fasting animal (Fig. 264,*A*) they are small, turbid, and poorly outlined. After a full meal (*B*) they enlarge and contain glycogen and shiny fat droplets. During the digestion of very fatty food they are distended with fat droplets. When such inclusions are removed, as by fixation and embedding, the cytoplasm presents a honeycombed appearance. There is also an increase in the fat content of the liver cells of the cow in late pregnancy. See Overbeck's discussion of the normal occurrence of fat in the liver cells of domestic animals.[12]

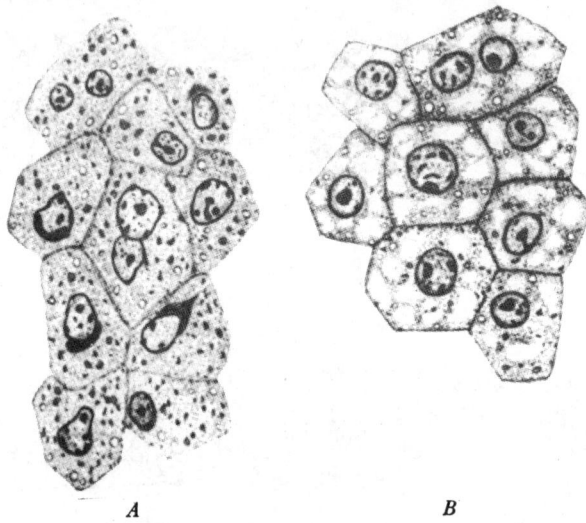

A   B

Figure 264. Hepatic cells of the ox. *A*, while fasting, *B*, after a meal.

Sinusoids. The interstices of the parenchymatous framework are filled by the network of hepatic sinusoids (Figs. 266,*d**; 268). The meshes of the network are of about the same size as one hepatic cell. The often wide, irregularly shaped sinusoids are not separated from the cells by a basement membrane, though a tissue space (of Disse) has been described between them. The cells lining the hepatic sinusoids have nuclei but no cell boundaries. This syncytial association gives rise to the *Kupffer cells*, which are fixed macrophages attached to the wall and projecting into the lumen of the sinusoid. The Kupffer cells have larger nuclei than the ordinary lining cells. They are directly exposed to the portal blood and able to remove foreign matter from it easily and quickly. Their marked phagocytic properties protect the liver and the whole organism against noxious substances. In herbivores and omnivores they nearly always contain fat droplets. They are part of the reticulo-endothelial system. As such they play an important part in erythrocyte destruction and iron metabolism. The ordinary endothelial cells which line the sinusoids are able to store some particulate matter but not vital dyes.[13]

---

[12] Elfriede Overbeck, Über physiologische und pathologische Fettablagerungen in der Leber bei Haussäugetieren, *Virchows Arch. 310* (1943): 458–492.

[13] Maximow and Bloom, p. 425.   *Fig. 266 is on p. 225.

Intrahepatic Ducts. Under favorable conditions, even without the application of special techniques, one may discern a fine round opening wherever the surfaces of two cells are apposed. These openings are well demonstrated by silver impregnation and represent the cross sections of bile capillaries (Fig. 266,e*). The bile capillaries are, like the intercellular secretory capillaries of other glands, very fine tubules. They are formed by troughlike indentations on two or three adjacent cells. Although their walls are too thin to be seen, they are more resistant to crushing or

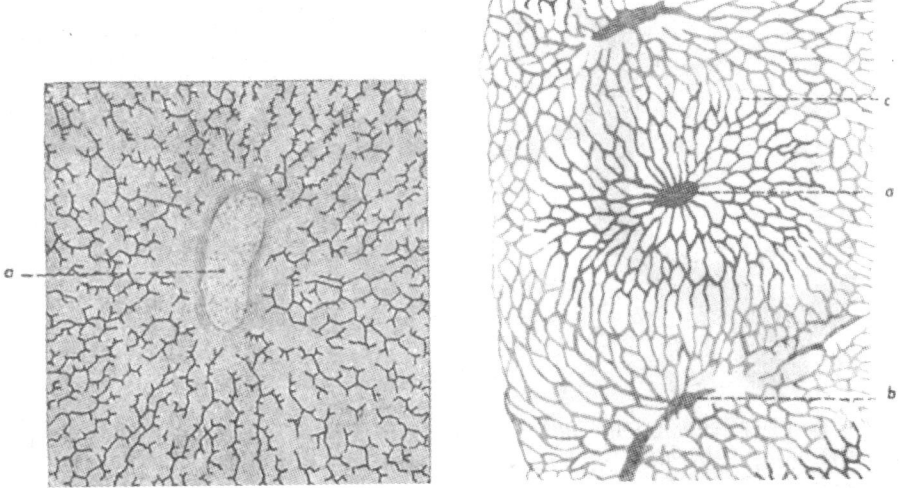

Figure 267 (left). Bile capillaries of the rabbit; silver impregnation (100×). *a*, center of the lobule (central vein). Hepatic cells and sinusoids are not shown.

Figure 268 (right). Cross section through lobules of the injected liver of the rabbit. *a*, central vein; *b*, portal vein (vena interlobularis); *c*, zone of contact of two injection masses.

maceration than the liver cells. The bile capillaries form continuous networks within the liver plates and interlaminar bridges. Because they are always enclosed between adjacent cells, they are as far removed as possible from the sinusoids (Fig. 266,c,d*). The hepatic cells therefore have two physiologically different surfaces through which they discharge their products. On the surface of the lobules the bile capillaries pass into the interlobular bile ducts. The transition from the hepatic cells surrounding the capillaries to the low epithelium of the ducts is abrupt. There are also small intralobular ducts which drain the capillaries.[14]

The interlobular bile ducts unite with others and run with the large vessels (branches of the hepatic artery and the portal vein) to the porta where they leave the organ in one or several trunks. The smallest interlobular ducts are lined by a low, simple epithelium on a thin basement membrane. Soon the cells become higher (Figs. 261; 262,c), until in the larger ducts the lining is a high columnar epithelium, in which single or multicellular intraepithelial glands give off an apocrine secretion (in the horse and goat). These ducts are characterized by a collagenous

---

[14] Elias, *Am. J. Anatomy 85* (1950): 379–456.   * Fig. 266 is on p. 225.

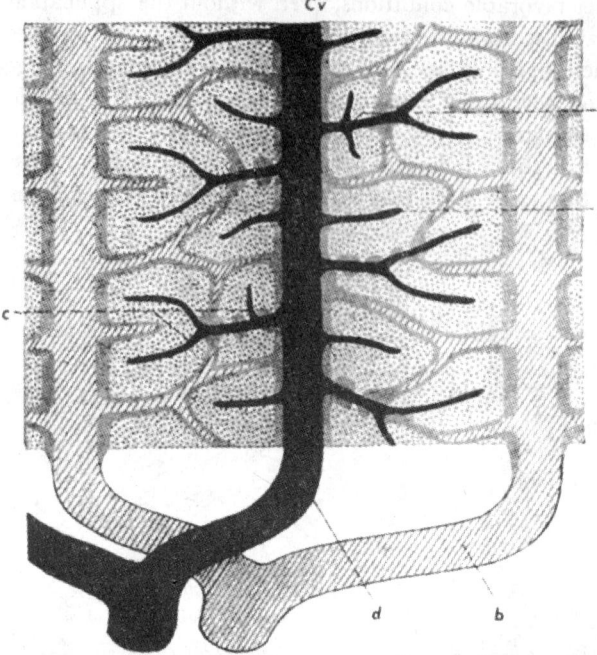

Figure 269. Diagram of the lobular arrangement and circulation of the pig's liver. *Cv*, collecting vein with two neighboring parallel branches of the portal vein. Black = hepatic veins; stippled = liver parenchyma; shaded = portal branches; gray = connective tissue sheaths. *a*, central vein without connective tissue envelope; *b*, branches of the portal vein; *c*, intercalated vein with incomplete envelope; *d*, branch of hepatic vein; *e*, intercalated vein running through a lobule. For the sake of simplicity branches of the hepatic artery and bile ducts, which accompany the portal veins, are not shown in the diagram. (After Pfuhl.)

lamina propria, which, especially in ruminants, contains smooth muscle fibers. Near the hilus of the liver the largest ducts also contain mucous glands.

Vessels and Nerves. Of the two afferent vessels the portal vein supplies mainly the parenchyma (functional circulation), while the hepatic artery is chiefly concerned with the nourishment of the interstitial tissue.

The portal vein divides in the liver into branches, which are accompanied by branches of the hepatic artery and bile ducts and are called interlobular veins (Figs. 261,*e;* 262,*b;* 268,*b*) because of their position in the interlobular connective tissue. These give rise to the capacious hepatic sinusoids (Figs. 266,*d**; 268). The portal vein thus supplies mainly the intralobular region. The sinusoids form, through their confluence near the apex of the lobule, the beginning of the central vein (Fig. 269,*a*), which at this point consists only of an intima. It continues along the axis of the lobule, receiving sinusoids in its course, and forms one of the radicles of the hepatic vein system. A few of the central veins open directly into a large *collecting vein* at the base of the lobule, but most of them join at acute angles to form *intercalated veins* with incomplete connective tissue sheaths. These in turn empty into collecting veins, which are enveloped by connective tissue. These pass into the larger hepatic veins, which leave the liver and finally empty into the caudal vena cava. Thus the entire ramification of the hepatic veins is separated from the arterial and portal branches and the bile ducts.

The hepatic artery (Fig. 261,*d*) supplies mainly the interstitial capillary nets, which nourish the liver capsule, the interstitial connective tissue, the nerves, the walls of the blood vessels, and, especially abundantly, the bile ducts. These capil-

---
* Fig. 266 is on p. 225.

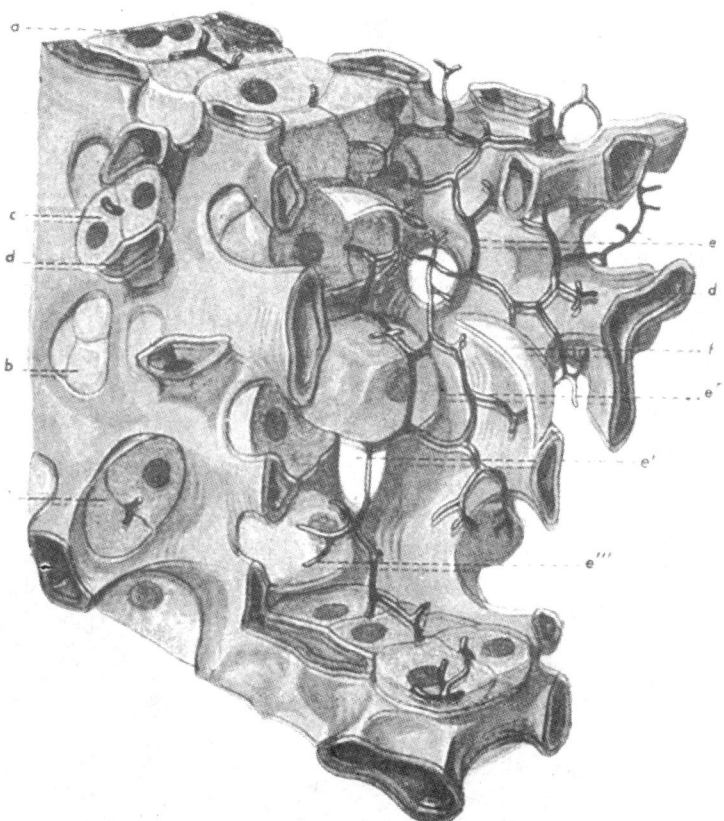

Figure 266. Spatial relationship of the liver sinusoids and bile capillaries to a liver cell plate or lamina hepatis. Hepatic cells, yellow; hepatic sinusoids, shown lying in two parallel planes, blue; bile capillaries (canaliculi) in black. *a*, hepatic cell plate between the anastomosing sinusoids; *b*, surface of plate, covered in life by connective tissue; *c*, interlaminar bridges (two-cell liver cords) cut across with bile capillaries projecting from them; *d*, cross sections through branches of sinusoids, *e*, network of bile capillaries; *e'*, bile capillary freed by removal of adjacent cells; *e''*, meshes in the net of bile capillaries, the hepatic cells having been removed; *e'''*, blindly ending bile capillary; *f*, reticular fibers shown as septa. (After Braus-Vierling.)

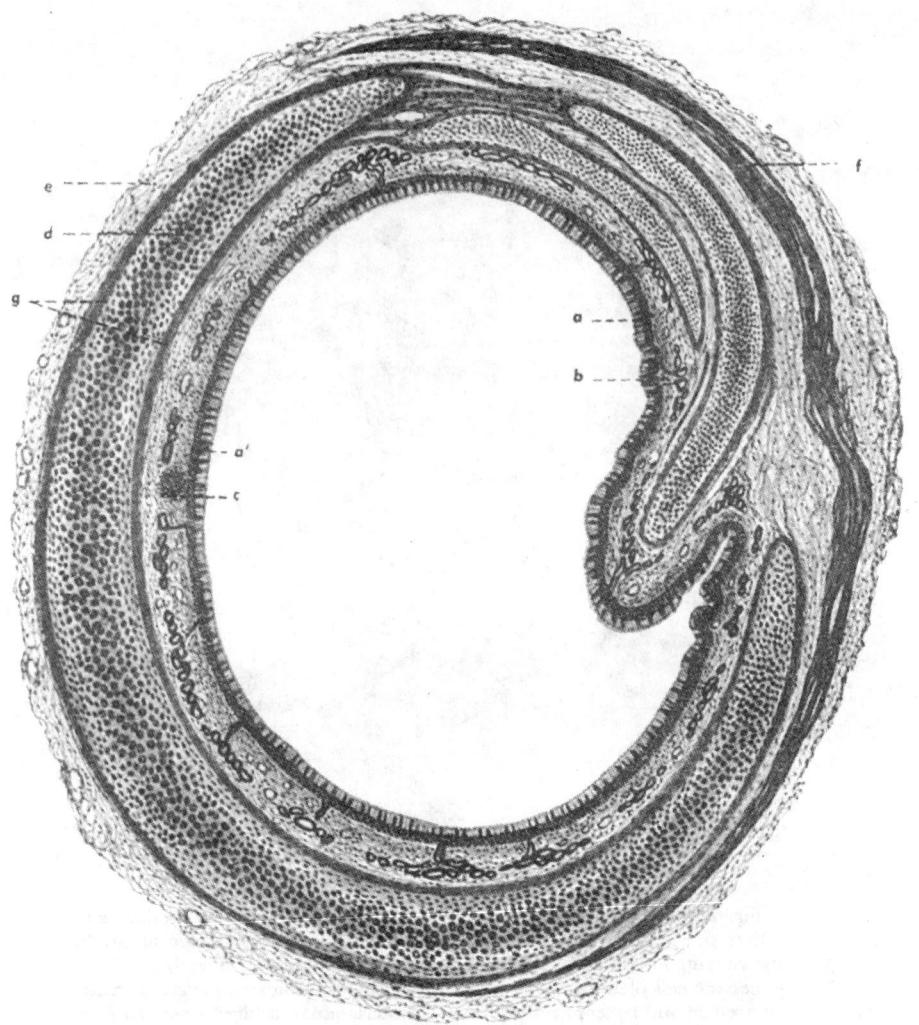

Figure 279. Cross section through the trachea of the cat; stained with hemalum-eosin. *a*, epithelium; *a′*, goblet cells in the epithelium; *b*, sections through glands; *c*, lymph nodules; *d*, tracheal ring; *e*, adventitia; *f*, m. transversus tracheae; *g*, fibrous membrane.

lary nets give rise to veins that empty into branches of the portal vein and therefore comprise the "internal radicles" of the portal vein. In addition, however, there are fine arterial capillaries that pass directly into the lobules and empty into the sinusoids, so that a portion of the blood of the hepatic artery benefits the lobule directly.

In sections of the liver the various vessels are easily identified microscopically. The arteries are distinguished from veins and bile ducts by their muscular coats (Fig. 261,d). The bile ducts are characterized by their epithelium (c), while the branches of the portal vein have wide lumina and occur near the arteries and bile ducts (e,e'). Those venous branches belonging to the system of the hepatic vein, on

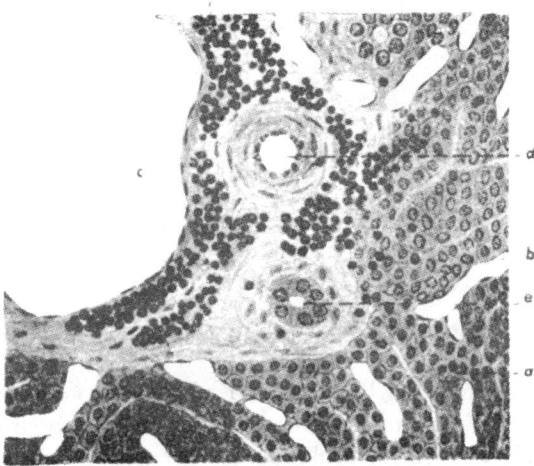

Figure 270. Section from the liver of a chicken. *a*, cells of the liver lobule; *b*, sinusoids; *c*, branch of the portal vein; *d*, artery; *e*, bile duct; *f*, lymphocytes.

the other hand, are found as isolated vessels surrounded by liver cells. They are also characterized by their width. In the smaller hepatic veins of the dog and some other mammals muscular thickenings have been discovered (throttle veins).

The liver contains superficial and deep lymph vessels, the deep ones accompanying the portal and hepatic veins. It has been claimed that lymph spaces between the sinusoids and the liver cells can be demonstrated by injection, but this is disputed.

The nerves of the liver are mostly unmyelinated and surround chiefly the hepatic artery and its branches. Very delicate fibers have also been found in the interior of the lobules.

LIVER OF BIRDS (Fig. 270). The structure is essentially the same as it is in mammals except that the lobulation is less distinct. The accumulation of lymphocytes around the vessels and between the cell cords is conspicuous. Lymphocytes may be intermingled with eosinophilic leukocytes, and the latter may form small foci of their own.

The Extrahepatic Ducts. The ductus hepaticus and ductus choledochus (Fig. 271) have a glandular mucous membrane, which is covered by high simple columnar epithelium (*a*) and contains lymph nodules (*c*). It consists further of a mid-

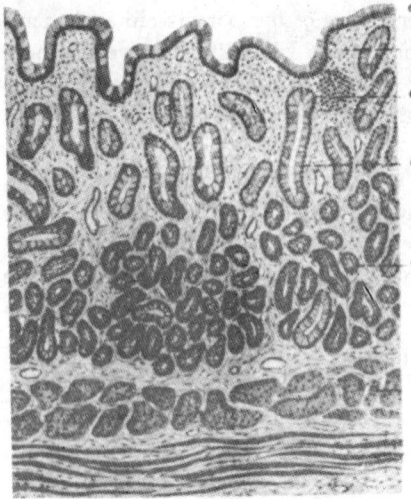

Figure 271. Section through the wall of the bile duct of the ox near its junction with the duodenum. *a,* columnar epithelium; *b,* lamina propria; *c,* lymph nodule; *d,* mucous, *e,* serous, glands; *f,f',* muscle layers of the wall.

dle layer, composed of mostly circular smooth muscle, and of a loose adventitia or serosa. Abundant elastic fiber nets are present in the wall of the duct. In the ox the musculature is thick and consists of a circular and a longitudinal layer. The muscles in carnivores are thinner. The remaining domestic animals have no continuous muscle layer.

The secretory epithelium is underlain by a delicate lamina propria. In ruminants it contains goblet cells. Tubular glands are present in the propria. They are predominantly mucous (*d*). Only a small proportion of them is serous (*e*).

The pars intestinalis of the common bile duct (ductus choledochus) perforates the intestinal wall at an angle and, in some species, forms with the pancreatic duct (of Wirsung) an ampullate enlargement, the diverticulum duodeni. Its mucous membrane is rich in glands except in the case of the pig. In the pig, ox, and horse goblet cells are present in the epithelium, but they are absent in other species. The muscular layer is heavier here than in the pars libera and forms, even in the sheep and goat, whose ducts are poorly muscled elsewhere, a continuous muscle layer capable of occluding the bile duct in the manner of a sphincter.

Gall Bladder. The gall bladder (Fig. 272), which is absent in the horse, exhibits a structure similar to that of the larger bile ducts. The folded mucosa contains lymph nodules and glands and is covered with high simple columnar epithelium,

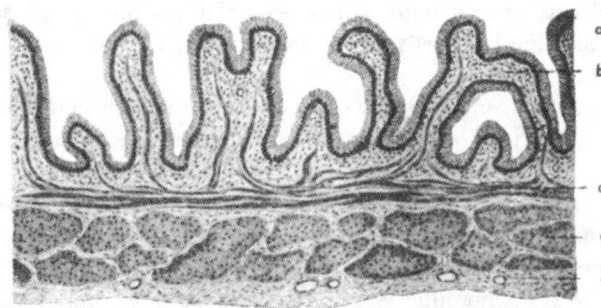

Figure 272. Section through the wall of the gall bladder of the dog. *a,* columnar epithelium; *b,* connective tissue of the lamina propria; *c,* inner muscle layer in longitudinal section; *d,* outer layer in cross section; *e,* serosa.

which, in the ox, contains goblet cells. The fibers of the muscular layer run in all directions, with a circular course predominating. The muscularis is covered by a serosa (e).

The number of glands varies with the species, region, and individual. Carnivores and swine have few, while ruminants have many, tortuous tubular mucous and serous glands.

The ductus cysticus resembles in structure the gall bladder and the other extra-hepatic ducts.

XII

The Respiratory System

THE air necessary for respiration passes through the conducting passages, most of which are characterized by rigid walls, and reaches the alveoli of the lung, where the oxygen-carbon dioxide exchange with the blood is carried on. The air passages consist of the nasal cavity, the pharynx, the larynx, the trachea, and the bronchi.

A. NASAL CAVITY

The nasal cavity is subdivided into the vestibular, respiratory, and olfactory regions. The mucosa is for the most part firmly fixed to the subjacent tissues.

1. Vestibular Region

The mucosa of the vestibule bears moderately pigmented, stratified squamous epithelium nourished by a papillary body. The propria, which contains many serous glands, is made up of compact collagenous tissue and is anchored to the underlying tissue by a similarly firm submucosa, in which there is an abundance of large vessels and nerves. Near the nasal opening it gradually passes into the external skin. In the horse the external skin, bearing hair and sebaceous and tubular glands, is continued into the vestibule and the diverticulum nasi.

2. Respiratory Region (Fig. 273)

The squamous epithelium of the vestibule changes gradually into stratified columnar and finally into ciliated pseudostratified epithelium (a), which is characteristic for the respiratory passages and contains varying numbers of goblet cells (a'). The basement membrane of this epithelium contains a feltwork of reticular fibers. The lamina propria has many elastic fibers in the deeper layers. It is also rich in leukocytes, which condense into lymph nodules in certain places. The propria contains tubuloalveolar glands (c) most of which are serous, although some mucous and mixed glands are encountered. The glandular end-pieces follow a tortuous course and may coil into a ball. Only in carnivores are the glands small in size and few in number. The normal nasal secretion is predominantly serous and serves to prevent the drying out of the epithelium.

The submucosa is composed of fairly regular collagenous tissue. It carries large vascular trunks (*e,d*) and, in certain areas, sizable venous plexuses, which are erectile and impart to the mucous membrane its cushion-like consistency and its pronounced red color. The submucosa passes directly into the periosteum, or into the perichondrium which invests the hyaline cartilage of the nasal septum.

3. Olfactory Region

The olfactory mucosa (Fig. 274) differs from that of the respiratory region mainly in that it is thicker and has a different color caused by pigment granules in the epithelium (in the horse and

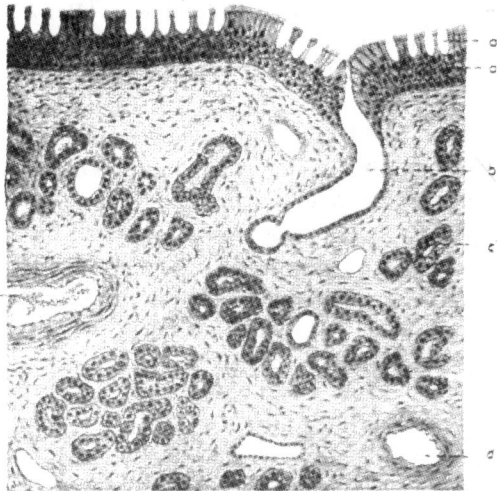

Figure 273. Section through the nasal mucosa of the horse near the vestibule (200×). *a*, pseudostratified ciliated epithelium containing *a'*, goblet cells; *b*, excretory ducts of *c*, nasal glands; *d*, vein; *e*, artery.

ox, yellowish; in sheep, yellow; in the goat, dark; in the pig, brown; and in carnivores, gray). It is also distinguished by the presence of peculiar tubular glands.

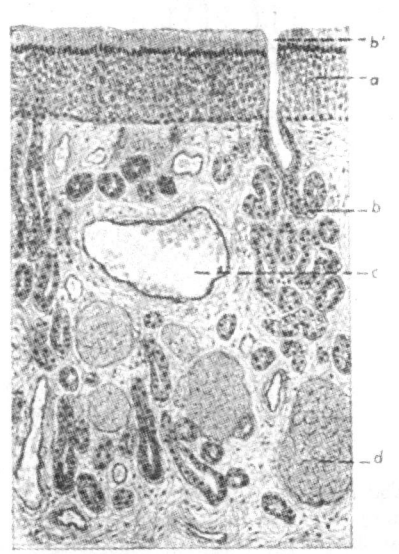

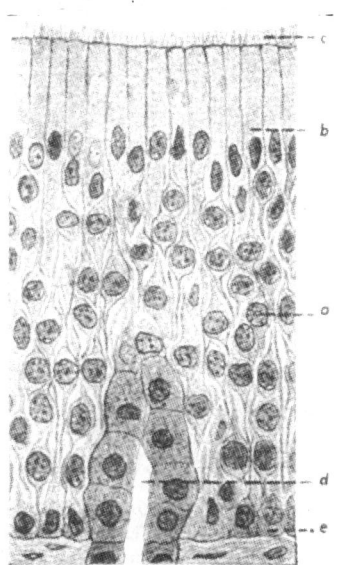

Figure 274 (left). Section from the olfactory region of the horse. *a*, olfactory epithelium; *b*, olfactory glands; *b'*, opening of a gland; *c*, vein; *d*, nerve.

Figure 275 (right): Section of olfactory epithelium of the sheep. *a*, olfactory cells; *b*, supporting cells; *c*, olfactory hairs; *d*, duct of an olfactory gland; *e*, basal cell of the olfactory epithelium.

The olfactory epithelium (Figs. 274,*a;* 275; 276) consists of three cell types: the supporting or sustentacular, the basal, and the olfactory cells. The *supporting cells* (Figs. 275,*b;* 276,*a*) are elongated columnar cells, whose cytoplasm is finely granular and often pigmented. They usually end in a bifurcated basal process, which is often connected with processes of neighboring cells. The deeper portion of the supporting cells bears many indentations caused by adjoining olfactory cells. The rather large oval nuclei are situated in the more superficial portion of the cell. They occupy about the same position in each cell, forming the zone of oval nuclei. The *olfactory cells* (Figs. 275,*a;* 276,*b*) are nerve cells and consist of a spheroid or ovoid cell body, which houses the nucleus, and a peripheral and a central process. The peripheral is rod-shaped and slender and bears on its free end the short, delicate olfactory hairs (Figs. 275,*c;* 276,*d*), which are stimulated by odoriferous substances dissolved in the secretions on the surface. The stimulus is then relayed through the cell body into the fine proximal cell process (Fig. 277,*b*), which is continued as an unmyelinated fiber of the olfactory nerve. The large spheroid nuclei of the olfactory cells lie somewhat deeper than those of the supporting cells. Since they do not occupy the same level in each cell they form a rather wide zone of round nuclei. There are also cell types intermediate in form between the two described. The stel-

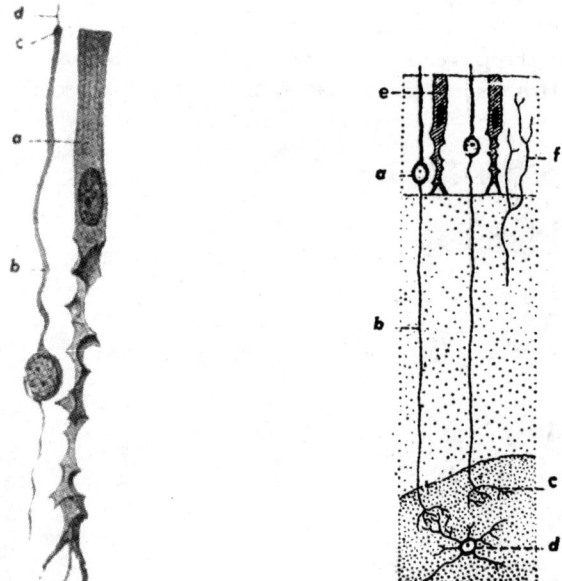

Figure 276 (left). Isolated supporting and olfactory cells from the olfactory epithelium. (After von Ebner.) *a,* supporting cell; *b,* olfactory cell, whose basal process is a nerve fiber while the end (*c*) of the peripheral process bears the olfactory hair (*d*).

Figure 277 (right). Diagram of the olfactory organ. *a,* olfactory cell; *b,* fiber of the olfactory nerve; *c,* olfactory glomerulus; *d,* mitral cell of the olfactory bulb; *e,* supporting cells; *f,* peripheral ending of a trigeminus fiber in the olfactory mucosa.

late *basal cells* (Fig. 275,*e*) border the tunica propria. Connected by their processes, they form a network around the basal portions of the supporting cells.

The free surface of the olfactory epithelium exhibits a thin, highly refractive cuticle with a well-developed network of terminal bars. The nonmotile olfactory hairs project beyond this surface and are surrounded by small quantities of mucus, which is secreted by the supporting cells.

The collagenous propria mucosae (Fig. 274) is rich in nuclei superficially, cavernous in its middle layer (*c*), and coarse-fibered in the deep layer. In addition to the olfactory plexus (*d*), the propria contains the tubular *olfactory glands* of Bowman (*b*), consisting of simple epithelium whose cells contain yellow pigment granules and elaborate a mucoserous secretion. The excretory ducts of the glands are lined with simple flat or cuboidal epithelium and extend through the olfactory epithelium (Fig. 275,*d*).

The submucosa of the olfactory mucous membrane resembles that of the other sections of the nasal cavity.

VESSELS AND NERVES. The arteries of the nasal cavity form a deep periosteal net and a superficial wide-meshed net with subepithelial capillaries. The arteries supply twigs that form periglandular capillary nets. The veins arising from the latter empty into a thick superficial venous plexus, while the remaining capillary nets furnish blood to the cavernous bodies, which consist of four or five layers of muscular, valveless veins. The lymphatics form a subepithelial and a deep capillary net. They communicate with the subdural and subarachnoid spaces. The entire nasal mucosa receives myelinated sensory fibers from the trigeminal nerve. Only Jacobson's organ (see below) and the olfactory region receive additional unmyelinated olfactory fibers. The axons arising from the olfactory cells pass into the olfactory tract as parts of the olfactory nerve. They terminate in the glomeruli of the olfactory bulb (Fig. 350).

The paranasal sinuses are lined by a mucous membrane which is little different from that of the nasal cavity. Its glands, however, are fewer and serous in nature.

The lateral nasal gland is a serous gland containing intercalated, striated, and excretory ducts. It is absent in the ox and man. The glandular body is located in the maxillary sinus (in carnivores) or near the nasomaxillary opening, and the excretory duct, which is lined with stratified epithelium, runs in the middle meatus nasi.

The mucosa of the nasopalatine duct (the ductus incisivus) is partially surrounded by a trough of hyaline cartilage and bears a stratified, nonciliated epithelium. It contains tubular serous and mixed glands, many leukocytes, and lymph nodules.

The vomeronasal organ (of Jacobson) has been credited with performing special olfactory functions. It consists of tubular hyaline cartilage lined with a mucous membrane which is rich in blood vessels and nerves (from the olfactory and trigeminal nerves) and contains serous glands. The structure of the mucosa resembles that of the nasal mucosa. Only a strip along the medial wall bears epithelium like that of the olfactory region.

THE NASAL CAVITY OF THE CHICKEN. The olfactory mucosa is similar to that of mammals. The nasal cavity opens into the oral cavity by way of the choana, a median slit in the roof of the mouth. Its mucosa bears pseudostratified ciliated epithelium, which contains numerous recesses lined with high mucous cells. The propria is uncommonly rich in lymphocytes. The epithelium of the respiratory region changes abruptly on the nasal side of the choanal margin into the stratified squamous epithelium of the oral cavity. The lateral nasal gland (glandula orbitonasalis) is found on the frontal bone near the medial canthus of the eye. Its secretory tubules are lined by cuboidal cells filled with acidophilic granules, and its two excretory ducts empty into the nasal cavity. Its function is to keep the nostrils from drying out during flight.

B. PHARYNX

The pharynx is subdivided into the nasopharynx (pars respiratoria) and the oropharynx (pars digestoria). With the exception of the soft palate and the dorsal wall, the latter of which consists only of mucosa applied to the skull, the wall of the pharynx is made up of (1) the mucosa, (2) the thin internal pharyngeal fascia, (3) striated muscle, (4) the outer pharyngeal fascia, and (5) a loose adventitia. The mucosa of the nasopharynx bears a ciliated pseudostratified epithelium with goblet cells, while that of the oropharynx is characterized by stratified squamous epithelium. The fibroelastic, glandular propria mucosae of the oropharynx has a papillary body and an abundance of lymphatic tissue (in the lymph nodules and pharyngeal tonsils, see p. 121). The tubular glands are mucous in the oropharynx and mixed in the nasopharynx, with the serous elements predominating. The inner pharyngeal fascia forms the deep boundary of the mucosa. It consists of elastic fiber nets, which are continued peripherally into the intermuscular connective tissue. The next layer is the striated muscle sheet, consisting partly of longitudinal, but mostly of circular, fibers. The muscle layer is followed by the outer pharyngeal fascia, a tough fibrous membrane containing elastic fiber nets. The outermost sheet is the adventitia, consisting of loose connective tissue.

The pharyngeal wall contains many blood vessels and lymphatics. The latter communicate with those of the nasal cavity. The nerves form superficial and deeper plexuses. Large and small groups of nerve cells are present, especially in the cat, between the pharyngeal muscles. The nerve endings resemble those in the nasal and oral cavity.

C. LARYNX

The laryngeal wall consists of (1) a mucosa, (2) a middle layer composed of cartilages, ligaments, and a connecting fibrous membrane, and (3) a muscular layer.

The mucosa of the vestibule down to the oral margin of the vocal folds bears stratified squamous epithelium. The remainder of the laryngeal epithelium is of the ciliated pseudostratified type. Thus the two surfaces of the epiglottis, the arytenoid cartilages, and the aryepiglottic folds are covered by stratified squamous epithelium. Taste buds have been found in the laryngeal portion of the epiglottic epithelium of ruminants, swine, and carnivores.

The propria mucosae is made up of connective tissue containing many elastic fibers and forms a low papillary body in the area of the squamous epithelium. It contains glands and much lymphatic tissue, including lymph nodules. The glands are serous, mucous, and mixed. They also extend into the submucosa and beyond, and often occur in large groups. The margin of the vocal folds and immediate surroundings are free from glands. The excretory ducts of the glands are ensheathed by smooth muscle cells and lined by cuboidal or, in large ducts, pseudostratified columnar epithelium. The lymph nodules are especially numerous in ruminants. Their number decreases progressively in horses, pigs, and carnivores.

The submucosa is thin, except at a few places, e.g., at the base of the epiglottis.

Of the cartilages making up the laryngeal skeleton, the thyroid, cricoid, and the main part of the arytenoid consist of hyaline cartilage, but the epiglottis with its cuneiform processes and the vocal and corniculate processes of the arytenoid cartilage are composed of elastic cartilage. The epiglottic cartilage may be partly or entirely replaced by adipose tissue. The hyaline cartilages ossify easily. In and around the cartilaginous articulations adipose tissue is often present, especially in the epiglottis of carnivores. The ligaments of the larynx, especially the inner ones, contain much elastic tissue.

The laryngeal muscles are composed of striated fibers.

The laryngeal saccules are absent in ruminants. In the horse they are lined by ciliated pseudostratified epithelium, in swine and carnivores by stratified squamous epithelium. Their propria contains a varying number of glands and lymph nodules.

The blood vessels form a coarse, deep submucous or perichondral plexus, a middle narrow-meshed periglandular network, and a dense subepithelial network. The lymphatics form a deep and a superficial net. The nerves contain microscopic ganglia. Some of them end freely in the epithelium, others in the taste buds.

D. TRACHEA

In the trachea (Figs. 278; 279*) the following layers are recognized:
1. Mucosa
   a. Ciliated pseudostratified epithelium
   b. Basement membrane (see *nasal mucosa*, p. 230)
   c. Propria
   d. Layer of longitudinal elastic fibers
   e. Submucosa with glands
2. Fibroelastic membrane containing and connecting the cartilaginous rings
3. Muscularis, present only dorsally
4. Adventitia

The mucosa is fixed to the underlying tissues smoothly and immovably. The ciliated pseudostratified epithelium (Fig. 278,a) contains numerous goblet cells and

* Fig. 279 is on p. 226.

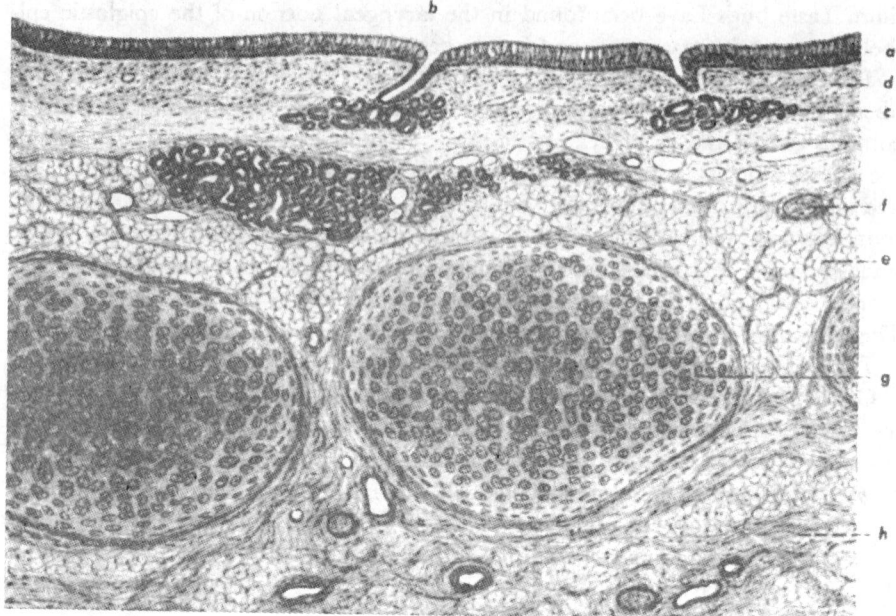

Figure 278. Longitudinal section through the wall of the trachea of the pig, *a*, ciliated pseudostratified epithelium; *b*, excretory duct of a gland; *c*, section of a gland; *d*, propria mucosae containing many lymphocytes; *e*, submucosal fat; *f*, nerve; *g*, tracheal ring in cross section; *h*, adventitia.

migrating leukocytes. The beat of the cilia, here as elsewhere in the respiratory system, is directed toward the outside and serves to remove dust particles. Many animals have only a rudimentary basement membrane. The lamina propria (*d*) consists of fine fibers and often contains many lymphocytes. It is separated from the submucosa by a fibroelastic membrane which consists of a latticework of collagenous and longitudinal elastic fibers and takes the place of a muscularis mucosae. The submucosa is rich in elastic fibers and fat and blends into the perichondrium in the region of the cartilaginous rings. The deeper layers of the propria and the submucosa contain mostly mixed, tubular glands (Figs. 278,*c*; 279,*b**), which are especially abundant ventrally and laterally. Some of these extend down to the interannular region and even outside the rings to the adventitia. Their excretory ducts are surrounded by muscle fibers and are lined by cuboidal or, in the larger ducts, pseudostratified epithelium (Fig. 278,*b*). Lymph nodules (Fig. 279,*c**) occur in the mucosa, especially of sheep.

The cartilaginous tracheal rings (Figs. 278,*g*; 279,*d**) are enclosed in a fibrous membrane. They prevent collapse of the trachea and interference with the air supply when the esophagus is distended by passing boluses. They consist of hyaline cartilage that often calcifies and ossifies in old animals. They are incomplete dorsally.

---

* Fig. 279 is on p. 226.

The musculature, m. transversus tracheae (Fig. 279,*f* *), is a dorsal strip of essentially transverse smooth muscle fibers. In the horse, ruminant, and pig, it lies inside the ends of the rings, between them and the mucosa, but in the dog and cat it lies outside the rings. In man it simply connects the ends of the rings.

The outer layers of the collagenous and elastic adventitia (Figs. 278,*h;* 279,*e* *) are loose and rich in adipose tissue, vessels, and nerves. Near the tracheal rings the adventitia blends into the perichondrium.

The blood vessels form a submucous, a periglandular, and a

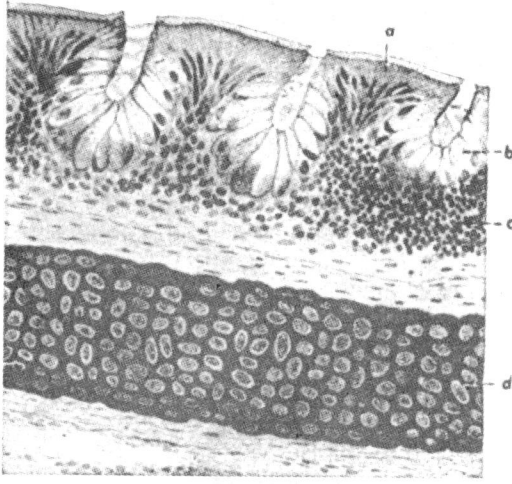

Figure 280. Cross section through the trachea of the chicken (300×). *a*, ciliated columnar epithelium; *b*, mucous glands; *c*, propria containing lymphocytes; *d*, cartilage.

subepithelial plexus, while the lymphatics make up a deep and a superficial network. The nerves possess microscopic ganglia and consist of both myelinated fibers and unmyelinated fibers, the latter ending on the smooth muscle cells.

THE TRACHEA OF THE CHICKEN (Fig. 280). The cartilages form complete rings (*d*) and largely ossify in aquatic birds. The mucous membrane bears pseudostratified ciliated epithelium (*a*), with numerous mucous crypts (*b*) resembling those of the nasal mucosa. The propria (*c*) is infiltrated by a large number of lymphocytes, which may displace parts of the mucous cells and occasionally reach the surface.

E. LUNGS

The lungs (Figs. 281-284) resemble in structure a compound alveolar gland. They consist of a supporting framework composed of the capsule and interstitial connective tissue, the air-conducting apparatus (bronchial tree), and the respiratory structures.

The lung capsule (Figs. 281,*k;* 282,*a*) is a sheet of visceral pleura. It is thickest in the ox and most delicate in carnivores. It contains smooth muscle fibers and, subepithelially, a dense network of elastic fibers separating the true serosa from the collagenous subserosa. The latter contains elastic fibers mainly on its deep surface, where they communicate with those of the lobules. Lymph nodules occur in the subserosa.

The subpleural tissue gives off processes to the interstitial tissue (Fig. 281,*l*) of the lungs. This constitutes the interlobular framework, which contains muscle fibers and divides the lung tissue into lobules of various orders. The lobulation, visible as polygonal fields on the surface and in sections of the lung, is well marked

* Fig. 279 is on p. 226.

in the ox because of the abundant interlobular tissue. The surface fields have an area of 1–2 sq. cm. They are not so distinct in other domestic animals.

The elastic fiber framework is under tension between the bronchi and the pulmonary pleura. Because of the negative pressure in the pleural cavity, the atmospheric pressure inside the lung presses the pulmonary pleura against the parietal pleura. When the thorax enlarges in inspiration, the negative pressure is increased and the lung is further expanded by an inflow of air. In expiration the negative pressure in the pleural cavity is reduced and the elastic framework contracts the lung, expelling part of the air.

The septa of the interstitial system contain the blood and lymph vessels, nerves, and bronchi (Figs. 282,d–g,i; 283,a,h,i). The interstitial tissue contains leukocytes

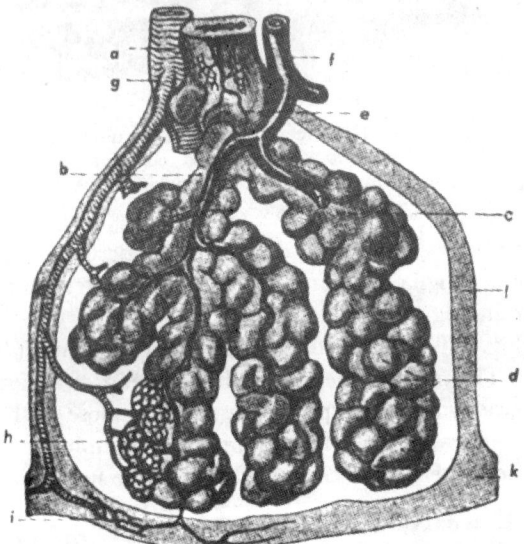

Figure 281. Diagram of a primary lung lobule. *a*, terminal bronchiole; *b*, respiratory bronchiole; *c*, alveolar duct; *d*, alveoli; *e*, bronchial·artery; *f*, branches of pulmonary artery; *g*, lobular branch of the pulmonary vein; *h*, pulmonary capillary net; *i*, subpleural capillary net; *k*, pleura; *l*, interlobular tissue.

and sometimes, especially in the pig, lymph nodules. Black or gray pigmentations occur in the interstitial tissue of horses and dogs, much as in man, especially in large cities. They are carbon particles concentrated here by phagocytic activity.

In addition to the delicate intralobular supporting framework, small vessels, and nerves, each lung lobule (Fig. 281) contains the respiratory structures. These arise from a terminal bronchiole (*a*) which enters the lobule and divides into two to four respiratory bronchioles (*b*). These branch into alveolar ducts (*c*) that in turn give rise to alveolar sacs. All of the respiratory structures bear alveoli (*d*). The bronchial tree itself arises through the bifurcation of the trachea into bronchi, which arborize into several orders of interlobular bronchi and bronchioles, down to the terminal bronchioles.

1. The Conducting System

The wall of the bronchi (Figs. 282,c; 283,a,f) consists of a mucosa, a muscularis, a fibroelastic membrane, which usually encloses cartilage, and a loose collagenous peribronchial layer.

The mucosa of the larger bronchi is nearly free from folds. With the decrease in caliber, however, longitudinal folds become more and more pronounced. The epithelium is of the ciliated pseudostratified type and contains goblet cells. As the mucosa decreases in thickness in the smaller bronchi and bronchioles, the epithelium becomes lower, until in the terminal bronchioles it is cuboidal. No goblet cells are present beyond the terminal bronchioles. The epithelium rests on a basement membrane, which gradually fades out in the smaller bronchi. The propria

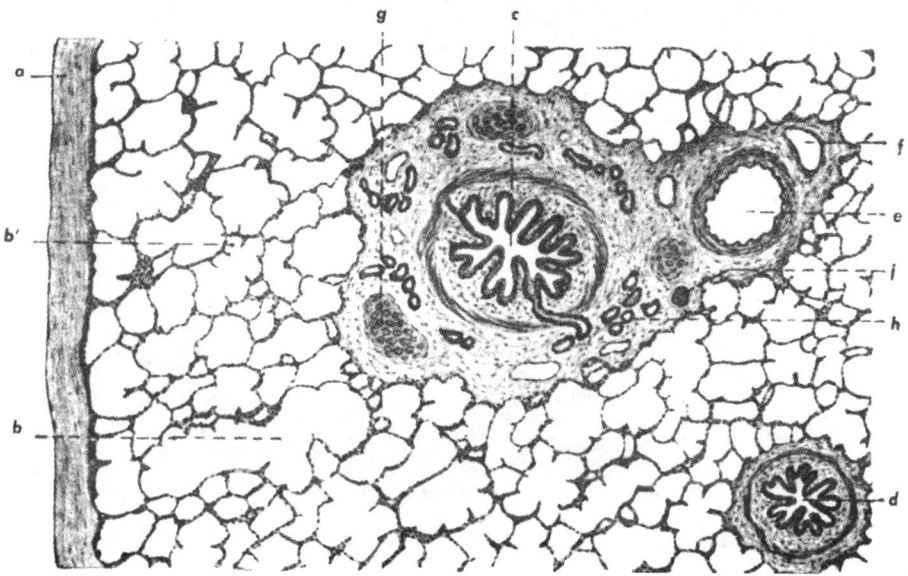

Figure 282. Section from the lung of the ox. *a,* pleura; *b,* alveolar duct; *b',* alveolus; *c,* small bronchus; *d,* bronchiole; *e,* artery; *f,* vein; *g,* plates of cartilage in the bronchial wall; *h,* glands in the bronchial wall; *i,* nerve.

mucosae is rich in cells superficially and contains muscle cells, glands, and sometimes lymph nodules. Nerves and vessels are abundant in its deeper layers. Its elastic fibers, like those of the trachea, follow mainly a longitudinal course and form a fine subepithelial and a coarser deep network. Only the large bronchi have a loose submucosa.

The smooth muscle layer (Fig. 283,*d*) adjoins the propria and may be discontinuous, as in sheep, for example. The fibers, which are predominantly oblique in direction, form a narrow-meshed latticework around the mucosa of the bronchi and regulate their caliber. The number of muscle fibers is gradually reduced toward the small bronchioles, but they remain highly conspicuous (Figs. 282,*d;* 283,*f*).

The fibroelastic membrane of the larger bronchi contains hyaline cartilage (elastic cartilage in man and cat), at first in rings, then in angular plates or strips (Figs. 282,*g;* 283,*i*). At a diameter of about 3 mm. there are only small widely separated strips of cartilage, which is occasionally elastic. In the smallest bronchioles (0.5–1

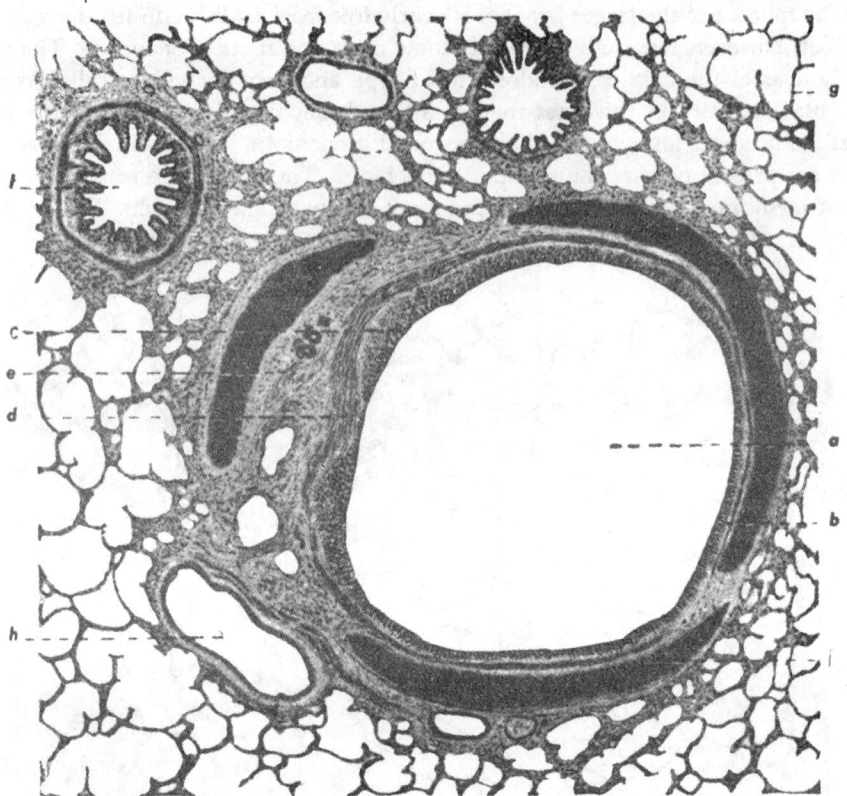

Figure 283. Section from the lung of the horse (70×). *a*, lumen of a bronchus; *b*, its ciliated epithelium; *c*, portion of wall cut obliquely; *d*, smooth muscle fibers; *e*, glands in the bronchial wall; *f*, bronchiole; *g*, alveoli in section; *h*, blood vessel; *i*, cartilaginous segments of the bronchial wall.

mm.) the cartilage is lacking. The fibrous membrane sometimes contains lymph nodules, especially near the points of division of the bronchi. (This occurs frequently in swine.) In the inner layers of larger bronchi this membrane also contains glands (Figs. 282,*h;* 283,*e*). These resemble the mixed tracheal glands and vary in number and size with the diameter of the bronchi. The smallest bronchioles are free from both glands and cartilage (Figs. 282,*d;* 283,*f*).

The peribronchial layer is loose connective tissue and contains vessels, nerves, and sometimes fat cells.

In the smaller bronchi (2 mm. and less in diameter) a dense plexus of veins and a few lymphatics is present between the muscularis and the fibroelastic membrane. This arrangement makes possible isolated contractions of the circular bronchial muscles without passive involvement of the surrounding lung tissue: the space created by the contraction is effectively filled by the engorging veins. The filling of the bronchial venous plexuses is accomplished through arteriovenous anastomoses from arteries that are equipped with blocking devices. These arteries arise from the pulmonary artery and anastomose with the bronchial arteries. The smaller bronchioles lack venous plexuses.

The *terminal bronchiole*, which enters the lung lobule, represents the transition from the conducting to the respiratory portion of the lung. It consists of a delicate collagenous and elastic membrane lined by cuboidal epithelium, which is still ciliated in its initial portions, and of a thin layer of interwoven muscle fibers.

2. Respiratory Structures

The *respiratory bronchioles* mark the beginning of the respiratory surface by virtue of a few alveoli opening directly from their walls. The cuboidal cells lose their cilia

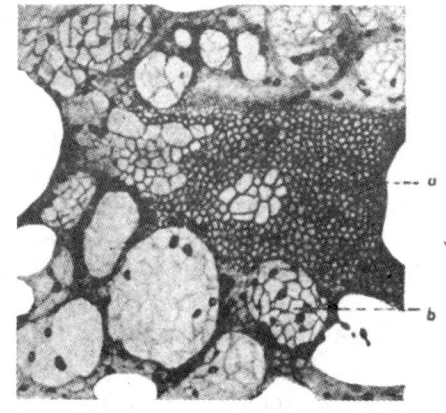

Figure 284. Section from the lung of the the horse; silver nitrate preparation (180×). *a*, simple cuboidal epithelium of a bronchiole (nuclei not shown); *b*, respiratory epithelium of the pulmonary alveoli (disputed, see text).

and finally become flattened. The theory that they are continued by a "respiratory epithelium" in the alveoli of normal mammals is disputed. The respiratory bronchioles branch into several *alveolar ducts*, the walls of which are honeycombed with the wide openings of alveoli (Figs. 281,*c*; 282,*b*). The arrangement provides a large respiratory surface. The diameter of the alveoli averages 0.3 mm. at inspiration and 0.1-0.2 mm. at expiration. The septa between adjacent alveoli have thickened margins at the lumen of the alveolar duct. These margins contain elastic fibers or smooth muscle bundles, which by their tone or by contraction prevent excessive dilation of the alveolar openings during inspiration. Every alveolar duct breaks up at an acute angle into three to five alveolar sacs, which in turn open into terminal or parietal alveoli. The alveolar ducts are separated by small quantities of interalveolar tissue.

The *interalveolar septa* consist mainly of a dense capillary network supported by fine reticular and elastic fibers. The reticular fibers are continuous with the collagenous fiber system of the interstitial tissue, permitting considerable mobility, but no great displacement of the septa. The elastic fibers are connected with the rest of the elastic fiber system. Fibroblasts and leukocytes occur in the thicker portions of the septa near the alveolar ducts and sacs. The capillaries weave back and forth throughout the fiber network of the ground membrane, bulging first into one alveolar cavity then into the other so that the gaseous exchange takes place on both surfaces. Peripherally, where neighboring alveoli do not come into contact, thin interalveolar tissue fills the space between the alveoli with their surrounding fibers and capillaries.

The question of the existence of a respiratory epithelium lining the alveoli is an old one. It is generally agreed that thick, nucleated *septal cells* occur in the niches between the bulging capillaries, usually at septal intersections, but these are too far apart to constitute a lining. According to some authors the intervening alveolar wall is lined with nonnucleated epithelial plates, which can be demonstrated only by staining their boundaries with silver nitrate (Fig. 284). According to Loosli,[1] the outlines stained with silver nitrate are those of the capillary endothelium; in the normal lung there is no continuous respiratory epithelium; and the capillaries are covered only by connective tissue ground substance and fine reticular and elastic fibers. Loosli considers the septal cells to be connective tissue elements.

The alveolar wall contains histiocytes, which phagocytose inhaled foreign matter. As "dust cells" they leave their place in the wall and pass through the lymphatics to the lymph nodes. The same protective function is ascribed to the septal cells, which are said to be able to detach themselves from the wall.

The intralobular supporting framework consists of a delicate collagenous fiber tissue that contains numerous elastic fiber nets, extremely fine vessels, nerves, and smooth muscle fibers. The latter combine with the elastic fibers to form rings around the openings of the alveoli. Therefore, cross sections through the thickened margins of the interalveolar septa show sections of smooth muscle fibers. These are especially common in the region of the alveolar ducts.

Pores in the alveolar wall, through which adjacent alveoli communicate, apparently occur only in older animals.

Vessels and Nerves. The vascular system includes an intralobular (perialveolar, respiratory, and functional) and an interlobular (interstitial and nutritive) system.

The intralobular system is derived from the pulmonary artery, which branches along with the bronchi without supplying capillaries to them. A terminal branch of the pulmonary artery enters the

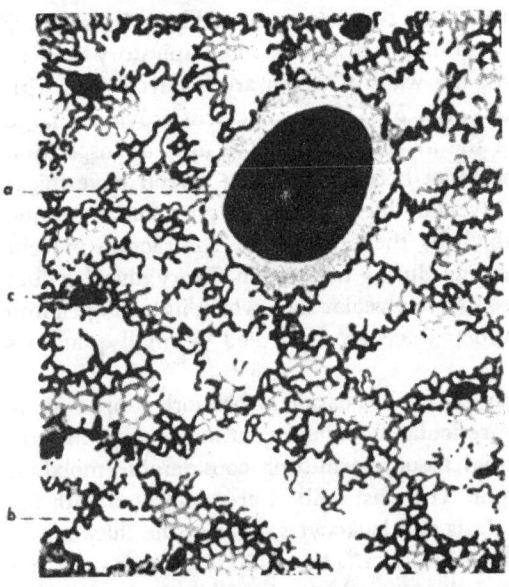

Figure 285. From the injected lung of the dog. *a*, artery; *b*, capillary; *c*, vein.

[1] "The Lung," in Maximow and Bloom, pp. 468 ff. See also C. G. Loosli, W. E. Adams, and T. M. Thornton, The Histology of the Dog's Lung Following Experimental Collapse, *Anat. Rec. 105* (1950): 697–721.

lobule with the terminal bronchiole and ramifies there (Fig. 281,*f*). These intra-lobular arterial branches give rise to the dense respiratory capillary net (Fig. 281,*h*) in the walls of the alveoli. Out of these partially intercommunicating plexuses arise the muscular pulmonary veins, some of which accompany the arteries and bronchi, while others run by themselves in the interlobular tissue (Fig. 281,*g*).

The bronchial artery is much smaller than the pulmonary artery. It also accompanies the bronchi and ramifies with them. Along its course, however, it gives off numerous twigs, which form interstitial capillary networks. These supply the bronchial walls, the framework of the lungs, the walls of the vessels, the lymph nodes, and the visceral pleura (Fig. 281,*e*). In the deeper portions of the bronchial mucosa the arterial branches form a network with longitudinal meshes made up of rather large vessels. They furnish the twigs supplying musculature and mucosa. The various capillary nets give rise to the radicles of the bronchial veins. Anastomoses exist between the pulmonary and bronchial arteries, and there are also communications between the interstitial capillary nets of the bronchial artery and the respiratory capillary nets of the pulmonary vessels.

The lymphatics of the lung form a deep net and a superficial one equipped with valves. The two nets anastomose. The former has its radicles in the interstitial tissue and the bronchial and vascular walls, while the latter is situated in and just below the pleura. The deeper lymphatics have many communications with the lymph nodules located at the points of division of the larger bronchi.

The nerves occur in bundles of myelinated and unmyelinated fibers. They enter the lungs and ramify with the bronchi and bear many ganglia. They end mainly on the smooth muscle fibers of the vessels and bronchi. Delicate plexuses have also been discovered on the alveolar surface and below the bronchial epithelium. Some of the pleural nerves end freely, while others bear lamellated corpuscles and spheroid terminal clubs.

THE LUNG OF THE CHICKEN (Fig. 286). The main bronchus does not ramify like the mammalian bronchus, but passes through the entire lung, giving off secondary bronchi in pennate fashion. It leaves the caudal end of the lung and enters the abdominal air sac. The secondary bronchi are connected with air sacs in the thoracic and cervical regions. There is no cartilage beyond the first portion of the main bronchus.

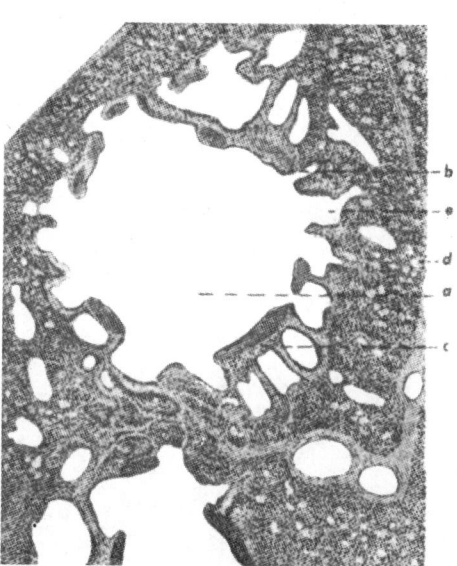

Figure 286. Section from the lung of a chicken (60×). *a*, parabronchus; *b*, epithelium; *c*, smooth muscle; *d*, respiratory capillaries in cross section; *e*, atrium.

The parabronchi (*a*) are parallel vertical tubules connecting the dorsal and ventral secondary bronchi. They also connect the secondary bronchi to the recurrent or saccobronchi, which return air to the lung from the abdominal and caudal thoracic air sacs. The parabronchi are 100–150 μ in diameter and are lined by an incomplete layer of flattened epithelial cells. These rest on a layer of circular smooth muscle fibers (*c*), which are in turn surrounded by elastic fibers. The wall is perforated by the openings of the saclike atria, which lead into branched, thin-walled respiratory capillaries, 5–15 μ in diameter.[2] These represent the mammalian alveoli. They are closely intertwined with blood capillaries, and the two networks appear to be part of the wall of the parabronchus. There is no continuous respiratory epithelium. The thin membranous wall of the air sacs is lined by simple ciliated columnar or by cuboidal epithelium.

---

[2] H. Grau, "Anatomie der Hausvögel," in W. Ellenberger and H. Baum, *Handbuch der vergleichenden Anatomie der Haustiere*, p. 1099.

XIII

The Urinary System

THE urinary system is composed of the kidneys and the excretory passages: renal pelvis, ureter, urinary bladder, and urethra.

A. KIDNEYS

The kidneys are the chief excretory organs of the body. They help to keep the composition of the blood nearly constant by removing foreign and waste material. The kidney is subdivided into cortical and medullary substance. The medulla projects into the renal pelvis or calyces with one or several papillae (one in the horse, sheep, goat, and carnivores; several in the ox and pig). The papillae are the apices of the renal pyramids, the bases of which are located at the corticomedullary junction.

The kidneys are compound tubular glands and consist mainly of excreting and conducting tubules and blood vessels. The kidneys are embedded in a deposit of fat and are covered by an easily removable connective tissue capsule, whose deeper portions in the sheep and ox contain smooth muscle fibers. At the hilus the capsule dips into the renal sinus and forms the adventitia of the renal pelvis. This adventitia is continuous with the interstitial tissue of the medulla. The supporting framework of the cortex and outer medullary zone is a latticework of delicate reticular tissue, which invests the tubules and blood vessels. It is more abundant in the remaining medullary substance. Fibrillar connective tissue accompanies only the larger vessels.

The densely packed uriniferous tubules, which number 200,000 to 300,000 in each kidney of the cat, follow a complicated course. That portion in which urine is produced is called the nephron.[1] It is composed of a renal corpuscle and a nonbranching, looped tubule. The nephron is comparable to the secretory end-piece of a gland. It is succeeded by an extensively branched system of collecting tubules. Nephrons and collecting tubules differ in their embryological derivation. Histologically the uriniferous tubules are seen to consist of convoluted and straight portions. The convoluted tubules occur, along with the renal corpuscles (see below)

---
[1] Gr. *nephros*, L. *ren* kidney.

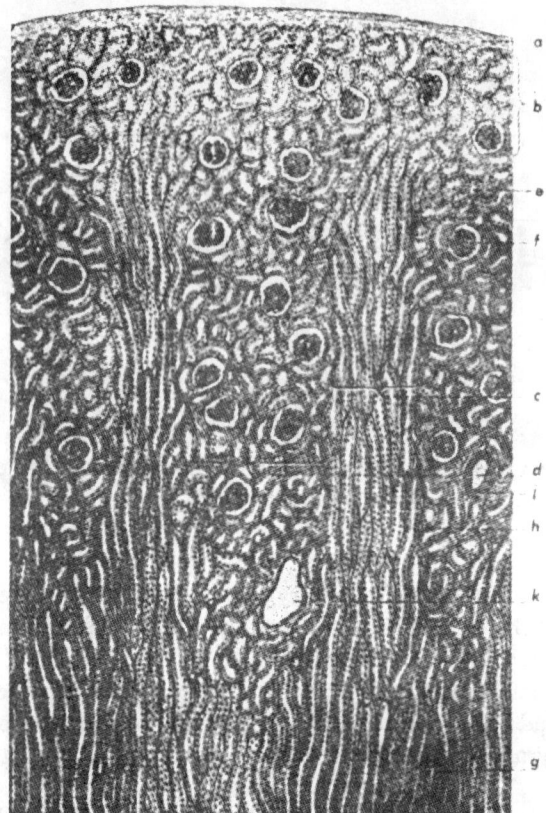

Figure 287. Radial section through the kidney of the horse. *a,* capsule; *b,* pars convoluta; *c,* medullary ray; *d,* pars convoluta between medullary rays; *e,* convoluted tubules in section; *f,* renal corpuscles; *g,* collecting tubules and loops of Henle in section; *h,* capillary; *i,* artery; *k,* vein.

in the pars convoluta of the cortex (Figs. 287,*b,d;* 288). The straight tubules are found in the medullary rays and in the medulla.

Topography of the Renal Corpuscles and Tubules. The *renal or Malpighian corpuscle* (Fig. 288,*a*) lies in the pars convoluta and consists of a ball of blood capillaries, the glomerulus (see also p. 247), and its two-layered envelope, the capsule of Bowman. The inner, or visceral, layer of this capsule invests the glomerulus very closely, but the outer, parietal layer is separated from the inner sheet by a slitlike space, which receives the secretion and is continuous with the lumen of the uriniferous tubule.

The uriniferous tubule is composed of several segments, which differ in their course and histological appearance. It begins with a short, constricted neck, whose wall is continuous with the parietal layer of Bowman's capsule. The neck soon widens into a larger passage, the *proximal convoluted tubule* (Fig. 288,*b,c*). After a tortuous course, this important part of the nephron straightens out and enters a medullary ray. Here it becomes narrower and continues as the U-shaped *loop of Henle* (*d,e*). This consists of a thin *descending limb* and a thicker *ascending limb*. The transition between the thin and thick segments rarely occurs at the crest of the loop.

The crest of the loop may lie either in the cortex, i.e., in a medullary ray, or in the medullary substance. The position is determined largely by the level of the renal corpuscle within the cortex. The human kidney has mostly short loops, while some species of domestic animals have predominantly (ox and pig) or even exclusively (cat) long loops. Especially where Henle's loop is short, the change from thin to thick segments often occurs before the crest is reached.

The ascending limb of the loop lies closer to the collecting tubule than the descending limb. Near the vascular pole of its corresponding renal corpuscle it widens and passes by way of a strongly curved segment into the short *distal convoluted tubule* (*f*), the last segment of the nephron. This is continued by the narrower initial portion of the collecting tubule, which is called the *connecting tubule* (*g*). It is particularly long in the horse, pig, and cat. It unites with other connecting tubules to make up a straight *collecting tubule* (*h*), which runs through a medullary ray and the medulla toward the renal pelvis. Along the way groups of them meet at acute angles and form larger tubules. In the medulla all the collecting tubules of one medullary ray combine into a single large collecting tubule. Finally the collecting tubules of adjacent medullary rays join and make up the large *papillary ducts* (*i*). These open into the renal pelvis through small pits, each of which receives two or three ducts (Fig. 296,*a*).

Structure of the Renal Corpuscles and Tubules. The *renal corpuscles* (Fig. 289) are 120–122 μ in diameter. The glomerulus (*e*) is a tuft of capillaries interposed in the arterial pathway and held together by delicate connective tissue. The capillary endothelium shows no cell boundaries and few nuclei. The glomerulus of young animals is covered by a single layer of cuboidal cells, the visceral layer of the capsule of Bowman. They are later transformed into flat cells, whose spherical nuclei bulge out into the lumen of the capsule. The visceral layer also dips in between the capillary loops. According to some authors the visceral layer is not continuous. The epithelial cells are separated from the endothelium by a delicate basement membrane. The outer layer of Bowman's capsule (*g*) is a simple epithelium consisting of flat, generally hexagonal cells with large oval nuclei. The capsule is surrounded by a thin basement membrane.

According to prevailing views the renal corpuscle acts passively as a filter, permeable to all the blood constituents of small molecular size. The substances that are useful to the body—chlorides, glucose, most of the water—are reabsorbed by various portions of the tubule.

The uriniferous tubule consists of a structureless basement membrane lined by simple epithelium, which has different characteristics in each segment of the tubule. On the outside the basement membrane is covered by spiral reticular fibers.

Opposite the vascular pole of the renal corpuscle, the squamous cells of the pa-

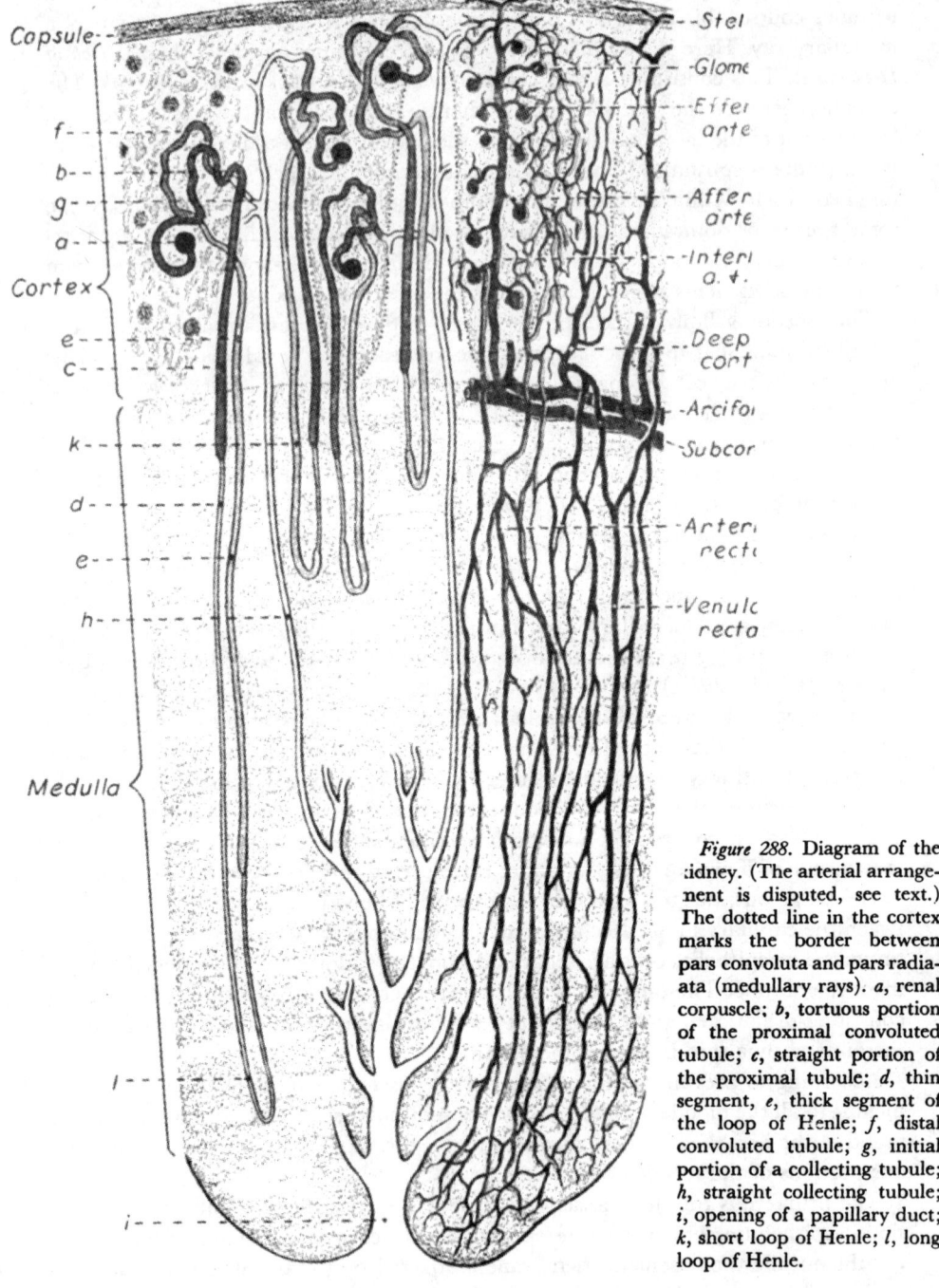

Capsule

f
b
g
a

Cortex

e
c

k

d

e

h

Medulla

l

i

Stel
Glome
Effer
arte

Affer
arte

Interi
a. t.

Deep
cort

Arcifor
Subcor

Arteri
recto

Venulc
recta

Figure 288. Diagram of the kidney. (The arterial arrangement is disputed, see text.) The dotted line in the cortex marks the border between pars convoluta and pars radiaata (medullary rays). *a*, renal corpuscle; *b*, tortuous portion of the proximal convoluted tubule; *c*, straight portion of the proximal tubule; *d*, thin segment, *e*, thick segment of the loop of Henle; *f*, distal convoluted tubule; *g*, initial portion of a collecting tubule; *h*, straight collecting tubule; *i*, opening of a papillary duct; *k*, short loop of Henle; *l*, long loop of Henle.

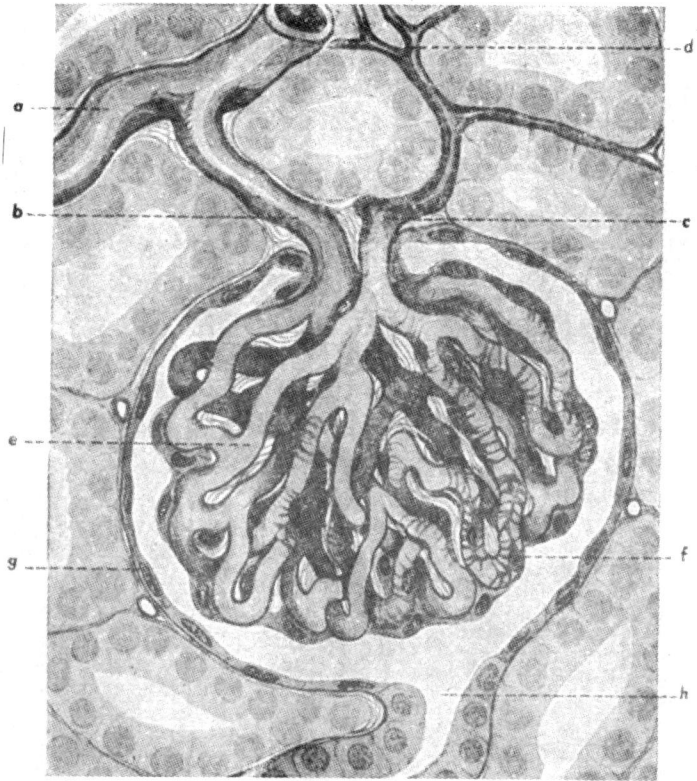

Figure 289. Renal corpuscle, schematic. *a*, interlobular artery; *b*, afferent arteriole; *c*, efferent arteriole; *d*, arteriolae rectae; *e*, glomerulus; *f*, epithelial cell of the internal layer, and *g*, of the external layer of Bowman's capsule; *h*, neck of the uriniferous tubule. Anastomosis of capillaries is controversial: see text.

rietal layer pass into the cuboidal cells of the neck of the tubule (Fig. 289,*h*). The neck has a diameter of about 34 μ.

The short neck is followed by the *proximal convoluted tubule* (Fig. 290). This is 45–60 μ in diameter and is lined by granular, somewhat cone-shaped cells. The cytoplasm shows a basal striation caused by rows of mitochondria. The nuclei of these cells are spheroid and varied in size. They are irregularly placed. Cell boundaries are indistinct and usually not visible. On the surface facing the lumen the cells bear a brush border, which degenerates rapidly postmortem and in common preparations has no distinct distal limit but gradually fades out toward the lumen. Basal striations and the brush border are most pronounced in the tortuous portion of the proximal tubule. In the straight part the basal striations grow less distinct.

The structure of the cells changes with their functional status. When active they are low; when they are not secreting they are high, the lumen is narrow, and the brush border is less distinct. Changes in cytoplasmic inclusions have been described.

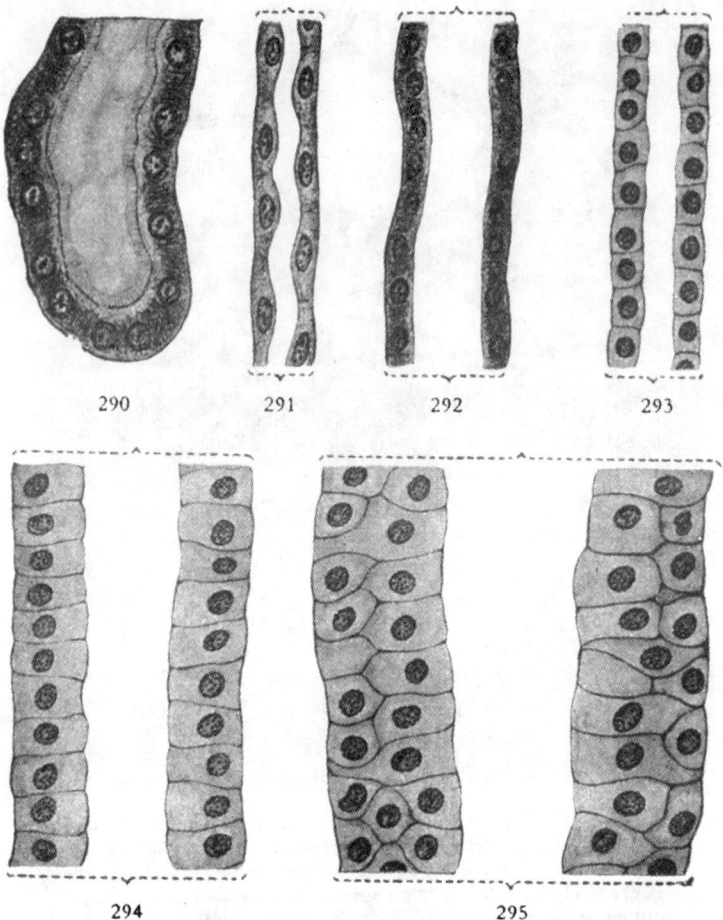

290   291   292   293

294   295

Figures 290–295. Epithelium of the various portions of the uriniferous tubules of the goat (450×). Fig. 290, proximal convoluted tubule. Fig. 291, descending (thin) segment. Fig. 292, ascending (thick) segment of Henle's loop. Fig. 293, connecting tubule (initial portion of the collecting tubule). Fig. 294, collecting tubule. Fig. 295, papillary duct.

In the cat the cells of the proximal convoluted tubules contain many fat droplets. This normal condition has been mistaken for fatty degeneration. The last tenth of the proximal tubule in the dog also contains much intracellular fat.

The *thin segment* of the loop of Henle is a lightly staining tubule of 10–17 μ in thickness. It is clearly marked off from the proximal convoluted tubule and contains flattened elongated cells (Fig. 291) with translucent cytoplasm and a spheroid nucleus, which causes the cell to bulge into the lumen.

The *thick segment* of the loop (Fig. 292) is 25–40 μ thick and has an epithelium resembling that of the proximal convoluted tubule except that the cells and their basal striations are shorter. A brush border is absent.

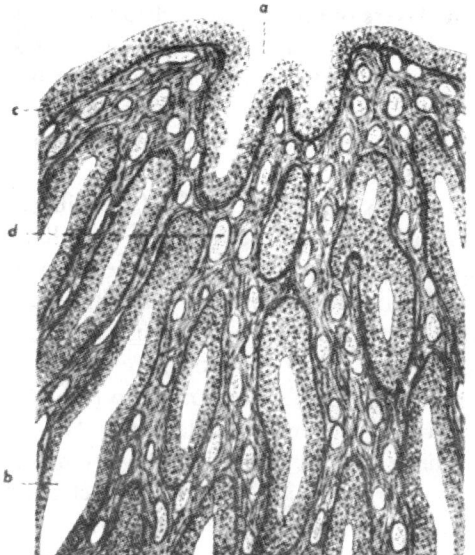

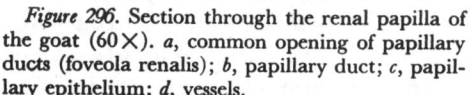

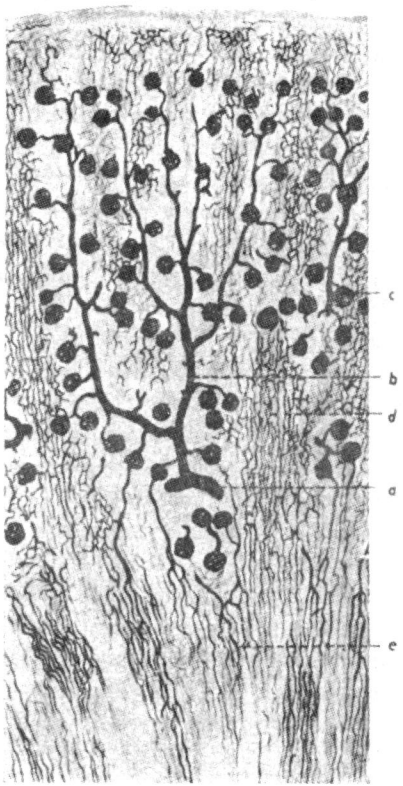

Figure 296. Section through the renal papilla of the goat (60×). *a*, common opening of papillary ducts (foveola renalis); *b*, papillary duct; *c*, papillary epithelium; *d*, vessels.

Figure 297 (*right*). Section from the kidney of the rabbit; injected through an artery (35×). *a*, subcortical artery; *b*, interlobular artery; *c*, glomerulus; *d*, capillaries in a medullary ray; *e*, arteriola rectae.

The *distal convoluted tubule*, 35–53 μ in diameter, has lighter, often shiny cells. These may begin to appear in the ascending limb of the loop. They show basal striations like those of the proximal convoluted tubules. Their nuclei are especially large in the horse.

The diameter of the *connecting tubule* ranges from 14 to 21 μ. This segment is composed of polygonal, light-colored elements, distinguishable only by their lesser height from the cells of the collecting tubules (Fig. 293).

The epithelium of the *smaller collecting tubules* (22–60 μ in diameter) consists of irregularly cuboidal cells with a central nucleus. Cell boundaries are distinct, and the cytoplasm is clear. Numerous fat droplets may be present, especially in older animals. In the larger tubules the epithelial cells grow higher (Fig. 294) until, in the *papillary ducts*, they become hexagonal columnar cells with more or less broad bases. The nuclei are often eccentrically located. In the papillary ducts the epithelium becomes two-layered (Figs. 295, 296) and, toward the opening, often transitional in type.

A network of terminal bars is present in all parts of the uriniferous tubules.

VESSELS AND NERVES (Figs. 288, 297). The arteries of the kidney are derived mainly from the renal artery, which enters at the hilus and divides into a number of branches. These give off branches to the layers of the capsule and to the pelvis and extend radially between the pyramids as the interlobar arteries. (Each pyramid represents a separate lobe of the fetal kidney.) At the corticomedullary junction they bend at nearly right angles and become the subcortical arteries (Figs. 288; 297,*a*). The old term arciform arteries gives the false impression that they are anastomotic arches between interlobar arteries.

The branches to the cortex arise on the convex side of the curve of the subcortical arteries and run a radial course at regular intervals between the medullary rays. They are called interlobular arteries (Figs. 288; 297,*b*). Along their course they give off many branches which either form glomeruli directly (as in the Carnivora) or divide into smaller twigs (as in the horse and ruminants), each of which forms a glomerulus. The afferent arteriole is provided with a cuff of epithelioid cells near the glomerulus. It divides in the larger glomeruli into five to eight, in the smaller into four, branches. These give rise to numerous capillary loops, which lie together in groups, giving the glomerulus a lobulated appearance. The capillary loops do not anastomose. (Fig. 289 is incorrect in this respect.) The efferent arteriole is narrower than the afferent vessel. It leaves the glomerulus close to the latter. Most of the efferent arterioles end in capillary nets which surround the uriniferous tubules and form polygonal or round meshes in the pars convoluta (Figs. 288, 297) and oblong ones in the medullary rays. The efferent arterioles of the glomeruli that lie close to the medulla form the arteriolae rectae, which supply the renal pyramids (Fig. 297). Thus the capillaries of the uriniferous tubules in cortex and medulla are supplied almost exclusively with blood that has passed through the glomeruli. Most authorities now agree that exceptions to this rule are rare.

The veins of the kidneys unite into the arciform veins, which lie in the outer medullary zone and run parallel to the surface. They anastomose freely and receive the interlobular veins from the cortex and the venulae rectae from the medulla. The arciform veins pass into larger trunks, which unite to form the renal vein. The interlobular veins arise from the capillaries of the cortex. The most peripheral radicles converge in starlike configurations visible from the surface as the stellate veins. In the cat they make up elaborate nets rather than star patterns before descending into the cortex as interlobular veins. The venulae rectae originate in the inner portion of the medulla. Direct communications between arterioles and venules are found here. The question of the prevalence and importance of arteriovenous anastomoses in the kidney is not settled.

The lymphatic plexus in the capsule is continuous with the one in the cortex. The deeper lymphatics arise from capillaries in the parenchyma. They are connected to interlobular plexuses which pass into trunks that leave the kidney at the hilus. The nerves, which still exhibit small ganglia at the hilus, contain both unmyelinated and myelinated fibers. They form abundant plexuses around the blood vessels on which they end. Some of them terminate on and in the walls of the renal tubules.

The urine is the excretory product of the kidney. It is an aqueous solution of in-

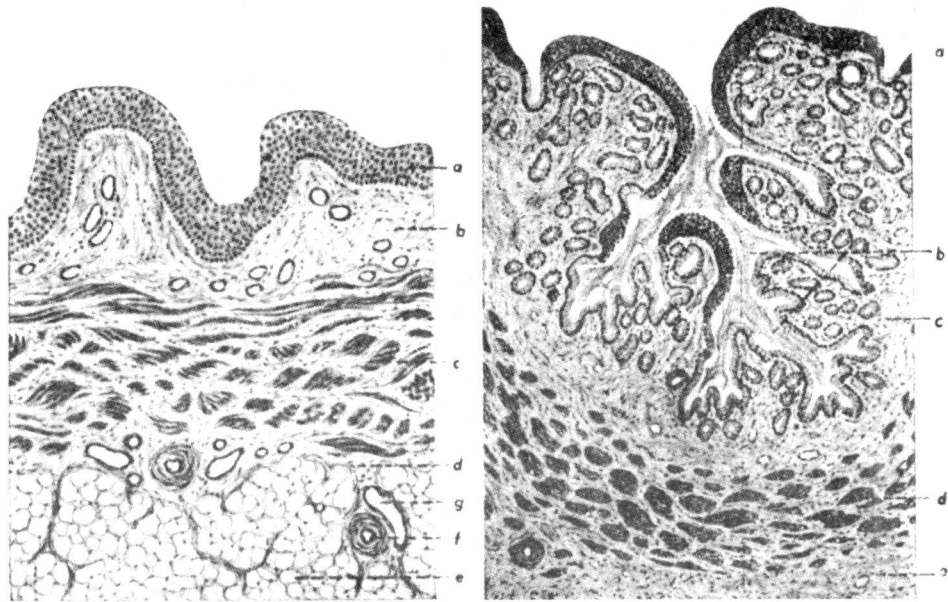

Figure 298 (left). Section through the wall of the renal pelvis of the pig. *a*, transitional epithelium; *b*, propria mucosae; *c*, muscularis; *d*, adventitia; *e*, adipose tissue; *f*, artery; *g*, vein.

Figure 299 (right). Section through the wall of the renal pelvis of a horse. *a*, transitional epithelium; *b*, lumen of mucous gland; *c*, interglandular tissue; *d*, muscularis; *e*, adventitia with vessel.

organic and organic substances, of which the latter are largely products of protein catabolism. With the exception of desquamated epithelial cells, the normal urine contains no organized sediments. The various histologically distinct portions of the renal tubules have been identified with certain steps in the formation of urine. The process is more complex than simple physical filtration or osmosis; there is active participation of the tubular epithelium. Most of this activity is reabsorption of water, glucose, chlorides, and phosphates. Tubular secretion (excretion) can be demonstrated with many foreign substances but is believed to be unimportant under normal conditions in mammals.[2]

THE KIDNEY OF THE CHICKEN. The pyramidal lobules, which correspond to the cortical lobules of the mammal, are separated by connective tissue. Their bases lie under the capsule and their apices project into the hilus. The glomeruli are smaller and the proximal tubules larger than in mammals. In the fresh state the cells of the tubules contain urate granules, which combine into larger pellets in the lumen. The collecting tubules, which end on the tips of the papillae, are lined by mucous cells of increasing height. The folded mucosa of the ureter bears a high pseudostratified epithelium with mucous cells. As in other avian organs, there are many

[2] H. H. Dukes, *The Physiology of Domestic Animals,* p. 407. See also Arthur M. Walker et al., The Collection and Analysis of Fluid from a Single Nephron of the Mammalian Kidney, *Am. J. Physiol.* 134 (1941): 580–595.

aggregations of lymphocytes in the kidney. The capillaries of the tubules are supplied by renal portal veins.[3]

B. THE EXCRETORY PASSAGES

From the renal papillae the urine passes into the pelvis; thence it flows through the ureter into the urinary bladder and leaves the body by way of the urethra. The wall of the excretory passages consists of a mucosa, a muscularis, and an adventitia. The mucosa is covered almost exclusively by transitional epithelium.

1. Renal Pelvis and Calyces

With the exception of the pig and goat (Fig. 296,c), the transitional epithelium is replaced on the renal papilla by two-layered cuboidal to columnar epithelium. In solipeds intraepithelial goblet cells occur. The propria mucosae (Figs. 298,b; 299,c) is composed of collagenous tissue which contains very few elastic fibers, except in the horse. Many tubuloalveolar mucous glands are present in the propria of the horse (Fig. 299,b). The propria becomes looser toward the periphery and is anchored in the interlobar connective tissue. In the horse and ox a distinct submucosa is present. The muscularis (Figs. 298,c; 299,d) consists only occasionally

[3] Rudolf Spanner, Der Pfortaderkreislauf in der Vogelniere, *Morph. Jahrb. 54* (1925): 560–632.

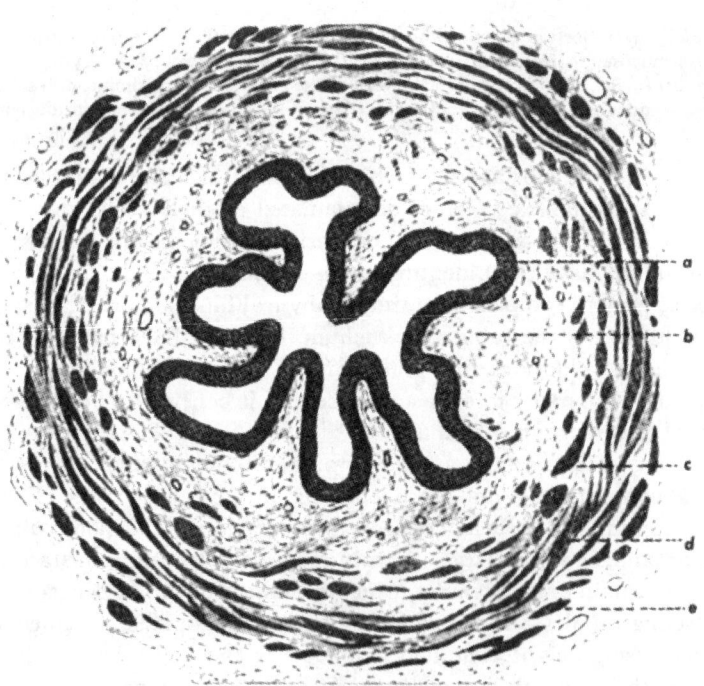

Figure 300. Cross section through the ureter of the pig. *a*, transitional epithelium; *b*, propria mucosae; *c*, inner longitudinal, *d*, middle circular, *e*, outer longitudinal, muscle layer.

(in the horse and ox) of clearly defined layers. In such cases there is an inner longitudinal layer and an outer circular layer with interconnecting strands. Isolated longitudinal fibers are often found outside the two main sheets. The collagenous adventitia contains fat cells, large vessels, and nerves, and sends processes from the renal papilla into the parenchyma. Loose collagenous and adipose tissue is present at the hilus between the capsule and the wall of the renal pelvis.

The wall of the renal calyces of the pig and ox contains less muscle than the pelvis of the pig and the corresponding main ducts of the ox. In these animals the muscle fibers form a sphincter-like circular layer at the base of each papilla. In the other species there is an additional sphincter at the beginning of the ureter.

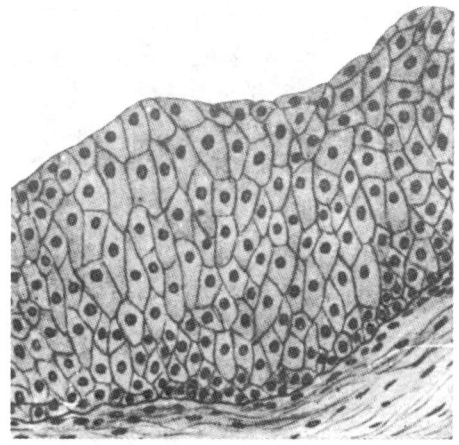

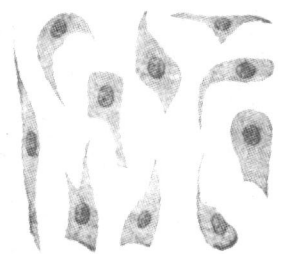

Figure 301 (left). Transitional epithelium from the ureter of the horse.

Figure 302 (right). Isolated epithelial cells from the ureter of the horse. Left, a cell from the distended ureter (lateral view).

The recessus terminales of solipeds are not evaginations of the pelvis but very large collecting ducts from the poles of the kidney, lined by stratified epithelium but devoid of musculature.

The blood vessels and lymphatics lie in the adventitia close to the parenchyma and form capillary networks in the mucosa. The numerous nerves are provided with ganglia, which are said to be absent in swine and carnivores in the proximal portion of the ureter.

2. Ureter

The folded mucosa bears a transitional epithelium with a wide variety of cell forms (Figs. 301, 302). In the distended ureter all cells appear in section to be narrow spindles. For a distance of 10 cm. from the pelvis, the collagenous propria of the horse contains tubuloalveolar mucous glands with wide lumina (Fig. 303,b). The musculature consists of thin bundles and forms an inner longitudinal (Fig. 300,c), a middle circular (d), and a thin outer longitudinal layer (e), which may occasionally be interrupted by collagenous bundles. Near the opening into the bladder the ureter contains only longitudinal muscle fibers. The loose adventitia contains the larger vessels and nerves.

The blood vessels are mostly directed longitudinally and form a dense subepi-

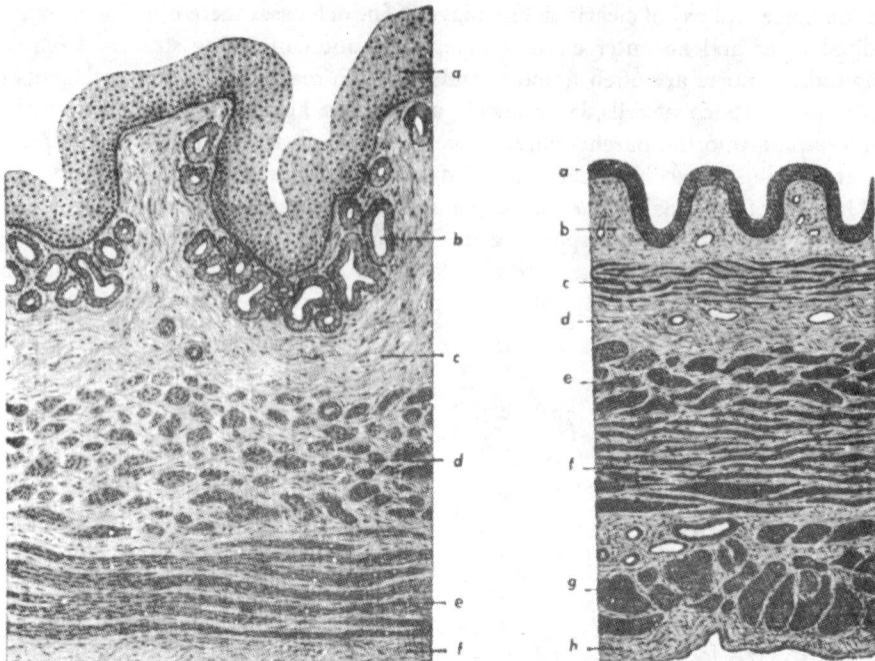

Figure 303 (left). Section through the wall of the initial portion of the ureter of the horse. *a*, transitional epithelium; *b*, mucous glands; *c*, propria mucosae; *d*, longitudinal, *e*, circular, muscle layer; *f*, adventitia.

Figure 304 (right). Cross section through the wall of the urinary bladder of the ox. *a*, transitional epithelium; *b*, propria mucosae; *c*, muscularis mucosae; *d*, submucosa; *e*, longitudinal, *f*, circular, *g*, outer longitudinal layer of the muscularis; *h*, serosa.

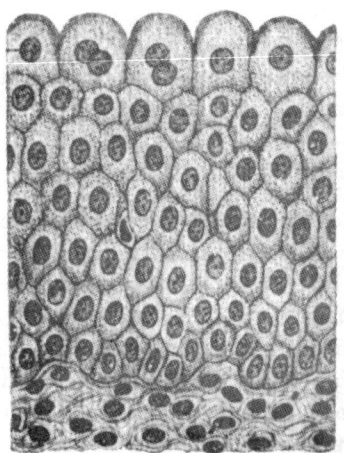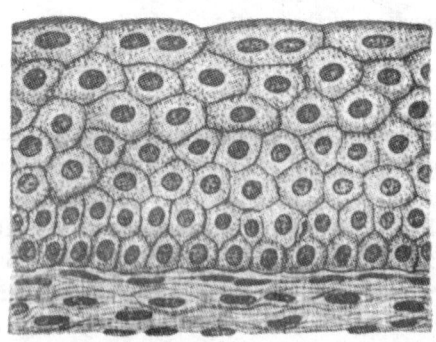

Figures 305 and 306. Epithelium of the undistended (*left*) and distended (*right*) urinary bladder of the sheep.

thelial capillary network. The lymphatics form a wide-meshed network, which is somewhat more deeply located. Ganglia are present along the nerves.

3. Urinary Bladder (Vesica Urinalis, Urocyst)

The bladder has the same layers as the ureter. The collagenous propria mucosae contains few elastic fibers and possesses a loose submucosa. Between these layers or in the submucosa there is usually a thin layer of longitudinal muscle comparable to a muscularis mucosae (Fig. 304,c). The propria bears transitional epithelium, whose cells flatten out when the bladder is distended (Figs. 305, 306). When found in urine sediment, they are indistinguishable from the epithelial cells of the ureter and renal pelvis, but are easily differentiated from those of the uriniferous tubules. The propria mucosae exhibits glandlike epithelial downgrowths and lymph nodules.

The muscularis of the bladder is made up of coarse bundles of fibers. Except for the random arrangement of the fibers in the apex of the bladder, the muscularis commonly consists of external and internal longitudinal layers and a middle circular layer. The latter is the thickest and shows the most continuity, while the outer longitudinal sheet may be modified or absent in some places. The layers are not separated by distinct intermuscular connective tissue strata but are connected by bundles of oblique muscle fibers, which often pass through the entire tunica muscularis and lend an interwoven appearance. There is a sphincter of smooth muscle at the neck of the bladder.

A serosa is present on the apex and body of the bladder; at the neck the muscularis is covered by an adventitia of the same structure as that on the ureter.

The arterial blood vessels form intermuscular and subepithelial capillary nets. Capillaries also enter the epithelium. The lymphatics make up a wide-meshed network on either side of the muscularis. The nerves usually accompany the vessels. Between the muscularis and mucosa they form a plexus which contains ganglia.

The urethra is described with the genital organs (see pp. 272, 304).

XIV

The Male Genital Organs

THE male genital organs consist of the testis, epididymis, ductus deferens, penis, and the accessory genital glands.

The testis produces the spermatozoa, but only after it reaches a mature and functional status under the influence of the gonadotrophic hormones of the hypophysis. Following castration the animal becomes impotent, and conspicuous changes occur in the secondary sex characteristics. These changes are to be ascribed to the absence of the endocrine activities of the testes, since implantation of testicular tissue restores the secondary sex characteristics. The sex hormones are therefore responsible for the body development typical of the sex and for the competence of the genital apparatus. The place of elaboration of the male sex hormone has not been definitely determined. Most of the evidence is in favor of the interstitial cells rather than the seminiferous epithelium.

A. TESTES

The testes (Figs. 307–312) are compound tubular glands. They are enveloped by a capsule—the *tunica albuginea*—and a layer of peritoneum, the *tunica vaginalis visceralis*. The latter is composed of collagenous tissue which is poor in blood vessels and elastic elements. Its free surface is covered by mesothelium (Fig. 309,b), while its attached surface blends into the underlying tunica albuginea. This is a fibrous membrane, which is so richly vascularized in certain places that it may be said to contain a stratum vasculare. The latter is in the middle of the tunic in the horse and boar and near the parenchyma in the ram and dog. At the margin of the testis where the epididymis is attached, the albuginea is connected to the mediastinum testis (Figs. 307; 308,g), a connective tissue cord that extends through the testis on its long axis and gives off collagenous sheets (in carnivores and pigs) or strands (in ruminants) radiating to the tunica albuginea. These *septula testis* divide the testicular parenchyma into pyramidal or cone-shaped lobuli testis. The mediastinum contains labyrinthine, communicating spaces of varying width and length, which make up the rete testis (Fig. 308,c; see also below).

There is no muscle in the interstitial tissue surrounding the seminiferous tubules,

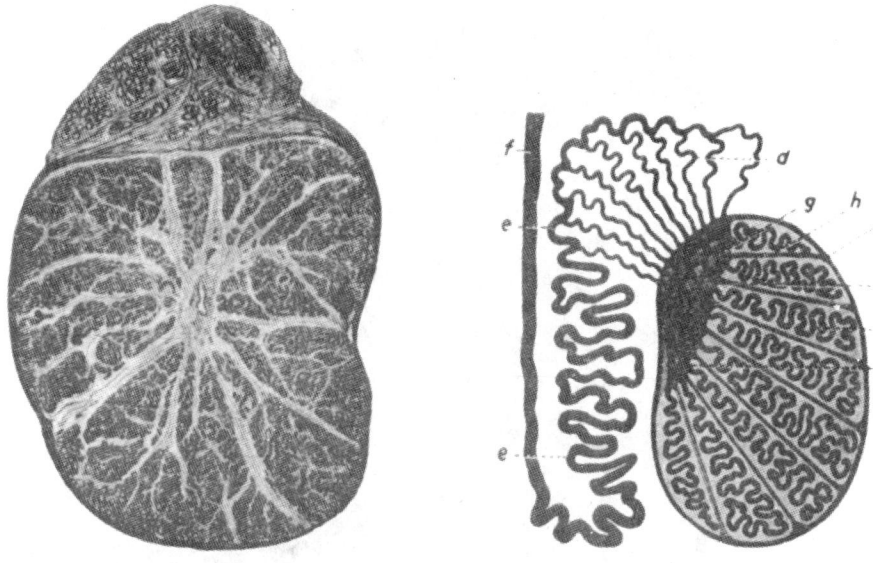

Figure 307 (left). Cross section through the testicle of the dog. In the center, mediastinum testis with radiating septa; between them, the parenchyma; on top, the epididymis. (After Schmaltz.)

Figure 308 (right). Diagram of the grosser structure of the testicle and epididymis. *a,* tubuli contorti; *b,* tubuli recti; *c,* rete testis; *d,* ductuli efferentes; *e,* ductus epididymidis; *f,* ductus deferens; *g,* mediastinum testis; *h,* septula testis; *i,* tunica albuginea testis.

and the spermia are nonmotile in the testis. Their movement through the tubules is attributed to secretory pressure and to the internal testicular pressure, which is regulated by the vascular system and becomes evident by the bulging of the parenchyma when the resistant capsule is incised. The movement is aided by a fluid probably secreted by the Sertoli cells (see below).

In the horse the albuginea is rich in smooth muscle fibers. These are derived from the m. cremaster internus and are continued in the septula testis. A compact mediastinum and rete testis are absent. Instead, the whole testis is traversed by thick, interconnected septa. The larger among these converge on a disc-shaped mass of connective tissue located at the fixed margin. The wider connective tissue strands contain, in addition to blood vessels, ducts corresponding to the retial spaces. These approach each other at the cranial pole of the testis and are continued as the ductuli efferentes (Fig. 308,*d*). Because of the irregularity of the framework the lobuli testis vary widely in shape and arrangement.

The testicular parenchyma consists of the seminiferous tubules, which are surrounded by delicate connective tissue. This interstitial tissue often shows a lamellar structure and contains vessels and nerves. The *interstitial cells* (of Leydig; Fig. 310,*c*) occur singly or in groups. They are more or less oval and have a large spherical nucleus with a distinct nucleolus. The cytoplasm contains yellow lipoid granules, protein crystalloids (in the horse and cat), and pigment deposits, which increase with age. The interstitial cells are probably derived from connective tissue

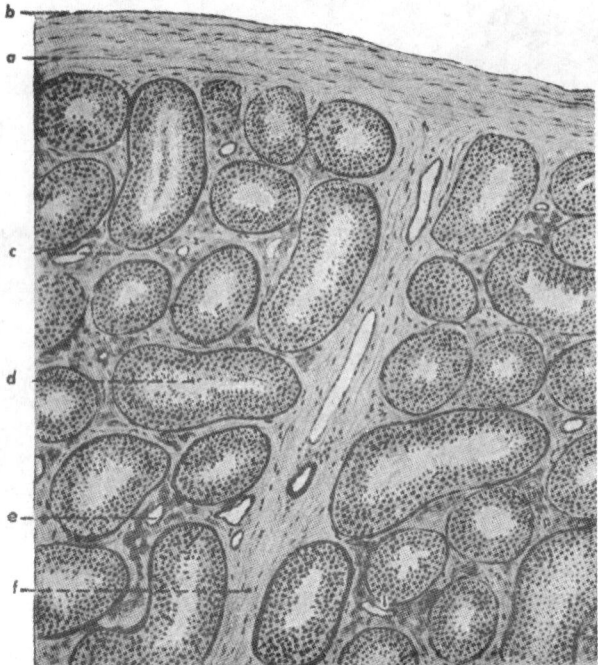

Figure 309. Section from the testicle of the tomcat (40×). *a,* tunica albuginea; *b,* tunica vaginalis, showing mesothelial cover; *c,* interstitial tissue, showing interstitial cells (of Leydig); *d,* seminiferous tubules; *e,* blood vessel; *f,* septulum testis.

cells. They are very labile elements and react to mild agents. They are most abundant in the boar and horse. Prior to the onset of spermatogenesis no typical interstitial cells are found in the horse. Large yellow richly pigmented xanthochrome cells are present. As mentioned previously, the interstitial cells are commonly credited with the production of testosterone, the male sex hormone.[1]

The *seminiferous tubules* (Figs. 309,*d;* 310) are 100–200 μ thick and 50–80 cm. long, with lumina of varying sizes. Usually there are two or three tubules in each lobule. They start blindly at the periphery and continue as tubuli contorti (Fig. 308,*a*) on their serpentine course toward the mediastinum, uniting along the way with other tubules. At the mediastinum they may pass directly into the rete testis or first into tubuli recti (*b*), which transmit the spermia to the rete.

The wall of the convoluted seminiferous tubule is composed of lamellar collagenous tissue containing elastic fibers and condensing into a thin basement membrane (Fig. 312,*g*) that is supported by reticular fibers. The basement membrane surrounds an epithelium consisting of Sertoli cells and spermatogenic cells.

[1] Charles W. Hooker, The Postnatal History and Function of the Interstitial Cells of the Testis of the Bull, *Am. J. Anatomy 74* (1944): 1–37. See also William F. Pollock, Histochemical Studies of the Interstitial Cells of the Testis, *Anat. Rec. 84* (1942): 23–30.

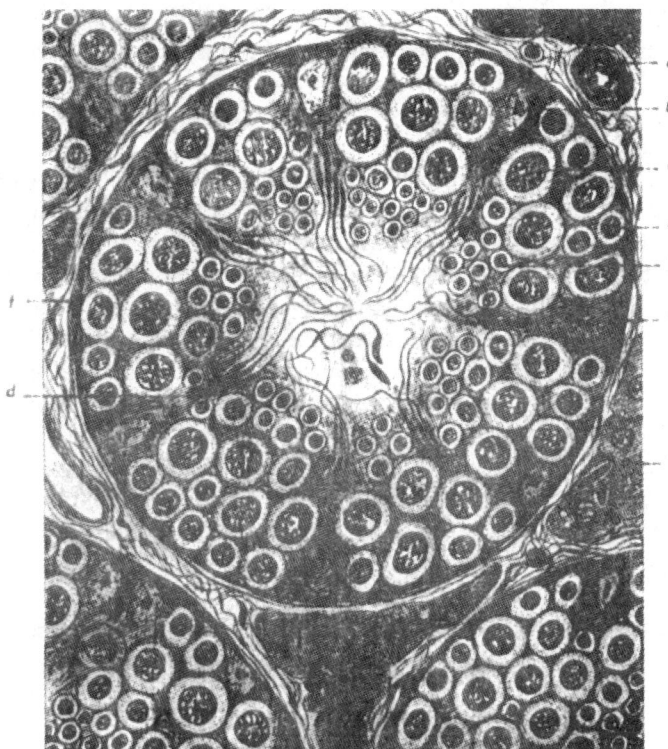

Figure 310. Cross section through a seminiferous tubule (tubulus contortus) of the stallion, at a high magnification. *a*, spermatogonium; *a'*, primary spermatocyte; *a''*, secondary spermatocyte; *a'''*, spermatid in the process of being transformed into a spermatozoon; *b*, Sertoli cell; *c*, interstitial cells, some of which contain crystalloid inclusions; *d*, cytoplasmic process of a Sertoli cell with embedded transforming spermatids; *e*, artery; *f*, membrana propria.

The *Sertoli cells* (supportive or sustentacular cells; Figs. 310,*b;* 312,*f*) are attached to the wall of the tubule and support and nourish the sperm cells. They are tall slender, radially arranged cells. The basal portion contains the nucleus and flares out into a thin basal plate, while the distal ragged end projects into the lumen. The spaces between them are filled by spermatogenic cells, which embed themselves at certain stages of their development into the cytoplasmic processes of the Sertoli cells. The latter have indistinct boundaries and apparently form a syncytium.

The *spermatogenic* cells (germ cells; Figs. 310, 312) lie in groups between the Sertoli cells in three to seven layers and include several generations produced by division. The stratification is such that the *spermatogonia* or mother cells make up the basal layer (Fig. 312,*a*). They may also form part of the second layer of cells. The next few layers are occupied by the *primary spermatocytes* (*b*), followed by the similarly spheroid, but smaller *secondary spermatocytes* (*c*). The remaining layers are made up of the minute *spermatids* (*d*), their transitional forms, and finally the *spermatozoa* (Figs. 311; 312,*e*).

The Sertoli cells are recognized by their basal, light-staining, vesicular nucleus, which has a distinct nucleolus (Fig. 312) and never shows signs of cell division. The cytoplasm often contains fat droplets and crystalloids. The spermatogonia in the basal layer are distinguished from the Sertoli cells by their round shape and their dark, spheroid nucleus, which is rich in chromatin and frequently seen in division. The same is true of the large dark-staining nuclei of the primary spermatocytes, which contain one or two nucleoli and a heterochromatic mass representing the sex chromosomes. The smaller secondary spermatocytes and spermatids have a light nucleus without nucleoli. Their cytoplasm, however, contains one or several dark-staining basophilic chromatoid accessory bodies. Spermatids show no meiotic figures (see *spermatogenesis* below).

The centrosphere of a spermatogenic cell is called an idiosome. Together with the centrioles, it plays an important part in the cell divisions and in the transformation of spermatids to spermatozoa. In the testes of young animals, the epithelium of the seminiferous tubules consists of large and small cells that show no differentiation.

The *spermatozoa* (spermia; Fig. 311) are 50–75 μ in length and consist of a head, middle piece, and tail. The head varies in shape with the species of animal, but is

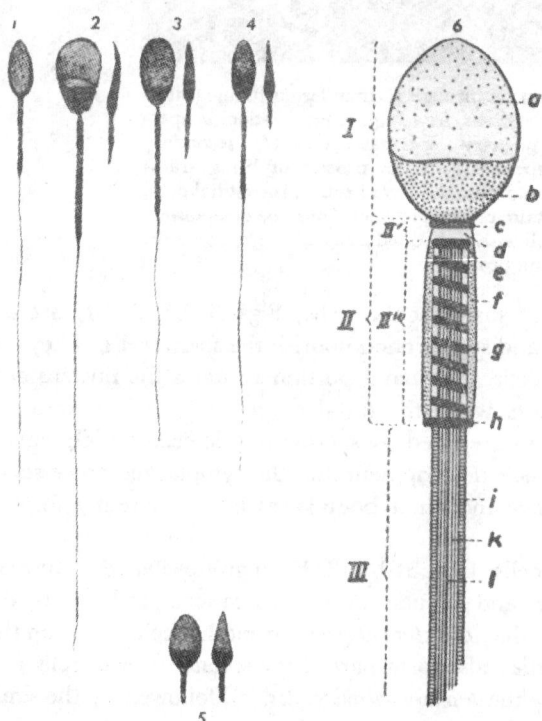

Figure 311. Spermatozoa of domestic animals and man. The heads are shown in surface and lateral views. *1*, stallion; *2*, bull; *3*, boar; *4*, cat; *5*, man; *6*, diagram of a human spermatozoon showing details. *I*, head; *II*, middle piece; *II'*, neck; *II''*, connecting piece; *III*, portion of the tail. *a*, head cap; *b*, pars posterior; *c*, anterior knob; *d*, intermediate mass; *e*, posterior knob; *f*, cytoplasm; *g*, spiral filament; *h*, terminal ring; *i*, plasma membrane; *k*, axial filament; *l*, central fibril.

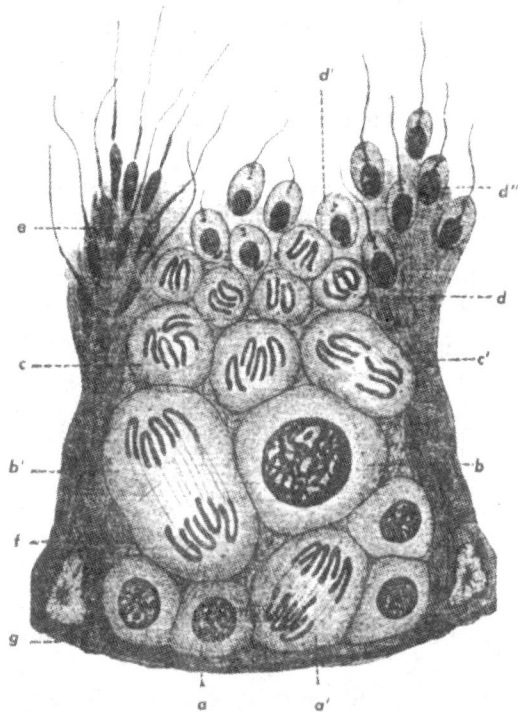

Figure 312. Diagram of the stages of spermatogenesis. *a*, spermatogonium; *a'*, spermatogonium in mitosis; *b*, primary spermatocyte, *b'*, in first meiotic division; *c*, secondary spermatocyte, *c'*, in second meiotic division (the division of the chromosomes is oversimplified, see text); *d*, spermatids, *d'*, undergoing spermiogenesis, and *d''*, having become attached to the cytoplasmic processes of Sertoli cells (*f*); *e*, mature spermatozoa; *g*, basement membrane.

usually flat and homogeneous, covered anteriorly with a head cap or galea. The middle piece is composed of the neck (*II'*) and the connecting piece (*II''*). The neck includes the anterior knob (*c*), the clear intermediate mass (*d*), and the posterior knob (*e*). From the latter arises the fibrillar axial filament (*k*) with its central fibril (*l*). In the connecting piece the axial filament is surrounded by a mitochondrial sheath or spiral filament (*3; 6,g*), which is enveloped by cytoplasm and ends at the terminal ring (*h*). The tail consists of the axial filament surrounded by a sheath. The connecting piece is considered to be the motor center.

Spermatogenesis. In the testis of the rat the phases of spermatogenesis are especially easy to follow. They occur in uninterrupted sequence along the course of the tubule, so that the same pictures are repeated at intervals. Therefore we may speak of spermatogenic waves. It should be noted, however, that new generations begin their development before the spermia of an earlier generation are fully developed. It is possible to see as many as four phases in different tubules in the same cross section. In man, dog, boar, and bull spermatogenesis is less regular. The process of spermatogenesis (Fig. 312), which involves multiplication, growth, maturation, and transformation, is as follows: In the sexually mature animal the spermatogonia (*a,a'*), which are the result of repeated mitotic divisions of the primordial germ cells, are located near the basement membrane. Their last generation develops through growth into the primary spermatocytes (*b,b'*). The next two cell divisions (of the primary and secondary spermatocytes) are called *meiosis*. The two meiotic divisions follow each other in rapid sequence while the chromosomes split only once, with the result that the four spermatids produced from one primary spermatocyte have only half the number of chromosomes characteristic for the species.

In cells that contain the whole (diploid) number of chromosomes, each chromosome has a mate, or homologue, derived from the opposite parent. In the prophase of the first meiotic division, which takes place in the primary spermatocyte, the two chromosomes of each pair become very closely associated (in synapsis) to form *bivalent* chromosomes. Each chromosome of the pair then splits into two chromatids in anticipation of the second meiotic division. While in the bivalent (tetrad) stage, the two original homologues exchange segments. This *crossing over* is the physical basis of important genetic phenomena. In the first meiotic anaphase, the homologous chromosomes separate (reductional division). In the second meiotic division, which takes place in the secondary spermatocyte, the two chromatids of each chromosome separate (equational division). Because of the exchange of segments between homologous chromosomes, the sequence of the reductional and equational divisions just described holds good only for the part of the chromosome that contains the kinetochore.[2] Genetic evidence based on a part of the chromosome in which a crossover had occurred would indicate a reversed sequence, as diagramed in Figure 312.

The spermatids usually occur in several layers. They are small and poor in chromatin. Although they have centrioles, they are no longer capable of division. After a rest period they embark upon a series of changes leading to the formation of spermatozoa (*e*). In this process of *spermiogenesis* they become oval, and their nucleus migrates into the part of the cell nearest the basement membrane. Groups of spermatids become so intimately attached to the cytoplasmic processes of the Sertoli cells that a cell boundary is no longer discernible. This association seems to provide the developing spermia with the nourishment necessary for transformation. In the process, the nucleus of the spermatid becomes the head, and the head cap is developed from the idiosome. The centrioles lie one behind the other at the posterior pole of the nucleus. The axial filament develops in association with the distal centriole, which becomes ring-shaped and in the late spermatid moves down the axial filament to the posterior limit of the middle piece.[3] The mitochondria form a sheath about the filament in the middle piece. Most of the cytoplasm is lost. During transformation the heads of the spermia become more and more deeply embedded in the Sertoli cells. Finally they are forced out into the lumen, tails first. The separation is probably brought about by the pressure of new generations of spermatogenic cells around the sides of the Sertoli cell. Full maturity is not reached

---

[2] Lester W. Sharp, *Fundamentals of Cytology* (New York: McGraw-Hill, 1943), p. 105.

[3] R. A. R. Gresson and I. Zlotnik, A Comparative Study of the Cytoplasmic Components of the Male Germ Cells of Certain Mammals, *Proc. Roy. Soc. Edinburgh* 62 (1945): 137–161. Also by the same authors, A Study of the Cytoplasmic Components during the Gametogenesis of *Bos taurus*, *Quart. J. Microsc. Sci.* 89 (1948): 219–228.

until after passage through the epididymis, and strong motility is acquired only on contact with the prostate secretion.

The shape of the spermatozoon shows its specialization for motility. In the uterus and oviduct, movement occurs rheotactically against the ciliary current, which is directed toward the outside. Motility remains good for relatively long periods of time in media isotonic to semen. Variations in viability and resistance to noxious agents exist among the species. Plain water and acid solutions quickly paralyze spermia, but they may survive for days in the alkaline secretions of the female genital tract.

The appearance of the spermatozoa varies widely among the species (Fig. 311). In the chicken the head of the spermatozoon is awl-like and comes to a fine point. The middle piece is absent, and the tail is 170 μ in length.

Atypical spermatozoa are not uncommon. They may be giant or dwarf forms, or have more than one head or tail.

Psychological conditions, e.g., a state of anxiety, are said to have a marked influence on the histological appearance of the testis.

The tubuli recti and the spaces and canaliculi of the rete testis receive the spermia produced in the seminiferous tubules. They possess a simple low columnar, cuboidal or squamous epithelium, which is considered to be a continuation of the Sertoli cells. Only in the ox do we find portions with stratified epithelium. A true basement membrane is found only in the tubuli recti. The transition from the seminiferous epithelium to that of the tubuli recti and retial passages is gradual.

VESSELS AND NERVES. The vascular trunks enter the tunica albuginea and the mediastinum. They are characterized by an especially long course through the albuginea. From here they enter the septula and form a dense capillary network around the seminiferous tubules. In the mediastinum the septal veins unite with the frequently sinus-like veins of the albuginea. The presence of arteriovenous anastomoses, which would regulate blood volume and thereby internal pressure, has been postulated. The lymphatics arise in the clefts between the seminiferous tubules and the interstitial connective tissue. A pair of them accompanies each blood vessel, and they form a plexus on the outer surface of the albuginea. In addition to vasomotor nerves there are nerve fibers that end with button-like terminations on the walls of the tubules or on interstitial cells. It is uncertain whether nerves actually enter the epithelium.

B. THE EXCRETORY DUCTS

At the cranial pole of the testis the mediastinum projects a little (2–10 mm.) beyond the testicular substance. At this point, six to twenty efferent ductules (Fig. 308,d) arise from the rete testis. At first they run a straight course; then they become narrower and form spiral coils, the turns of which are joined together by connective tissue to make up the *vascular cones*, whose apices point toward the testis. Taken together they constitute the head of the epididymis in the stallion, or a part of it in other animals. They unite to form the ductus epididymidis (epididym'idis; e). As this duct follows its spiral course, its walls thicken and it forms cone-shaped lobules, which collectively are called the body of the epididymis. A decrease in the amount of coiling marks the beginning of the tail of the epididymis, which passes into the ductus deferens (*f*).

1. Epididymis

The epididymis (Figs. 313, 314) is enveloped by a collagenous or, in the horse, a muscular tunica albuginea, whose inner layer gives off collagenous leaflets between the lobules of the epididymis.

The *ductuli efferentes* (Fig. 313) are 0.1–0.3 mm. in diameter and have delicate walls. The lumen is uneven because of the alternation of groups of high ciliated columnar cells with cells of a more cuboidal type. The epithelium rests on a base-

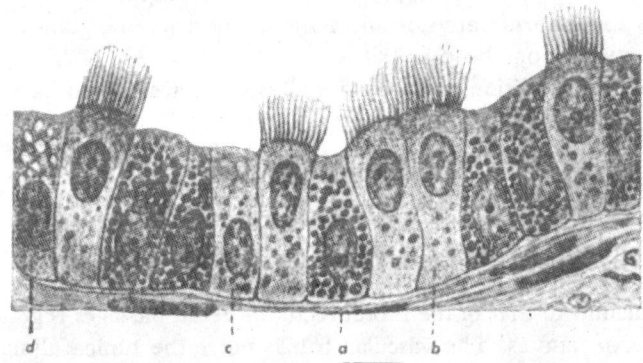

Figure 313. Surface epithelium from the ductuli efferentes of the epididymis. *a*, nonciliated cells; *b*, cells with kinocilia; *c*, cell containing little secretion; *d*, cell with vacuoles.

ment membrane surrounded by a thin collagenous propria. In the transport of spermia, the secretion originating in the seminiferous tubules is probably of importance in addition to fluid produced by the duct cells.

The ductus epididymidis (Fig. 314,*a*) is usually full of spermatozoa. It has a rather wide lumen and a collagenous wall, which increases in thickness and contains layers of circular smooth muscle fibers (*e*). Its epithelium is pseudostratified and usually has two rows of nuclei. It consists of small basal cells, which contain fat in ruminants and boars, and very high columnar cells, whose free surface bears a matted tuft of long stereocilia. In the tail of the epididymis the epithelium becomes lower (*c*) and usually simple, while the predominantly circular muscle layer grows heavier. Muscular contractions are important in the further movement of the spermia. At this point the wall begins to show the longitudinal folds characteristic of the ductus deferens (*b,c*).

The epithelial cells of the ductuli efferentes and the ductus epididymidis are the sites of active secretory processes. The evidence for this is in the various secretory granules present in the cells and the peculiar secretory droplets on the free surface. The nonciliated cells of the epithelium of the ductuli efferentes are especially rich in granules (Fig. 313). Vital dye experiments indicate that the epithelium of

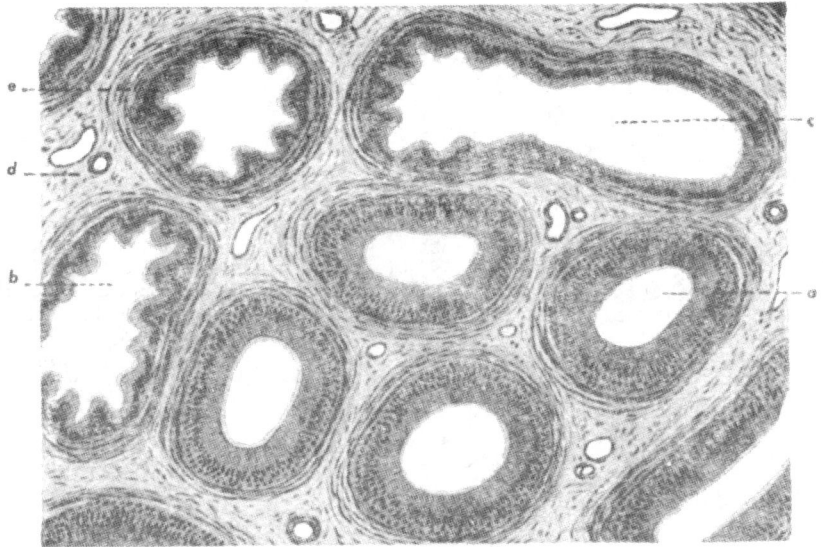

Figure 314. Section from the epididymis of the guinea pig. *a*, ductus epididymidis; *b*, cross section through the initial portion of the ductus deferens; *c*, junction of the ductus epididymidis with the ductus deferens; *d*, interstitial tissue; *e*, circular muscle layer of the epididymal duct and the ductus deferens.

the ductuli efferentes may be concerned with resorption. The epithelium of the ductus epididymidis also contains vesicular intraepithelial glands filled with secretion and surrounded by cuboidal or flat epithelium. These glands are absent in ruminants. In the horse the tail of the epididymis shows epithelial villi containing muscle and vessels.

The epididymis serves for the slow transport and storage of spermia. Its length provides an opportunity for them to complete the process of maturation. The secretion of the epididymal epithelium probably furnishes nutriment to the spermatozoa. A slight degree of motility is attained in the epididymis.

2. Ductus Deferens

The very thick wall of the ductus deferens (Figs. 315, 316) consists of a mucosa and an adventitia or, in part of its course, a serosa composed of peritoneum. A nonglandular and a glandular portion are recognized. The mucosa (Fig. 315,*b*) shows longitudinal folds and contains many elastic fibers. Its surface epithelium is simple columnar or pseudostratified with two rows of nuclei, and shows little evidence of secretory activity. Spermatozoa are often found adhering to it. The muscularis makes up the heaviest layer of the wall. In the boar and ram it consists of an inner, predominantly circular layer and an outer longitudinal layer of smooth muscle bundles. In the stallion, bull, and carnivore the fibers are interwoven and the layers less distinct. Sometimes there is an inner longitudinal layer, so that a total of three layers is present. The loose collagenous adventitia or subserosa contains numerous nerves and vessels and also branched longitudinal muscle fibers.

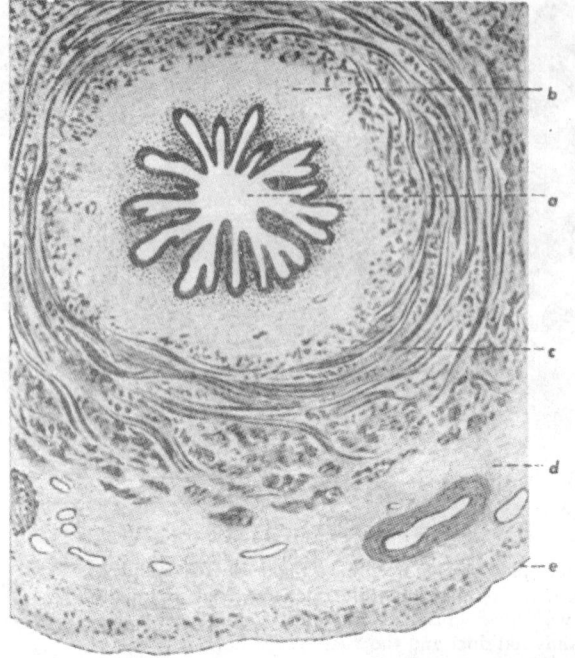

Figure 315. Cross section through the nonglandular portion of the ductus deferens of the horse. Only a portion of the upper and lateral walls is shown (24×). *a*, lumen with epithelium; *b*, propria mucosae; *c*, musculature; *d*, subserosa; *e*, serosa.

Figure 316. Cross section through the wall of the glandular portion of the ductus deferens of the goat. *a*, lumen of the duct; *b*, propria mucosae; *c*, submucosa; *d*, interglandular connective tissue showing many muscle bundles; *e*, section through a gland containing secretion, spermatozoa, and crystals; *f*, musculature.

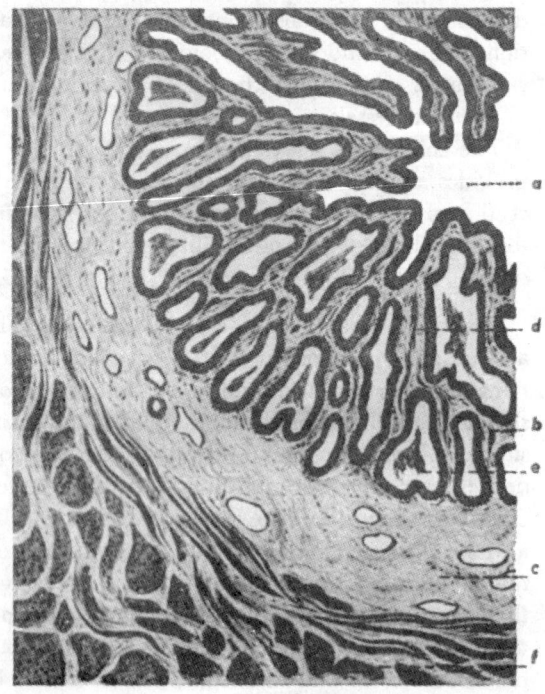

Prior to its entrance into the urethra the deferent duct undergoes a fusiform thickening, resulting in what is called the ampulla, (Fig. 316). This glandular portion of the ductus deferens shows the same structure as the accessory sex glands; i.e., it contains branched tubular glands (Fig. 316,*e*), which exhibit saclike dilatations. In the ampulla they open on the mucosal surface without special excretory ducts. Their lumen often contains a secretion. Sometimes it contains crystals and stratified concretions, which are occasionally calcified (as in horses and ruminants). The epithelium of the glands and duct is of the simple columnar type. The cells vary in height with their functional state. The muscularis is arranged in circular and longitudinal layers or, in ruminants, in interlacing bundles (*f*). It gives off radial fiber bundles into the collagenous interglandular tissue. Large fat cells are found subepithelially in the bull. The ampulla of the cat lacks glands. They are smallest in the boar; they are best developed and show the most branching in the solipeds. In the dog the glands extend into the initial portion of the urethra.

The spermatic cord is covered by a fold of peritoneum and includes numerous vessels and nerves, the ductus deferens, and a few bundles of smooth muscle fibers.

C. THE ACCESSORY GENITAL GLANDS

The accessory glands open into the urethra and include the ampullary glands (see above), the seminal vesicles, the bulbo-urethral or Cowper's glands, and the prostate gland. They are branched tubular glands of generally lobular structure. The tubules often have vesicular dilatations and variously shaped, more or less alveolar pockets along the walls and at the ends. A characteristic feature of the lobules is the collecting sinus (Fig. 317,*a*). This is usually centrally located, is often large, even vesicular, and sends out branched diverticula (*b, c*) in all directions. Collecting sinuses are absent from the seminal vesicles of the stallion and the pars disseminata of the prostate of the boar and ruminants. The glandular epithelium and that of the collecting sinuses lie on a basement membrane and consist of simple columnar cells that show secretory phenomena and surround a rather wide lumen, which is filled with secretion. The collecting sinuses lead directly into excretory ducts, which bear simple or stratified columnar epithelium and occasionally give rise to glandular outpocketings. The accessory sex glands are characterized by the occurrence of smooth muscle in the interstitial and interlobular tissue as well as in the capsule. The connective tissue is usually thick and the muscle abundant. Another characteristic is the presence of concretions (corpora amylacea) which calcify in older animals.

The accessory glands may be distinguished from other glands on the basis of the characteristics described. It is difficult, however, to tell one accessory gland from another histologically because of the great variation among the species. In general the following can be said: The glands of the ampullae are not very densely packed. They show saclike dilatations and outpouchings and open into the ampulla without excretory ducts. Spermatozoa, concretions, and crystals are often present. Concretions and crystals also occur in the seminal vesicles, which may be differentiated by the greater width of their glandular end-pieces from the prostate and bulbo-

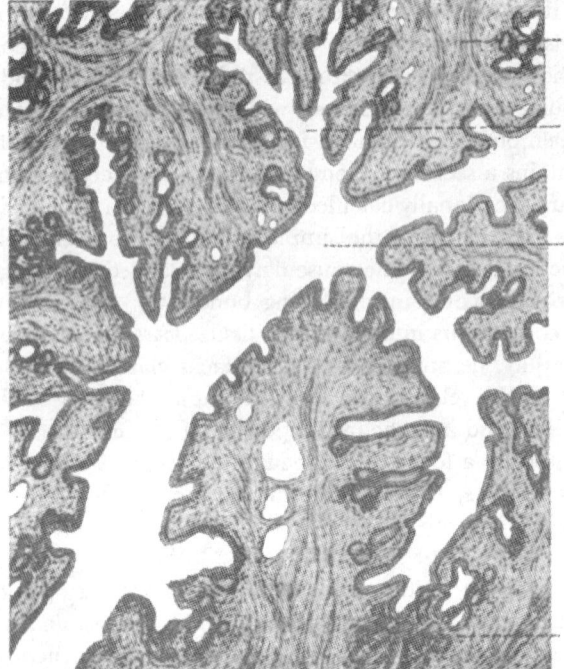

Figure 317. Section from the prostate of the stallion. *a*, central collecting sinus; *b*, its branches; *c*, cross sections through the terminal branches of the larger glandular tubules; *d*, smooth muscle.

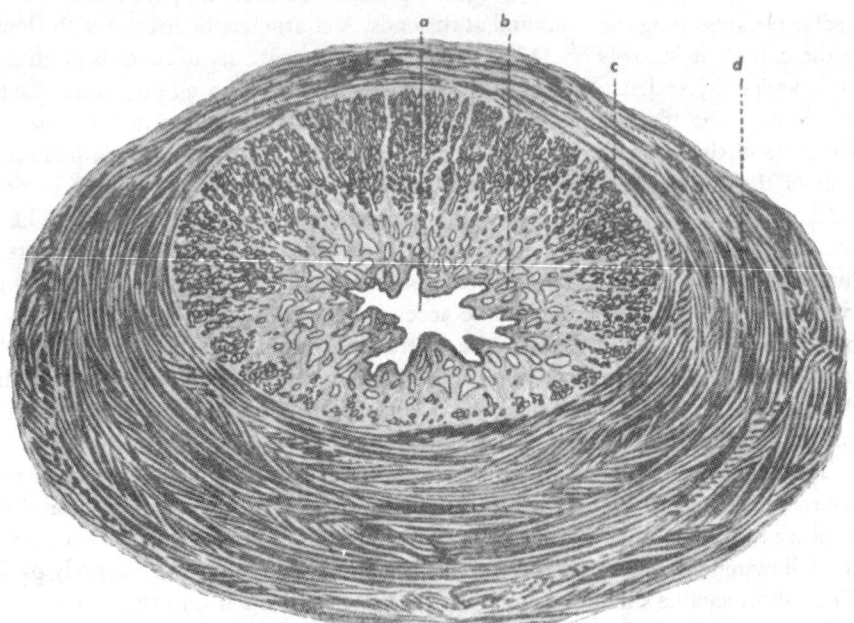

Figure 318. Cross section through the pelvic urethra of the bull showing the pars disseminata of the prostate. Surrounding the lumen (*a*) lies the stratum cavernosum (*b*). The lobular pars disseminata of the prostate is wide dorsally but sparse ventrally (*c*). Surrounding the glandular zone is the striated urethral muscle (*d*), which is very thick ventrally.

urethral glands. In the bull there are peculiar fat cells between the epithelium and the basement membrane in the ampullary glands and the seminal vesicles. The prostate and bulbo-urethral glands greatly resemble each other. In the bulbo-urethral, however, the glandular tissue is denser, there is less interstitial tissue, and lobulations are often not very distinct (in the stallion and bull). Both glands have collecting sinuses. The prostate often contains concretions while the bulbo-urethral does not. The epithelium of the bulbo-urethral glands gives a mucin reaction.

In castrated animals the accessory glands are considerably smaller than normal, and the amount of interstitial tissue is much greater in comparison to the glandular tissue. The glandular tissue is often represented only by undeveloped forms.

The secretions of the accessory sex glands make up most of the volume of the semen. The secretion of the seminal vesicles is gelatinous, that of the bulbo-urethral glands is viscous and mucoid. The prostate secretion is watery and the motility of the spermatozoa is greatly increased in it.

1. Seminal Vesicles

The seminal vesicles are branched tubular glands, whose ducts show greater or lesser dilatations depending on the species of animal. The glandular epithelium and the epithelium of the intraglandular excretory ducts is always simple columnar and shows various functional stages. The main excretory duct has a stratified epithelium. An abundance of smooth muscle is present in the capsule and in the septa that invade the gland.

The seminal vesicles are absent in carnivores. In ruminants and swine they make up a compact, lobulated gland, but in man and solipeds they are true vesicles made up of mucosa, muscularis, and adventitia.

The wall of the seminal vesicles of the stallion is permeated by wide, branched secretory tubules with alveolar outpouchings. The seminal vesicles of ruminants consist of rather large lobules separated by heavy, muscular septa. Each lobule consists of wide, saclike, branching passages. These open centrally into sacculated but narrower excretory ducts, which give rise to the main excretory duct in the caudal part of the gland. In the boar the gland is divided into very small lobules separated by heavy strands of connective tissue. The axial ducts of the lobules open into oblong, somewhat sacculated spaces, which are located in the center of the gland and pass into the large collecting duct. In the boar only the walls of the glandular spaces contain muscular elements and elastic fibers; the capsule is non-muscular.

2. Prostate Gland

The prostate gland (Figs. 317, 318) in ruminants and swine consists mostly of a pars disseminata, which forms a glandular layer in the wall of the entire pelvic urethra. In the bull and the boar there is a small dorsal *corpus prostatae* near the bladder. In horses and carnivores the body of the prostate is much larger, and the pars disseminata is represented only by scattered small glands (the urethral glands of Littré). The pars disseminata is always covered by the striated urethral muscle, but the body is exposed at the cranial border of the muscle. In the dog the large prostate surrounds the origin of the urethra.

The prostate is a lobulated compound tubular gland, which is surrounded by a capsule and contains abundant muscular interstitial connective tissue. The glandular epithelium is underlain by a collagenous propria and may be high or low columnar. It shows signs of active secretion, and secretory droplets often adhere to the surface of its cells. Intercellular secretory canaliculi have been seen in the stallion and bull. In the horse the epithelium of the excretory ducts resembles that of the glandular portion, but in other animals it changes after it leaves the lobule and gradually comes to resemble that of the urethra. Concretions are frequent, especially in old boars.

There is an abundance of vessels, nerves, and ganglia. The latter can be found throughout the entire supporting tissue; in the cat, they are especially prominent in the connective tissue between the two lateral lobes. Lamellar corpuscles have been found in the capsule of the prostate of the stallion and the cat.

3. Bulbo-urethral Glands

The paired bulbo-urethral or Cowper's glands, which are lacking in the dog, are covered by striated musculature. The underlying capsule is purely fibrous in the bull, but it contains smooth muscle in other animals. Continuous with it are the interlobular connective tissue septa which contain smooth musculature extending into the lobules. In the stallion the muscular tissue is striated. The glandular lobules contain a central collecting sinus, from which narrow, coiled, and ramifying branches radiate in all directions. The glandular epithelium and that of the collecting sinuses are columnar (especially high in the bull) and show the mucin reaction as well as various functional stages. The excretory ducts bear a similar epithelium except that no mucin is present. In the horse, the cat, and especially the pig, the ducts are surrounded by glandular tissue. In the adult boar the gland lumina are so distended with thick secretion that the tubular structure is obliterated.

D. THE MALE URETHRA

The urethra is divided into a pelvic portion, into which the ductus deferens and all the accessory glands open, and a penile portion.

1. Pelvic Urethra

The pelvic urethra (Fig. 319) is lined by a longitudinally folded mucosa, which bears transitional epithelium showing evidence of secretory activity. The surface of the epithelium is irregular and marked by recesses called the lacunae of Morgagni. The thin propria is collagenous and poorly vascularized.

Next to the mucosa lies the stratum vasculare or cavernosum, which is present in all species, though in varying degrees of development. In the tomcat it is absent between bladder and prostate. It is composed of a dense plexus of veins, which are connected in a labyrinthine manner and have the character of erectile tissue. The trabeculae between the veins are rich in smooth musculature.

The adjoining glandular layer contains the prostatic tissue (or urethral glands) and shows varying degrees of development in the different species (see p. 271). The

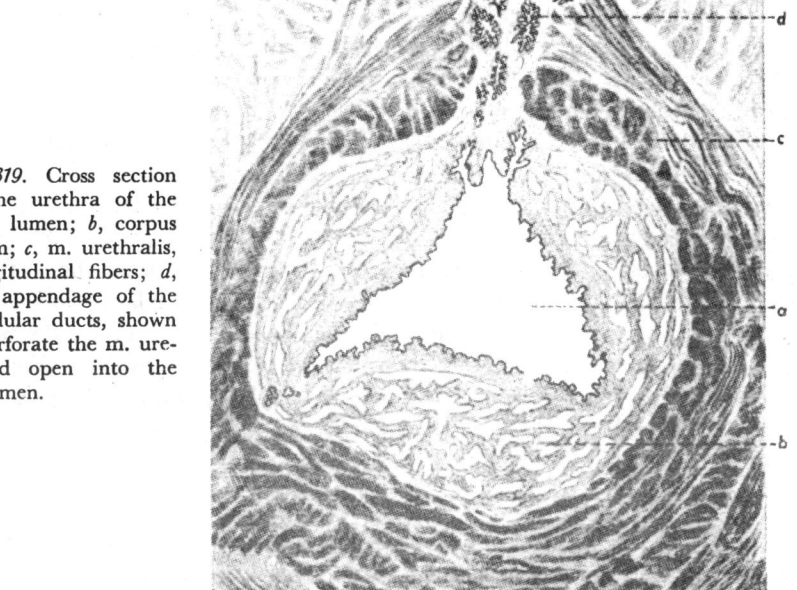

Figure 319. Cross section through the urethra of the stallion. *a*, lumen; *b*, corpus cavernosum; *c*, m. urethralis, inner longitudinal fibers; *d*, glandular appendage of the bulboglandular ducts, shown as they perforate the m. urethralis and open into the urethral lumen.

next layer is a sheet of thin bundles of smooth muscle, followed by the striated urethral muscle (*c*).

The colliculus seminalis is the prominent continuation of the urethral crest, which arises in the bladder. It shows in general the same structure as the urethral mucosa. It bears the openings of the ductus deferens and the seminal vesicles. Ganglia are present here in the cat and boar.

The prostatic utricle is an elongated vesicle lying in the colliculus seminalis. It occurs more or less regularly in all domestic animals. It is lined with simple or stratified epithelium, which shows secretory and degenerative phenomena. The lumen contains secretion and detritus. The mucosa is usually surrounded by musculature. The prostatic utricle represents the fused ends of the Müllerian ducts and is the homologue of the uterus or vagina.

The semen is the combined product of the testes, their excretory ducts, and the accessory sex glands. In addition to the spermatozoa (up to 300,000 per cc. or 10 billion per ejaculate in the horse) we find the following normal admixtures: urethral epithelial cells, columnar epithelial cells from the accessory glands, leukocytes, hyaline bodies, and small concretions from the seminal vesicles. As the semen cools, the characteristic crystals of Böttcher make their appearance. The microscopic examination of semen is of great practical importance in artificial insemination.

2. Penile Urethra

The penile urethra (Fig. 320) has fewer glands but more erectile tissue than the pelvic portion. The folded mucosa bears transitional epithelium, which changes at the urethral opening to stratified squamous epithelium on a papillary body. The propria mucosae varies in thickness, In the bull it has the character of lymphatic tissue, but in the stallion and boar it contains the small scattered glands of Littré, and in the stallion, the lacunae of Morgagni, as in the pelvic urethra.

The cavernous tissue (c) adjoining the mucosa is composed of connective tissue trabeculae which are continuous peripherally with the tunica albuginea that limits the erectile tissue. The trabeculae contain many elastic fibers and blood vessels, and in the horse and bull, longitudinal smooth muscle fibers. Between the trabeculae there are spaces increasing in size toward the albuginea, which are lined with endothelium and usually filled with blood. Toward the mucosa these spaces pass into an extensive venous plexus which occupies the deeper layers of the mucosa. The cavernous spaces receive their blood from these veins and from the capillaries of the trabecular system. Thus the erectile tissue has a purely venous character. An exception is the erectile tissue of the bulbus urethralis, which is especially rich in muscular tissue. Here the artery of the urethral bulb opens directly into the cavernous sinuses.

E. THE PENIS

The penis (Fig. 320) may be divided into body and glans. The body consists of the erectile corpus cavernosum penis (f), whose two crura are attached to the ischial arch; the urethra (a,b) surrounded by the corpus cavernosum urethrae (c); and the mm. bulbocavernosus (d) and retractor penis (e). The tip of the penis is made up of the glans, which may be indistinct in some species.

1. The Body of the Penis

The portion of the urethra that runs along the ventral surface of the body of the penis has already been described. The corpora cavernosa (Figs. 320,f; 321), which

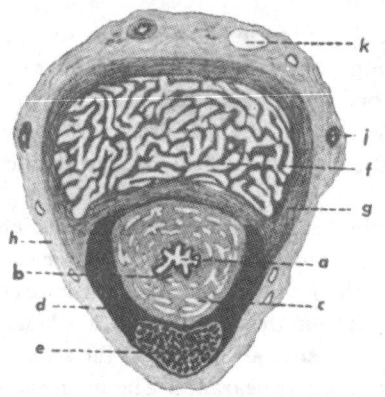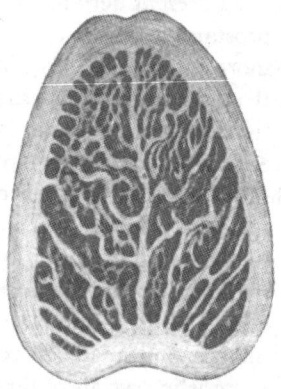

Figure 320 (left). Cross section through the penis of a colt. *a,* lumen; *b,* mucosa; *c,* corpus cavernosum urethrae; *d,* m. bulbo-cavernosus; *e,* retractor penis; *f,* corpus cavernosum penis; *g,* tunica albuginea penis; *h,* adventitia of the penis; *i,* artery; *k,* vein.

Figure 321 (right). Cross section through the corpus cavernosum of the collapsed equine penis. The shallow groove for the urethra is seen basally.

make up the body, consist of an envelope, a system of trabeculae, and the true
erectile tissue. The fibrous envelope, *tunica albuginea*, is a relatively thick membrane
composed of dense collagenous tissue and elastic fibers. It gives off similarly con-
structed trabeculae, which are interconnected to make up a coarse trabecular
framework. The trabeculae form a median septum, which is present only near the
root of the penis of ruminants and boars, but is continuous throughout the body
in the dog. In the stallion and tomcat the septum is not continuous.

Between the trabeculae lies the spongy *erectile tissue proper*. This consists of a fine
framework of lamellae and cords, continuous with the trabeculae and albuginea,
and of variously shaped communicating spaces—cavernae. The spaces are mostly
longitudinal and are largest and most abundant in the crura. In most species they
have no special wall outside the endothelium. They are bounded by the inter-
cavernous lamellae and trabeculae, which carry vessels and nerves and are composed of fibroelastic tissue (in ruminants and the boar) and smooth muscle fibers
(especially in the stallion and carnivores). Scattered adipose tissue is present in the
corpora cavernosa of all domestic mammals. Distal to the insertion of the m. ischio-
cavernosus the corpus cavernosum of the bull consists largely of fibrous tissue, but
this never entirely displaces the erectile tissue, which serves to stiffen the penis
rather than enlarge it.

BLOOD VESSELS. There are species differences, as well as conflicting opinions on
the arrangement of the blood vessels. In man and the stallion there is a capillary
net, the superficial cortical plexus, immediately subjacent to the albuginea. It communicates with a deep cortical plexus of veins, which are connected to the cavernous spaces of the erectile tissue.

The main arterial supply of the corpora cavernosa penis comes through the deep
artery of the penis, which enters the crura. Branches of the dorsal artery penetrate
the tunica albuginea. The arteries course along the trabeculae but may also traverse the erectile tissue. They give off numerous branches, part of which furnish
capillaries to the trabeculae and albuginea, while the greater number pass into
the capillaries of the superficial plexus. Other arterial branches open into the deep
plexus or into the cavernous spaces directly. These *helicine arteries*[4] form groups of
two to ten arterial twigs, held together in bundles by connective tissue. They are
characterized by their tortuous course, the cushion-like thickenings of their walls
formed by longitudinal muscle bundles, and the presence of epithelioid cells in
their intima. These structures serve to occlude the arteries in the collapsed penis.
The cavernous spaces and the deep venous plexus are drained by the deep and
dorsal veins of the penis and the veins of the urethral bulb. The veins that correspond to the nutrient arteries penetrate the albuginea to neighboring venous trunks.

Erection of the body of the penis is caused by dilation of the helicine arteries.
The increased arterial flow compresses the cortical veins against the albuginea and
retards drainage. According to Deysach,[5] animals that do not have a long os penis

---

[4] Gr. *helix* coil.

[5] The Comparative Morphology of the Erectile Tissue of the Penis, *Am. J. Anatomy 64* (1939):
111.

have thick-walled venae profundae. By contraction these veins close the small tributaries penetrating their walls and thus prevent drainage. Erection is terminated by constriction of the arteries and a slow emptying of the cavernous spaces by contraction of the smooth muscle and elastic fibers.

Following castration of young animals the erectile tissue of the penis fails to develop fully.

2. Glans Penis

The end of the penis is covered by a special kind of tissue. It is richly vascularized and in some species contains a true erectile body, which forms a terminal enlarge-

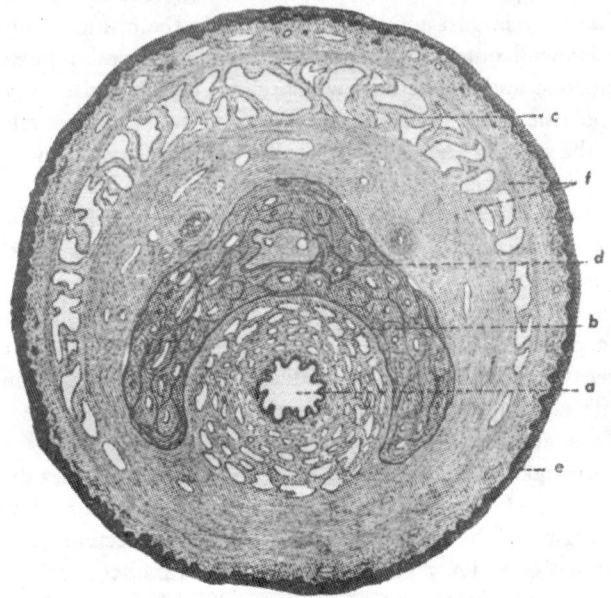

Figure 322. Cross section through the glans penis of the dog.
a, urethra; *b*, corpus cavernosum urethrae; *c*, corpus cavernosum glandis; *d*, os penis; *e*, squamous epithelium; *f*, tunica albuginea.

ment of the penis, the glans (Fig. 322). It is prominent only in man, stallion, and dog. The glans is covered by the penile prepuce. This cutaneous, nonglandular cover has a papillary body and stratified squamous epithelium and is rich in nerves and special nerve endings.

The erectile tissue of the glans is separate from the corpus cavernosum penis. In animals other than the boar it communicates with the corpus cavernosum urethrae. In carnivores this continuity is extensive. The structure of the venous erectile tissue of the glans resembles that of the corpus cavernosum urethrae.

The *bulbus glandis* of the dog is a thick corpus cavernosum, which is rich in elastic tissue and contains muscle fibers. In carnivores the glans covers the *os penis* (Fig. 322,*d*), which is the ossified terminal portion of the corpora cavernosa penis. In the stallion, ram, and goat the urethra projects beyond the end of the penis, forming the urethral process, which is ensheathed in a thin layer of cavernous tissue. In the stallion it is rich in lymphatic tissue. In the tomcat the cutaneous coat of the glans bears rows of small spines, which are cornified at their tips. Small projections are also seen in the stallion and goat.

3. Prepuce

The prepuce consists of an external part, which is continuous with the abdominal skin, a parietal part, and a visceral part. The external layer meets the parietal layer at the preputial orifice. The parietal layer is reflected inward and forward at the preputial fornix to cover the end of the penis as the visceral layer. The stal-

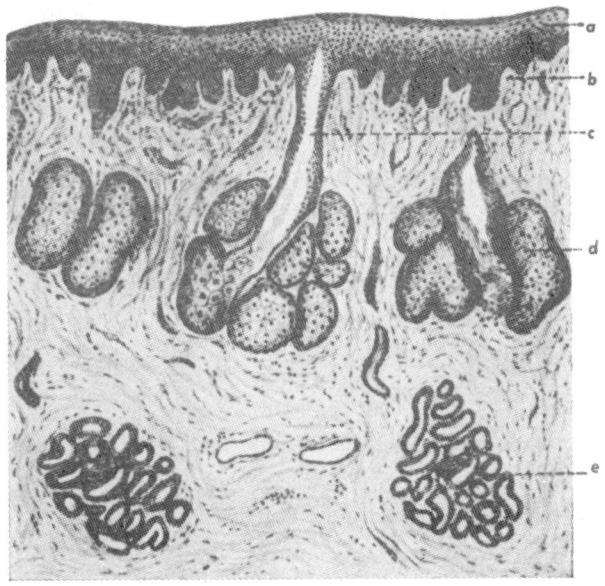

Figure 323. Section from the parietal layer of the prepuce of the horse. *a*, squamous epithelium; *b*, papillary body; *c*, excretory duct of an independent sebaceous gland; *d*, secretory portion; *e*, tubular preputial gland.

lion has an additional internal fold (prepuce proper) which extends from the fornix toward the glans and ends at the preputial ring.

The external part of the prepuce has the same structure as the skin. The abundance of hair varies with the species of animal. The parietal layer (Fig. 323) is connected to the external layer by loose connective tissue, which contains, in addition to large vessels, smooth muscle bundles derived from the tunica dartos scroti and also bundles of striated muscle (except in the horse and cat). It possesses a papillary body and stratified squamous epithelium. Hair and skin glands (Fig. 323,*d*,*e*) extend only a short distance inside the preputial orifice (the preputial ring in the horse), where the glands are especially well developed. Sebaceous glands that open on the surface rather than into a hair follicle occur here (*c*). The remainder of the parietal layer and the visceral layer lack hair and glands. The visceral (penile) prepuce is continuous at the urethral orifice with the urethral mucosa.

At the fornix of the prepuce peculiar epithelial evaginations are present. Lymph nodules are seen in the parietal layer of the ram and boar, in the fornix of the bull, boar, and dog, and in the layer covering the glans in the bull. As for nerve endings, terminal bulbs and genital corpuscles have been found in the visceral preputial layer of all animals. In the cat Pacinian corpuscles have also been described.

F. THE SCROTUM

The scrotum is composed of the common integument and the tunica dartos. The scrotal skin differs from the rest of the integument in that it is thinner, has less hair, and has better-developed glands. Both sebaceous and tubular skin glands are present, and both are large. The boar, however, has only few and small glands. On the inside the scrotal skin is attached to the tunica dartos by a thin layer of loose connective tissue. The dartos consists of bundles of smooth muscle fibers running in various directions and of collagenous and elastic fibers. In the boar adipose tissue is also present. At the scrotal raphe the muscle bundles turn in to form the septum scroti.

XV

The Female Genital Organs

THE entire adult female genital apparatus—ovaries, oviducts, uterus, and vagina—is the scene of regularly recurring processes of growth and involution, which constitute the sexual cycle. They are interrupted only by pregnancy and old age. The gonadotrophic hormone of the anterior lobe of the hypophysis stimulates the ovary and the formation of the ovarian hormones (estrogen and progesterone), which exert a specific influence on the rest of the reproductive apparatus and the mammary gland.

A. THE OVARIES

The ovary performs both an exocrine function (oögenesis and ovulation) and an endocrine one. Its hormones influence the development of primary and secondary sex characteristics and govern the sexual cycle. The process of egg cell production causes a continuous rhythmic alteration in the gross and microscopic architecture of the ovary. The histological picture varies considerably depending on the plane of section and the phase of the cycle.

The ovaries (Figs. 324–330), except those of the mare (see p. 288), are subdivided into a cortex or zona parenchymatosa (Fig. 324,e) and a medulla or zona vasculosa (d). At the hilus, where the mesovarium is attached, the medullary substance extends through the cortex and the tunica albuginea to the surface. The connective tissue framework or *stroma* of the cortex condenses on the surface of the ovary to form the tunica albuginea, which is covered by germinal epithelium.

In young animals the germinal epithelium (Figs. 325; 326,a) consists of a single layer of cuboidal or columnar cells, which are flattened in the adult and become interrupted by scar tissue. It is continuous with the epithelium of the oviduct and with the peritoneal mesothelium.

The tunica albuginea (Fig. 325,b) may be up to 100 μ in thickness. It is richer in collagenous fibers and somewhat poorer in cells than the cortical stroma, into which it blends. Usually the fibers are irregularly interwoven, but occasionally they are arranged in lamellae as in man. The albuginea lacks elastic and argyrophil fibers.

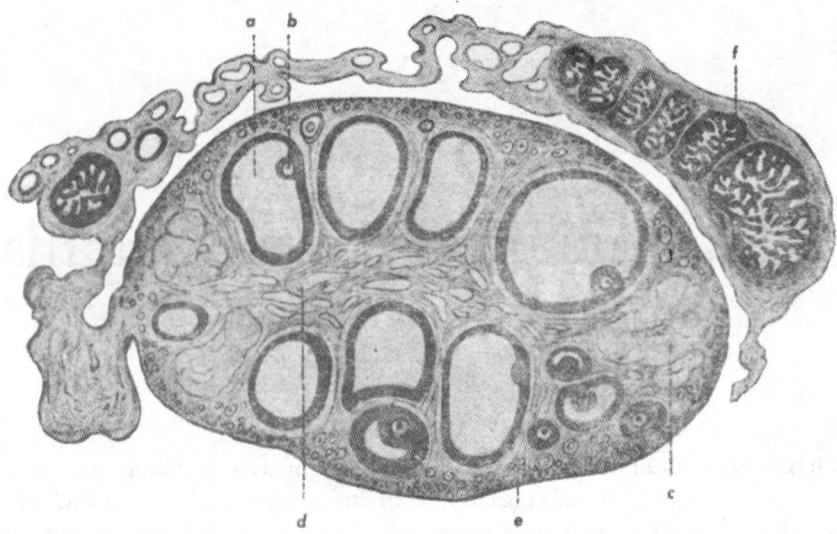

Figure 324. Section through the ovary and oviduct of the cat (70×). *a*, Graafian follicle; *b*, oöcyte in its cumulus oöphorus; *c*, corpora lutea; *d*, medullary substance; *e*, primary follicle in the cortical substance; *f*, oviduct with fimbria, sectioned in several places. On the left, the mesovarian attachment.

The cortical stroma is very rich in cells but is free from elastic tissue. It must be considered a specialized, highly adaptable form of supportive tissue. The cellular structure is reinforced by reticular fibrils, which cannot be demonstrated by the usual stains. The fusiform cells have elongated nuclei and occur in dense strands. Their direction is parallel to the surface of the ovary or the follicles and blood vessels which they enclose. The cortical fibroblasts are auxiliary cells subservient to the developing ova. They are probably not ordinary fibroblasts.

It has been demonstrated on the sow's ovary, which is most suitable for such observations, that the cortical stroma is a highly reactive tissue. The stroma fibroblasts are capable of further differentiation, dye storage, and proliferation. In response to certain stimuli they may leave their cellular association and differentiate into wandering macrophages. They may round up, store lipids, and assume an epithelioid character, performing nutritive and secretory functions in the follicles and occurring singly or in clusters in the stroma as the interstitial cells (of the bitch and cat). These various functional forms may revert to stroma fibroblasts at any time. In the mare pigmented cells are present. These decrease in number with age.

The cortical stroma contains the ovarian follicles, in various stages of development and regression (Fig. 326). The follicles are very numerous (in swine, about 60,000 in each ovary) and are of varying size, usually becoming larger from the periphery inward. They occur in two main layers. Immediately below the tunica albuginea the small primary follicles are evenly distributed (in ruminants) or clustered in groups (in carnivores). In the deeper layers, which are more favorable to their development, lie the larger Graafian follicles (Figs. 324,*a,b;* 326,*e*).

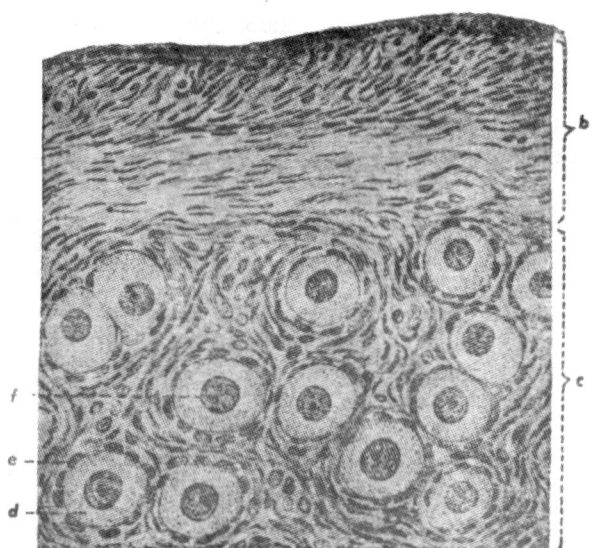

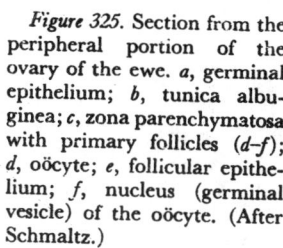

Figure 325. Section from the peripheral portion of the ovary of the ewe. *a*, germinal epithelium; *b*, tunica albuginea; *c*, zona parenchymatosa with primary follicles (*d–f*); *d*, oöcyte; *e*, follicular epithelium; *f*, nucleus (germinal vesicle) of the oöcyte. (After Schmaltz.)

In the embryo the germinal epithelium covering the genital ridge contains the primordial sex cells. It forms cordlike proliferations which invade the underlying mesenchyme to form the inner epithelial mass of the developing ovary. This epithelium, which contains primitive ova surrounded by smaller cells, degenerates early and is replaced by the connective tissue medulla. The cortex is formed by a new proliferation of germinal epithelium in which there are large sex cells multiplying mitotically, the oögonia. These finally stop dividing and begin to grow into primary oöcytes. The mesenchyme growing toward the periphery breaks up the epithelium into primary follicles consisting of an oöcyte surrounded by smaller cells. These are more numerous in young animals. In the sow they are often hard to recognize because of their delicate structure. The mesenchyme continues to proliferate and forms the cortical stroma and the tunica albuginea, the latter of which separates the germinal epithelium from the cortex. It has been claimed that no new primary follicles are formed after the tunica albuginea. There is evidence, however, that new follicles are formed throughout life, at least in some species (e.g., the bitch), by ingrowth of epithelial cords through the albuginea.

The microscopic (30–50 μ) *primary follicles* (Fig. 325,*d*) consist of an oöcyte, an enveloping single layer of follicular cells (*e*), and a basement membrane. The follicular epithelium is flat at first, later becoming cuboidal to columnar. In somewhat older follicles we find several layers of follicular epithelium. Such follicles are called growing, or secondary, follicles (Fig. 326,*d*). The oöcyte has also grown and assumed an eccentric position. A homogeneous envelope, the zona pellucida, appears between the oöcyte and the surrounding follicular cells. The basement membrane between the epithelium and the stroma becomes more distinct.

In older, usually macroscopic follicles the cells of the follicular epithelium separate to form clefts, which later become confluent. The cavity thus formed is lined by stratified follicular epithelium, the *membrana granulosa*. The liquor folliculi, which fills the cavity, is rich in protein and estrogen.

The largest follicles, with a diameter that varies greatly among the species, are called *Graafian follicles*. The stroma cells surrounding them have formed an envelope of 60–250 μ in thickness. This *theca folliculi*[1] (Fig. 326) is composed of two layers.

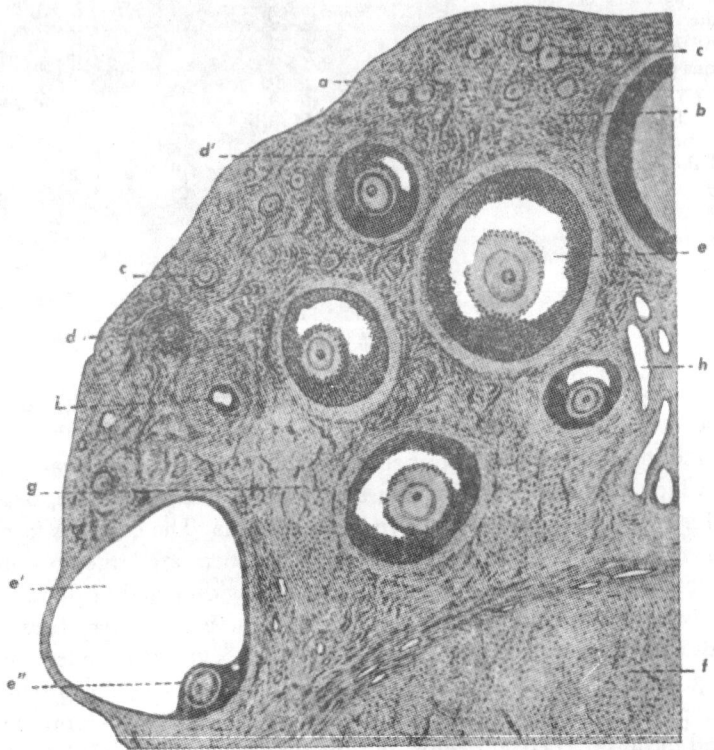

Figure 326. Section from the ovary of the bitch, somewhat diagrammatic (45×). *a*, germinal epithelium; *b*, stroma ovarii; *c*, primary follicle; *d*, growing follicle; *d'*, follicle beginning to show a cleft in the follicular epithelium; *e*, early Graafian follicle; *e'*, large Graafian follicle prior to rupture; *e''*, cumulus oöphorus; *f*, corpus luteum; *g*, groups of interstitial cells; *h*, vessels of the medullary substance; *i*, atretic follicle.

The theca interna is well supplied with capillaries, and its stroma cells become modified into epithelioid, lipid-containing, spheroid, or polymorphic cells located in the meshes of a delicate fiber net. There is physiological evidence that the cells of the theca interna are the chief source of ovarian estrogens,[2] which enter the blood stream through the walls of the abundant thecal capillaries. Some of the

[1] Gr. *theke* a case.
[2] Frederick L. Hisaw, Development of the Graafian Follicle and Ovulation, *Physiol. Rev. 27* (1947): 95.

hormone also passes through the membrana granulosa into the liquor folliculi. The theca externa consists of fusiform stroma cells, which are arranged concentrically around the follicle. The division between the two laminae is not distinct, nor is there a sharp line of demarcation between the theca and the surrounding stroma. The theca externa is looser on the side toward the surface of the ovary.

Adjoining the theca interna centrally is the follicular epithelium (Fig. 326), which is composed of a layer of columnar cells next to the thin basement membrane and of several layers of spheroid to polyhedral cells. These surround the oöcyte, forming a mound of cells, the cumulus oöphorus, which projects into the follicular cavity (Fig. 326,e''). The follicular epithelial cells which immediately

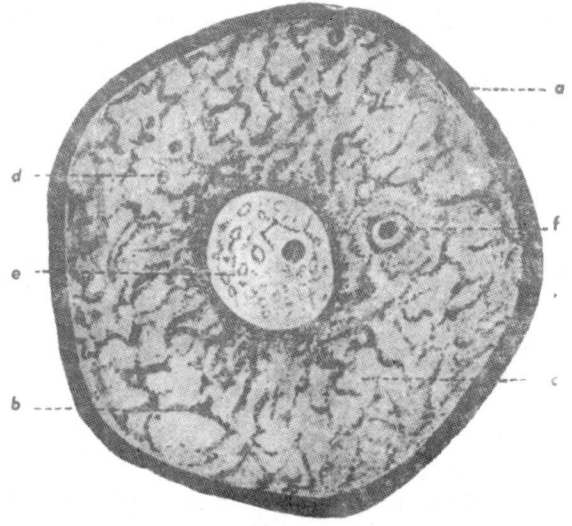

Figure 327. Section through an oöcyte of a twenty-six-year-old woman. The epithelia adjacent to the oölemma are not shown. *a*, oölemma; *b*, mitochondria; *c*, yolk; *d*, fat globules; *e*, nucleus; *f*, cytocentrum. (After van der Stricht.)

surround the oöcyte are columnar and radially arranged and are called collectively the corona radiata (Fig. 328,a). They are separated from the oöcyte by a hyaline membrane of about 10 μ in thickness, the oölemma or zona pellucida (Figs. 327,a; 328,b). In carnivores, the sow, and the ewe some follicles contain two to six oöcytes. The deepest portions of the largest follicles reach the vicinity of the medulla. When they are ripe, they extend to the surface of the ovary and often project beyond it (Fig. 326,e').

The number of Graafian follicles that ripen in one estrual cycle is more or less fixed for each species; i.e., the uniparous animals usually produce only one. Large but immature follicles are found in larger numbers. In ruminants and the sow there are about forty in one ovary. The diameter of ripe follicles in the various species is as follows: woman—9 to 12 mm.; mare—up to 70 mm.; cow—up to 15 mm.; ewe, goat, sow—5 to 8 mm.; bitch and cat—about 2 mm.

The Oöcyte. The oöcytes (Fig. 327) show progressive growth stages. These consist of the formation of envelopes and cellular inclusions (yolk) which lead to an enlargement of the oöcyte and make possible the first developmental processes in the fertilized egg. At the end of their growth period the primary oöcytes have a diameter of 100–150 μ and are spherical in shape. The enveloping oölemma is perforated by radial pores through which the cells of the corona radiata send delicate processes to the surface of the oöcyte. These are supposedly of nutritional significance to the developing egg cell. The oöcyte consists of the cytoplasm and a large vesicular nucleus containing a nucleolus. The cytoplasm consists of stringy protoplasm with inclusions of fairly large, dark yolk granules. The latter increase in quantity as the oöcyte grows. Near the nucleus we find an area of condensed cytoplasm containing one or two centrioles. This cell center is not present in advanced oöcytes.

Following the growth period the oöcytes undergo a process of maturation. The first stage of maturation takes place during estrus, while the egg is still in the fol-

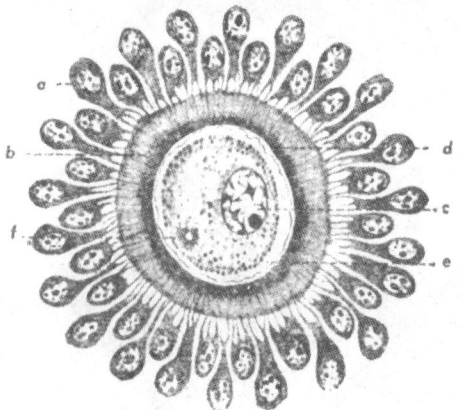

Figure 328. Primary oöcyte of a hedgehog. *a*, corona radiata; *b*, oölemma; *c*, germinal vesicle; *d*, vitelline membrane; *e*, hypolemmal space; *f*, cytocentrum. (After Bonnet.)

licle. At the first meiotic division each daughter cell receives the same amount of nuclear material, but one of them acquires nearly all the cytoplasm, while the other becomes the tiny first polar body, which may be seen for a time between the egg cell and the oölemma.

The large daughter cell is the secondary oöcyte. The first meiotic division is usually followed by ovulation. (The order is reversed in the bitch.) The liberated egg immediately begins the second meiotic division. This is not completed unless fertilization takes place. It results in the extrusion of another polar body and in the formation of a female pronucleus, which, like the male pronucleus from the spermatozoon, contains the haploid number of chromosomes. Actually the stage of the "ovum" never exists in mammals because the cell is an oöcyte still in the process of maturation until it is fertilized, when it becomes a zygote. The term ovum is used quite generally to refer to an egg cell, however. From the foregoing it can be seen that oögenesis closely parallels spermatogenesis, except that the latter results in the formation of four spermatozoa from one spermatogonium, while each oögonium gives rise to but one functional ovum.

The mature ovum has a diameter of 150–300 μ. It contains fat, pigment, vacuoles, and miscellaneous inclusions and has often, in addition to the zona pellucida, another envelope, the vitelline membrane. This lies next to the ovum (Fig. 328,*d*).

Ovulation. The discharge of the ova from the ovary is associated with pronounced vascular engorgement of the genital organs and increased activity of their glands. It begins with the growth of the Graafian follicle, due mainly to the increase of follicular fluid. The follicle pushes through the tissue separating it from the surface of the ovary until it projects beyond the ovarian surface. Meanwhile the granulosa cells have undergone a kind of lipoid degeneration, and the adhesion

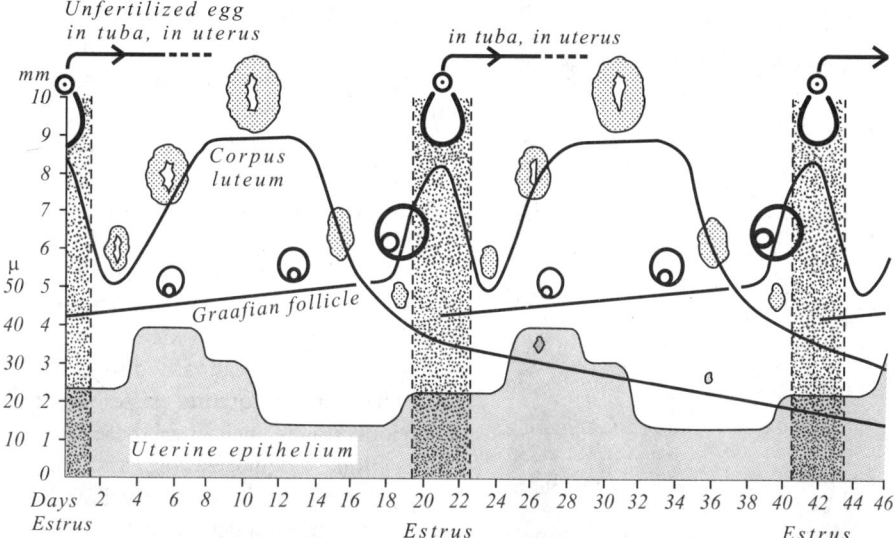

Figure 329. Ovarian cycle of the sow for forty-six days following an ovulation. The figures in mm. indicate the diameter of the Graafian follicle and the corpus luteum. The figures in micra apply to the height of the uterine epithelium at the same time. (After Hirsch.)

of the cumulus oöphorus to the remaining follicular epithelium has been reduced to narrow cytoplasmic bridges, which finally break: the follicle is ready to rupture. This takes place during estrus. A thin avascular spot in the generally hyperemic wall of the follicle gives way and the follicular fluid flows out, carrying the ovum surrounded by the corona radiata. The ovum is received by the funnel-shaped abdominal end of the oviduct, which is closely applied to the surface of the ovary. Follicular rupture is followed by hemorrhage, which is slight in carnivores, sheep, and goats—more extensive in the mare, cow, and sow—and fills the follicular cavity.

Corpus Luteum. After ovulation the follicular wall collapses in folds and the granulosa cells undergo exuberant proliferation and hypertrophy. In the mare, cow, and carnivores, a yellow pigment associated with lipids, lutein, appears in the cells. As the blood clot is resorbed, a solid yellow body or corpus luteum (Fig. 330) is rapidly formed. In the ewe, goat, and sow, however, it is grayish-white or flesh-colored because of the absence of lutein from the proliferated granulosa cells.

The corpus luteum is organized by highly vascular connective tissue sprouts from the theca interna, whose cells penetrate between the lutein cells. The thecal cells may be recognized as smaller, epithelioid elements (theca lutein cells) between the much larger granulosa lutein cells. They make up part of the framework of the corpus luteum and may assume the shape of fibroblasts. The corpus luteum, now an endocrine gland, consists of a capsule, radial septa extending into the interior, an extensive capillary network, and, closely associated with the capillaries, the lutein cells. The latter are filled with yellow or colorless lipoid granules, which are mixtures of phosphatides and cerebrosides in the case of the granulosa lutein cells and of cholesterol compounds in the case of the theca lutein cells.[3] The spherical nuclei of the lutein cells are rich in chromatin. Centrally there is often a connective tissue core that lacks lutein cells. This encloses a small cavity which contains hematoidin or coagulated protein. It is a vestige of the follicular cavity and gradually disappears.

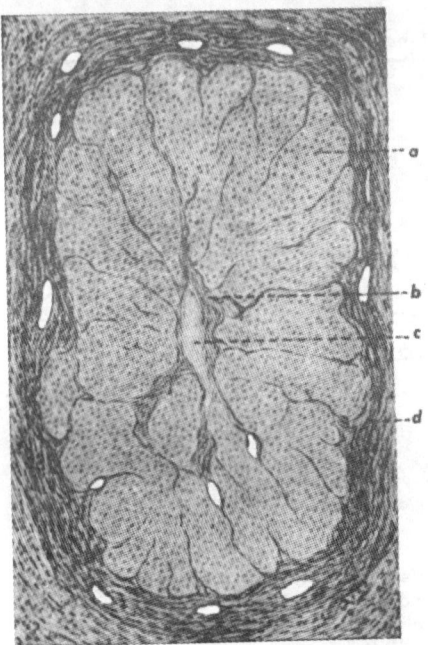

Figure 330. Section through the corpus luteum from the ovary of the cat (90×). *a*, lutein cells; *b*, supporting framework; *c*, connective tissue core containing a cavity; *d*, capsule.

The corpus luteum passes through various stages including those of proliferation, vascularization, and maturity. During the latter, the yellow body attains its highest degree of development and has the appearance of an endocrine gland. If fertilization does not take place, the corpus luteum becomes smaller and degenerates sooner or later. This corpus luteum "spurium" is still present when the one arising at the next heat develops. The two may be differentiated on the basis of their color. The yellow body finally becomes paler and smaller and persists for varying lengths of time in the form of a white, gray, or (in the ox) red connective tissue, scar, which steadily decreases in size, becoming the corpus albicans or fibrosum. When conception occurs, the degeneration of the yellow body is delayed, usually until the birth of the young, but not necessarily this long. The corpus luteum of pregnancy (corpus luteum verum) prevents the animal from coming into heat and, with the possible exception of the mare, also prevents ovulation. Following parturition the corpus luteum of pregnancy, like the shorter-lived corpus luteum spurium, regresses. The theca lutein cells undergo proliferation and transformation into fibroblasts and histiocytes. These resorb the granulosa lutein cells, which have meanwhile under-

---

[3] Maximow and Bloom, p. 553.

gone fatty degeneration, until finally the corpus luteum has been replaced by ovarian stroma. The regression of the corpus luteum again permits the maturation of one or more Graafian follicles. In the cow the weight of the corpus luteum increases up to the third month of pregnancy, during which its activity and progesterone content reach their peak. At that time one gram of corpus luteum tissue contains an average of thirty micrograms of progesterone. This hormone serves in the preparation for and the maintenance of pregnancy. The phase of uterine proliferation caused by the follicular estrogens is succeeded after ovulation by the phase of secretion induced by progesterone. After fertilization progesterone is largely responsible for the implantation of the embryo. Together with estrogens and anterior pituitary hormones, it stimulates the development of the mammary gland.

Atretic Follicles. Comparatively few egg cells reach maturity. Most of the oöcytes produced, together with their follicles, undergo the process of atresia.[4] This may set in at any stage of their development. It begins with signs of degeneration (fatty changes, pyknotic nuclei) in the oöcyte and the follicular epithelium. The cells of the theca interna proliferate and invade the degenerating follicular epithelium. Finally there is only a mass of lipid-containing cells which is broken up by connective tissue and scattered in the stroma as interstitial cells. The process of atresia varies among the species.

Medulla. In the medullary substance (the zona vasculosa; Fig. 324,d) the cortical stroma passes into loose fibroelastic tissue containing many blood vessels, large bundles of nerve fibers, and strands of smooth muscle continuous with the musculature of the suspensory apparatus. The ovarian arteries are remarkable for their spiral course. The similarly convoluted veins form a dense plexus in the medullary substance. In carnivores and ruminants one often finds, especially near the mesovarium, a netlike arrangement of medullary tubules, which are lined by flat or columnar, sometimes ciliated epithelium and represent the vestiges of the rete ovarii. Solid cellular cords also occur. Near the ovary we find remnants of the mesonephros—the epoöphoron and paroöphoron—which consist of blindly ending, tortuous tubes. Their collagenous lamina propria bears simple epithelium, which in the epoöphoron is of the ciliated columnar type. They often undergo cystic dilatation.

VESSELS AND NERVES. The arteries of the ovary are derived from the ovarian branch of the utero-ovarian artery and from the uterine artery. They enter from the hilus into the medullary substance, where they give off numerous branches supplying the entire stroma and especially the thecae of the follicles. The periodic changes occurring in the ovary after the onset of puberty exert an influence on the ovarian vessels. In the immediate vicinity of the growing follicle there is a progressive development of the cortical vascular system. With the formation of the two layers of the theca, a double basket-like vascular meshwork develops around the follicle. The portion of the Graafian follicle that bulges out on the surface of the ovary loses its veins and arteries but retains its capillaries. As the corpus luteum develops, it is permeated by capillary loops, which disappear during its regression to

---

[4] Gr. *atretos* not perforated. i.e., the follicular cavity is obliterated.

be replaced by the diffuse cortical capillary network. Arteriovenous anastomoses and occlusive mechanisms in the vessels occur in the cortex, and apparently also in the medulla (in the cow and cat). The changing demands on the vascular system during the development and regression of the follicle and corpus luteum often cause marked changes in the walls of the ovarian arteries (ovulation sclerosis). These involve an increase in the elastic components, which may be associated with proliferations of the intima. Lymphatics are present in great numbers and demonstrable also in the theca externa of the follicles. Their trunks are found at the hilus. The nerves, which enter by way of the medulla, are largely unmyelinated and terminate in part on the walls of the vessels. Other nerve fibers form dense plexuses and run mostly to the follicular walls but also to the tunica albuginea and germinal epithelium. In the corpus luteum the nerve fibers are distributed intercellularly throughout the entire gland. Sensory fibers and ganglia have been reported.

The Ovary of the Mare. In this species there is no subdivision into cortical and medullary substance. Only the ovulation fossa, located at the free border, is covered by germinal epithelium, the remainder being invested by peritoneum (mesovarium). Beneath the peritoneum is a thicker layer, which is free from follicles and contains tortuous blood vessels, vestiges of the rete ovarii, and some muscle. This peripheral layer corresponds roughly to the zona vasculosa of other animals. Heavy tracts of connective tissue with rather large blood vessels are continued into the interior, where the follicles are distributed. This mixed tissue seems to be the equivalent of the cortex of other animals. The delicate primary follicles are hard to find, however.

The shape and structure of the fetal ovary is much like that of other animals. It is ovoid and covered by germinal epithelium, and the follicles lie near the surface. The germinal epithelium recedes toward the free border, however, and is followed by the peritoneum with its underlying connective tissue and blood vessels. The original cortex is thus covered, and the follicles become mixed with the central stroma. In the young animal ovulation may take place anywhere on the surface of the ovary, but especially at the poles.[5] It is only in old mares that unequal growth causes a bending of the ovary which deepens the ovulation fosssa. Because of the thick peripheral layer of connective tissue everywhere except under the germinal epithelium in the fossa, the follicles rupture into the fossa in old animals.

THE OVARY OF THE CHICKEN. Only the left ovary of the chicken develops to maturity. In the sexually mature animal the organ resembles a bunch of grapes. It is subdivided into numerous larger and smaller lobes. It contains a large number of egg cells in various stages of development embedded in a collagenous and highly vascular stroma. In the youngest stages the cells are about 40 μ in diameter and have a large vesicular nucleus. A delicate vitelline membrane separates the egg proper from the follicular epithelium. The surrounding connective tissue makes up

[5] Max Kupfer, The Ovarian Changes and the Periodicity of Oestrum in Cattle, Sheep and Goats, Pigs, Donkeys, and Horses, *Union of S. Africa Dept. of Agr., Vet. Res. Reports 13–14* (1928): 1251. See also F. N. Andrews and F. F. McKenzie, *Estrus, Ovulation, and Related Phenomena in the Mare* (Mo. Agr. Exp. Sta. Res. Bull. 329, 1941, 41.

the theca folliculi. By the addition of yolk the eggs develop into the large berry-like spheres which correspond to the future egg yolk. The stroma contains accumulations of lymphocytes and eosinophilic cells.

The parts of the *chicken egg* (Fig. 331) recognized by the layman are the yolk, the white, and the shell with its membranes. On the surface of the yolk, which represents the actual cell, lies the round, whitish, 1–2 mm. wide germinal disc (the blastodisc; *a*) composed of cytoplasm and containing a nucleus. From this animal pole a flask-shaped cord of white yolk (latebra; *b*) extends into the center of the yolk. Around this white center, concentric layers of yellow and white yolk are deposited. The former contain coarser yolk masses and exceed the latter considerably in thickness. The entire yolk is enclosed by the tough oölemma, which has formed

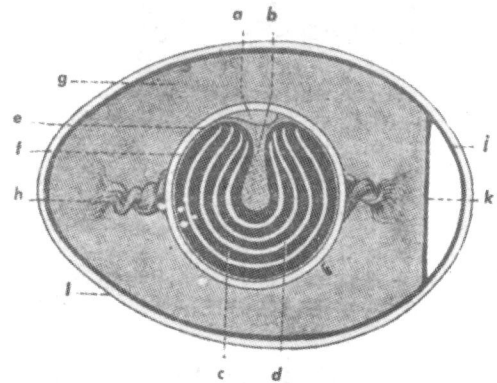

Figure 331. Longitudinal section through a chicken egg. *a*, germinal disc (nucleus not shown); *b*, latebra; *c*, yellow, and *d*, white, yolk; *e*, vitelline membrane; *f*, oölemma; *g*, albumen; *h*, chalazae; *i*, outer, and *k*, inner, shell membrane, enclosing the air cell; *l*, calcareous shell.

in the ovary. Fertilization takes place at the ovarian end of the oviduct. The albumen (*g*) is secreted by the first part of the oviduct (magnum). The layer of albumen immediately adjoining the oölemma remains fluid, allowing the yolk to rotate so that the germinal disc remains uppermost when the egg is turned. The chalazae (*h*) are condensations of albumen between the oölemma and the shell membrane at either end of the egg. In the isthmus of the oviduct the egg receives the two shell membranes (*i,k*), which are fused except at the blunt pole, where they part to form the air space. The calcareous shell is secreted by the epithelium of the uterus. It is perforated by fine canaliculi, which make respiratory exchange between the air and egg possible.

B. UTERINE TUBES

The wall of the uterine tube (the oviduct or Fallopian tube; Fig. 333) is composed of a mucosa, muscularis, and serosa. The mucosa bears simple columnar epithelium, parts of which are pseudostratified (as in ruminants and swine). Only part of its cells are ciliated. During heat the epithelium assumes a secretory character. Before parturition it also exhibits great secretory activity. The propria lacks glands and consists of connective tissue containing many cells, vessels, and muscle fibers.

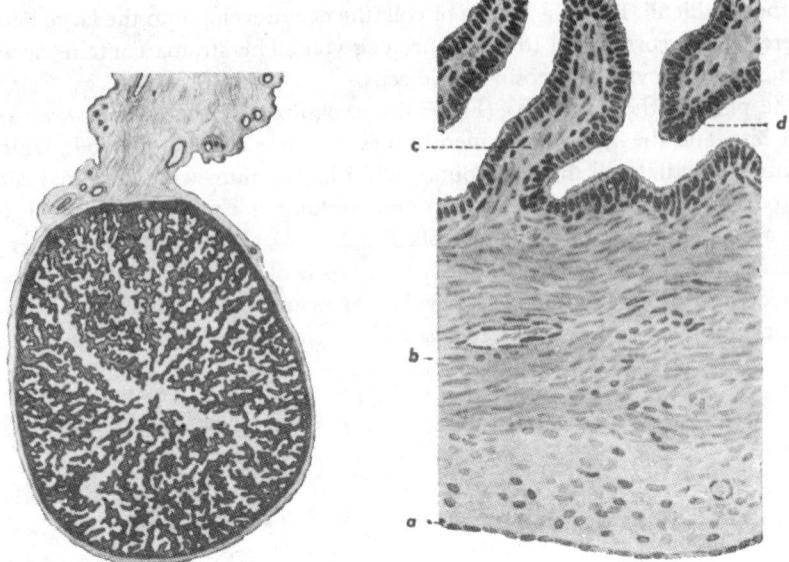

Figure 332 (left). Cross section through the ampulla of the oviduct of the sow.(After Schmaltz.)

Figure 333 (right). Section through the wall of the oviduct of the sow (270×). *a*, serosal mesothelium; *b*, tunica muscularis; *c*, fold of mucosa, covered by high simple columnar epithelium, which is partially ciliated; *d*, nonciliated cells.

A submucosa is absent. The mucosa forms large primary and smaller secondary folds (Figs. 324,*f*; 332).

The folding of the mucosa is negligible in the isthmus but increases greatly in the ampulla toward the ostium abdominale. The mucosal folds are most pronounced in the sow and mare, less so in ruminants, and subject to individual variation in carnivores.

The tunica muscularis is rich in elastic tissue and gives off numerous radial strands into the neighboring mucosa. It is made up chiefly of circular fiber bundles, but isolated longitudinal and oblique bundles also occur. It becomes thicker toward the uterus and blends into the circular uterine muscle layer. It undergoes special contractions during estrus, which probably serve to propel the ovum toward the uterus.

The subserosa contains many vessels (stratum vasculare) and, peripheral to these, a continuous layer of longitudinal muscle fibers.

The highly vascular mucosa of the fimbriae shows the same structure as the tubal mucosa but contains few or no muscle fibers.

Blood vessels are especially numerous during pregnancy. They generally follow a longitudinal course and form dense subepithelial plexuses. The intermuscular lymph vessels receive the lymph from the subserous and mucosal capillary nets and drain into the lymphatics in the mesosalpinx. The nerves are made up partly

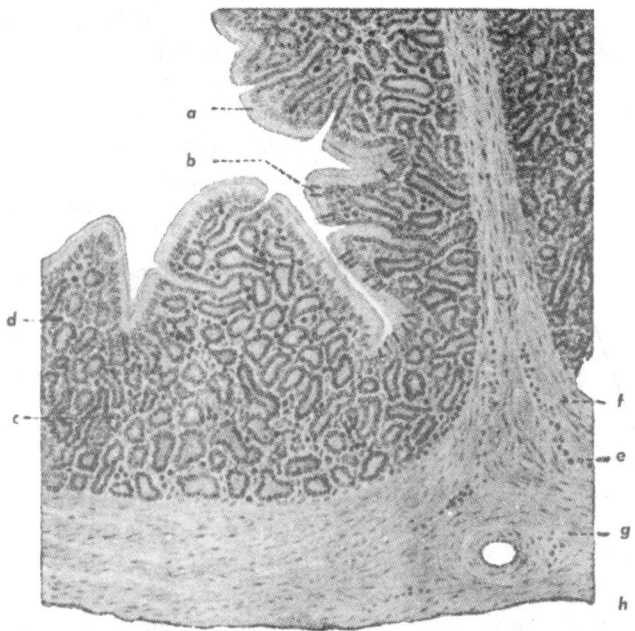

Figure 334. Part of a cross section through the oviduct of the chicken (130✕). *a*, nonciliated columnar cells; *b*, ciliated cells; *c*, glandular layer; *d*, plasma cells; *e*, lymphocytes; *f*, inner, *g*, outer muscle layer; *h*, serosal mesothelium.

of myelinated and partly of unmyelinated fibers, which send their branches close to the epithelium.

OVIDUCT OF THE HEN. Only the left oviduct (Fig. 334) persists in the chicken. It is greatly dilatable and begins with an open funnel (infundibulum), in which fertilization takes place. It is continued as the magnum, which eventually narrows down into the isthmus, only to widen again at the thick-walled uterus. This is followed by a narrower part, called the vagina, which opens into the cloaca. The tubal wall has a serous coat, a tunica muscularis, and a folded mucosa. The fibers of the muscular layer form a latticework and in places show two layers. The inner one (*f*) is carried into the folds. The mucosa is covered by simple ciliated columnar epithelium. The propria is rich in coiled, branched tubular glands (*c*), which are lined by cuboidal epithelium. The glands of the various segments furnish first the layers of albumen, then the shell membranes, and finally the calcareous shell. Nodular aggregates of lymphocytes and also many plasma cells are found in the wall of the oviduct.

C. UTERUS

The changes that recur in a definite sequence in the uterine cycle serve to facilitate reception and implantation of the embryo. They consist of proliferation of the

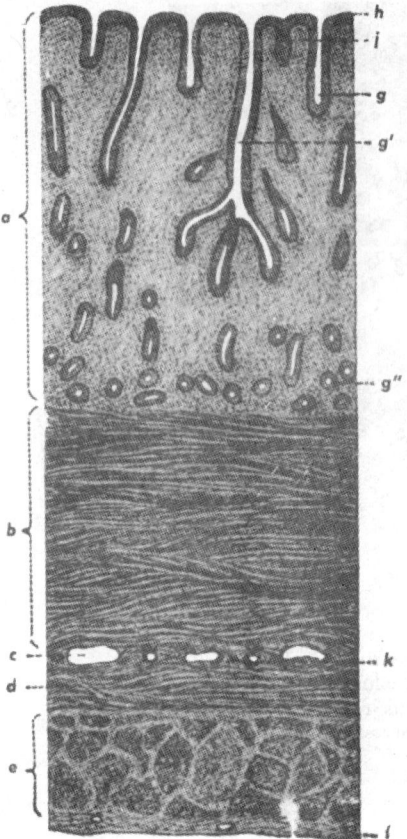

Figure 335. Cross section through the uterine wall of a bitch during anestrus. *a,* endometrium; *b,* circular muscle layer; *c,* vascular layer within the circular musculature, which is continued for a short distance peripherally (*d*); *e,* longitudinal muscle layer; *f,* serosa; *g,* uterine crypt; *g',* uterine glands, *g'',* in cross section; *h,* nonciliated columnar epithelium; *i,* tangential section through the opening of a uterine gland; *k,* artery.

mucous membrane and the musculature and occur regardless of whether fertilization takes place or not.

The uterus of domestic mammals is of the bicornuate type. It consists of a mucosa, a tunica muscularis, and a serosa. The following description applies generally to the resting stage.

The mucosa (endometrium; Figs. 335,*a;* 336,*b,d*) bears a columnar epithelium whose cells are only temporarily ciliated. The simple secretory epithelium is high in the horse and man and low in carnivores. In the sow and ruminants the epithelium is stratified.

The lamina propria contains the uterine glands. The deepest layer has a fibrillar structure and often contains an abundance of blood vessels (in the mare, ruminants, sow). It gives off connective tissue sheaths containing elastic fibers to the glands. At times pigment deposits are present in the propria, especially of sheep.

The *uterine glands* or crypts (Fig. 335,*g*) are simple branched tubular glands, which are more or less coiled, especially toward their ends. The glands possess a lamellar connective tissue sheath and are lined by simple, sometimes ciliated columnar epithelium. Tissue spaces are found between the fibroelastic gland sheath and the lamina propria.

The glands of carnivores (Fig. 335) show the least branching and coiling. Between the long uterine crypts there are shorter ones (*g*), which measure only 0.1–0.2 mm. and are present only at certain times. These are absent in other domestic animals and man. The glands of the horse are greatly coiled and branched, while those of ruminants (Fig. 336,*c*) and swine are much wider superficially than in the deeper portions, where they are narrow and strongly coiled and branched. The number of glands decreases toward the cervix. In young animals the glands are scarcer, short, and show less branching and tortuosity then they do in older ones.

The mucosa of ruminants contains nonglandular portions, the caruncles (Fig. 336,*k*), which are small prominences in virgin animals but develop into large com-

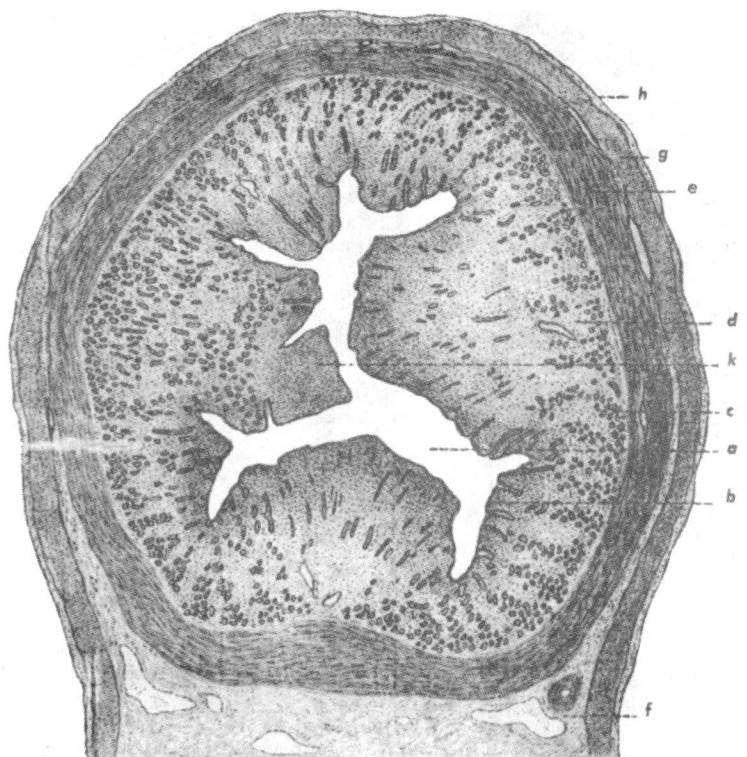

Figure 336. Cross section through a uterine horn of the ewe (stage of regression). *a*, lumen; *b*, epithelium; *c*, uterine glands in cross, oblique, and longitudinal sections; *d*, interglandular tissue of the propria mucosae; *e*, circular, *g*, longitudinal, muscle layer; *f*, stratum vasculare; *h*, serosa; *k*, caruncle.

plex structures in pregnant animals (see p. 298). They consist of highly cellular connective tissue comparable to the ovarian stroma. Their deeper portions are unusually rich in blood vessels. The glands lying deep to the caruncles open close to the caruncular base.

The uterine mucosa lacks a submucosa. The glands extend down to the tunica muscularis. Their blind ends may even lie within it. Occasionally, however, a subglandular stratum separates them from the musculature (in the cat and older animals of other species).

The muscularis (myometrium) is divided into a thick inner circular layer (Fig. 335,*b*) and a thinner outer longitudinal layer by the stratum vasculare, which contains numerous large vessels and nerves. The stratum vasculare is not very distinct in man and swine and is sometimes, especially in the cow, located within the outer half of the circular muscle layer so that a thin layer of circular muscle is found outside the stratum vasculare.

The serosa (perimetrium; Fig. 335,*f*), the stratum vasculare, and the layer of longitudinal muscle are all continuations of the broad ligament, which invests and

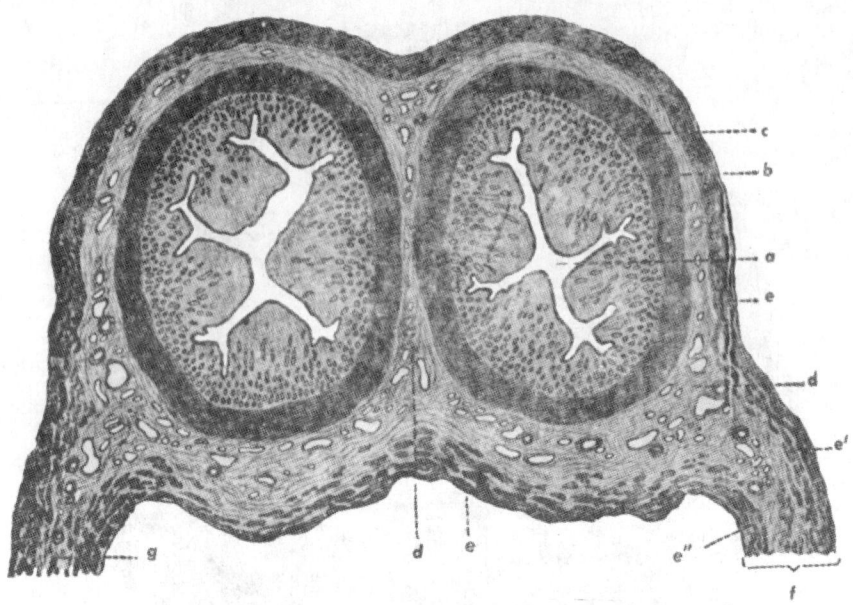

Figure 337. Cross section through the uterine horns of the ewe. *a*, lumen; *b*, uterine glands; *c*, circular muscle layer; *d*, stratum vasculare; *e*, longitudinal muscle layer; *f*, broad ligament with muscle layers *e'*,*e''*; *g*, vascular subserosa, which passes into the stratum vasculare uteri.

suspends the uterus (Fig. 337,*f*,*g*). The stratum vasculare corresponds to the subserosa. The longitudinal muscle layer should be interpreted as a muscularis serosae.

The Cervix. Toward the cervix uteri the uterine glands fade out. Only in carnivores does the cervical mucosa contain glands to the level of the external os. The mucosa is thrown into high folds, which bear secondary folds. The corresponding deep, branched furrows have small glandlike accessory furrows. The surface epithelium contains mucigenous cells, which secrete increasing quantities of mucus during estrus and pregnancy and pass into the epithelium of the vagina at the external uterine orifice. In sheep and swine solid or hollow epithelial cones extend into the underlying tissue. The collagenous propria contains few elastic fibers. In the mare the deep part contains plexuses of large veins. The cervical musculature is rich in elastic fibers and highly developed. This is true especially of the circular layer, which forms the body of the annular folds of sheep, goats, and swine and of the portio vaginalis uteri of the mare and cow (see p. 301).

VESSELS AND NERVES. The blood vessels enter the uterus from the broad ligament. They are very numerous, thick-walled, and follow a tortuous course in the stratum vasculare, giving off branches to the other layers. The mucosal twigs form periglandular and subepithelial capillary networks. The veins lack valves. In animals that have gone through a pregnancy, arteries and veins exhibit cushion-like intimal thickenings, and in all layers of the wall they show a great increase of elastic tissue, which forms clumps in old subjects. Lymphatics are numerous and form a subserous network. Their trunks lie in the stratum vasculare. The nerves end partly on the muscle fibers and partly in the mucosa.

Uterine Cycle. As in the ovary, so in the uterus each sexual cycle brings on a typical build-up of the tissues followed by involution. This is especially true of the mucosa. There is a basic similarity among the species in the periodic uterine changes, which recur at intervals characteristic for each species. Only quantitative differences of considerable degree are met with. The uterine cycle of domestic animals shows several distinct phases: proestrus, estrus, metestrus, diestrus, and anestrus. The various stages are naturally of shorter duration in the cow, where the cycle is completed in twenty-one days, than in the bitch, where the cycle lasts six months. The corresponding conditions will be briefly described for these two species. (See also Dukes's *Physiology*.)

During estrus (heat), which lasts 8–30 hours with an average of 14 hours in the cow and 4–13 days in the bitch, the endometrium is hyperemic, edematous, and, in the bitch, covered with a bloody mucous secretion. The vascularity of the mucosa has been increased under the influence of follicular estrogen. The surface epithelium is columnar. The uterine glands show some growth. Ovulation occurs in the cow on the day after heat; in the bitch, on the first or second day of heat.

Following estrus there is a period of *metestrus* (not very clear in the bitch) when the corpus luteum is developing and the hormonal control changes from estrogen to progesterone.

During the first part of *diestrus*, or the stage of glandular hyperplasia (in the cow: 2nd to 14th day of the cycle; in the bitch: 2nd to 4th week of the cycle), the development of the glands reaches its peak. They become longer and more coiled and secrete actively. The glandular epithelium becomes high columnar. The hyperplasia is especially marked in the bitch.

In case fertilization has not taken place the uterine mucosa now enters the stage of regression—the latter part of diestrus (cow: 15th to 19th day; bitch: 4th to 12th week). The thickened mucosa shrinks, secretions cease, and the glands become shorter. The stage of uterine regression, however, is not characterized as in man, by the sloughing of whole sections of mucosa accompanied by hemorrhage (menstruation). In the ovary the corpus luteum degenerates.

In the bitch a long period of rest (anestrus) now follows, during which the uterine mucosa is low, the glands are straight, and the epithelium cuboidal. This stage is succeeded by proestrus, leading up to the next heat period. In the cow, on the other hand, there is no anestrous period, and the stage of mucosal congestion and edema coincident with the maturation of another follicle begins on the nineteenth day.

Gravid Uterus

The fertilized ovum of domestic mammals is propelled by the ciliary beat and the peristaltic waves of the tubal muscle into the uterus, where it develops into the blastocyst. This effects an intimate union with the endometrium by means of its external envelope, the trophoblast. Soon the ectodermal trophoblast is lined by extraembryonic mesoderm and the two tissues comprise the *chorion*. The

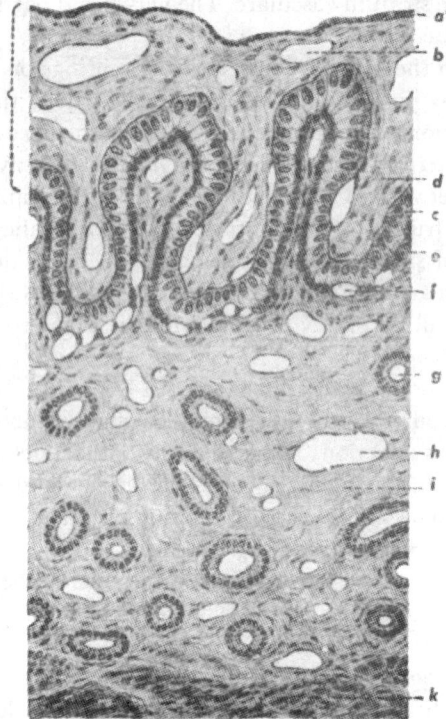

Figure 338. Section through the placenta of the pig (140X). *a*, allantochorion; *a'*, allantois epithelium; *b*, fetal blood vessel; *c*, chorionic epithelium (trophoblast); *d*, chorionic ridge; *e*, uterine epithelium; *f*, intraepithelial capillaries; *g*, uterine glands; *h*, maternal blood vessel; *i*, propria mucosae; *k*, myometrium.

chorion is vascularized by the vessels of the allantois, a sac that fills the extraembryonic coelom and fuses to the inside of the chorion. Thus the fetal portion of the definitive placenta is formed by the allantochorion (Fig. 338,*a*). In the simple forms of placentae there is merely an apposition of fetal and maternal tissues. This is called an indeciduate placenta because there is little or no loss of uterine tissue at birth (e.g., in the sow, mare, and cow). In the deciduate placenta there is a fusion of fetal and maternal tissues, and more than half the thickness of the uterine mucosa is lost, (e.g., in carnivores, primates, and rodents).

Diffuse Placenta. On the surface of the elongated, tubular blastocyst of the pig, circular folds several millimeters in width are formed. These bear smaller secondary folds or ridges ("villi" in cross section) and are distributed over the entire chorion (Fig. 338,*d*). Only the ends of the fetal envelope remain free from them. The simple columnar chorionic epithelium (trophoblast; *c*) on the folds and ridges is apposed to the cuboidal or flat epithelium lining the grooves in the endometrium.

In both of these cellular layers blood capillaries (*f*) invade the epithelium, providing close contact between the two vascular systems. The uterine lamina propria, which was already well vascularized during estrus, is relatively poor in cells because of the intensive edema. There is abundant secretion by the uterine glands, which are much more active than those in the nonpregnant animal. The glands open on the surface in groups, and the accumulated secretion (uterine milk) raises the chorion off the endometrium in cup-shaped areolae. The myometrium also undergoes changes during pregnancy. Its connective tissue appears edematous. The muscle fibers themselves become longer and thicker, while the nuclei retain their shape and size.

The diffuse placenta of the horse is similar in structure to that of the pig, except that it has true villi, which are 2–3 mm. long and arranged in tufts.

Cotyledonary Placenta. In the domestic ruminants the elongated chorionic

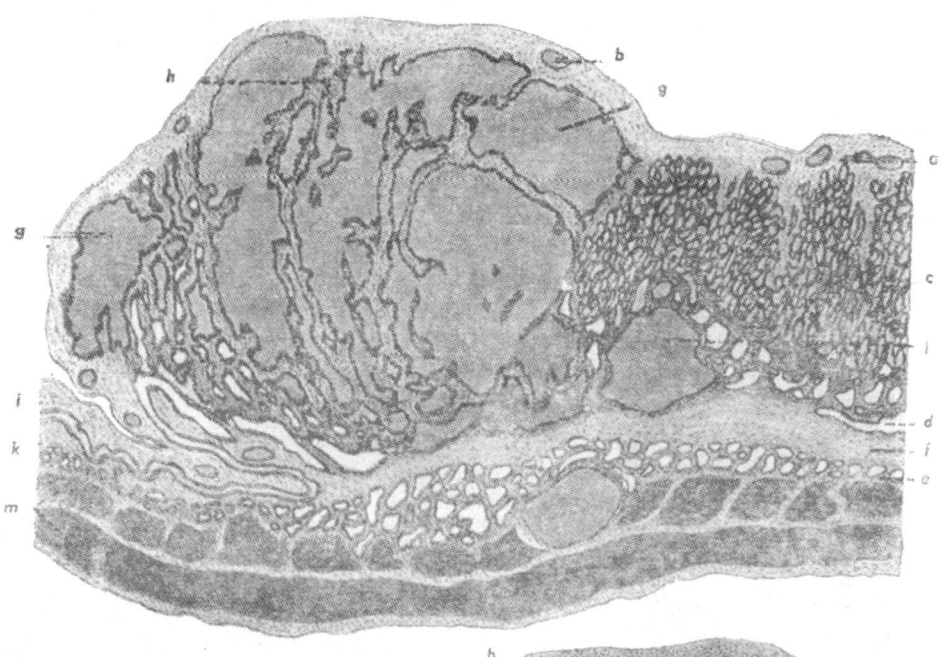

Figure 341. Cross section through the zonary placenta of the dog (near term). *a*, allantochorion; *b*, fetal blood vessel; *c*, placental labyrinth; *d*, spongy layer; *e*, deep glandular layer; *f*, supraglandular layer; *g*, blood spaces of the green border and, *h*, its chorionic villi; *i*, chorion laeve; *k*, uterine glands, overlain by uterine epithelium; *l*, blood-filled cavity of the spongy layer; *m*, myometrium.

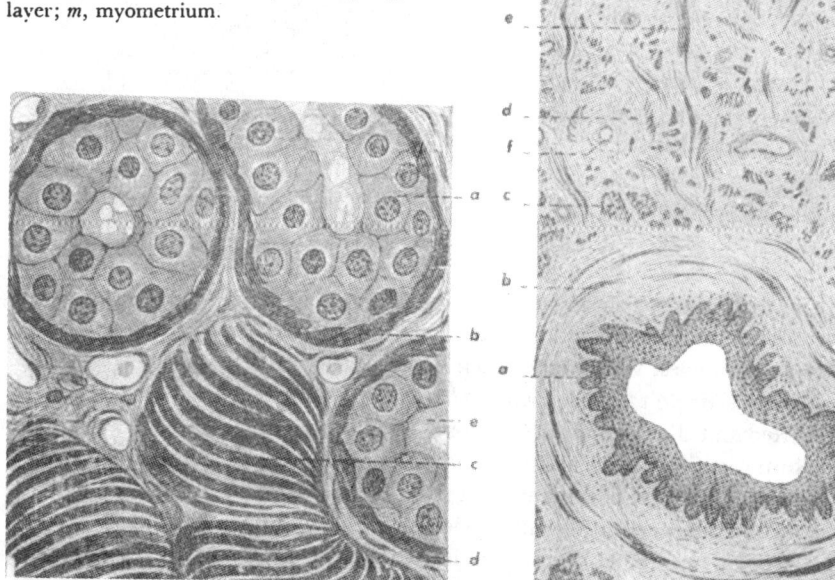

Figure 392 (*left*). Section through the secretory portion of a merocrine tubular gland from the metacarpal pad of the dog (500×). *a*, secretory cells; *b*, smooth muscle fibers (red) in oblique section; *c*, the same in longitudinal section; *d*, basement membrane; *e*, lumen.

Figure 397 (*right*). Cross section through the teat of the cow in the region of the papillary duct. All muscle cells are shown in red. *a*, squamous epithelium of the papillary duct; *b*, circular muscle of the papillary duct; *c*, longitudinal muscle strands of the teat; *d*, oblique, *e*, radial muscle strands of the teat; *f*, artery; *g*, corium; *h*, epidermis.

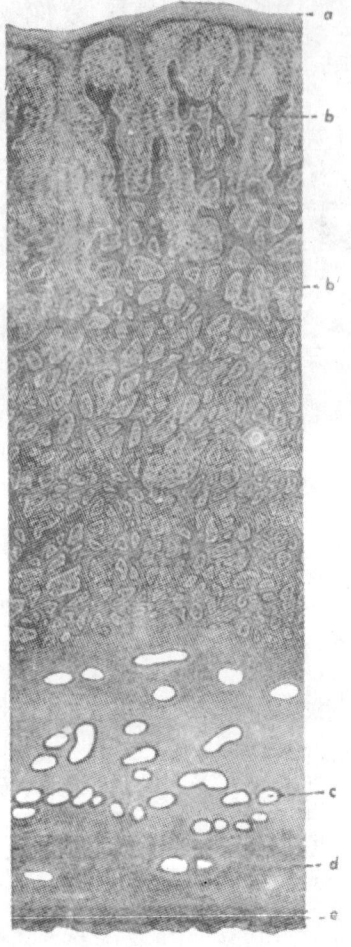

Figure 339 (left). From the bovine placenta; section through a cotyledon and the uterine wall (20×). a, allantochorion; b, chorionic villi; b', sections through parts of villi; c, uterine glands; d, myometrium; e, serosa.

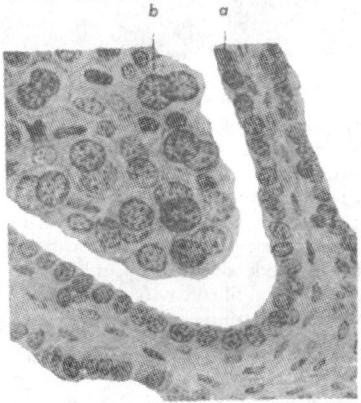

Figure 340. Chorionic villus and uterine crypt of the ox (500×). a, epithelium of the uterine glands; b, trophoblast, showing diplokaryocytes.

sac gives rise to about 100 clumps of villi (Fig. 339,b,b')—the cotyledons, between which the chorion may be smooth or bear short, single villi. The cotyledons attach to the uterine caruncles, which have been described (see p. 293; also Fig. 336,k). Cotyledon and caruncle together form a *placentome*. These structures are convex in the cow, flatter and disc-shaped in the goat, and concave in the ewe. In the cow the epithelium remains intact in the placentomes, degenerating only on the intercaruncular mucosa.[6] In the sheep and goat the uterine epithelium of the caruncular crypts is destroyed. Regeneration takes place after the fetal portion of the placenta is expelled. In all ruminants the chorionic epithelial cells of the villi are mostly transformed into binucleate giant cells (diplokaryocytes; Fig. 340,b). These have

[6] Ray D. Hatch, Anatomic Changes in the Bovine Uterus during Pregnancy, *Am. J. Vet. Res.* 2 (1941): 411–416.

strong resorptive powers and adjoin the caruncular connective tissue wherever the epithelium is absent.

Zonary Placenta. In the dog the deciduate placenta develops in a belt around the middle of the chorionic sac. The chorioendometrial fusion takes place during the stage of gland hyperplasia. The uterine wall and placenta of the bitch form six layers in the region of the placenta.

1. The allantochorion bears simple epithelium on the side facing the allantoic cavity. Its mesenchymal layer contains the blood vessels (Fig. 341,*b**) of the embryonic circulatory system.

2. During development the epithelium of the chorionic villi proliferates and forms a syncytium (syntrophoblast). The same is true of the uterine epithelium (symplasma), which obliterates the uterine gland openings and causes the glands to become distended with secretion (see layer no. 3). The villi penetrate into the maternal tissue and destroy it, except for the capillaries and isolated connective tissue cells, which become rich in cytoplasm, join the syncytium, and are then called decidual cells. (According to Wislocki and Dempsey[7] true decidual cells occur in the cat but not in the bitch.) The chorionic villi fuse into lamellae, in which the central layer of fetal mesoderm is covered on both sides by cellular trophoblast, and this in turn by syntrophoblast. In immediate contact with the syntrophoblast is the intact endothelium of the maternal capillaries. The uterine edges of the lamellae are thickened so that they are club-shaped in cross section, and firmly anchored in the uterine tissue. This entire layer is called the placental labyrinth.

3. The spongy layer (*d*) is made up of occluded gland tubules in the middle depths of the mucosa. They are distended with secretion and extravasated blood.

4. Under the spongy layer is a clearly defined connective tissue sheet, which is penetrated only by the ducts of the deep glands. This is the supraglandular layer (*f*).

5. The deep glandular layer is made up of the ends of the uterine glands, which have multiplied during early diestrus and secrete actively in the region of the zonary placenta.

6. The uterine musculature is edematous and the vessels in the stratum vasculare are engorged and greatly increased in number.

At parturition the placenta separates from the rest of the endometrium through the spongy layer. The regeneration of the lost portion of the mucosa proceeds from the sides and from the deep glandular epithelium.

At the margins of the zonary placenta we find extensive hematomata between endometrium and chorion, which are stained by a blood pigment (green border in the bitch, Fig. 341,*g**; brown border in the cat). On either side of the placenta the chorion is free from villi (*i*) and is apposed to the unchanged uterine epithelium (*k*).

---

[7] Histochemical Reactions in the Placenta of the Cat, *Am. J. Anatomy* 78 (1946): 1–45.
* Fig. 341 is on p. 297.

In laboratory rodents—mouse, rat, rabbit, and guinea pig—the maternal blood capillaries in the discoidal placenta are destroyed by the proliferating syntrophoblast, so that the maternal blood circulates through labyrinthine sinuses in the syntrophoblast. According to Mossman,[8] fetal capillaries penetrate the trophoblast and enter into direct relation with the maternal blood.

Following parturition the uterus undergoes *involution*. This consists of regression of the musculature and the mucosa and, in animals with deciduate placentation, of regeneration of the uterine mucosa. The uterus does not revert completely to the virginal state. Traces of pregnancy and parturition persist, such as thickening of the wall and stratum vasculare, pigment deposition, and increase in elastic tissue. For about two weeks after parturition there is a normal discharge of *lochia*, consisting of blood-tinged mucus and decomposed tissue shreds. In the bitch the early discharge contains green clotted blood.

D. VAGINA

The wall of the vagina consists of a mucosa, a tunica muscularis, and an adventitia or, cranially, a serosa with a muscularis serosae. The nonglandular mucosa exhibits longitudinal folds and bears a stratified epithelium whose appearance is altered more or less in the various species by the sexual cycle. The epithelium is thickened by an increase in the number of layers during proestrus and estrus in all species. With the exception of the cow, the surface layers are stratified squamous. They are cornified during heat in the carnivores and rodents. Intraepithelial glands have been found in the bitch during heat. The appearance of cornified scales in the vaginal smear of rodents is diagnostic of estrus. In the mare most of the epithelium is made up of polyhedral cells, with only a thin layer of flattened, occasionally cornified cells on the surface. In the cranial part of the vagina in the cow the surface cells are high columnar and secrete mucus. The absence of cornification in the cow is associated with a low estrogen output. Leukocytes appear in the vaginal mucosa during heat in most species and appear in the vaginal discharge in metestrus. The epithelium reverts to a low stratified cuboidal or columnar epithelium in metestrus.

The lamina propria forms little or no papillary body. Its connective tissue is rich in cells near the epithelium and contains lymph nodules. There is a loose submucosa.

The tunica muscularis usually consists of a thick inner circular layer and a thin outer longitudinal layer. The latter is continued for a short distance in the wall of the uterus. In the sow and bitch, and to a lesser degree in the cat, a thin layer of longitudinal muscle is found inside the circular layer.

The collagenous adventitia contains large vessels, nerves, and ganglia. Cranially it is continuous with the subserosa. As in the case of the uterus, the serosa carries its own longitudinal muscularis serosae. Dorsally the serosal musculature

---

[8] Comparative Morphogenesis of the Fetal Membranes and Accessory Uterine Structures, *Carnegie Contrib. Emb.* 26 (1937): 129–246.

is absent between the lines of insertion of the broad ligaments. Ventrally it blends with the proper vaginal muscle.

In the zone of transition from the vagina to the uterus the arrangement of the musculature varies according to the development of the cervix. The conditions are simplest in the ewe and sow, in which there is no demarcation between the uterine and vaginal muscles except that the circular layer thickens considerably in the region of the cervical prominences, whose basis it forms. In the mare and cow the heavy muscular wall of the intravaginal portion of the cervix is formed by a thickening and infolding of the circular, and to a lesser extent also of part of the longitudinal, muscle sheet. Most of the longitudinal muscle is fused with the muscularis serosae and passes directly into the uterine wall. In the bitch, where the vaginal portion of the cervix is fused to the dorsal wall, the inner longitudinal and the circular layers of vaginal muscle form a loop around the external uterine orifice. The external longitudinal muscle of the vagina continues into that of the uterus.

E. VULVA

The vulva in domestic animals consists of the vestibule, the labia, and the clitoris.

(1) **The Vestibule.** The cutaneous mucosa is covered by stratified squamous epithelium, which is often infiltrated by leukocytes. The epithelium of the mare and sow often shows tubular evaginations similar to the lacunae of Morgagni in the human urethra. The propria forms a papillary body and is much richer in elastic tissue than that of the vagina. It contains numerous lymph nodules. In the deeper layers a dense cavernous plexus of large veins is found. In certain places the vestibular mucosa contains *vestibular glands*, which are branched tubular glands resembling in structure the male accessory glands. Their end-pieces are lined with simple columnar epithelium, showing different functional stages, and their excretory ducts with stratified epithelium.

Man, ruminants, and cats have a lobulated *major vestibular gland* (of Bartholin), located in the submucosa or in the m. constrictor vestibuli and homologous to the bulbo-urethral gland in the male. Its excretory duct opens on the lateral wall caudal to the urethral opening. The *minor vestibular glands* are scattered in the cat and ewe and concentrated in the median ventral groove cranial to the end of the clitoris in the cow. Swine and solipeds have only small isolated glands with usually long and wide excretory ducts. The bitch has small lobular glands, which are deeply embedded in the constrictor vestibuli and which open by way of long excretory ducts.

The outer vestibular wall is made up of circular and longitudinal striated muscle (constrictor vestibuli), which is incomplete dorsally and passes ventrally into the urethral muscle. The smooth muscle inside the constrictor is a continuation of the vaginal musculature. In swine and carnivores, however, this is distinct only in the dorsal gap in the constrictor.

In the mare and bitch a well-defined corpus cavernosum is present between

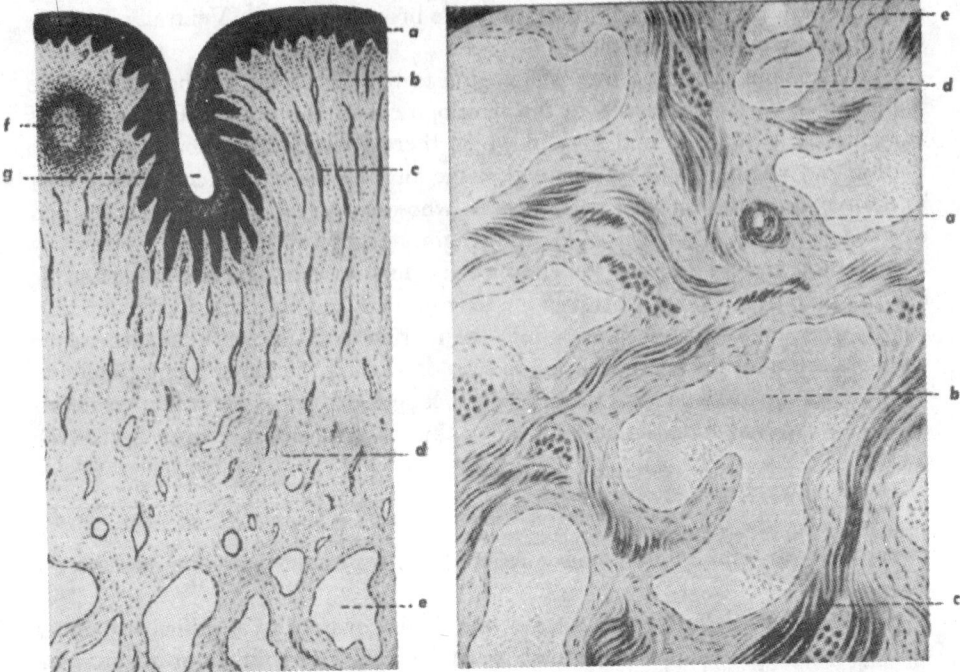

Figure 342 (left). Section from the glans clitoridis of the mare. *a,* squamous epith lium with papillary body; *b,* connective tissue of the visceral layer of the prepuce; *c,* capillaries; *d,* connective tissue of the clitoris; *e,* distal end of the corpus cavernosum (see Fig. 343); *f,* lymph nodule; *g,* fur-row of the clitoris.

Figure 343 (right). Portion of the corpus cavernosum clitoridis of the mare (80×). *a,* artery; *b,* cavernous spaces containing blood corpuscles; *c,* smooth muscle; *d,* lymphatic; *e,* nerve.

mucosa and tunica muscularis near the labia. It has the structure of the male corpus cavernosum urethrae and is called the *bulbus vestibuli.* The *hymen* is an annular fold of mucosa that marks the boundary between vagina and vestibule in virgins. It varies in development with the species.

On either side of the urethral orifice of the cow and sow, and more rarely of the mare and carnivores, we find the openings of the vestigial mesonephric ducts, called the ducts of Gartner. Their wall consists of a collagenous lamina propria covered by columnar epithelium. The paraurethral ducts, which occur in man, sheep, swine, and cat, have a similar structure and may have glandular appendages, the paraurethral glands.

(2) **The Clitoris** (Figs. 342–344). The clitoris is rich in elastic tissue and consists of the corpus cavernosum clitoridis, the glans, and the prepuce, the latter of which is a continuation of the vestibular mucosa.

The corpus cavernosum clitoridis (Figs. 343; 344,*c*) is homologous to the corpus cavernosum penis. It possesses a heavy tunica albuginea with many vessels and nerves.

The corpus cavernosum clitoridis of solipeds and woman is well developed and equipped with abundant musculature. In ruminants there is less cavernous tissue. In the cat and sow varying quantities of fat cells are present in the trabeculae and cavernous tissue. They are also found to a slight extent in solipeds and in larger quantities in ruminants. In the bitch the axial part of the corpus clitoridis has been transformed into a fatty structure. A septum is present in solipeds and dogs. In the other domestic animals the tapering end of the corpus cavernosum terminates in a corpus fibrosum. Venous plexuses lie on the dorsal surface of the tunica albuginea.

The end of the corpus cavernosum clitoridis is capped by the richly innervated glans or a rudiment of it. The glans clitoridis resembles structurally the glans penis. A true erectile body is present in the glans clitoridis only in the bitch and mare. Ruminants have only a fibroelastic cover on the distal end of the corpus. This contains a venous plexus in the ewe. In the sow and cat the cover corresponds closely to the highly vascular propria of the vestibular mucosa.

The preputium clitoridis, composed of the nonglandular cutaneous mucosa of the vestibule, has parietal and visceral parts as in the male. The membrana visceralis or glandis (Fig. 342,a) contains an abundance of terminal nerve corpuscles —bulbs of Krause, genital corpuscles, and Pacinian corpuscles (in the cat and sow).

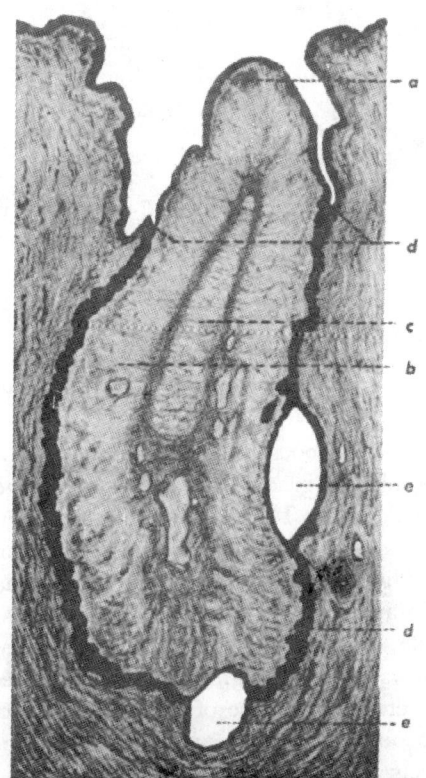

Figure 344. End of the clitoris of the cow. a, lymph nodule in the visceral layer of the prepuce; b, substance of the glans; c, end of the corpus cavernosum clitoridis; d, epithelial lamina, which has failed to split into the parietal and visceral preputial layers; e, separation of the two layers due to the intervention of a blind duct. Similar splits are seen next to the tip of the clitoris. The inner layer (visceral prepuce) covers the tip of the clitoris, while the outer (parietal prepuce) passes into the surrounding skin. (After Schmaltz.)

It also contains lymph nodules. The space intervening between the parietal and visceral layers of the prepuce is the fossa clitoridis.

The fossa is distinct in solipeds and the bitch. In the ewe and cat there is only a slight indication of it, and it is absent in the cow and sow. In these four species the epithelial lamina that grows down around the clitoris in the embryo fails to split into parietal and visceral preputial epithelium (Fig. 344, d). The epithelial lamina sends variously shaped projections into the connective tissue.

(3) **The Labia.** The integument of the labia vulvae shows the same structure as the external skin (Figs. 345, 388). It is rich in sebaceous and tubular glands

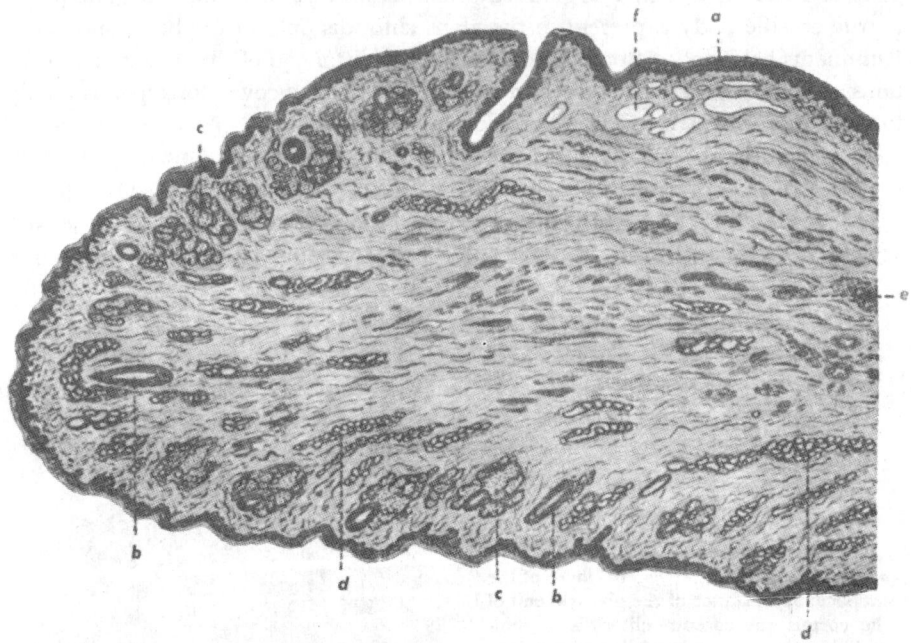

Figure 345. Cross section through the labium vulvae of the cow. *a*, mucosa; *b*, integument with hairs in cross section; *c*, sebaceous, *d*, tubular, glands; *e*, muscle fibers; *f*, lymphatics.

(*c*,*d*). Sebaceous glands not connected with hair follicles are also present. The external skin gradually passes into the vestibular mucosa. Both possess abundant elastic tissue. The labia contain fat. There are smooth muscle fibers in the mucosa, and striated muscle surrounds the vulvar cleft (m. constrictor vulvae).

The Female Urethra. The mucosa is nonglandular, rich in elastic tissue, and contains many cavernous veins. It shows a papillary body near the external orifice only, and is covered by stratified epithelium, which in the mare, cow, and sow shows tubular evaginations as in the vestibule. Lymph nodules are present. The cavernous structure of the mucosa becomes more and more evident toward the opening. In woman and the cow single branched tubular glands (of Littré) also occur.

An inner circular and outer longitudinal layer of heavy smooth muscle surrounds the mucosa. The mare and bitch have an additional inner longitudinal muscle layer. Near the external orifice the musculature fades out, dorsally at first, and disappears at the vestibule. Lateral and ventral to the smooth muscle lies the striated urethral muscle, which blends into the constrictor vestibuli.

THE CLOACA OF THE CHICKEN. The colon and the urinary and genital passages open into the cloaca. An annular fold separates it from the rectum, and it communicates with the outside through the vent. The cloaca is lined by simple columnar epithelium, which contains many goblet cells.

The *bursa of Fabricius* opens on the dorsal wall. It consists of a cavity lined by simple columnar epithelium, into which numerous branching tubular glands open. Between these we find unusually large quantities of small lymph nodules, which undergo marked enlargement with increasing age at the expense of the glandular elements.

XVI

The Nervous System

A. THE CENTRAL NERVOUS SYSTEM

THE brain and spinal cord are covered by the meninges, and their cavities are lined by the ependyma.

Meninges

The meninges serve to protect the central nervous system and to carry its blood vessels. We distinguish the tough dura mater, or pachymeninx, from the delicate leptomeninges, the arachnoid and pia mater.

The *dura mater* is a tough collagenous membrane with elastic fiber nets. It contains blood vessels, including venous sinuses in certain parts. The free (inner) surface is covered with mesenchymal epithelium. In the cranial cavity, where there is no movement of the surrounding bones, the dura is fused with the periosteum. In the spinal canal, however, it adapts itself to the changing topographical relations of the spinal cord and is not fused with the periosteum. Between them is the extradural (epidural) space, which is filled with venous plexuses, lymph spaces, and fat.

The dura mater is separated by the subdural space from the *arachnoid*, a delicate, collagenous membrane, which is somewhat similar in structure to the omentum. The free surfaces of the arachnoid and the numerous trabeculae it sends to the pia are covered by mesenchymal epithelium. Under the arachnoid is the subarachnoid space. This is filled with the *cerebrospinal fluid*, which also fills the cerebral ventricles and the central canal of the spinal cord. The central nervous system is thus suspended in liquid which protects it against mechanical insult. The cerebrospinal fluid also receives wastes from the nervous tissue, which are passed on to the venous sinuses of the dura by way of the *arachnoid villi*. These consist of arachnoid tissue covered by epithelium. They project through the subdural space into the dura and the venous sinuses. They form, along with delicate trabeculae of connective tissue, the connection between dura and arachnoid and are the points at which the cerebrospinal fluid enters the venous circulation.

The *pia mater* consists of delicate, lamellar connective tissue, the free surface of which is covered by the mesenchymal epithelium. It is the carrier of the main blood vessels and gives off small arterial branches with collagenous sheaths into the underlying nervous tissue (Fig. 348,*d*). The adventitia of the vessels is always separated from the nervous tissue by a glial membrane.

Pial lamellae (telae chorioideae) project into the ventricles and, by means of foldings, give rise to the *chorioid plexuses*, which are rich in vascular loops and covered by simple cuboidal epithelium. The epithelial cells are separated only by delicate connective tissue from the underlying vessels. They may contain various inclusions, such as fat and pigment, and possibly regulate the composition of the

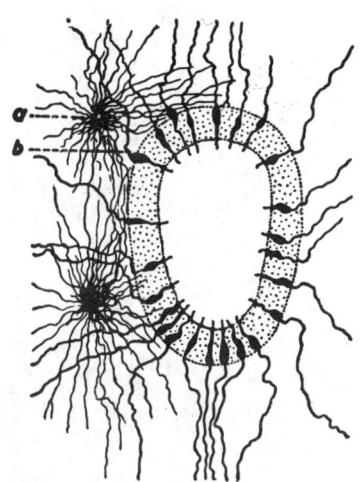

Figure 346. Neuroglia cells of the spinal cord. *a*, neuroglia cells (astrocytes) in the substantia gelatinosa centralis; *b*, ependymal cells surrounding the central canal. (After Lenhossék.)

cerebrospinal fluid or contribute to its formation. Numerous mast cells are present in the collagenous stroma of the plexuses.

Ependyma. The ependyma (Figs. 115; 346,*b*) lines the cavities of the central nervous system. It is part of the neuroglia and consists of a single layer of cells, which in young animals bear cilia. The height of the cells varies with the location. In the embryo the ependymal cells taper basally into a long, branching process, the ependymal fiber, which persists only partially and in certain regions.

In the floor of the fourth ventricle and the central canal of the spinal cord, nerve cells and fibers occur between ependymal cells. The nerve endings lie between the ependymal cells or free in the lumen and are well adapted to react to pressure changes or displacement of the cerebrospinal fluid.

Substance of the Brain and Cord. The nervous tissue consists of gray and white matter. Both contain a peculiar, delicate, lattice-like supporting framework and accessory tissue, the neuroglia, which has been described on p. 81. Within the glial framework are the true nervous elements—nerve cells and fibers in the gray substance and nerve fibers only in the white matter. On parts of the outer and inner surfaces of the brain and cord are thin layers of neuroglia, which are free from nerve cells and fibers, e.g., the marginal glia of the spinal cord. The nervous tissue is separated from the mesenchymal tissue by a limiting membrane, where glia and connective tissue meet.

In addition to the neuroglial framework, brain and cord also have a coarser, vascular, connective tissue framework formed by processes from the pia. In the white matter of the spinal cord they form a system of septa. The invading processes surround the entering blood vessels in the form of adventitial sheaths containing lymph spaces.

The gray substance, which performs the central functions and shows local structural peculiarities, contains cell bodies or entire neurons. These are surrounded by

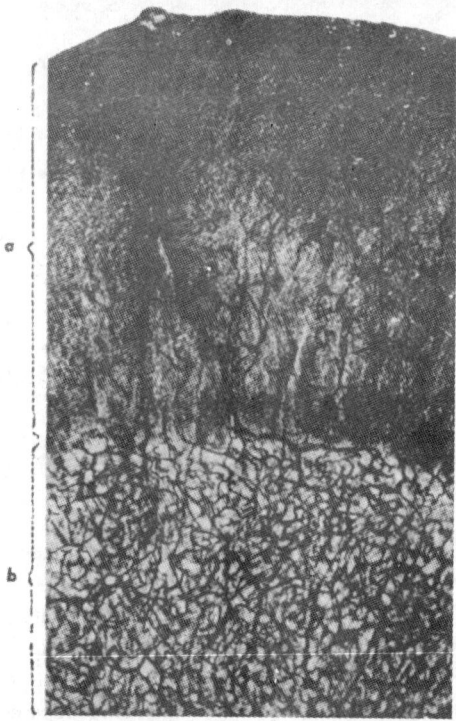

Figure 347. From the spinal cord of the cat. The blood vessels have been injected (40×). a, white matter with a bifurcating artery and wide-meshed capillary nets (right); b, gray matter showing abundant narrow-meshed capillary nets.

neuroglia composed of protoplasmic astrocytes (Figs. 349,f; 353,g). The dendrites of the nerve cells form feltlike networks (neuropil) with the usually unmyelinated axons. The nerve cell processes end in the form of telodendra on neighboring nerve cells or in more distant parts of the gray matter. They may also enter the white matter and form tracts leading to other parts of the gray matter. The gray matter is characterized by a great abundance of capillaries. The plexuses these form are more or less round-meshed (Fig. 347,b). The nerve cell bodies are scattered, or clustered in groups called *nuclei*. Layers containing few nerve cells and consisting mostly of neuropil and a fine glial network are called molecular layers. Layers consisting of glia alone also appear gray and are included in the gray matter.

As a rule the white matter contains no nerve cell bodies or neuropil. It is composed almost entirely of myelinated fibers without a neurilemma. The myelin sheaths cause its white appearance. Its glia cells are mostly fibrous astrocytes (Figs. 349,g; 353,h). The capillary nets have long, wide meshes (Fig. 347,a). The white matter is less vascular than the gray. Most of its nerve fibers form bundles that are separated from each other by connective tissue septa.

Often one finds in the brain substance or ventricles stratified corpora amylacea, which, like starch, stain violet with iodine.

THE BLOOD VESSELS OF THE CENTRAL NERVOUS SYSTEM. Cerebrum and cerebellum are permeated by dense capillary networks, which are derived from the arteries that enter from the pia. The various regions show differences in arrangement and density of the capillary nets. These are especially dense near the nuclei. In the spinal cord the arteries enter with the nerve roots and form a network in the pia. Ventral to the ventral fissure lies the unpaired ventral spinal artery (Fig. 354). From this the gray matter receives a number of branches, which enter by way of the fissure. Over the entire surface of the spinal cord the pial vessels supply branches to the white matter. Within the substance of the cord the arteries break up into capillary nets, which give rise to veins that return to the pia. All vessels are separated from the nerve tissue proper by connective tissue and glia. The glial fibers are often radially attached to the capillary walls by means of terminal thickenings. The substance of the central nervous system lacks lymphatics, but perivascular lymph spaces are encountered in the adventitia surrounding the vessels.

1. Cerebrum

In the cerebrum the gray matter occurs as the cortex, as the central gray matter surrounding the ventricles, and as well-defined nuclei, such as those of the thalamus, the corpora quadrigemina, and corpus striatum. All these parts are interconnected by tracts of white matter, the main mass of which is formed by the medullary center and the internal and external capsules.

a. Cerebral Cortex

Four poorly defined layers may be differentiated in the cerebral cortex on the basis of the shape of their nerve cells:

(1) Directly under the pia lies the molecular or plexiform layer (Figs. 348; 349, I), which is poor in cells and is especially well developed in the horse. It is covered by a thin layer of glia cells and has as a framework a fine reticulum formed by glial processes and the dendrites of the pyramidal cells. In addition to horizontal myelinated nerve fibers (tangential fibers) and glia cells, this layer contains the Cajal cells (Fig. 349,c). These are fusiform or stellate structures with horizontally directed processes, which send numerous branches at right angles toward the surface and are said to be equivalent to axons.

(2) The layer of small pyramidal cells (Figs. 348; 349,II) contains cells with their apices directed toward the surface. Their size is about 10–12 μ. At their apex these cells taper into a long main dendrite, which gives off small lateral branches on its way to the molecular layer, where it ramifies, forming an inextricable feltwork in the most superficial layers. Laterally and basally short dendrites are given off from the pyramidal cells. The myelinated axon arises at the base and gives off

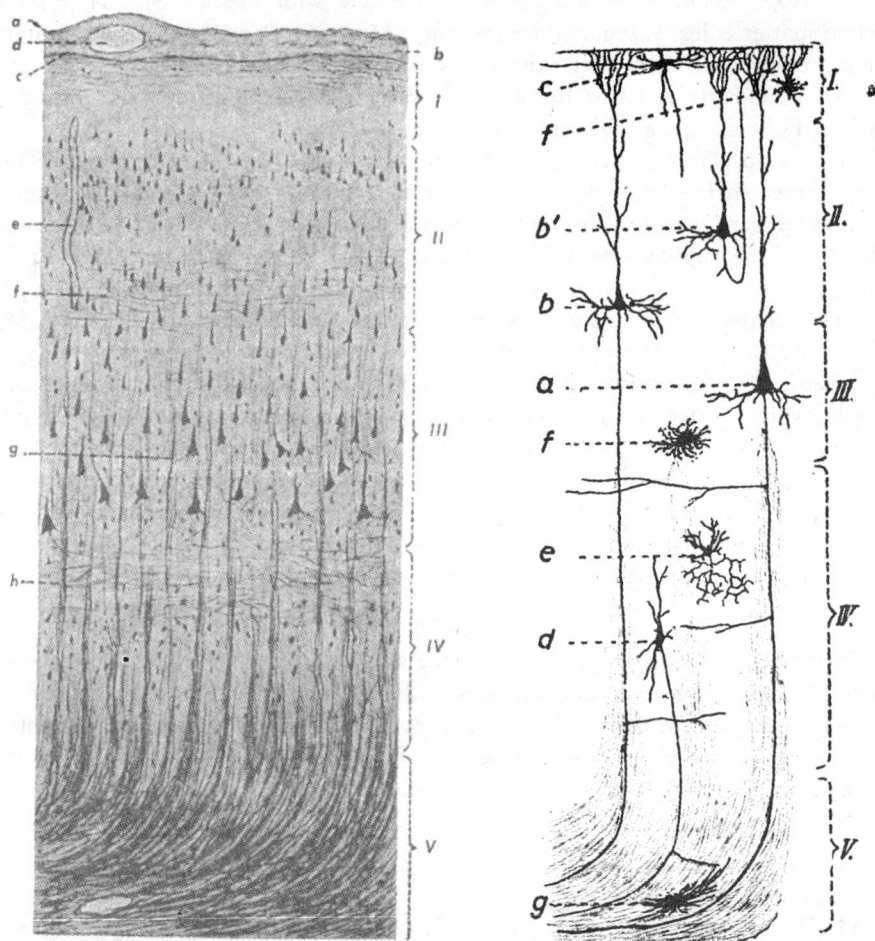

Figure 348 (left). Vertical section through the cerebral cortex of the cat; myelin stain (65×). *I*, molecular layer; *II*, layer of small, and *III*, large, pyramidal cells; *IV*, layer of polymorphous cells; *V*, white matter; *a*, pia mater; *b*, superficial glial layer; *c*, tangential fibers; *d,e*, blood vessels; *f*, supraradial network; *g*, radial bundles; *h*, interradial network.

Figure 349 (right). Diagram of the structure of the cerebral cortex; Golgi impregnation. *I*, molecular layer; *II*, layer of the small, and *III*, large, pyramidal cells; *IV*, layer of polymorphous cells; *V*, white matter; *a*, large, *b*, small, pyramidal cell; *b'*, Martinotti's cell (small pyramidal cell with ascending axon); *c*, Cajal cell; *d*, polymorphous cell; *e*, Golgi type II nerve cell; *f*, glia cell (protoplasmic astrocyte); *g*, glia cell (fibrous astrocyte). Red = myelinated fibers. The stratum of glia which lies on top of the molecular layer is not shown.

numerous horizontal collaterals on its way toward the white matter. The axon of some of the small pyramidal cells—Martinotti's cells (Fig. 349,*b'*)—makes a 180° turn toward the surface, bifurcates, and enters the network of tangential fibers.

(3) Toward the white matter the small pyramidal cells are replaced by the layer of large pyramidal cells (Figs. 348; 349,*III*). These measure 20–30 μ and more. They give origin to the fibers of the pyramidal motor pathways.

(4) In the layer of polymorphous cells (Figs. 348; 349,*IV*) the cells are smaller again (5–8 μ) but more irregular and varied in shape. Their relatively short dendrites ramify in all directions, and their axons extend into the white matter.

The outer part of the fourth layer is sometimes called the granular layer. In the motor areas still another zone, that of the giant pyramidal cells, intervenes between the granular and polymorphous layers. The various areas of the cortex show differences in the number of layers and their cellular composition.

In the three deeper layers a few Golgi type II cells (Fig. 349,*e*) are present. Their processes, which are commonly short, but may sometimes extend into the molecular layer, ramify throughout the cortical substance.

Some of the myelinated nerve fibers of the cortex are axons of the pyramidal and polymorphous cells, as well as their collaterals. The remainder are fibers that extend from the white matter into the cortex (corticipetal fibers). Large numbers

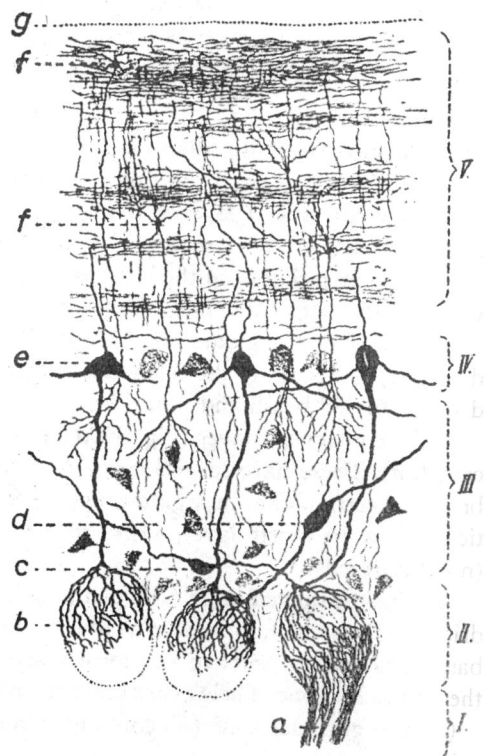

Figure 350. Diagram of the structure of the olfactory bulb. *I*, layer of superficial olfactory fibers; *II*, layer of the olfactory glomeruli; *III*, molecular layer; *IV*, mitral cell layer; *V*, granular zone and white matter (layer of the deeper olfactory fibers); *a*, olfactory nerve bundles; *b*, glomerulus olfactorius; *c*, small brush cell; *d*, large brush cell; *e*, mitral cell; *f*, granular cell; *g*, ependyma (shown as dotted line). Red = myelinated nerve fibers. (After Koelliker.)

of these enter the cortex from the white matter, either grouped into radial bundles (Figs. 348,*g*; 349, in red) or more diffusely distributed. Their number decreases toward the surface so that the radial bundles fade out as they approach the zone of small pyramidal cells. In addition to these vertically ascending fibers and the tangential fibers of the molecular layer there are also other myelinated fibers, which run horizontally across and above the radial bundles. These form the inter-radial and supraradial networks. Toward the ends of the radial bundles the inter-radial network is formed by a denser layer of fibers, which are mostly collaterals of the pyramidal cell axons.

In the white matter of the cerebrum (Figs. 348; 349,*V*), bundles of myelinated fibers converge radially from the cortex toward the cerebral peduncles. They pass around the lateral ventricles, which are bordered by a thin layer of neuroglia and lined by ependyma. In the cerebral peduncles the myelinated nerve bundles lie parallel and continue to the white matter of the pons and cerebellum. The cerebral hemispheres are connected by transverse fiber bundles running in the commissures, of which the corpus callosum is the largest.

Nuclei composed of nerve cells are distributed in the white matter of the brain. One of these, the red nucleus of the midbrain, is of special importance in the control of motor activities in domestic animals.

The cells of the cortical gray matter are the material basis of consciousness. The cortex is the seat of the psychic functions of sensation and will. The various activities of the cerebrum, such as motor functions and sensory perceptions and their evaluation, take place in definite cortical areas.

b. Olfactory Bulb

In the olfactory bulb, the subcortical center of the olfactory nerve, the following layers are recognized, starting at the periphery:

(1) The superficial layer is formed by interwoven unmyelinated fibers (Fig. 350,*I,a*) which are the axons of the olfactory cells in the nasal mucosa (p. 231). The fibers emerging from the deep surface of this layer break up into telodendra, which contribute to the formation of the olfactory glomeruli.

(2) The olfactory glomeruli (Fig. 350,*II,b*) are oval or round balls, 10–30 μ in diameter, composed of the telodendra of the olfactory fibers and those of the more deeply situated brush and mitral cells.

(3) The molecular layer (Fig. 350,*III*) contains the fusiform or pyramidal brush cells (*c,d*). These have several basal dendrites and a main dendrite, which has a brushlike termination in a glomerulus. The axons of the brush cells descend vertically into the fourth layer, where they turn horizontally into the olfactory tract (not illustrated).

(4) The mitral cell layer (*IV*) contains large tetrahedral cells. Their main dendrite has the same termination as that of the brush cells. Their smaller lateral and basal dendrites interweave and form a layer of horizontal fibers at the margin of the molecular zone. Their axons enter the olfactory tract.

(5) The granular zone (*V*) contains numerous fusiform granule cells (*f*). These

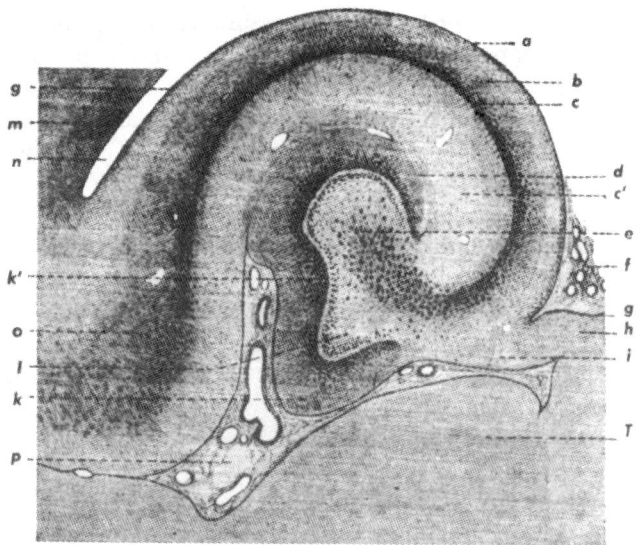

Figure 351. The right hippocampus of a dog (16×). The section is cut through the dorsal part and is viewed from behind. *a*, endoventricular alveus; *b*, layer of polymorphous cells of the hippocampus; *c*, layer of the small and large pyramidal cells; *c'*, lacunar layer (between *c* and *c'* is the stratum radiatum); *d*, molecular layer; *e*, margin of the hippocampus; *f*, chorioid plexus of the lateral ventricle; *g*, ventricular ependyma; *h*, fimbria; *i*, extraventricular alveus; *k*, stratum radiatum of the dentate gyrus; *k'*, its pyramidal cell (granular) layer; *l*, its polymorphous cell layer; *m*, tapetum; *n*, lateral ventricle; *o*, gyrus hippocampi; *p*, hippocampal fissure; *T*, thalamus.

give off a long peripheral axon,[1] which extends into the molecular layer, where it arborizes. This layer is interwoven with nerve fibers running in all directions (Fig. 350, in red). Therefore it has been called the layer of deeper olfactory fibers.

The remaining white matter, which also contains granule cells and still belongs to the fifth layer, contains large numbers of myelinated and unmyelinated nerve fibers, that run mostly parallel to the surface. These are in part axons of the brush and mitral cells and their collaterals. The rest are conducting toward the olfactory lobe. They ramify extensively and terminate in this layer as well as in the mitral cell and molecular layers.

The ependymal cells (*g*), which line the olfactory cavity and represent the sixth layer, have basal processes extending into the bulbar substance.

c. Hippocampus

Knowledge of the microscopic structure of the hippocampus (Ammon's horn) is important in the diagnosis of rabies, because the Negri bodies, which are pathognomonic of this disease, occur mainly here.

[1] Stephen W. Ranson and S. L. Clark, *The Anatomy of the Nervous System*, p. 284.

The hippocampus is formed where the cerebral cortex is rolled into the lateral ventricle along the hippocampal gyrus. The gyrus is visible on the medial surface of the cerebral hemisphere, but the hippocampus itself is concealed within the ventricle. It curves around the thalamus from dorsal to caudal to ventral. The turned-in edge is folded under the slender dentate gyrus. We distinguish the following layers, starting from the lateral ventricle (Figure 351):

(1) The ventricular ependyma (g).

(2) The alveus layer, composed of myelinated nerve fibers (a).

(3) The next layer (stratum oriens, b) contains relatively few polymorphous nerve cells, which send a tangle of fibers to surround the pyramidal cells.

(4) The layer of pyramidal cells (c). Large and small pyramidal cells occur here in one layer. The abundant apical dendrites make up a stratum radiatum. The basal axon passes into the alveus.

(5) The lacunar layer (c').

(6) The molecular layer (d).

The layers of the gyrus dentatus are much reduced. There is a layer of polymorphous nerve cells (l) and a prominent layer of pyramidal cells, also called the granular layer (k').

d. The Basal Ganglia and the Central Gray Matter

The basal ganglia (corpus striatum, claustrum, and amygdaloid nucleus) and the thalamus and corpora quadrigemina consist of strata and nuclei of gray matter. Their multipolar nerve cells vary in size and may have long or short axons.

The central gray matter forms a subependymal layer surrounding the lateral and third ventricles and the aqueduct of Sylvius and continuing into the wall of the infundibulum. It consists of neuroglia, nerve fibers, and nerve cells, which are mostly multipolar. On the ventral side of the aqueduct nearest the lumen lie nuclei and longitudinal fiber bundles and, further toward the periphery, layers of nerve fibers with nerve cells interspersed singly or in groups.

2. Cerebellum

The cerebellum is connected to the cerebrum and spinal cord by numerous pathways. It governs the maintenance of equilibrium and the co-ordination of body movements. The cerebellum is divided into a cortex consisting of gray matter, a white corpus medullare, and some gray nuclei contained in the white matter.

The cortex is subdivided into three layers, whose minute structural relations are best demonstrated by means of the Golgi method:

a. The outer molecular layer (Figs. 352,a; 353,I) is poor in cells and is covered on its surface by a thin limiting membrane. It contains two kinds of multipolar nerve cells: the peripheral small cortical cells and the deeper large cortical cells, commonly called basket cells. The dendrites of the small cells (Fig. 353,c) spread out in the same plane as those of the Purkinje cells (see below), while the axon may arborize in the vicinity of the cell body or extend for a considerable distance. It gives off numerous branches close to its origin. The dendrites of the more deeply situated basket cells (b) are usually directed peripherally. Their axon runs paral-

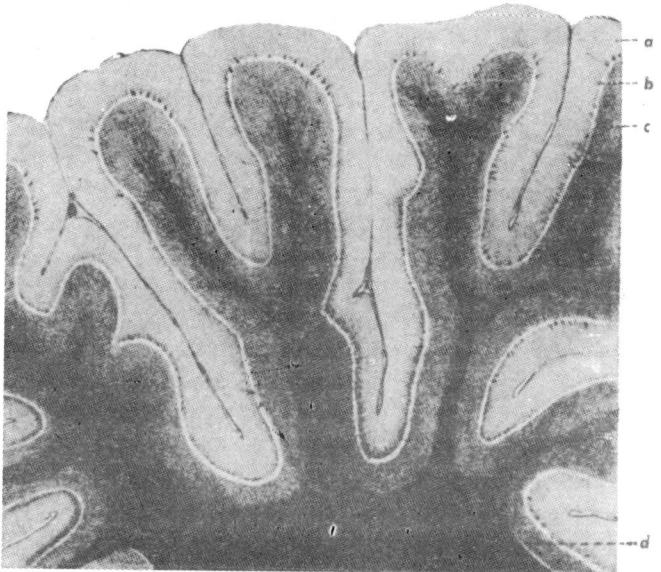

Figure 352. From the cerebellum of the horse; white matter dark, gray matter light. *a*, molecular layer; *b*, ganglionic layer of Purkinje cells; *c*, granular layer; *d*, white medullary substance.

lel to the surface at right angles to the direction of the gyrus. It gives off vertically descending branches, whose telodendra form a basket around the Purkinje cells (Fig. 353,*a*, *left*).

b. The ganglionic layer consists of the Purkinje cells (Figs. 352,*b*; 352,*a*), which are large, usually pyriform nerve cells. Their primary antler-like dendrites arise from the peripheral cell pole and soon break up into a great array of branches, which extend to the surface of the cortex. The processes spread out in one plane only, at right angles to the long axis of the gyrus. The dendrites of neighboring cells are interconnected. The axons arise from the basal (medullary) cell surface. They soon receive a myelin sheath and traverse the granular layer on their way to the medullary substance. While in the granular layer they give off numerous recurrent myelinated collaterals, which break up into terminal twigs partly in the granular and partly in the ganglionic layer.

c. The inner, rust-colored granular layer (Figs. 352,*c*; 353,*II*) varies in thickness and contains Golgi type II cells and the small granule cells. The granule cells, which predominate, are spheroid and poor in cytoplasm. They have three to six short dendrites ending in clawlike processes. Their axon remains unmyelinated and ascends vertically into the molecular layer, where it undergoes a T-shaped bifurcation. The branches run parallel to the convolutions, crossing the dendritic branches of the Purkinje cells. The cells of Golgi type II (*e*) give off several dendrites, some of which ramify in the granular layer while others spread out in the

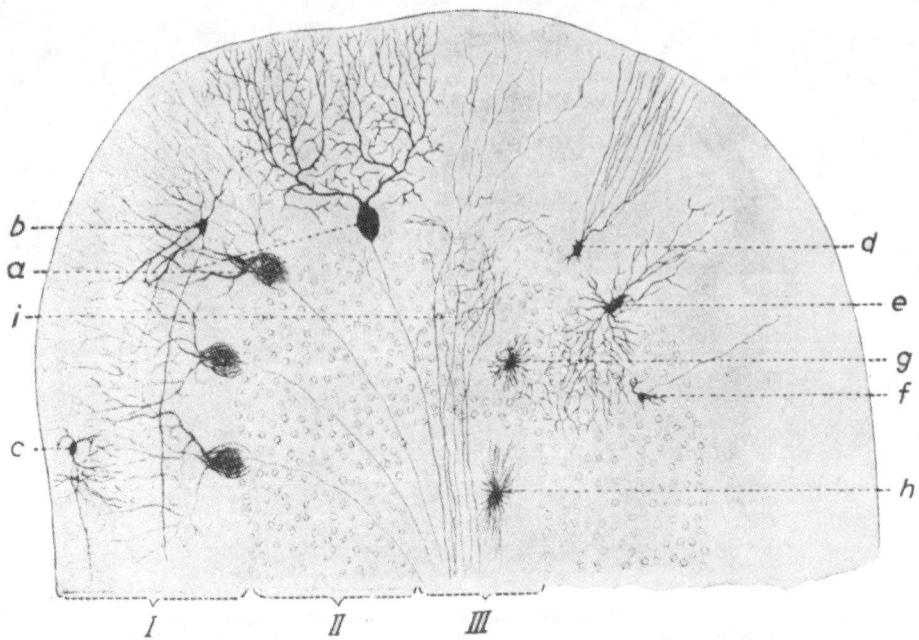

Figure 353. Diagram of the structure of the cerebellum. *I,* molecular and ganglionic layers; *II,* granular layer; *III,* white medullary substance; *a,* Purkinje cells; *b,* large cortical (basket) cell; *c,* small cortical cell; *d,* glia cell; *e,* large granule cell; *f,* small granule cell; *g,* protoplasmic astrocyte; *h,* fibrous astrocyte; *i,* nerve fiber plexus in the granular layer (afferent fibers).

molecular layer. Their axon breaks up near the cell body into an abundant arborization which extends through the whole thickness of the granular layer.

In addition to the nerve cells, their processes, and the neuroglia, the cerebellar cortex also contains myelinated nerve fibers which enter the cortex from the medullary substance and form a plexus around the cells of the granular layer. The *mossy fibers* originate from the spinal cord (nucleus dorsalis, p. 317). In the granular layer they give off numerous branches bearing characteristic tufts which synapse with the dendrites of the granule cells. The *climbing fibers* are said to include those from the vestibular nerve. They lose their myelin sheaths in the ganglionic layer and wind their way up on the dendrites of the Purkinje cells. The granular layer also contains Purkinje cell axons, which have acquired a myelin sheath.

In addition to the usual forms of neuroglia cells (Fig. 353,*g,h*) the outer part of the granular layer also contains glia cells with numerous long processes, which extend in a straight line to the cortical surface (*d*), where they spread out to form the superficial glial membrane.

3. Spinal Cord

Surrounding the central canal of the spinal cord (Fig. 354) lies an axial strand of gray matter, the cross section of which shows the familiar H-shaped pattern.

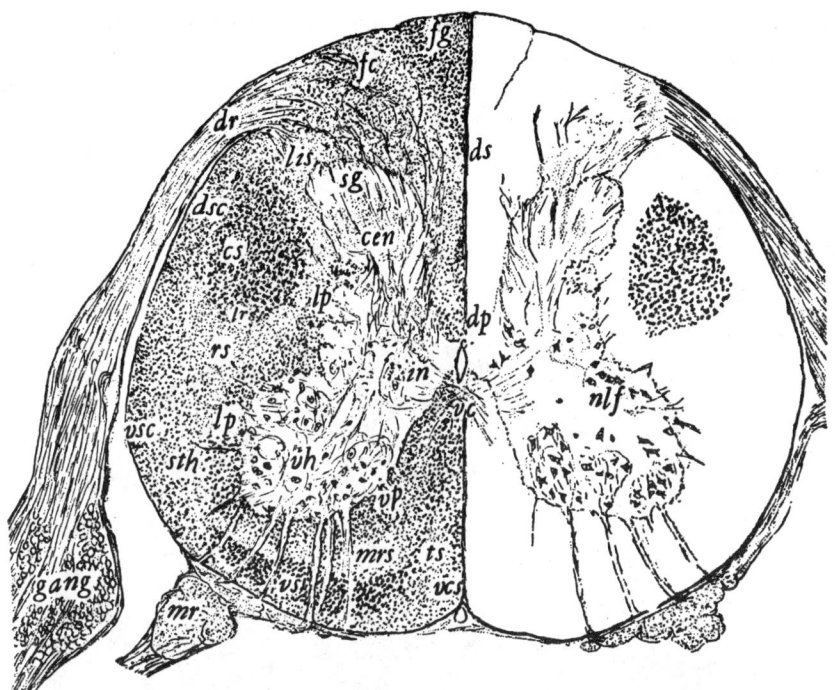

Figure 354. Transverse section of the seventh cervical segment of the spinal cord of the cat (Marchi method, 12×). *cen,* central nucleus of dorsal horn; *cs,* corticospinal (pyramidal tract); *dp,lp,vp,* fasciculi proprii; *ds,* dorsal septum; *dsc,* dorsal spinocerebellar tract; *fc,* fasciculus cuneatus; *fg,* fasciculus gracilis; *lis,* fasciculus dorsolateralis (Lissauer); *lrs,* lateral reticulospinal tract; *mrs,* medial reticulospinal tract; *rs,* rubrospinal tract; *sg,* substantia gelatinosa dorsalis; *sth,* spinothalamic tract; *ts,* tectospinal tract; *vc,* ventral commissure; *vcs,* ventral corticospinal tract; *vh,* ventral horn; *vs,* vestibulospinal tract; *vsc,* ventral spinocerebellar tract. (From Papez.)[2]

The lateral halves are connected by a thin transverse bridge, called the gray commissure. The central canal is lined by ependyma and enclosed by a layer of glia, the substantia gelatinosa centralis. The gray matter is covered on all sides by a coat of white matter.

In cross sections of the gray matter we recognize the ventral horn (cross section of the ventral gray column), the more slender dorsal horn (dorsal gray column in cross section), and, connecting the two, the pars intermedia. At the tip of the dorsal horn is the lighter substantia gelatinosa dorsalis (Fig. 354,*sg*), which consists of a mass of glia with nerve cells interspersed. Adjoining this peripherally is a narrow zona spongiosa, followed by the fasciculus dorsolateralis (*lis*), which contains fine nerve fibers in oblique and transverse sections. In the thoracic and cranial lumbar cord there is a sharply defined group of nerve cells on the medial side of the dorsal horn near the commissure. This is the *nucleus dorsalis* or Clarke's column. In the caudal part of the cervical cord and the adjoining thoracic cord of man the pars

[2] James W. Papez, *Comparative Neurology,* Fig. 114.

intermedia bears the intermediolateral column, rudiments of which are present in the most cranial part of the cervical cord of carnivores and solipeds.

The white matter, which encloses the gray matter on all sides, is divided into two lateral halves by the median ventral fissure, which contains a sheet of pia mater, and by the dorsal median septum formed by neuroglia. Each of these halves is further divided by the outgoing, ventral, motor root and the entering, sensory, dorsal root into ventral, lateral, and dorsal funiculi.

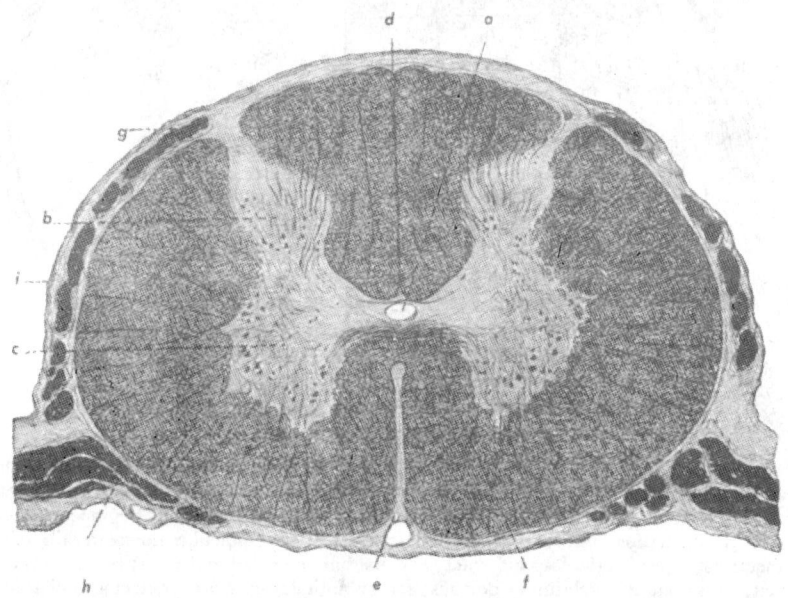

Figure 355. Cross section through the lumbar spinal cord of the cat. *a*, central canal; *b*, dorsal gray column; *c*, ventral gray column; *d*, dorsal septum; *e*, ventral fissure; *f*, white commissure; *g*, dorsal, *h*, ventral root of the spinal nerve; *i*, meninges.

The funiculi are divided into tracts and fasciculi, the boundaries of which are not visible in ordinary preparations. The location of the tracts is determined by degeneration studies. An incision is made into the central nervous system of a live animal. The fibers that are thus separated from their cell bodies degenerate, and can be demonstrated in sections with special stains. The functions of the tracts cannot be discussed here, but their positions are indicated in Figure 354. In most instances the connections and the direction of conduction are revealed in the name. The fasciculi gracilis and cuneatus are afferent tracts. The corticospinal tract is not so important in domestic animals as it is in man. It disappears a short distance caudal to the section illustrated in the cat, and is much shorter in herbivores. The rubrospinal tract from the red nucleus is well developed in the lower mammals. The fasciculi proprii are composed of short ascending and descending fibers close to the gray matter. The reticulospinal fibers originate in the reticular formation of the medulla. Tectospinal fibers come from the roof of the midbrain. The two ventral funiculi are connected by a bridge of white matter, the white commissure (Fig. 354,*vc*).

The gray substance sends fine processes (septa medullaria) into the white substance. These are especially well developed lateral to the base of the dorsal gray column, where they interweave with the myelinated fiber bundles in the reticular formation. The cross sectional appearance of the spinal cord and the proportion of gray to white matter vary from one region of the cord to another.

The gray matter of the cord consists of nerve cells and fibers, held together by neuroglia. The following groups of nerve cells are distinguished on the basis of the distribution of their axons:

a. The motor cells (Fig. 356,*e*) are characterized by their large size (up to 150 μ) and the length and abundance of their processes. They are distributed throughout the ventral column. Their number within a certain region is dependent upon the size, number, and function of the muscle groups that they supply. Often, especially at the point of origin of the nerve roots, they unit into segmental, more or less sharply circumscribed groups, nuclei.

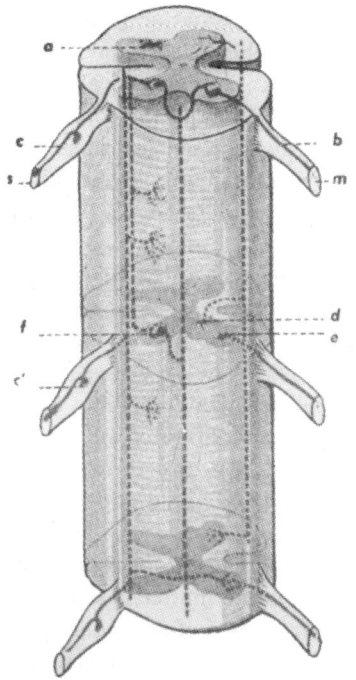

Figure 356. Diagram of the spinal cord showing position and branching of the nerve cells. *a*, Golgi type II cells; *b*, motor fiber of the ventral root; *c*, sensory fiber of the dorsal root; *c'*, spinal ganglion cell; *d*, commissural fibers; *e*, motor cell; *f*, column cell; *m*, motor root; *s*, sensory root.

These, however, are not so distinct in the horse and ruminants as in man. Their dendrites extend into the dorsal gray columns and into the ventral and lateral funiculi of white matter. Their axon traverses the white matter, where it receives a myelin sheath and enters the ventral root (*m*) of a spinal nerve, in which it travels to a voluntary muscle.

The ventral roots of the spinal nerves also carry other efferent fibers, which are derived from smaller, autonomic motor cells in the gray matter (especially abundant in the intermediolateral cell column). These are the preganglionic fibers of the autonomic nervous system.

b. The column cells (Fig. 356,*f*) make up the great majority. They are usually smaller than the motor cells and, although distributed singly or in groups throughout the gray matter, are most abundant in the dorsal columns. The dendrites of the column cells show little branching. Their axons give off numerous collaterals in the gray matter and pass out into the white matter (especially the funiculus lateralis). They usually divide into cranial and caudal branches. Some of the cranial branches reach the brain. The others run a long or short course and turn back into the gray matter of the cord. While still in the white matter, they give off collaterals, which also enter the gray and terminate in synapse with nerve cells. These fibers and their collaterals mediate reflexes involving more than one segment of the cord. Some of the column cells that lie in the dorsomedial portion of the ventral gray column send their axon through the white commissure into the ventral or lateral funiculus on the other side (Fig. 356,d). A special group of column cells are the relatively small, pigmented cells of the dorsal nucleus. These cells have but few processes, and their axons enter the spinocerebellar tracts and continue to the granular layer of the cerebellar cortex, where they end as mossy fibers.

c. The Golgi type II cells are small cells whose short axon ends within the gray substance (Fig. 109). Apparently they occur only in the dorsal gray columns. They have been called reflex cells, and possibly they play a part in the transmission of a stimulus from a dorsal root fiber to the motor cells.

The nerve fibers of the gray matter occur singly or in bundles and follow a longitudinal or a transverse course. Included among them are axons and collaterals of cord cells, spinal ganglion cells (see below), and brain cells. The parts of the gray commissure dorsal and ventral to the central canal are taken up mainly by fiber bundles that cross the mid-line. They are often arranged in layers.

The white matter is separated from the spinal meninges by the marginal glia. It is composed of predominantly myelinated fibers of varying thickness, with only a few unmyelinated fibers. Most of the myelinated fibers are directed longitudinally, except in the region of the nerve roots and in the white commissure, where they pursue a radial or transverse course.

Three main kinds of fibers may be distinguished:

a. Fibers of the column cells.

b. Nerve fibers derived from brain cells. For example, fibers from cells in the red nucleus cross to the opposite side in the midbrain and descend in the rubrospinal tract of the lateral funiculus to end in contact with motor cells of the ventral column.

c. Axons of the spinal ganglion cells entering the cord (see pp. 74, 323; also Fig. 356,c) make up two bundles. One of these, the medial division, enters the dorsal funiculus, while the thinner, lateral division joins the dorsolateral fasciculus. Each axon divides into a cranial and a caudal branch which run with the funiculi and give off collaterals into the gray matter, where they terminate in a free arborization. They form one dense plexus in the tip of the dorsal horn and in the substantia gelatinosa dorsalis and another one around the cells of the dorsal nucleus. Thick bundles of collaterals, called reflex bundles, continue to the ventral gray columns, where they surround the motor cells. They form part of the direct reflex arc and are the shortest route of transmission of a stimulus from a sensory area to the motor cells of the same cord segment. Other bundles cross the median plane dorsal to the central canal and participate in the formation of the dorsal gray commissure. The white commissure (Fig. 354,vc) consists of fibers derived from the ventral gray columns. They run obliquely across the most dorsal portion

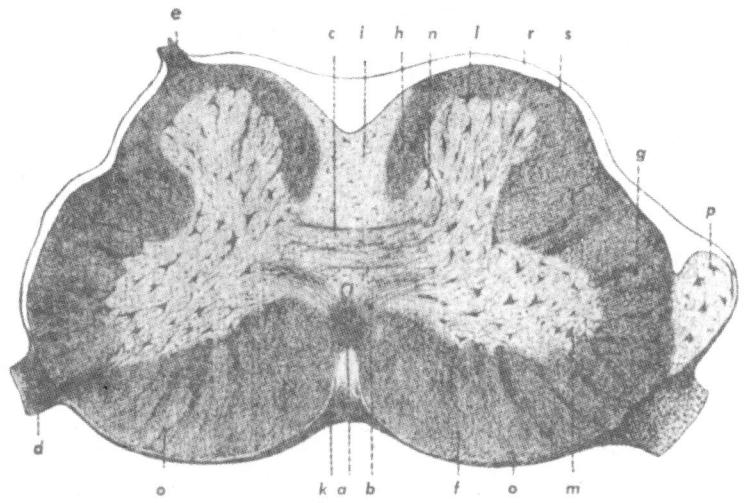

Figure 357. Cross section through the lumbar cord of the chicken (20×).
a, central canal; *b*, ventral, *c*, dorsal gray commissure; *d*, ventral, *e*, dorsal
root; *f*, ventral, *g*, lateral, *h*, dorsal funiculus; *i*, sinus rhomboideus; *k*, ligamentum longitudinale dorsale and the vertebral artery; *l*, column cell;
m, motor cells of the ventral gray column; *n*, cell of Clarke's column; *o*, ectopic
nerve cells in the white matter; *p*, nucleus of Hoffmann-Kölliker, sectioned
only on one side; *r*, dura mater, *s*, pia mater.

of the ventral funiculi, over the ventral fissure, and into the ventral funiculus and
gray matter of the other side.

SPINAL CORD OF BIRDS. The lumbar enlargement of the cord is very wide (Fig.
357). This is associated with a wide ventral fissure and a thick dorsal glial septum
(*i*). There is a dorsal groove called the rhomboid sinus. Clarke's columns (*n*) are
distinct. There is a remarkable occurrence of ganglion cells (root cells) in the white
substance (*o*). Joined to the lateral funiculus at the emergence of the ventral roots
is an elongated mass (*p*) of ganglion cells (Hoffman-Kölliker nuclei).

4. Medulla Oblongata

In the medulla the neural tube is opened dorsally and spread flat, so that the
sensory areas are lateral and the motor areas closer to the mid-line. The fourth
ventricle, corresponding to the central canal of the spinal cord, is covered by
ependyma and pia mater. The complexity is increased over that of the cord by
the presence of additional nuclei. The motor nuclei are distinguished by their large
cells. The substantia gelatinosa centralis is spread out under the ependyma covering the floor of the fourth ventricle and is very thin. The substantia gelatinosa dorsalis forms here the spinal nucleus of the trigeminus. The fiber bundles of the white
matter follow a complex course between the gray nuclei and envelop them.

The medulla is a vital organ because of the important regulatory centers for the
respiratory, circulatory, and digestive systems located in it. It contains nuclei of

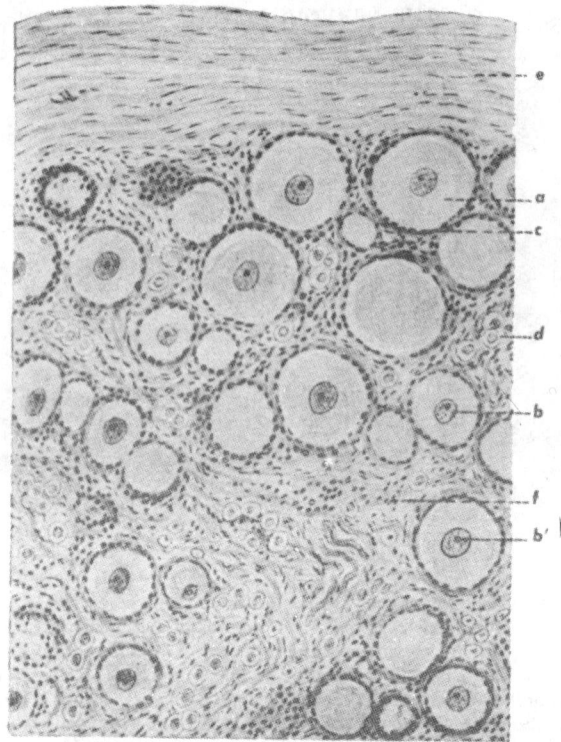

Figure 358. From the spinal ganglion of a horse (120×). *a*, nerve cells; *b*, nucleus of a nerve cell showing a large nucleolus (*b'*); *c*, cellular envelope of the nerve cell; *d*, myelinated fibers in cross section; *e*, capsule; *f*, connective tissue.

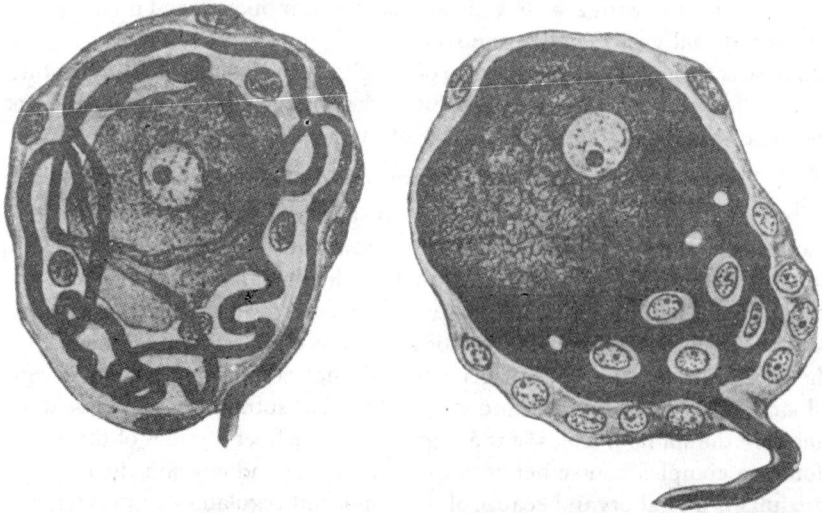

Figure 359. Spinal ganglion cells; silver impregnation. *Left:* unipolar nerve cell, showing spiral turns of the axon inside the cell capsule. *Right:* fenestrated nerve cell. (After Schaffer.)

all but the first four cranial nerves; it is not merely an organ of conduction but mainly a reflex center.

B. THE PERIPHERAL NERVOUS SYSTEM

The peripheral nervous system is composed of the peripheral ganglia, the peripheral nerves, and the peripheral nerve endings.

1. The Ganglia

The ganglia are accumulations of nerve cells that have left the central nervous system early in embryonic development. They are divided into cerebrospinal and autonomic ganglia. The ganglia are surrounded by a sheath of regular connective tissue, which is the continuation of the perineurium (see p. 326; also Fig. 358,e). Their vascular connective tissue framework contains numerous nerve cells and fiber bundles running in various directions.

(a) **The cerebrospinal ganglia** include the spinal ganglia, which are located on the dorsal roots of the spinal nerves, and the ganglia of the sensory branches of the cranial nerves. The ganglia of the vestibular and cochlear nerves show the same structure as the other cerebrospinal ganglia, but their nerve cells are bipolar.

In the cerebrospinal ganglia the nerve cells (Fig. 358,a) lie in the connective tissue framework between tracts of nerve fiber bundles. They are surrounded by a layer of flat satellite cells of a glial nature, which are comparable to the Schwann cells of the peripheral nerves. Outside the satellite cells is a homogeneous membrane, followed by a delicate capsule of cellular connective tissue that represents the endoneural sheath of Henle (p. 326). This capsule is absent in the horse. The great majority of the spheroid and pyriform nerve cells belong to the unipolar type (p. 74). Their axon may leave the capsule directly, as is often the case in the cranial sensory ganglia, or it may perform several spiral turns around the cell body inside the satellite layer. This is most often the case in the spinal ganglia (Fig. 359, left). Upon its emergence from the cell capsule the axon divides into two branches. One of these enters the spinal cord by way of the dorsal root and ends in the gray matter of the cord or brain. The other is the sensory branch, which comes from the periphery. Most of the processes of the ganglion cells are myelinated, but there are some small cells with unmyelinated processes. There are also visceral afferent cells whose processes may or may not be myelinated.[3] The peripheral branches of these reach the spinal ganglia via rami communicantes from the sympathetic trunk. In the horse and dog we also find the so-called fenestrated nerve cells, whose cytoplasmic processes return to the cell body (Fig. 359, right).

(b) **In the autonomic ganglia** (Fig. 360) the nerve cells are of varying size, sometimes binucleate, and predominantly multipolar. Their unmyelinated axon, the postganglionic fiber, leaves the ganglion and courses in a visceral nerve to its end organ (smooth muscle or gland). Many postganglionic fibers pass into the cerebrospinal nerves via gray rami communicantes. They supply the skin glands and the smooth muscle of the skin and somatic vessels. The dendrites form a dense network within the ganglion. The preganglionic myelinated nerve fibers entering

[3] Ranson and Clark, pp. 112, 124.

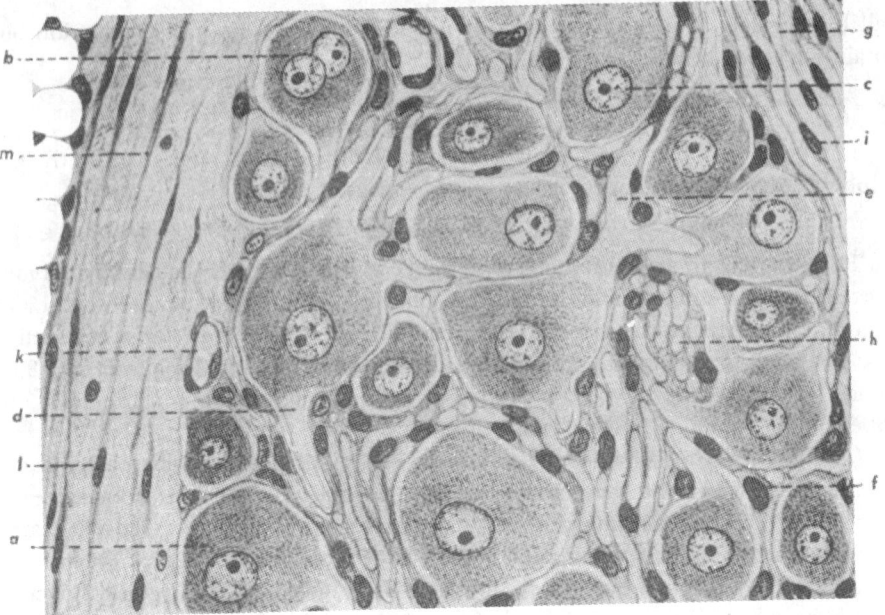

Figure 360. Section from a sympathetic ganglion (celiac ganglion) of the horse (400×). *a*, nerve cell; *b*, nerve cell with two nuclei; *c*, nucleus with nucleolus; *d*, origin of an axon; *e*, dendrite; *f*, cell of the connective tissue envelope; *g*, sympathetic (unmyelinated) fibers in longitudinal and, *h*, cross section; *i*, nuclei of neurolemmal cells; *k*, capillaries; *l*, fibroblast; *m*, fibrous lamella of the connective tissue capsule of the ganglion.

the ganglion come from the central nervous system. They may pass through the ganglion or end on the ganglion cells after losing their myelin sheath. Myelinated and unmyelinated visceral sensory fibers pass through the autonomic ganglia on their way to cell bodies in the spinal ganglia.

2. Peripheral Nerves

The peripheral nerves contain sensory fibers arising from the cells of the cerebrospinal ganglia, as well as motor fibers from the motor cells of the brain and cord. Both types possess a myelin sheath and a neurilemma. In addition, most peripheral nerves also contain unmyelinated autonomic fibers. In the visceral nerves the autonomic fibers predominate.

(a) **The cerebrospinal nerves** are composed of fibers that vary greatly in size and in the thickness of the myelin sheath. The motor fibers of skeletal muscles are thick and heavily myelinated. They are mostly responsible for the white appearance of the nerve trunk. There are also many unmyelinated autonomic and pain fibers, especially in cutaneous nerves. Each nerve is protected against its environment by a collagenous epineurium (Fig. 361,*a*), which contains elastic fibers, blood vessels, and fat cells. Within this sheath the nerve fibers are collected into fiber bundles. The spaces between the bundles are filled by loose, vascularized connective tissue, which is continuous with the epineurium. On the surface of the fiber

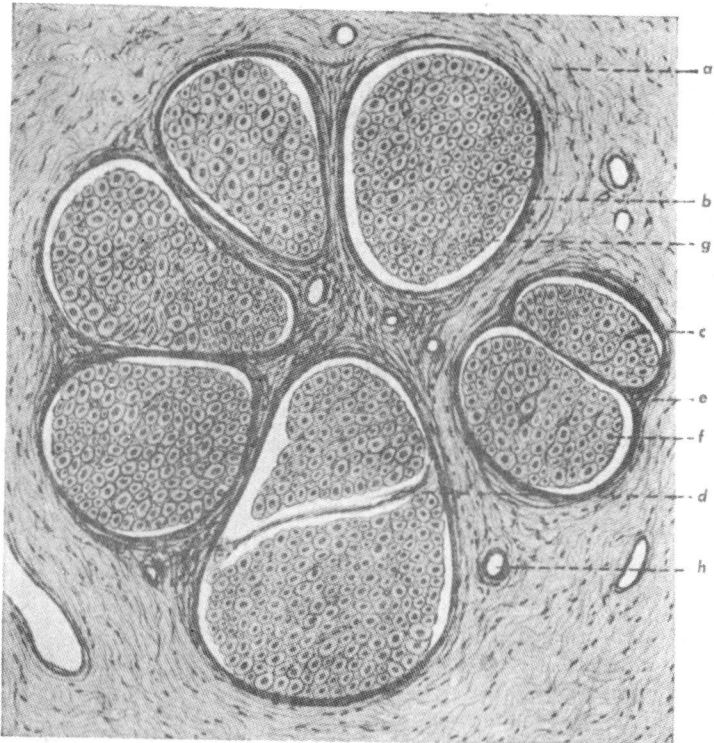

Figure 361. Cross section through the facial nerve of the horse. *a*, epineurium; *b*, perineurium; *c*, endoneurium; *d*, endoneural septum; *e*, perineural septum; *f*, myelinated nerve fibers; *g*, axons; *h*, artery in the interfascicular tissue.

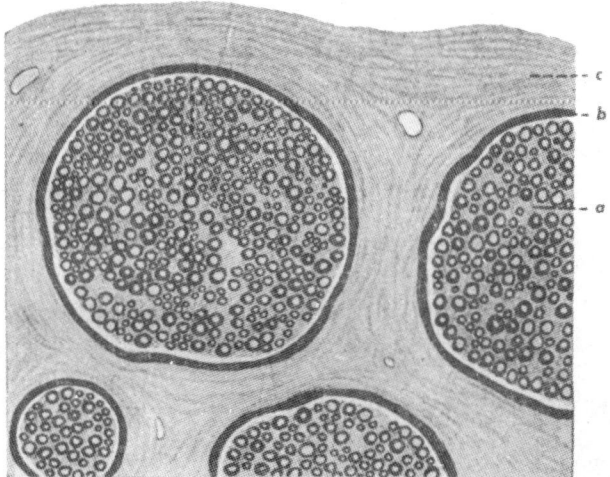

Figure 362. Portion of a cross section through a myelinated nerve of the horse; osmic acid treatment (80×). *a*, endoneurium; *b*, perineurium; *c*, epineurium.

bundles the connective tissue condenses into a varying number of concentric membranes made up of longitudinal fibers. Each component membrane bears flattened connective tissue cells on its inner surface. This system of membranes forms a sheathlike perineurium (Fig. 361,*b*) around each fiber bundle and gives off delicate septa, the endoneural lamellae, into the interior of the bundle. In addition, each nerve fiber is enveloped by an endoneural sheath (of Henle), which bears latticeworks of reticular fibers. On the outside of the membrane are longitudinal collagenous fibers of uneven distribution. The endoneural sheaths and lamellae are collectively called the endoneurium (Fig. 361,*c*). The neurilemma is inside the endoneural sheath.

The perineurium and endoneurium are interpreted as the peripheral continuations of the dura and pia respectively. The neurilemma is glial in nature and isolates the nerve fiber from the surrounding connective tissue.

(b) The sympathetic trunks and the visceral nerves derived from them (Fig. 363) contain a varying number of fine, myelinated fibers of cerebrospinal origin (*c*), but they are made up mainly of unmyelinated postganglionic, autonomic fibers (*a,b*) and therefore appear more or less gray. Some of the myelinated fibers in the sympathetic trunks are preganglionic fibers; the others belong to visceral sensory neurons. The fibers are commonly grouped into bundles and separated by connective tissue. The grouping is absent in the sympathetic trunks of the cat.

The old sympathetic system of the gross anatomists is often confused with the sympathetic or thoracolumbar division of the autonomic system. The two terms are not synonymous. The autonomic system is a physiological concept—not an anatomical entity that can be separated physically from the rest of the nervous system. It is made up of visceral efferent fibers forming two-neuron chains between the central nervous system and smooth muscle or glands. Autonomic fibers are carried in most of the peripheral nerves. In addition to the thoracolumbar divi-

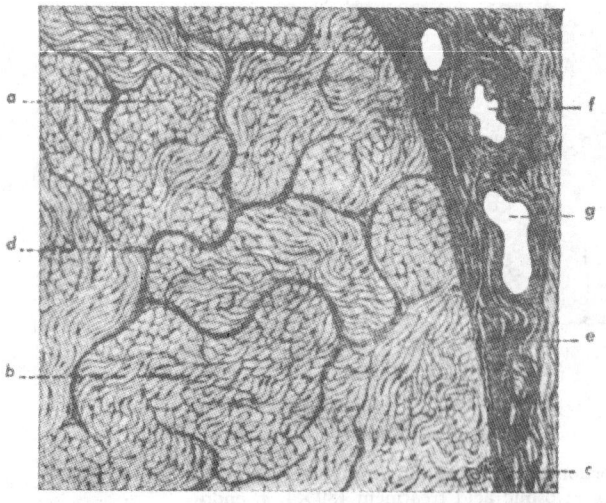

Figure 363. Cross section through a portion of the splenic nerve of the ox; osmic acid preparation (100×). *a,b,* bundles of unmyelinated nerve fibers in cross section; *c,* myelinated nerve fibers; *d,* perineurium; *e,* epineurium; *f,* arteriole; *g,* venule.

sion there is also a craniosacral, or parasympathetic, division with generally antagonistic action.

The gross anatomical sympathetic system, composed of the sympathetic trunks, their ganglia, and the attached nerves, includes myelinated visceral afferent fibers as well as thoracolumbar autonomic fibers. The visceral afferent fibers have their cell bodies in the dorsal root ganglia and do not differ materially from somatic afferents. Both types of afferent impulses can elicit autonomic response.

The larger blood vessels of the nerves are situated in the epineurium and form elongated capillary nets in the perineurium and endoneurium The smallest nerves lack blood vessels and, like all nerve fibers are merely bathed in tissue fluid. Between the lamellae the perineurium and within the fiber bundles are tissue spaces which communicate only with the subdural and subarachnoid spaces, but not with the lym-

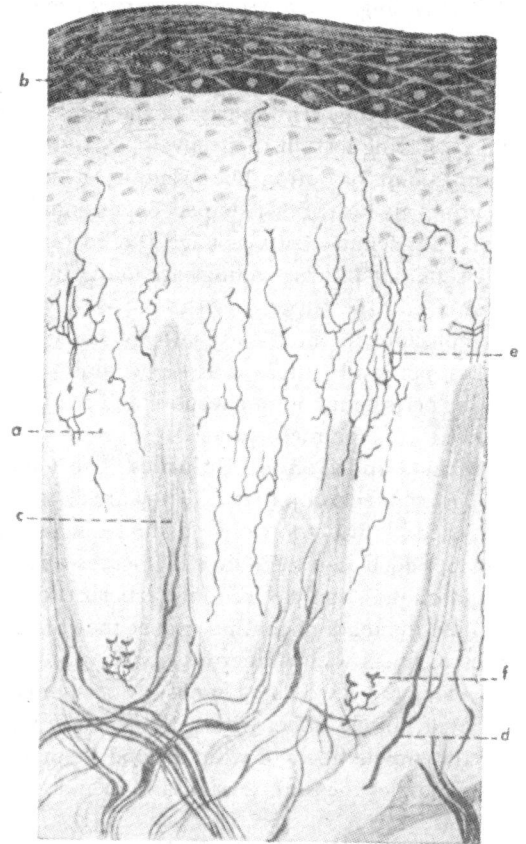

Figure 364. Section through the planum rostrale of the pig. a, squamous epithelium; b, its stratum corneum; c, papillary body; d, myelinated nerve fibers; e, free intraepithelial nerve endings; f, Merkel's corpuscles. (After Szymonowicz.)

phatics, which are present in the interfascicular connective tissue but are completely enclosed. The nerves (nn. nervorum) end partly on the vessels and partly in the connective tissue. Isolated nerve cells often occur along the course of the cerebrospinal nerves.

3. Peripheral Nerve Endings

The peripheral nerve endings act as intermediaries between tissues and organs on the one hand and the nervous system on the other. Upon reaching their destination, the nerve fibers divide, distal to a constriction of Ranvier, into several twigs. These may or may not be myelinated. Among the terminations of nerve fibers we distinguish free endings, endings in spindles, and terminal corpuscles. At this point only the general sensory endings and motor endings on muscle will be dealt with.

The endings of the secretory nerves are described on p. 32, the special sensory endings under their respective organs.

a. Sensory Nerve Endings

Free Endings. In the case of the free endings (Figs. 110,*e;* 364; 365) the nerve fibers, having lost all their envelopes and having split into neurofibrils, terminate in fine points or button-like swellings formed by fine nets. Sometimes the thickened neurofibrils form bowl-shaped expansions attached to the base of an epidermal cell. Intracellular endings have also been described.

OCCURRENCE. Free endings are found in the stratified epithelia of mucous membranes and the cornea; in the deeper layers of the epidermis up to the stratum granulosum; in the root sheaths of hairs; in the connective tissue of skin, hoofs, claws, epi- and endocardium, and muscles; in the ciliary body and the iris; and in the periosteum, joint capsules, and dental pulp. The free nerve endings are considered to be pain receptors.

Muscle and Tendon Spindles. The tendon spindles are usually located near the muscle-tendon junction. They are fusiform swellings on the fiber bundles, surrounded by firm connective tissue capsules. Each is supplied by one to four nerve fibers, which lose their myelin sheaths and break up on the surface of the fiber bundle into a netlike terminal arborization. The muscle spindles (Fig. 366,*e*) resemble the tendon spindles except that the swelling is made up of a group of fine muscle fibers with numerous nuclei, which is surrounded by a connective tissue envelope (*a*). Two kinds of nerve fibers enter the spindle; motor nerves supply the striated muscle fibers within the spindle, while sensory fibers form arborizations on the muscle fibers or wind around them as rings or spirals. The muscle and tendon spindles measure tension and degree of contraction. They are proprioceptive organs.

Endings on Tactile Cells. These include Merkel's tactile cells, Grandry's corpuscles, and Meissner's corpuscles.

(a) **Merkel's cells** (Figs. 364,*f;* 367,*c*) of mammals are oval nucleated cells, 6–12 μ in size. They are approached by extremely fine nerve fibers, which lose their myelin sheaths and become attached to the base of the tactile cells by means of terminal expansions, the tactile menisci or discs (*b*). The tactile meniscus is a dense network of neurofibrils, which often gives off bundles of fibrils for the formation of additional menisci. Still other nerve fibers form a terminal network around the tactile cells.

OCCURRENCE. These cells are found in the deepest layers of the epidermis and in the outer root sheath of hairs.

(b) **Grandry's corpuscles** of birds are compound tactile corpuscles composed of a collagenous capsule and from two to four vesicular tactile cells, which are larger than those of mammals. The entering nerve fibers lose their myelin sheaths and terminate between two tactile cells as flat tactile discs. The compound tactile cells are also surrounded by pericellular terminal nets from other fine nerve fibers.

OCCURRENCE. Grandry's corpuscles are encountered in the skin of the beak and in the tongue and palate of birds.

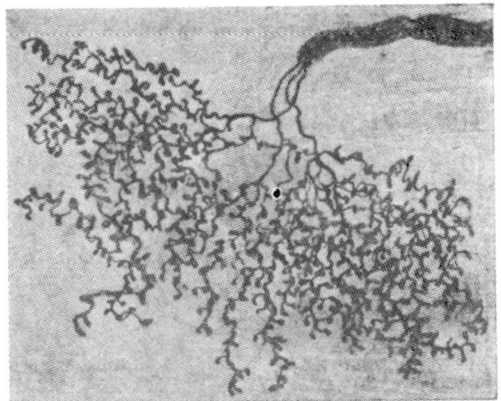

Figure 365. Sensory nerve endings from the atrial endocardium of the dog.

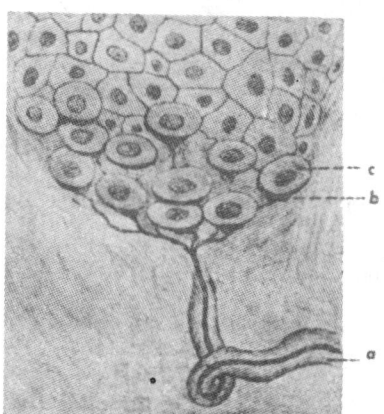

Figure 367. Merkel's corpuscles in the epithelium of the snout of a pig. *a,* Myelinated nerve fiber, which loses its myelin sheath and enters the epithelium; *b,* tactile disc (meniscus); *c,* tactile cell.

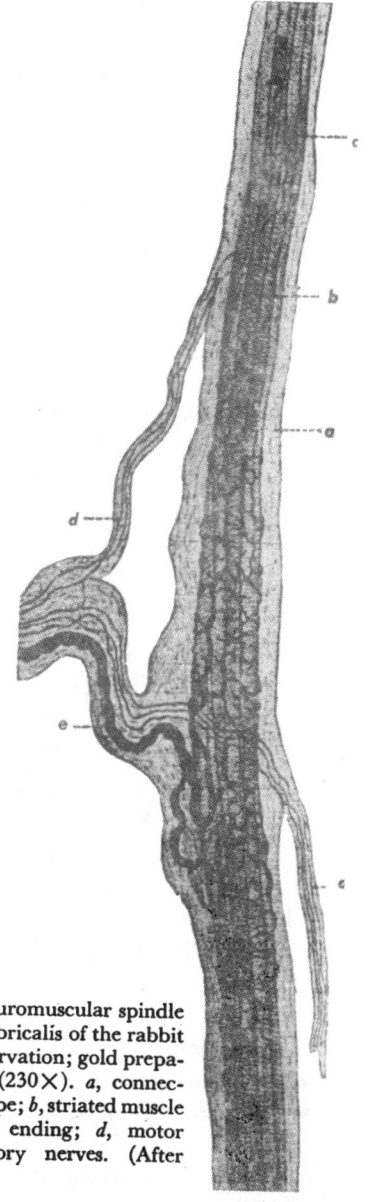

Figure 366. Neuromuscular spindle from the m. lumbricalis of the rabbit showing the innervation; gold preparation, isolated (230×). *a,* connective tissue envelope; *b,* striated muscle fiber; *c,* motor ending; *d,* motor nerves; *e,* sensory nerves. (After Kerschner.)

(c) Meissner's corpuscles (Fig. 368) are up to 100 μ in length and 25–30 μ wide and are found in the papillary body of the corium. In shape they resemble a fir cone. Their thin connective tissue capsule, which is continuous with the perineural sheath of the nerve fibers, contains flat, transversely arranged tactile cells. The striated appearance of the corpuscles is due to the arrangement of the nuclei and to the spiral turns of one to five myelinated nerve fibers (*c*). These lose their sheaths

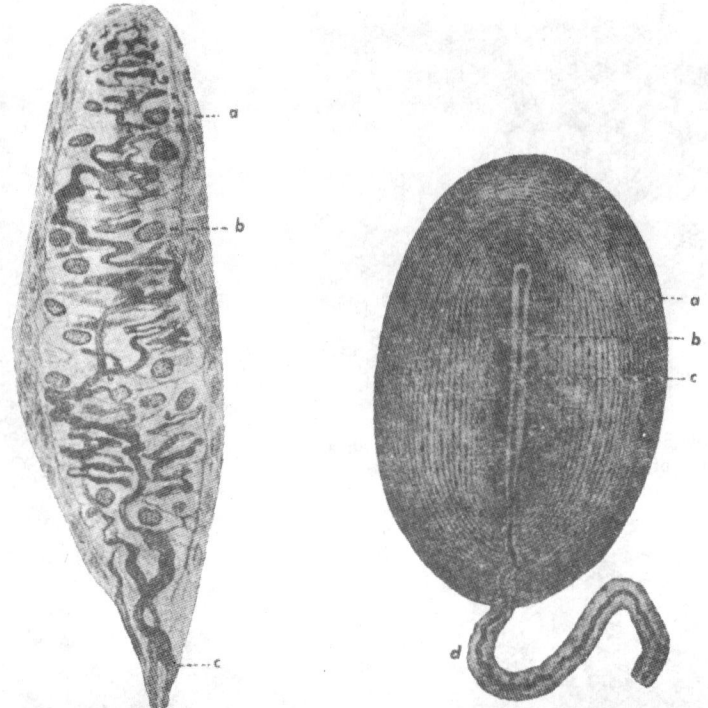

Figure 368 (left). Longitudinal view of a tactile corpuscle from a dermal papilla. *a*, connective tissue; *b*, tactile corpuscle with its cells; *c*, nerve fiber.

Figure 369 (right). Longitudinal section through a lamellar corpuscle (75×). *a*, external, *b*, internal lamellar system; *c*, inner bulb and axis cylinder; *d*, nerve fiber with myelin sheath.

and terminate as branched naked axis cylinders with expansions on the tactile cells. Bundles of fibrils sometimes emerge from the corpuscle and terminate intraepithelially or join with neighboring corpuscles.

OCCURRENCE. We find Meissner's corpuscles in the papillae of the papillary body of the human skin, especially on the palms and soles. They also occur in the domestic mammals.

Lamellar Corpuscles. The lamellar corpuscles, or terminal bulbs, are structures of varying size and shape, which consist of an inner bulb and a lamellar capsule. The inner bulb may be cylindrical, bulbar, or spheroid in shape. It contains the endings of the nerve fibers, which have lost their myelin sheath and enter as naked axis cylinders, while their neurilemma passes into the capsule. Variations in the number of enveloping lamellae and in the arrangement of the nerve fibers give rise to several kinds of terminal bulbs, the most important of which are listed below:

(a) **The end bulbs of Krause** are cylindrical. Their nerve fiber, on entering the bulb, loses its myelin and penetrates almost the entire length of the finely granular and concentrically striated inner bulb. Its ending is either rounded off or expanded into a button consisting probably of a dense network of neurofibrils. The capsule consists of two to five concentric connective tissue lamellae with flat nuclei.

OCCURRENCE. Krause's end bulbs occur in the skin and in adjoining mucous membranes, especially in the conjunctiva and the tongue. They are considered by some to be cold receptors.

(b) **The Vater-Pacini corpuscles** (Figs. 369, 370) are larger (2 mm.) than the end bulbs of Krause and are distinguished from them by the presence of an external system of double lamellae, consisting of twenty to sixty layers (Fig. 369,*a*). Each of the collagenous lamellae has two compact fibrous layers, the surfaces of which bear fibroblasts with flattened nuclei (Fig. 370,*e*). These two layers enclose

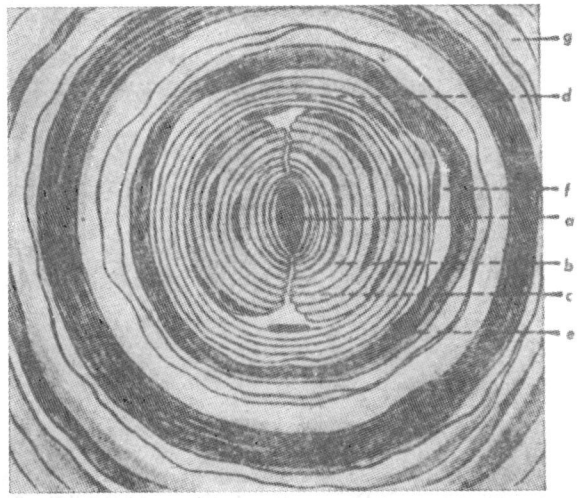

Figure 370. Central portion of a cross section through a lamellar corpuscle from the mesentery of a cat (680×). *a*, axis cylinder; *b*, semilamellae of the inner bulb; *c*, common space, enclosed by the edges of the semilamellae; *d*, innermost complete lamella; *e*, nucleus; *f*, interlamellar space; *g*, lamellar space filled with fluid.

the lamellar space (*g*), which is filled with serous fluid and crossed by collagenous fibrils. The lamellae become thinner toward the center. As a rule they are apposed to one another, but they may be partially separated by interlamellar spaces. The inner lamellar system surrounds the axon and makes up the inner bulb. Unlike the outer system it consists of lamellae (*b*) that are only troughlike half-tubes, composed of two layers each. The nerve fiber supplying the corpuscle (369,*d*) loses its myelin sheath on entering and runs the length of the inner bulb. It remains undivided or may bifurcate toward the end. The axis cylinder and its terminal branches give off along their entire course numerous extremely fine twigs which form an elongated coil. This is surrounded by the terminal arborization of a second thin nerve fiber.

Opposite the point of entrance of the nerve fiber a longitudinal strand connecting all the lamellae is often found. Each lamellar body is invaded by small blood vessels which form glomeruli. With an increase in blood pressure a greater quantity of fluid enters the lamellar spaces and distends the lamellar corpuscles. The Pacinian corpuscles are probably concerned with the regulation of blood pressure, as well as the sensation of local pressure.

OCCURRENCE. The Pacinian corpuscles are present in the periosteum and the subcutaneous tissue, around joints, on the sympathetic trunks, in the mesentery and pancreas of the cat, in the parathyroids, in the penis, clitoris, muscle sheaths, planum nasolabiale, and corium of hoofs and claws, in the foot pads of carnivores, near the coccygeal artery of long-tailed mammals and the glomus coccygeum of man, in the vicinity of the thoracic aorta and its large branches, in the follicles of tactile hairs, etc.

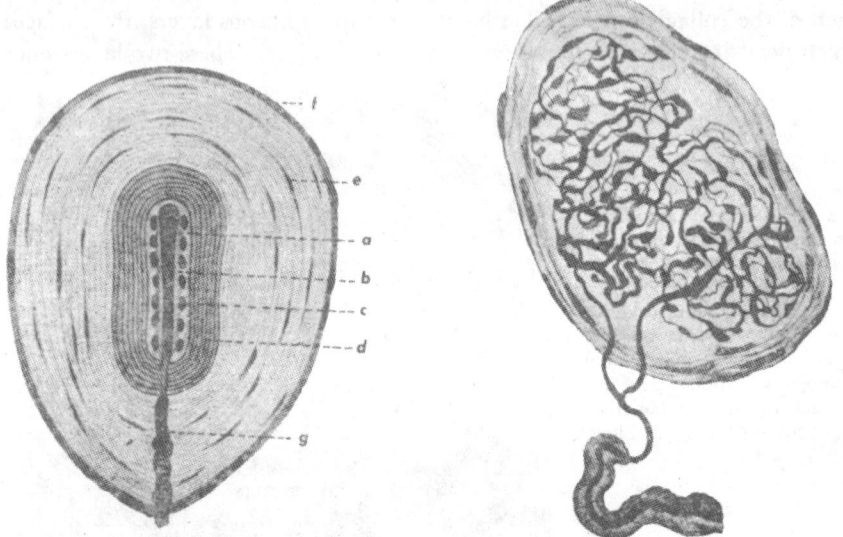

Figure 371 (left). Herbst's corpuscle from the skin of the beak (cere) of the duck; longitudinal section (360×). *a,* axis cylinder; *b,* inner bulb; *c,* cells of the inner bulb; *d,* inner lamellae; *e,* fibroblasts of the outer lamellae; *f,* capsule; *g,* myelin sheath.
Figure 372 (right). Genital corpuscle. (After Dogiel.)

(c) **Herbst's corpuscles** (Figs. 371, 386) are smaller (80–140 μ) and have fewer lamellae than the Pacinian corpuscles. Their inner bulb bears on its external surface a single row of round cells (*c*).

OCCURRENCE. They occur in the tongue and in the waxy skin of the beak (ceroma; p. 346) of many birds, especially aquatic ones.

(d) **The Golgi-Mazzoni corpuscles** differ from the Pacinian corpuscles in that they are smaller and have only two or three lamellae in their capsule. The inner bulb is represented by a core consisting of nucleated, finely granular masses. In it the axis cylinder undergoes extensive ramification and convolution and forms a network in which the neurofibrils often terminate in knobs.

OCCURRENCE. Golgi-Mazzoni corpuscles are found in the papillae of the lip, tongue, and buccal mucosa; on the penis; in the glans, the digital skin of the cat, and the hoof corium.

(e) **The genital corpuscles** (Fig. 372) have a structure resembling that of the Golgi-Mazzoni corpuscles. They frequently have a thicker sheath consisting of from three to eight lamellae and an unusually dense network of neurofibrils, which is derived from the arborization of one to ten axis cylinders.

OCCURRENCE. These corpuscles are present in the clitoris of swine, cat, etc.

(f) Ruffini's corpuscles are elongated structures, up to more than a millimeter in length. The entering nerve fiber loses its myelin sheath and divides into numerous varicose branches, which anastomose and end in little buttons. A strong fibroelastic capsule envelops the corpuscle.

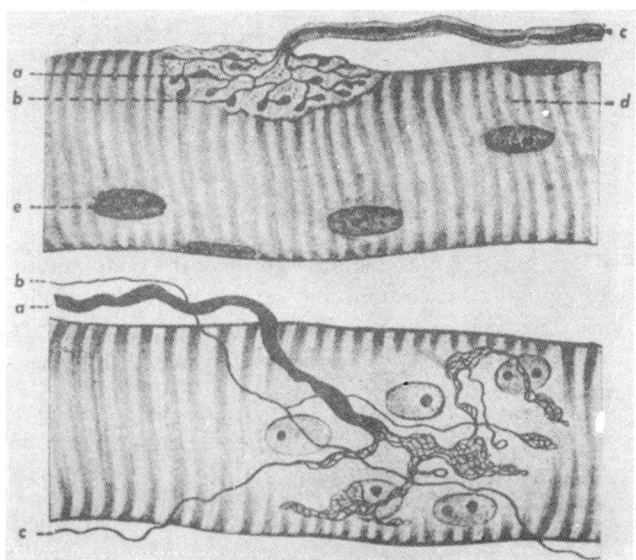

Figure 373. Motor nerve ending. *a,* motor end plate; *b,* terminal expansions; *c,* nerve fiber; *d,* muscle fiber; *e,* nucleus of the muscle fiber.

Figure 374. Motor end plate in striated musculature; silver impregnation (1800×). *a,* myelinated cerebrospinal motor nerve fiber, whose neurofibrils form terminal networks; *b,* unmyelinated fiber; *c,* nerve fiber that arises from the end plate and terminates on a neighboring fiber without forming an end plate. (After Boeke.)

OCCURRENCE. Ruffini's corpuscles occur in the connective tissue of skin and subcutis, in the finger tips of man, the digital pads of carnivores, and the hoof corium. Some authorities consider them to be heat receptors.

b. Motor Nerve Endings

The endings found in smooth and cardiac musculature are similar. The nerve plexuses give rise to unmyelinated fiber bundles, which form secondary plexuses. These in turn give off extremely fine branches, which penetrate between the muscle fibers, divide, and give off short collateral twigs. These are attached to the muscle fibers, often with a slight terminal swelling. Fibers forming terminal loops within the cytoplasm have also been described.

The endings in skeletal muscle are different (Figs. 366, 373, 374). The nerve trunk of each muscle divides into branches, which give rise to the intramuscular nerve plexus. From this arise isolated terminal fibers, each of which attaches to a muscle fiber. At the junction the nerve fiber loses its myelin and the neurilemma becomes continuous with the sarcolemma. The axon passes beneath the sarcolemma into a mass of sarcoplasm with many nuclei.[4] Here it breaks up into winding terminal branches with bulbous swellings. The whole structure is called a motor end plate.

---

[4] Maximow and Bloom, p. 200.

XVII

The Skin

THE function of the skin is to protect the body and to serve as an organ of heat regulation, excretion, and sensation. It also produces certain special secretions. The skin, or *cutis*, is divided into the epithelial *epidermis* and the connective tissue *corium* or *dermis*. The underlying *subcutis* attaches the skin to the subjacent organs.

A. EPIDERMIS

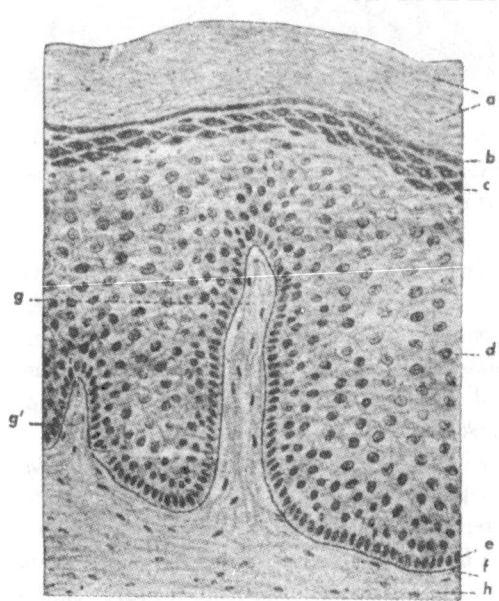

Figure 375. Cross section through the epidermis. *a*, stratum corneum; *b*, stratum lucidum; *c*, stratum granulosum; *d*, stratum spinosum; *e*, stratum cylindricum; *f*, basement membrane (disputed); *g*, papilla (*g'*, cut off); *h*, corium.

The epidermis (Fig. 375) is a stratified squamous epithelium covered by a stratum corneum and resting on the papillae of the corium. The epidermis is characterized by a high degree of elasticity. Its free surface may appear smooth or show elevations caused by the underlying papillae. In certain locations, as on the nose and footpads of the dog, the epidermis forms independent elevations.

The epidermis is divided into two main layers: the succulent deep layer (stratum germinativum or Malpighii; Fig. 375,*d,e,*) and the superficial horny layer (Fig. 375,*a,b,c*). These are further subdivided—the deep layer into two, the superficial layer into three, secondary layers. Starting from the corium, we distinguish the following layers:

1. The stratum cylindricum (Fig. 375,*e*) consists of a layer of more or less columnar cells with basal processes. Most contemporary authors deny the existence of a basement membrane. Mitotic figures are sometimes seen here.

2. The stratum spinosum or prickle cell layer (Fig. 375,*d*) is composed of stratified prickle cells, which fill in all the depressions between the dermal papillae. These cells are connected by intercellular bridges (pp. 21, 25, and Fig. 26). The cells and intercellular bridges of the Malpighian layer are traversed by cytoplasmic fibrils (tonofibrils), which possibly reinforce the epithelium. The fact that mitoses also occur in the prickle cells makes it necessary to include both of these layers in the stratum germinativum.

3. The stratum granulosum (Fig. 375,*c*) consists of one to five layers of fusiform, finely serrated cells. They show the first signs of cornification in

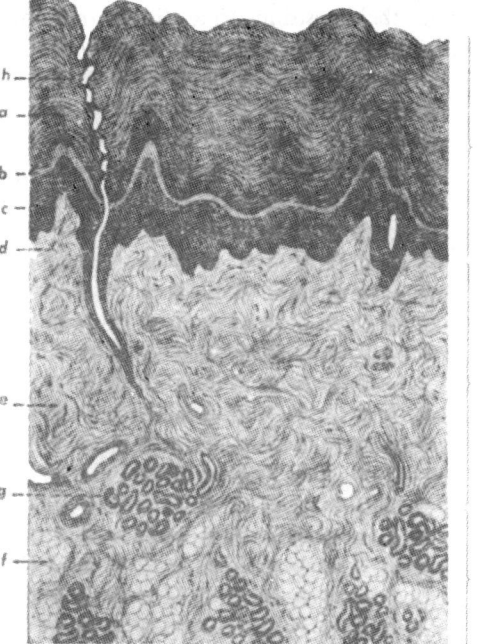

Figure 376. Section through the metacarpal pad of the dog (30×). *1*, epidermis; *2*, corium; *3*, subcutis; *a*, stratum corneum; *b*, stratum lucidum; *c*, stratum profundum; *d*, papillary body; *e*, stratum reticulare; *f*, adipose tissue; *g*, tubular glands; *h*, their excretory duct.

the form of shiny basophilic keratohyalin granules, which increase in size and number toward the surface and lend a granular appearance to this layer. The nuclei shrink and undergo chromatolysis. Cytoplasmic fibrils are hard to demonstrate.

4. The stratum lucidum (Fig. 376,*b*) is a shiny acidophilic layer of homogeneous appearance. Here the keratohyalin granules have liquefied and are uniformly dispersed throughout the cells, obscuring the boundaries of the nonnucleated and greatly flattened cells. The liquefied keratohyalin, which has also undergone chemical changes, is now called eleidin. In places where the epidermis is thin, this layer is absent, and the stratum granulosum also is thin and discontinuous.

5. The stratum corneum proper (Fig. 376,*a*) consists of cells that are usually flat but may at times be swollen and vesicular. They exhibit short toothlike processes in place of the intercellular bridges and contain in their cornified peripheral layer the true horny substance, keratin.

A nucleus is absent, and the interior of the cell often appears empty or dried to a fine meshwork. The cells are dead and are shed as scales.

The epidermis of our domestic animals, except albinos, bears pigment either diffusely or in patches (see p. 9). The pigment granules are found largely within and between the deep epidermal layers, which are the more highly pigmented the deeper their position. In addition, there often exists a diffuse coloration of the cytoplasm, which may extend into the stratum corneum. The stratum corneum, however, is usually nonpigmented.

B. CORIUM OR DERMIS

The most superficial layers of the corium are condensed into a feltwork of delicate reticular fibers with an admixture of fibroelastic elements. The remainder of the corium consists of bundles of collagenous fibers. They vary in thickness, may be flat or round, follow a wavy course, and interweave in the three dimensions.

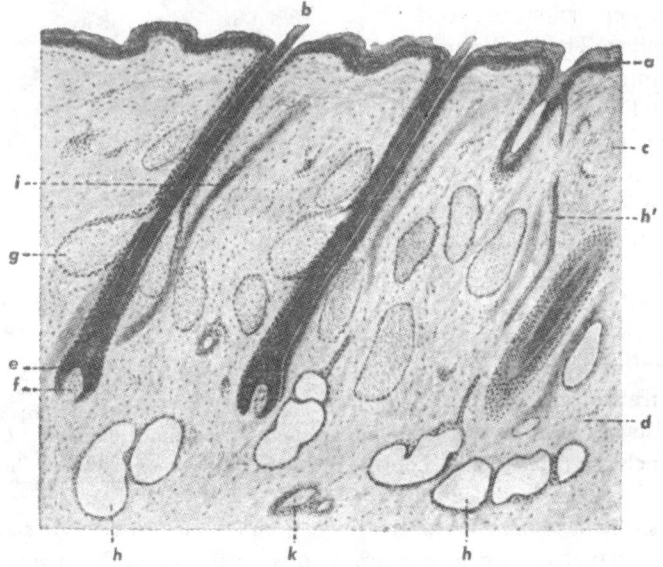

Figure 377. Section through the abdominal skin of the ox.
a, epidermis; b, hair; c, corium; d, deep layer of the corium;
e, hair bulb; f, hair papilla; g, sebaceous gland; h, tubular
gland; h', its excretory duct; i, m. arrector pili; k, vessels.

Some elastic fibers join the collagenous bundles, while others form fine networks, especially in the more superficial layers of the corium (as in the ox, sheep, and dog). Other nets surround the smaller vessels and the hair follicles. On the basis of the direction of their bundles, two intergrading layers are recognized.

1. In the papillary layer or papillary body (Fig. 375,g) the fine collagenous bundles are densely interwoven. The surface of this layer bears cone-shaped papillae, which usually contain capillary loops (Fig. 126). These papillae are small and poorly differentiated in the hairy portions of the skin. Wherever the hair coat is dense, the dermal surface between the hairs is either perfectly smooth or shows only slight elevations and a few small folds (Fig. 377).

The shape of the papillae varies. There are simple papillae, which may be long and slender or short and thick. Others are large and have a bifurcated end (e.g., in the external genitalia and the planum nasale). Some papillae branch into more than two cone-shaped processes, giving rise to compound papillae, as in the foot pads of the dog (Fig. 376). Large slender papillae are present in all hairless areas and those having but little hair. They are especially prevalent at the various muco-cutaneous junctions: diverticulum nasi, planum nasale, planum rostrale, labial margins, foot pads, teats, udder, glans penis, clitoris, and the tip of the tail. Many papillae of man contain Meissner's corpuscles.

2. The stratum reticulare is not sharply marked off from the stratum papillare. It is the deeper and heavier layer of the corium. Here the fiber bundles interweave mainly in a horizontal plane (Fig. 376,e).

The thickness of the skin varies with age, sex, species, and body region. The ox has the thickest, the sheep the thinnest, skin. It is thicker on the back and on the extensor surfaces of the limbs than on the belly and the flexor surfaces. The skin is very thick on the tail of the horse, on the dewlap of the ox, and on the ventral aspect of the neck of the pig.

C. SUBCUTIS OR HYPODERMIS

The subcutis (Fig. 376,3) consists of loose collagenous trabeculae, which contain many elastic fibers and cross each other to form a meshwork, the spaces of which are subdivided further by smaller bundles. A homogeneous adhesive ground substance converts the fiber nets to thin membranes. Between the membranes are narrow tissue spaces. These may, under pathological conditions, contain fluid (as in edema and anasarca) or air (in emphysema). The degree to which the skin can be folded or displaced depends on the development of the subcutis, i.e., the extensibility, length, and thickness of the fiber bundles. The spaces of the subcutis are often filled with adipose tissue. This may take the form of small clusters of cells or larger masses. Often it makes up a cushion of fat (panniculus adiposus; Fig. 376,f), which in well-finished animals extends to the deep surface of the cutaneous muscles. Subcutis and corium contain fibroblasts and histiocytes, pigmented cells (melanophores), plasma cells, and eosinophilic granulocytes (see p. 91).

The panniculus adiposus is heaviest in the pig, where it forms the bacon, fat back, clear plate, etc. The foot pads of carnivores contain a thick pad of fat. Wherever the skin is anchored tightly to subjacent tissues, the subcutis and adipose tissues are absent or sparse. This is the case in the inner surface of the ear, the lips, eyelids, nose, glans penis, etc. Fat is never present in the scrotal skin. The subcutaneous fat serves as filler, a shock absorber (as in foot pads), a sheath for easily injured parts (e.g., nerves and vessels), and, because it is a poor conductor of heat, it protects the body against excessive heat loss.

The wattles of the goat are appendages consisting of skin and subcutis. They include a striated muscle, a bar of elastic cartilage, and vessels and nerves. Wattles are sometimes seen in pigs, but here the proper muscle is absent. The subcutis contains glands that resemble the tubular glands of the external auditory meatus. Wattles are still rarer in sheep, where they contain neither muscle nor cartilage.

D. HAIR

Except for a few areas (the end of the nose, foot pads, and all mucocutaneous junctions) the skin of domestic animals is covered with hairs. These are epidermal structures—flexible, elastic horny threads, the free portion of which is called the hair shaft. The proximal part, or root, is almost always set obliquely in the skin (it is vertical in the sheep). This angle and the direction of the hair vary with the species and body region. The hair root is attached to an underlying dermal papilla by means of its knoblike, hollow proximal end, which is called the hair bulb. The papilla causes the end of the bulb to be invaginated much like the bottom of a champagne bottle.

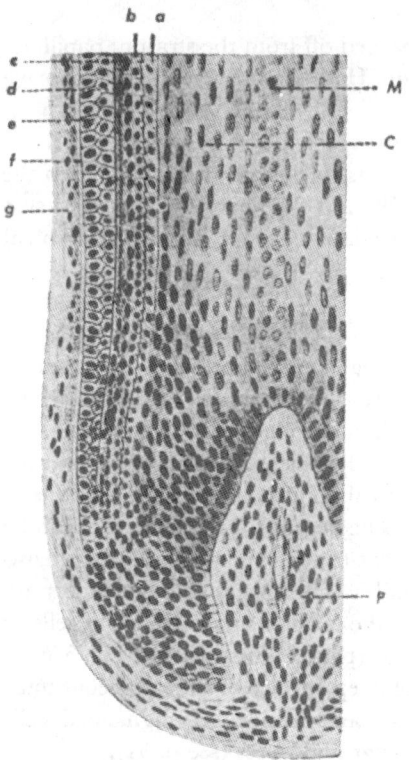

The hair roots are inserted into pits in the skin, the hair follicles. These have a saclike fundus, a narrow neck, and a wider funnel-shaped opening. The follicle consists of a peripheral connective tissue portion, or follicle proper, and an inner epithelial part, the root sheaths.

(1) Hair Shaft. The hair is composed of medulla, cortex, and cuticle. The *medulla* (Figs. 380,a; 382) is an axial cord of one or more longitudinal rows of cells, which are either cuboidal or flattened from top to bottom. In the region of the root the medulla is solid, but in the shaft it contains air vacuoles. It gradually disappears toward the tip of the hair. As the distance from the papilla increases, the cells shrink and admit air between them or even into their interior. The nuclei also shrink, and near the mouth of the follicle they can hardly be demonstrated.

Figure 378. Longitudinal section through a hair root (400×). *C*, cortex, *M*, medulla of the hair; *P*, hair papilla containing a capillary; *a*, hair cuticle; *b*, cuticle of the sheath; *c*, Huxley's layer; *d*, Henle's layer; *e*, outer root sheath; *f*, glassy membrane; *g*, dermal follicle.

The *cortex* (Fig. 378,*C*) consists of completely cornified, fusiform cells with elongated nuclear remnants. Their longitudinal axis is parallel to that of the hair, and they are held together by means of cornified intercellular bridges—much more firmly in the longitudinal than in the transverse direction. Toward the bulb the cells become shorter and softer, until finally they are oval and contain spheroid nuclei. These cells contain the pigment which gives the hair its color. It may be finely dispersed or in granules. Medullary pigment has little influence on the hair color. The air spaces in the medulla play a part in the graying of hair.

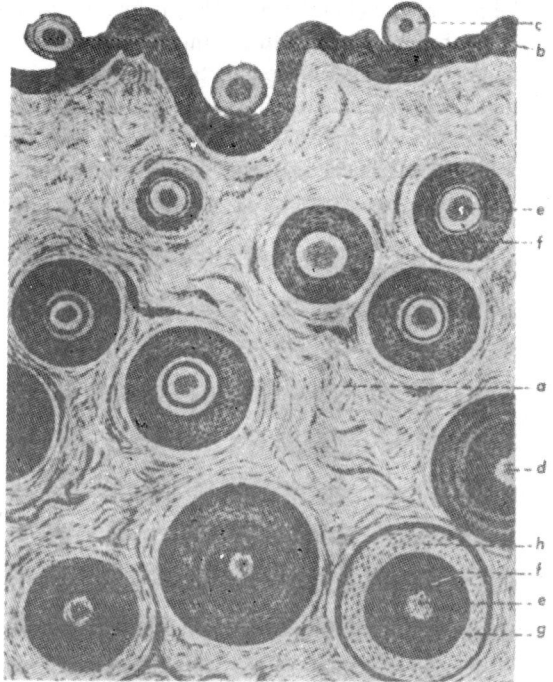

Figure 379. Oblique section through the skin of the pig. The hairs are sectioned transversely at various levels (70×). *a*, corium; *b*, epidermis; *c*, hair shafts; *d*, papilla; *e*, medulla; *f*, cortex; *g*, inner, *h*, outer root sheath. The cross section marked *h,f,e,g*, is again shown in Fig. 380 under high magnification.

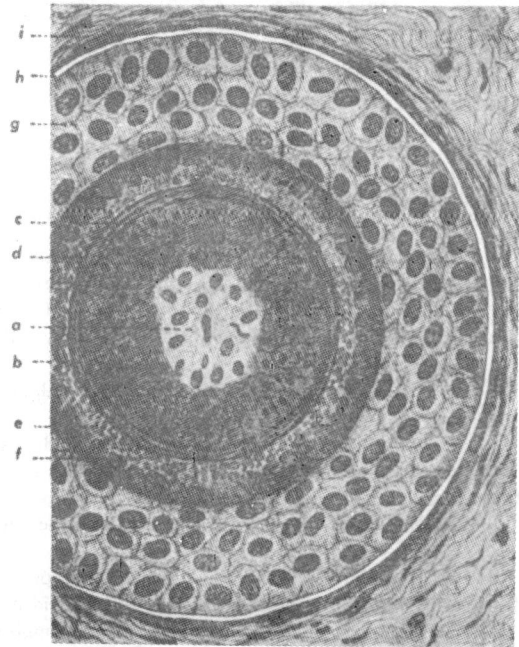

Figure 380. Cross section through a hair root of the pig (400×). *a*, medullary substance; *b*, cortical substance; *c*, hair cuticula; *d*, cuticle of the sheath; *e*, Huxley's, and *f*, Henle's, layer of the inner root sheath; *g*, outer root sheath; *h*, glassy membrane; *i*, dermal hair follicle (internal layer).

The hair *cuticle* (Figs. 378,*a*; 382) is formed by flat, cornified, and nonnucleated cells, which are arranged like shingles with their free edge directed toward the tip of the hair. The edge of the hair therefore appears slightly serrated in profile.

The *cover hairs* just described are the most common in domestic animals other than sheep. Another important type is the fine, crimped *wool hair*, or lanugo hair, which forms the fleece of sheep. It also forms the undercoat in goats, some breeds of swine, and carnivores. It is prominent in very young animals. In man it is lost

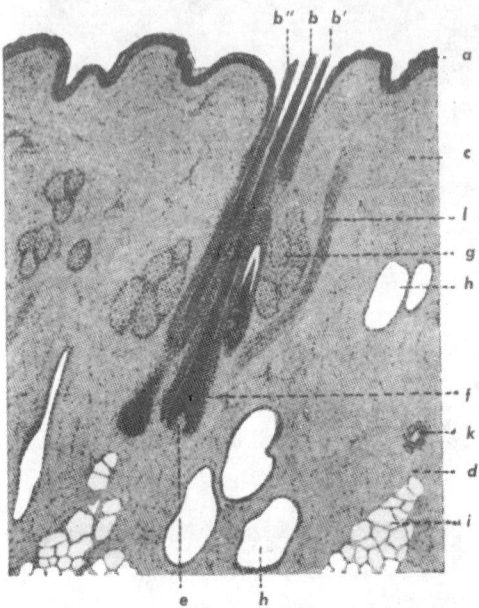

Figure 381. Section through the skin of the dog. *a*, epidermis; *b*, main hair; *b'*,*b''*, accessory hairs; *c*, corium; *d*, deep layer of the corium; *e*, hair papilla; *f*, hair bulb; *g*, sebaceous gland; *h*, apocrine tubular gland; *i*, adipose tissue; *k*, blood vessel; *l*, m. arrector pili.

in utero. The medulla is lacking in the finer cover hairs, the wool hairs of ungulates, and the hair of the human scalp.

KEY FOR THE IDENTIFICATION OF THE COVER HAIRS OF DOMESTIC ANIMALS (FIG. 382)

[The hairs should be defatted with ether and examined in glycerine and water.]

  I. Cortex very thick, medulla no more than $\frac{1}{3}$ of the width of the hair or absent........Man
 II. Cortex thick, at least $\frac{1}{2}$, but no more than $\frac{2}{3}$ of the width
     a. Medullary cells rectangular, separated by rather wide, lighter streaks; borders appear rough...Horse (1)
     b. Medullary cells much wider than high, edges smooth, forming a fine, flat meshwork ....Ox (2)
     c. Medullary cells higher, almost square, edges smooth....................Dog (5)
     d. Medullary cells indistinct, very granular, often higher than wide...........Pig (3)
 III. Cortex of moderate thickness, $\frac{1}{6}$ of the width of the hair
     a. Medullary cells often triangular, with the base bulging out toward the hair root ....Goat (4)
     b. Medullary cells in rows of one to three, profile of hair distinctly serrated....Cat (6)
 IV. Cortex very thin, no more than 1/10 of the width
     a. Medullary cells rectangular, in several longitudinal rows.........Rabbit (7), Hare

b. Medullary cells polygonal, thin-walled, honeycomb-like arrangement, contain vacuoles......................................European Red and Roe Deer, Chamois
Wool hairs, crimped, medulla absent, cuticle cells like cups stacked into each other, edges projecting...Sheep (8)

The hairs are either evenly distributed (as in the horse and ox) or occur in groups (as in the pig, dog, and cat). There are usually three hairs in a group, of which one is the main hair and is larger than the other two. In carnivores each of these three cover hairs is surrounded by six to twelve wool hairs, the follicles of which branch

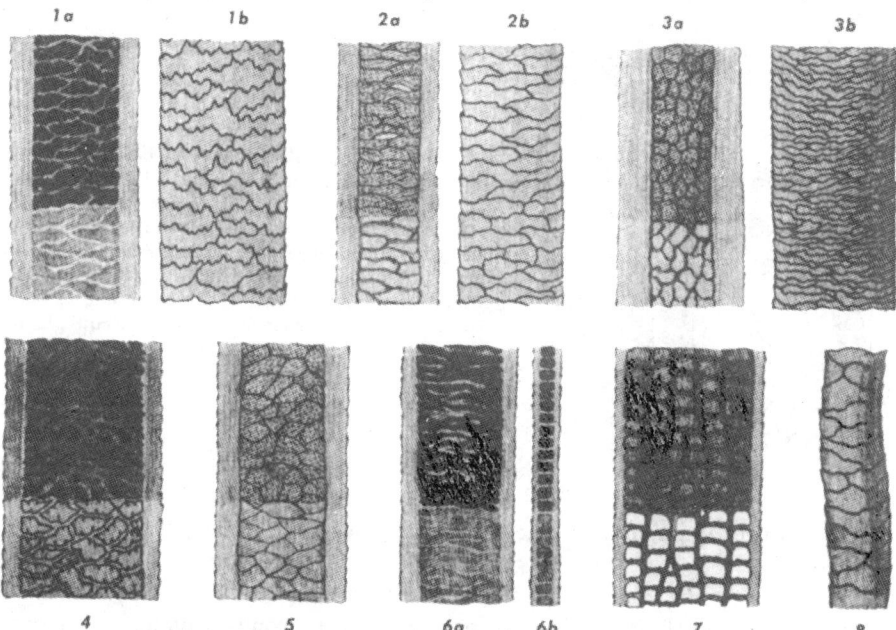

Figure 382. Hairs of domestic mammals. 1, horse; 2, ox; 3, pig; 4, goat; 5, dog; 6, cat (cover and wool hair); 7, rabbit; 8, sheep (wool fiber); a, showing the medulla partially cleared; b, cuticular pattern.

off from the follicle of the cover hair at the opening of the sebaceous glands (about the middle of the root). Thus, in carnivores a whole bundle of hairs projects from a common follicular opening (Fig. 381).

(2) Hair Follicle. The follicle is formed by corium and epidermis. The former furnishes the dermal follicle, the latter, the epithelial root sheaths.

The *connective tissue follicle* consists of an outer and an inner layer and the glassy membrane. The outer layer is composed of longitudinal bundles of collagenous fibers and of delicate elastic fibers. It is rich in vessels and nerves and blends without any sharp line of demarcation into the neighboring corium. The inner layer (Fig. 380,*i*) is made up of circular collagenous fibers and reaches only to the neck of the follicle. Inside this layer is the glassy membrane (basement membrane).

An inner and an outer root sheath are recognized in the epithelial part of the follicle. The *outer root sheath* (Fig. 378,*e*) adjoins the glassy membrane and is the continuation of the Malpighian layer of the epidermis. The *inner root sheath* grows upward with the hair from the papilla as far as the opening of the sebaceous gland, where it disintegrates. It is firmly connected to the outer sheath. It consists of a single outer layer of nonnucleated cells, the layer of Henle (Fig. 378,*d*) followed centrally by a one- to three-layered stratum of nucleated cells, the layer of Huxley. The innermost layer is the cuticle of the sheath (*b*), a membrane similar in structure to the adjacent hair cuticle. The free edges of the cells, however, are di-

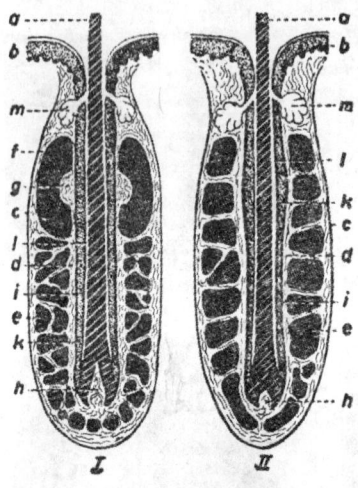

Figure 383. Hair follicles of sinus hairs in longitudinal section, semidiagrammatic (150×). *I*, cat; *II*, horse; *a*, hair; *b*, epidermis; *c*, outer, *d*, inner, layer of the dermal follicle; *e*, the blood sinus (in *I* this sinus has been differentiated into a nontrabecular annular sinus *f*, into which projects the sinus pad *g*); *h*, hair papilla; *i*, glassy membrane of the follicle; *k*, outer root sheath; *l*, inner root sheath; *m*, sebaceous glands.

rected toward the papilla, so that the two cuticles interdigitate. Both are unpigmented.

(3) **Hair Papilla.** The papilla (Fig. 378,*P*) contains vessels, but apparently no nerves. In the case of pig bristles it occasionally bears secondary papillae. It is connected to the rest of the corium by means of the constricted papillary neck and is covered by a thin continuation of the glassy membrane. The outer root sheath ends at the neck of the papilla in a tapered edge. The inner root sheath and the hair grow from a layer of plump, nucleated cells which cover the papilla. These cells regularly exhibit mitosis and are called the hair matrix.

Cross sections through hair roots, taken at various levels, show a quite variable picture, as may be gathered from the description and Figure 379.

The connective tissue portion of the follicle of the finer cover hairs and wool hairs consists only of a few fibers. In the case of *tactile hairs*, however, it is highly developed and rich in elastic fibers. Here a blood sinus, lined with endothelium, intervenes between the outer and inner layers of the dermal sheath. Therefore these hairs are also called *sinus hairs* (Fig. 383). The two layers of the connective tissue sheath are heavier and tougher than those of ordinary hairs. In ungulates they are connected by numerous fibroelastic trabeculae so that the sinus (*e*) has a cavernous structure. In carnivores these trabeculae are absent in the upper part. Thus a smooth-walled annular sinus (*f*) is formed, into which projects a cushion-like thickening of the inner layer. The term *vibrissae* is best restricted to the hairs in the nostrils. They are not sinus hairs.

Hair Development (Fig. 384). At the point where a hair is about to develop, the epidermis thickens and forms a cylindrical hair germ, or epithelial peg, which grows down into the corium and shows a bulbous enlargement on its free end. The corium proliferates and forms the connective tissue follicle and the papilla, the latter invading the enlarged end of the hair germ. A central hair cone (*c*) is differentiated in the cellular mass near the papilla. This eventually gives rise to the

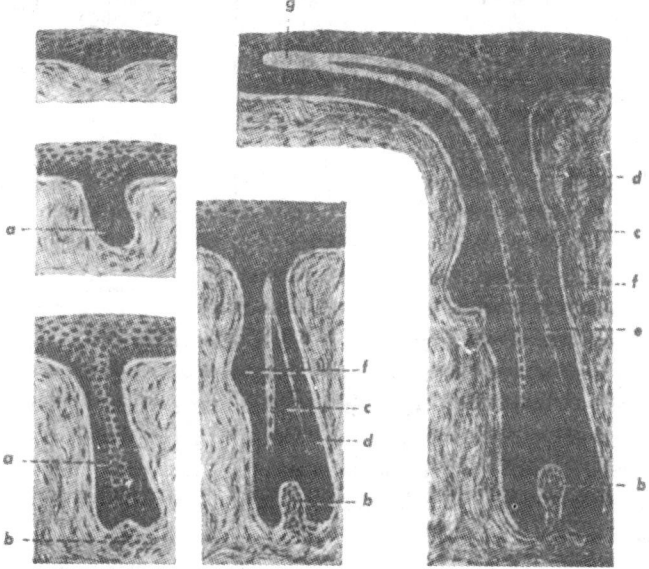

Figure 384. Diagrammatic representation of hair development. *a*, hair germ; *b*, hair papilla; *c*, hair cone; *d*, outer root sheath; *e*, inner root sheath; *f*, primordium of a sebaceous gland; *g*, hair canal.

hair proper, the two cuticles, and the inner root sheath, while the surrounding epithelial cells furnish the outer root sheath. The entire hair is at first surrounded by the inner root sheath. The axial hair germ cells that lie distal to the tip of the hair cornify and later disintegrate. Thus a canal is formed, through which the hair grows to the surface. In the process it breaks through the inner root sheath. Meanwhile hair bulb and follicle have developed further. The sinus hairs develop and break through earlier than ordinary hairs.

Shedding. In the process of hair replacement (Fig. 385) the hair bulb cornifies and separates from the papilla. The hair is then pushed toward the surface by proliferation of the cells immediately surrounding the papilla. The lower end becomes frayed like a broom. At the same time the hollow bulb becomes filled with cells and turns into a solid club (*b*), which remains near the opening of the sebaceous gland for some time. Proximal to it the empty root sheaths form a thin epithelial

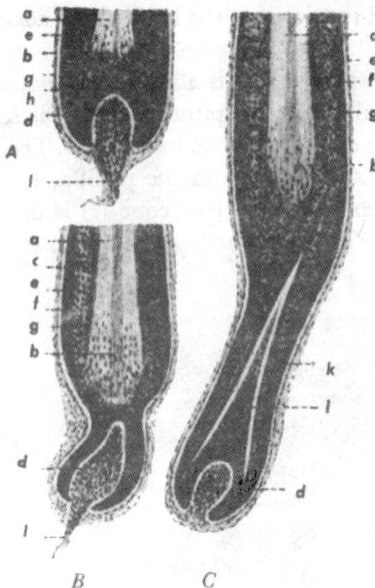

Figure 385. Replacement of hair, semidiagrammatic. *a,* hair about to be shed; *b,* frayed, clublike root; *c,* loosened root sheath; *d,* papilla; *e,* stratum spinosum of the hair follicle; *f,* glassy membrane of the follicle; *g,* dermal follicle; *h,* primordium of the new hair in *A; i,* new hair in *C; k,* root sheath of the new hair; *l,* hair stalk.

cord (*c*), at the bottom of which lies the atrophied papilla (*d*). The papilla has moved toward the surface, but it remains connected with its former site by means of the hair stalk, which is the collapsed dermal hair sheath (*l*). Even before the old hair has been completely pushed out, the papilla begins to grow again (*B,d*). The matrix cells, which surround the papilla, form a new hair (*i*), while the papilla descends to its former position. The new hair grows out alongside the old hair (*a*), which it finally dislodges.

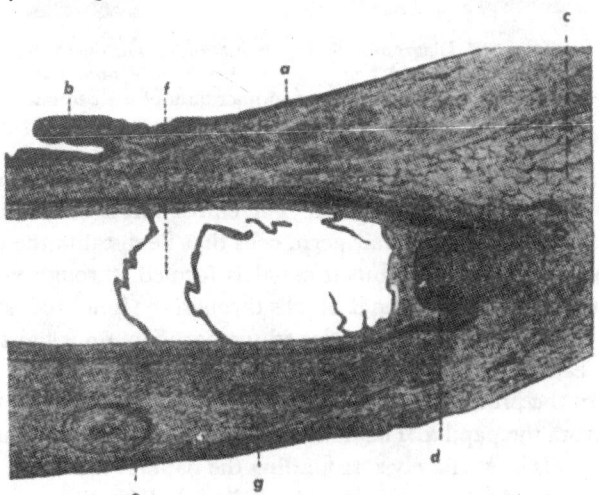

Figure 386. Section through the skin of the chicken (35×). *a,* epidermis; *b,* cutaneous fold; *c,* fat; *d,* feather papilla; *e,* Herbst's corpuscle; *f,* quill; *g,* muscle of the feather.

THE SKIN OF THE CHICKEN. In the feathered areas the skin is thin, easily displaced, and shows small folds (Fig. 386). The epidermis consists of a few layers of epithelial cells, which are superficially cornified and partly desquamated. A papillary body is absent. The corium shows a superficial layer composed of delicate collagenous fibers and a deeper layer made up of tougher fiber bundles, which are interwoven like a mat. The subcutis is much thicker. It contains an abundance of fat in its loose connective tissue. The skin is obliquely penetrated by the feather follicles, which extend deeply into the subcutis. The feather follicles are tubular invaginations from the skin. The blind end is invaginated by the feather papilla (d), which consists of finely fibered connective tissue containing vessels and nerves. The follicle is lined by several layers of epithelium.

Like the hairs, the feathers are epidermal structures. They consist of the shaft and the vane. The proximal part of the shaft is the quill or calamus, the tapering point of which has an opening at the end, the umbilicus. This houses the feather papilla. The quill is hollow. It contains air and cellular debris, called the medulla. The following types of feathers are recognized: (1) the contour feathers, which include the cover feathers and the large flight and tail feathers, (2) down feathers, and (3) filoplumae or hairlike

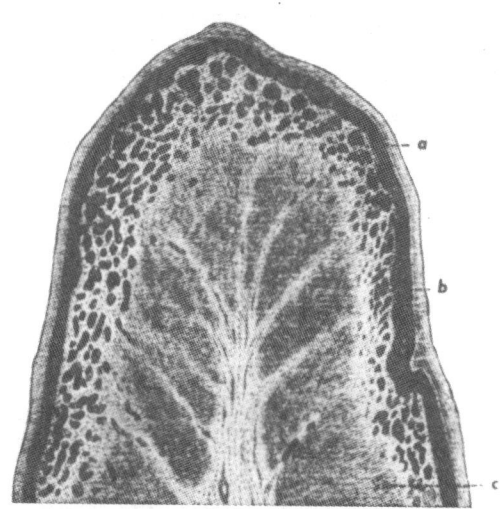

Figure 387. Section through the comb of the chicken (55×). a, epidermis; b, capillaries; c, mucous connective tissue.

feathers. The medulla is the product of the proliferating epidermal cells located on the top of the papilla. The horny substance of the shaft is formed by the cells on the sides of the papilla. The feather follicles are connected with smooth muscle bundles or their elastic tendons, which cause erection of the feathers. Often several muscles are attached to one follicle. Collectively they make up the subcuticular stratum musculare (g). The skin of birds contains no glands, except for the uropygeal gland (see p. 357).

Special skin characteristics are found in the following parts: On the feet the skin is tightly attached and bears scales. The scales are formed by flat processes of the dense corium, covered on both sides by very thick epidermis. The thick stratum corneum is especially conspicuous. Aggregates of lymphocytes are occasionally found in the subcutis. The toe pads are characterized by the presence of a heavy cushion of adipose tissue in the subcutis. This cushion shows clearly its composition of plurivacuolated fat cells. It is subdivided into compartments by strands of connective tissue and is amply supplied with blood vessels. The toe pad is covered by thick epithelium, into which high papillae project. It shows a stratum lucidum and a thick stratum corneum. The claws, spurs, and beak are horny structures resembling the claws of carnivores (p. 366). In the duck and goose the beak is not covered by hard horn but by a soft waxy variety called the ceroma. In the chicken the ceroma is limited to the base of the beak around the nostrils. The comb and wattles are skin appendages, the color of which indicates their rich vascularization. The comb (Fig. 387) shows in the center of its broadened base a deposit of fat, which is crossed by connective tissue strands and also ensheathed in connective tissue. The fat fades out toward the edge of the comb. The central connective tissue sheet is covered on either side by a thick layer of mucous connective tissue containing small stellate cells. Toward the surface there is a fine-fibered connective tissue with numerous lymphocytes. Below the epidermis lies a network of capillaries, which increase in number toward the margin of the comb and are distended with red blood corpuscles. The comb is covered by a superficially cornified, thick epidermis (a).

E. THE SKIN GLANDS

1. Sebaceous Glands

The sebaceous glands (Figs. 388,a; 389) arise in the fetus by proliferation of the outer hair root sheath. They make up the superficial layer of glands and occur in the middle depths of the corium. They usually open into the neck of a hair follicle. Only in a few places on the body do they occur as independent sebaceous glands not associated with hairs. This is the case in the glans penis, prepuce, labia vulvae, anus, external ear canal, and the tarsal glands of the eyelids.

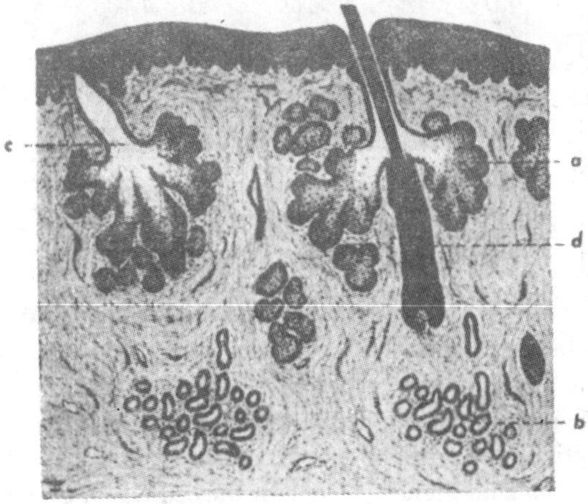

The sebaceous glands are simple alveolar holocrine glands and appear as evaginations of the follicle, the glassy membrane of which is continuous with the basement membrane of the gland.

Figure 388. Section through the cutis of the sheep near the labia vulvae. a, sebaceous gland opening into a hair follicle; b, apocrine tubular gland; c, independent sebaceous gland opening directly on the surface; d, hair.

The glandular body is filled with epithelial cells. Of these, the ones nearest the periphery are small and low, and the central ones are larger and polygonal. The cells show all gradations of secretory activity from the deposition of single fat globules to the disintegration of the cells. (See holocrine glands, p. 31). The nuclei shrink in the process and finally disappear altogether. Cells lost in secretion are replaced by the peripheral cells. If the fat of the cells is extracted by means of solvents, the cytoplasm becomes honeycombed in appearance. The excretory duct of the larger glands (Fig. 390) bears an epithelium resembling the epidermis and covered by a stratum corneum. The excretory ducts of the small glands have stratified squamous epithelium, which blends into the stratum spinosum of the outer root sheath.

Wherever the hair is dense, the sebaceous glands are long and narrow. Where the distance between hairs is greater, they are spheroid. In the dog they are often club-shaped and coiled. They are branched in the horse and dog. Their size and number depends on the species, size of hairs, and region of the body. The smaller the hairs, the larger the sebaceous glands. The horse and the dog have the largest glands, while those of the pig are rudimentary. In ungulates as a rule two to six sebaceous glands empty into one hair follicle. In carnivores several hair follicles unite into a group with one common opening. With this follicle complex is associated a complex of about the same number of sebaceous glands. A ring of sebaceous glands also opens into the follicles of the tactile hairs. The largest sebaceous glands usually occur in the areas around mucocutaneous junctions. Sebaceous glands are absent from foot pads, hoofs, claws, horns, the planum nasolabiale and the teats of the ox, and the planum nasale of sheep, goats, and carnivores.

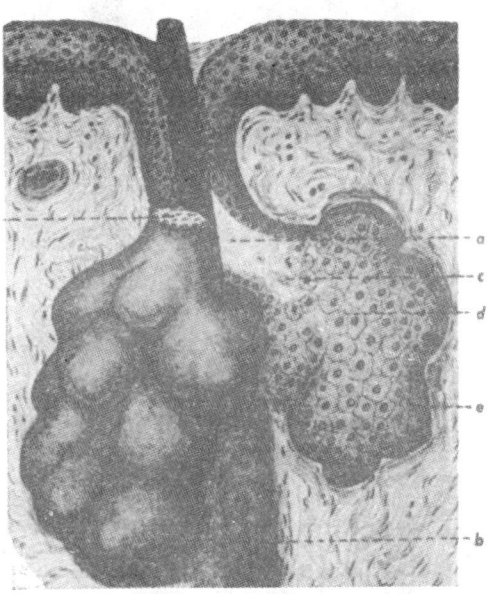

Figure 389. Sebaceous gland opening into a hair follicle, semidiagrammatic. *a*, excretory duct; *b*, hair follicle; *c*, secretion; *d*, secretory cells undergoing fatty transformation; *e*, newly formed secretory cells.

The secretion of the sebaceous glands, sebum, consists of cellular debris and a lipoid mixture high in cholesterol. It keeps the skin and hairs pliable and protects them against drying and moisture. The sebum is discharged by the contraction of the follicular muscles (p. 358).

2. Tubular Skin Glands

Two kinds of tubular skin glands (Figs. 376,*g;* 377,*h;* 388,*b;* 391; 392*) are recognized: merocrine and apocrine. The secretory tubule of either type has a basement membrane containing circular reticular fibers. Longitudinal or spiral smooth muscle fibers (myoepithelial cells) are interposed between the basement membrane and the single layer of secretory cells (Fig. 392,*b,c**).

The secretory portion of the *merocrine tubular glands* consists of a narrow tube of

---

* Fig. 392 is on p. 297.

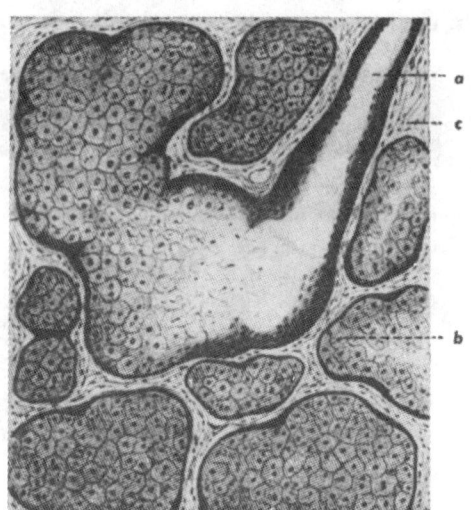

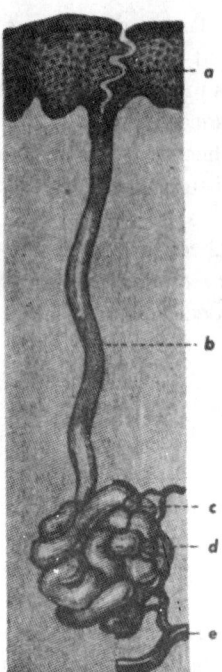

Figure 390 (left). Section through a sebaceous gland from the prepuce of the horse. *a*, excretory duct; *b*, body of the gland; *c*, interlobular tissue.

Figure 391 (right). Merocrine tubular gland, semidiagrammatic. *a*, excretory duct as it penetrates the epidermis; *b*, excretory duct; *c*, capillary network; *d*, body of the gland; *e*, artery.

uniform diameter, which is generally rolled into a ball (the glomiform glands). The cuboidal to columnar cells elaborate a watery secretion (sweat). In the region of the excretory duct there is a layer of longitudinal collagenous bundles outside the basement membrane. The excretory duct is lined by a double layer of cuboidal cells with cuticular border, which become lower toward the epidermis. The duct passes between dermal papillae to the surface—not into a hair follicle. Where the epidermis is thick the duct is continued to the surface by a spiral canal walled only by epidermal cells (Fig. 376,*h*).

The *apocrine tubular glands* usually have much wider secretory tubules than the preceding. In cattle they may be 150 μ in diameter. They are serpentine or rolled into a ball, and may show saclike diverticula (e.g., in the dog; Fig. 381,*h*). Where they pass into the excretory duct, they suddenly become narrower (20 μ in the ox). During secretion the cells show budlike apical projections. The finely granular, basophilic cytoplasm contains fat droplets, brown pigment granules, and a spheroid nucleus. The apical portion is detached into the lumen during secretion. The lumen thus becomes larger again and is lined by low cells with flattened nucleus (Fig. 393). The myoepithelial cells form a denser layer here than in the merocrine glands. The excretory duct opens into a hair follicle above the ducts of the sebace-

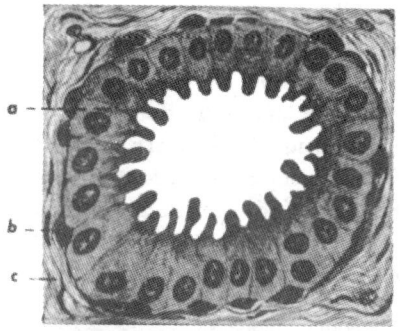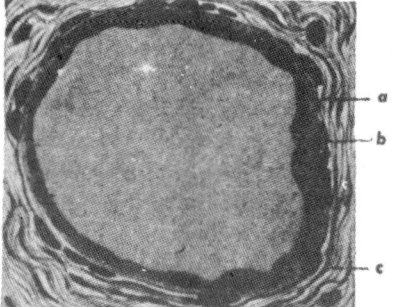

Figure 393. Cross sections of apocrine tubular glands from the anal sac of the dog. *Left:* cells filled with secretion; *right:* emptied cells. *a* (left), high columnar cells with lobed processes; *a* (right), flat cells; *b*, transverse sections of muscle cells; *c*, periglandular tissue.

ous glands. There is only one apocrine gland per follicle (Fig. 377,*h*). The tactile hair follicles usually have none. The apocrine glands, like the sebaceous glands, develop as outgrowths of the hair follicles, whereas merocrine glands are downgrowths from the surface epithelium. The secretion of the apocrine glands is fatty. Their secretory portions are always deep to the sebaceous glands.

Both merocrine and apocrine tubular glands were formerly designated as sweat glands. This name, however, actually applies only to the merocrine glands of man and other primates.[1] In these species the true sweat glands are distributed over the entire skin surface. The apocrine glands of man are restricted to only a few areas of the skin (e.g., the axilla). In domestic mammals, on the other hand, the apocrine glands make up by far the majority of the tubular skin glands. Numerous transitional forms and peculiarities are met with, however, in the various species and regions of the skin. Some apocrine skin glands produce odoriferous substances. The mammary gland is included in the apocrine skin glands.

In the horse, sheep, pig, and cat the secretory tubule is wound up (glomiform), whereas in the ox, goat, and dog it is serpentine. In the horse it is frequently filled with proteinaceous particles. The poorly developed tubular glands of the cat are present in only a few body areas (oral region, anus, lower jaw, and foot pads); the dog has small tubular glands that are better developed in some regions (as the back, mouth, and anus).

The tubular glands are largest at the margins of the haired skin, in the cutaneous sinuses (in the sheep and pig), on the nose and lips, on the ventral surface of the tail of the sheep, and around the teats of the sow. They are absent from the glans penis and from the teats and interdigital skin of cattle.

In accordance with the morphological findings, the dog does not normally produce liquid sweat; the horse produces albuminous sweat that lathers easily; and the ox, sheep, and goat produce a fatty secretion with characteristic odor.

---

[1] Josef Schaffer, Zur Einteilung der Hautdrüsen, *Anat. Anz. 57* (1924): 353–372.

3. Mammary Glands

The mammary gland of a lactating animal (Figs. 394–396) is a compound tubuloalveolar gland. Its component parts are the capsule, the interstitial framework with vessels and nerves, the parenchyma, and the lactiferous ducts.

The udder is surrounded by a fibroelastic capsule (mammary fascia) and the skin. From the capsule tough connective tissue septa containing elastic fibers, smooth muscle, and adipose tissue enter the gland and separate the lobes and lobules (Fig. 394,e). At the height of lactation the septa between adjacent glandular end-pieces are often so thin that the alveolar walls seem to touch each other.

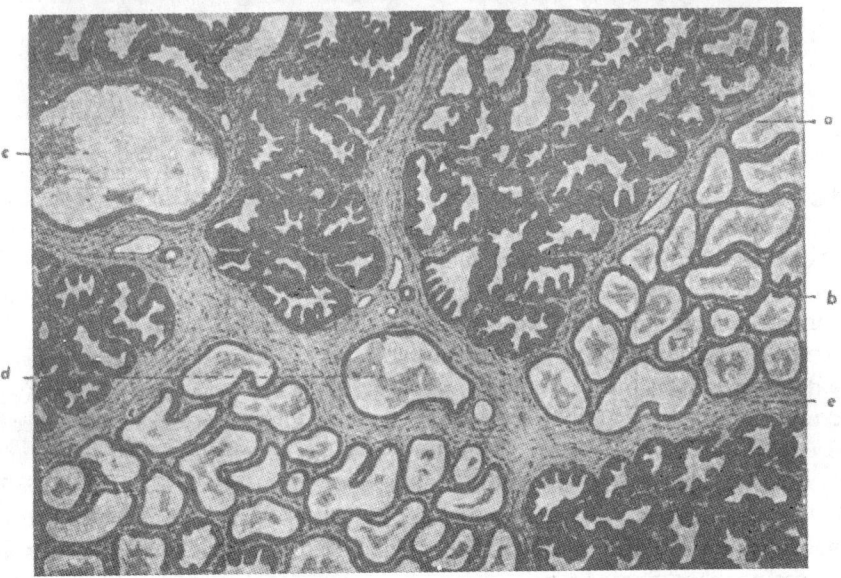

Figure 394. Section from the mammary gland of a lactating goat. *a*, mammary lobule with distended alveolar epithelium; *b*, another lobule with empty epithelial cells; *c*, initial section of a lactiferous duct; *d*, cross section through an interlobular duct; *e*, interlobular connective tissue.

The quantity of interstitial tissue varies with the constitution, condition, and age of the animal. In the "fleshy udder" the collagenous and elastic tissue predominate, while in fat animals the adipose tissue is well developed.

The *parenchyma* consists of secretory tubules with alveoli, capillary nets, and delicate connective tissue, which contains a fine network of elastic fibers. The tubular end-pieces of animals in advanced pregnancy or during lactation bear large numbers of bulblike alveoli. The alveoli are surrounded by branched, stellate, myoepithelial cells, the contraction of which supposedly aids in the emptying of the alveoli. The basement membrane is indistinct. The epithelial lining of the alveoli (Figs. 394, 395) shows extreme variation with the secretory stages of the gland. Immediately preceding and during the onset of milk formation the cells are high columnar or prismatic with the free end protruding into the lumen. The cell borders are usually indistinct, and the position of the nucleus is quite variable (Fig. 395, *left*).

In the distal portion of the granular cells shiny fat droplets soon appear, some of which become confluent. They are finally cast off into the lumen, usually with the distal portion of the cell. The separation may be delayed until the entire cell is filled by a single large fat globule, which displaces the nucleus basally or to the side. After the extrusion of the secretion the cells are much lower because of the loss of the distal cell portion and sometimes even of the nucleus. The flattening of the cells is increased by distention of the alveolus with secretions (Fig. 395, *right*). After the alveoli have been emptied, the cells become higher again by regeneration of their secretory portions. Many secretory cells perish and their debris is included in the alveolar contents. Not all alveoli are in the same stage of secretion at one time. Even adjacent alveoli may present a contrasting appearance.

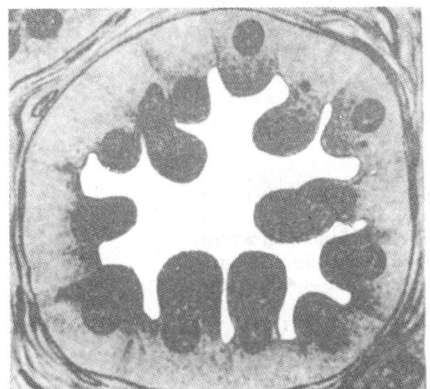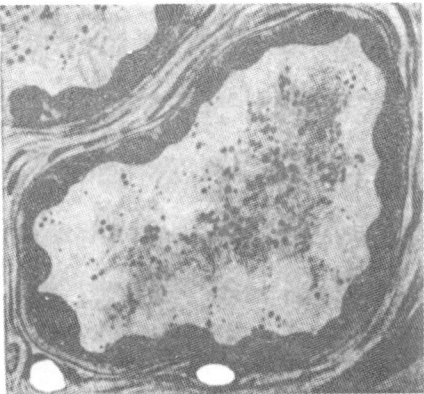

Figure 395. Section through mammary alveoli of the bitch with distended (left) and empty (right) cells. The intracellular and intra-alveolar fat globules have been stained with osmic acid.

The lactating mammary gland frequently contains islands of parenchyma that are rich in leukocytes. The islands show alveoli with narrow lumina containing colloid-like clumps. Structurally they resemble a gland in the colostrum-producing stage and are considered to be nonfunctioning parts of the gland. Often one finds in the alveoli of older animals spheroid concretions, called corpora amylacea. These vary in size, are concentrically stratified, and consist of casein (Fig. 396,*c*). During the lactation period the homogeneous or granular Nissen's bodies appear in the epithelium and in the secretion. These are small lymphocytes or pinched off nuclei of epithelial cells.

Up to the age of puberty the mammary gland shows a rudimentary structure. (Shortly after birth the mammary gland undergoes temporary stimulation, which results in the secretion of the so-called witch's milk.) In the nonfunctional gland of young animals the abundant pliable connective tissue contains ducts and glandular tissue consisting only of epithelial buds with or without rudimentary lumina. During puberty there is an increase in parenchymatous tissue. The cyclic hormonal activity of the ovary causes a regularly recurring hypertrophy and regression of the mammary gland. During pregnancy the placental hormones and progesterone

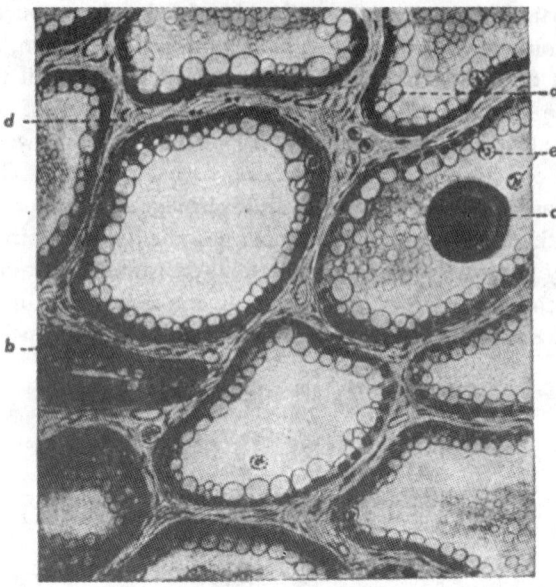

Figure 396. Lactating mammary gland of a mature cow (210×). *a*, active secretory epithelium; *b*, resting secretory epithelium; *c*, corpus amylaceum in an alveolus filled with secretion; *d*, interalveolar connective tissue; *e*, leucocytes.

furnish a strong stimulus for proliferation of the mammary tissue, resulting in a complete transformation and maturation of the gland. The budding epithelium crowds out the connective tissue and gives rise to a growth of secretory tubules and alveoli, which cause an enlargement of the whole organ. Increased multiplication of cells is evidenced by numerous mitoses in the epithelium, which also increases in height. The glandular epithelium and the connective tissue are infiltrated with leukocytes. The appearance of fine granulations and fat droplets in the cells and the presence of many leukocytes indicate the onset of secretion in animals in advanced pregnancy. The product of this secretion is at first colostrum. After a few days, under further influence of the anterior pituitary hormone prolactin, milk secretion is set into full motion. This stage is recognized by the appearance of the cells as described above, the disappearance of the leukocytes, and the reduction of interalveolar connective tissue.

During the involution of the mammary gland after lactation, the processes described above are reversed. The glandular tissue gradually ceases its activity and regresses. The interstitial connective tissue proliferates and fills in the spaces that have been formed by the reduction of the alveoli. Isolated patches of parenchymatous tissue may retain their secretory ability for a longer time. In the resting phase the mammary gland shows branched tubules with small alveoli, which are lined by low, nongranular, fat-free epithelium. Numerous leukocytes appear in the alveolar lumen. They are also present intraepithelially and in the interstitial tissue.

The various periods of maturation and regression of the mammary gland are not so strictly defined in the cow and goat as they are in woman and other mammals, because dairy breeding and management practices have prolonged the lactation period.

Milk contains dissolved proteins (mostly caseinogen), lactose, minerals, and small (2–5 μ) fat globules held in emulsion. Disintegrating cells and nuclei are also present.

Colostrum contains, in addition to the normal milk constituents, the spheroid colostrum corpuscles (up to 45 μ in diameter). They are considered to be leukocytes in which the nucleus has become masked by masses of intracytoplasmic fat globules. According to an older view, they are swollen epithelial cells filled with fat. Colostrum differs chemically, physically, and biologically from ordinary milk. It is secreted for only a short time following parturition. Colostrum is high in globulin, the protein with which antibodies are associated. The globulin content of the blood of the newborn is very low before the first feeding. Colostrum also has a laxative effect and aids in the expulsion of the intestinal waste (meconium) accumulated during intra-uterine life.

The system of *lactiferous ducts* begins with small intralobular tubules. The larger ducts show many ampullate dilatations (Fig. 394,*c,d*). The lactiferous ducts are not evenly distributed throughout the mammary tissue. The larger ones course just beneath the skin. The smallest ducts bear low simple secretory epithelium, which becomes columnar and finally two-layered in the larger ducts. The epithelium rests on a lamina propria of collagenous tissue interspersed with elastic fibers, smooth muscle cells, and blood vessels. The musculature of the duct walls is mostly longitudinal.

Unlike the arrangement in other glands (e.g., salivary), the secretory tissue of the mammary gland is not confined to the terminal branches of the ducts. It also grows from the sides of the ducts as far down as the base of the teats and is firmly anchored to the duct wall by the interstitial tissue. The larger lactiferous ducts, the walls of which are perforated by the openings of smaller ducts, possess more or less annular folds that project into the lumen at various intervals. The portions of the duct between these folds form the ampullate dilatations. The folds are reinforced by connective tissue tracts derived from the interstitial tissue. They contain elastic fibers and smooth muscle. The folds create collecting spaces in which the milk is allowed to accumulate between milkings or nursing periods.

In the more primitive mammary gland, such as that of the bitch, several large lactiferous ducts converge on each teat and dilate to form *lactiferous sinuses*, each of which is drained to the surface by a teat canal. In the cow, however, there is only one lactiferous sinus or milk cistern in each gland (quarter). The sinus receives about ten lactiferous ducts. Part of the sinus is in the body of the gland and part of it is within the teat. The division between gland sinus and teat sinus is marked by an annular fold, which is often incomplete or absent. It contains a venous circle and smooth muscle. The mucosa of the lactiferous sinus bears a usually two-layered columnar epithelium. Only in the sheep, in the region of the annular fold at the base of the teat, is there a zone of stratified squamous epithelium with a stratum corneum. The lamina propria of the mucous membrane contains dense networks of elastic fibers and, in the teat sinus, usually also accessory lobules of mammary tissue. The mucosa of the cistern often forms, especially in cows, a network of folds and niches, which give the cistern a spongy appearance.

The arrangement and function of the smooth muscle in the lactiferous ducts and sinus are of great physiological interest. It is possible to demonstrate muscle bundles in cross section in the edges of the folds surrounding the openings of the lactiferous ducts into the sinus. Similar muscle cross sections have been demonstrated in the (inconstant) fold between the gland and teat sinus.[2] These muscles have been interpreted as sphincters which hold the milk in the gland between milkings. It was claimed on purely morphological grounds that they relaxed to "let down" the milk. Gaines,[3] however, published direct experimental evidence thirty-five years ago that intramammary pressure is increased when the milk is "let down." It does not seem likely that relaxation of muscle sphincters could cause such an increase of pressure. Attempts to explain the let-down by accelerated secretion or increased local blood pressure were unsuccessful. It has since been demonstrated by a long series of experiments[4] that the milk is secreted continuously and stored between milkings, mostly in the alveoli and dilated lactiferous ducts. The capacity of the sinus is relatively small. When the teat is stimulated by handling or suckling, the posterior lobe of the hypophysis secretes oxytocin, a smooth muscle stimulant, which causes the milk to be forced down, presumably by contraction of the myoepithelial cells around the alveoli and the muscles of the ducts and sinus. The reflex is said to be independent of any efferent nerves to the udder. The apparent contradiction between the physiological and morphological findings may be explained by a more complete study of the musculature. One cross section does not make a sphincter. It has not been shown that the muscle strands in the folds around the openings of the lactiferous ducts actually close the openings. They may serve to contract the whole sinus. The presence of circular muscle fibers in the constrictions between ampullae in the upper part of the lactiferous ducts is doubtful.[5] According to Mainzer,[6] these folds are caused by elastic fibers. Such an arrangement would be in agreement with the contraction-expulsion theory: when the muscle in the wall of the duct is relaxed, it dilates to form ampullae; when stimulated by oxytocin to contract, it forces the milk out through the elastic constrictions.

The *teat* (papilla; Fig. 397*) consists of the mucosa of the teat sinus and canal,

---

[2] Hermann Ziegler, Zur baulichen Eigenart der Milchgänge, *Schweizer Arch. Tierhlk. 83* (1941): 47–52.

[3] W. L. Gaines, A Contribution to the Physiology of Lactation, *Am. J. Physiol. 38* (1915): 285–311.

[4] Fordyce Ely and W. E. Petersen, Factors Involved in the Ejection of Milk, *J. Dairy Sci. 24* (1941): 211–223.

[5] Eric W. Swanson and C. W. Turner, Evidence for the Presence of Smooth Muscle Elements Surrounding the Alveoli of the Mammary Gland, *J. Dairy Sci. 24* (1941): 635–638.

[6] Gerhard Mainzer, Ein Beitrag zur Morphologie der Milchgänge im Euter der Kuh, *Zeitschr. f. mikrosk. anat. Forschung. 45* (1939): 443–460.   * Fig. 397 is on p. 297.

the fibromuscular, vascular middle layer, and the skin, which contains much elastic tissue. The middle layer is absent in carnivores. The columnar epithelium in the teat sinus passes gradually (in the mare, bitch, and sow) or abruptly (in ruminants and the cat) into the stratified squamous epithelium of the teat canal, or papillary duct. The epithelium of the teat canal rests on a papillary body. The propria contains an extensive network of elastic fibers.

The middle layer is rich in longitudinal blood vessels, especially thick-walled veins. The smooth muscle fibers in the connective tissue stroma form an inner thin longitudinal layer, a middle circular layer (*b*), and an outer layer of longitudinal (*c*), radial (*e*), and oblique (*d*) bundles. The individual muscle layers vary in degree of development with the species. The inner longitudinal layer is absent in the bitch. In the cow, goat, and bitch the circular stratum condenses at the beginning of the papillary duct into the sphincter papillae. The other species have a dense annular network of elastic tissue around the teat canal.

The skin of the teat (*g,h*) is hairless and nonglandular in the cow and sow. The mare, cat, and bitch have fine or microscopic hairs and abundant sebaceous glands on the teat. The glands are especially large around the orifices in the mare.

Ruminants have one duct in each teat, the sow 2–3, the mare 2–4, the cat 4–7, the bitch 8–20, and woman 15–24 ducts.

The male mammary gland has small teats, which are occasionally canalized. Vestiges of glands are usually present.

VESSELS AND NERVES. The mammary gland contains many blood vessels. Narrow-meshed nets of capillaries surround the alveoli and ducts. The veins are valveless and do not always run with the arteries. The venous system is more extensive than the arterial system. The large lymphatics form plexuses in the parenchyma, teats, and subcutis. Vasomotor and sensory nerves are present. Nerve endings on the secretory cells have been described. Krause's end bulbs and Meissner's corpuscles occur within the interstitial connective tissue.

4. Special Glandular Structures of the Skin

The glands of the planum nasolabiale of the ox are serous glands with intercellular secretory canaliculi (Fig. 170). Their convoluted secretory tubules represent highly specialized and modified tubular glands. The glands of the planum nasale of sheep and goats have the same structure. The glands opening on the planum rostrale of the pig are tubular. The planum nasale of carnivores is free from glands. (See *lateral nasal gland*, p. 233.)

The wall of the *anal sac* (Fig. 398) of carnivores bears a cutaneous mucosa covered by stratified, pigmented, and superficially cornified epithelium. The propria (*b*) forms no papillary body. It contains lymph nodules (some are intraepithelial) and is composed of a loose subepithelial layer and a deeper fibroelastic sheet, which also contains smooth muscle fibers. These are also present in the glandular layer (*c*), which in the dog contains many apocrine tubular glands. Their epithelium is often sloughed off and either passes out with the secretion or remains as detritus, filling the glandular lumen. The cat also has sebaceous glands in addition to apocrine glands. In both species tubular and alveolar glands are always found in the excretory ducts of the anal sacs. The glandular stratum is surrounded by a fibro-elastic layer with striated muscle (*d*).

The glands of the frog in the horse are found mainly in the region of the frog-stay. In the donkey they are scattered throughout the entire frog. They are simple or branched coiled glands and open between the horn tubules. The glands of the foot pads of carnivores are coiled glands, which elaborate a fatty secretion.

The wall of the interdigital pouch of the sheep contains, in addition to fine hairs,

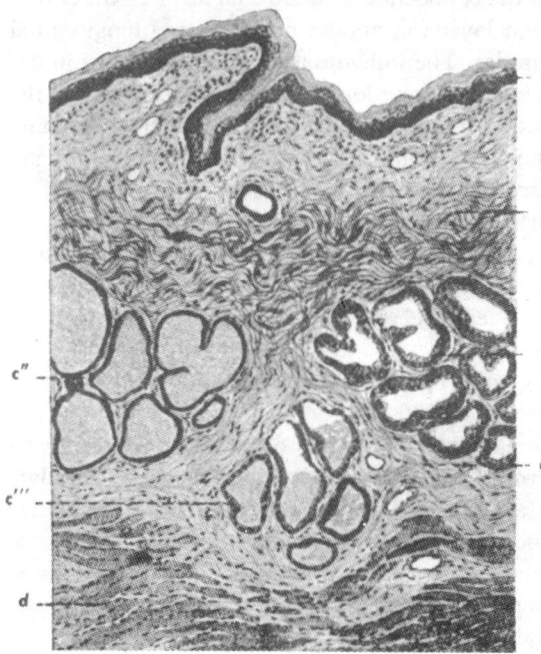

Figure 398. Section through the wall of the anal sac of the dog. *a*, squamous epithelium; *b*, propria mucosae; *c*, glandular layer; *c'*, gland lobule with high columnar, distended secretory cells; *c''*, lobule with flat, empty glandular epithelium; *c'''*, lobule with low columnar secreting glandular cells; *d*, striated muscle in the collagenous outer stratum.

well-developed sebaceous glands and large, compound, muscular apocrine glands.

The horn gland, which lies in the corium caudomedial to the base of the horn in the goat, is composed of branched alveolar glands, which are arranged in several layers. They usually open into hair follicles and they vary in development with age and sex.

The wall of the infraorbital sinus of the sheep has few hairs and no papillae but contains large sebaceous glands and large muscular apocrine glands.

The skin of the inguinal folds of sheep contains branched sebaceous glands and large yellow-brown apocrine glands, which are rich in musculature.

The carpal glands of the pig comprise one to twelve cutaneous invaginations containing greatly branched brownish merocrine mucous glands with many muscle fibers.

The skin of the preputial pouch of the boar is nonglandular and possesses high papillae and numerous lymph nodules. Large sebaceous and tubular glands lie at the entrance to the pouch.

The circumoral gland of the cat is composed of sebaceous glands. A group of large sebaceous glands is found on the dorsal surface of the root of the tail and is called the supracaudal organ.

For descriptions of other special glandular structures of the skin, such as the tarsal, ceruminous, circumanal, and preputial glands, consult the index.

UROPYGIAL GLAND. This is the only cutaneous gland of poultry (Fig. 399,*I*). It is at first a paired organ, which unites to form one pear-shaped structure of the size

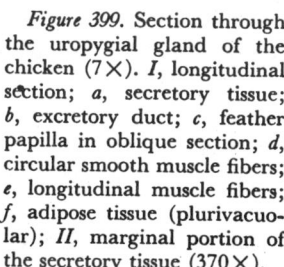
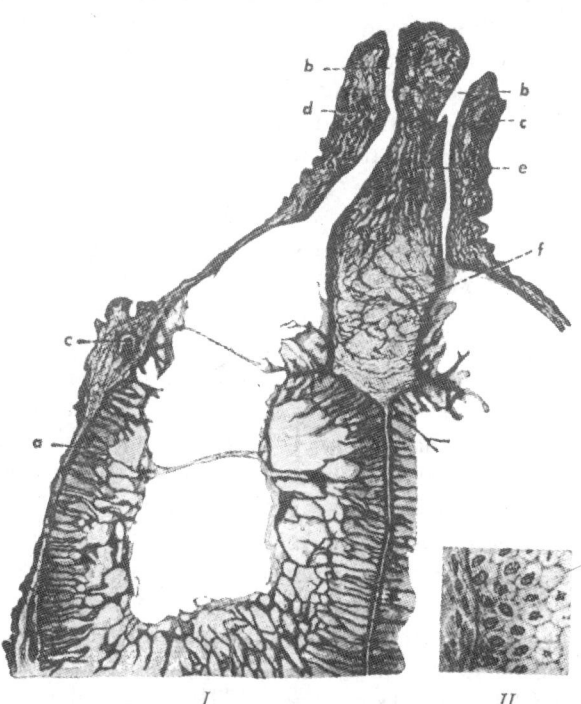

Figure 399. Section through the uropygial gland of the chicken (7×). *I*, longitudinal section; *a*, secretory tissue; *b*, excretory duct; *c*, feather papilla in oblique section; *d*, circular smooth muscle fibers; *e*, longitudinal muscle fibers; *f*, adipose tissue (plurivacuolar); *II*, marginal portion of the secretory tissue (370×).

I   *II*

of a hazelnut. It rests on the last coccygeal vertebrae just under the skin. Its excretory ducts (*b*) end at the apex of a papilla. The tough collagenous capsule of each half bears on its inner surface trabeculae which divide the peripheral part of the gland sinus into niches (*a*). The surface epithelium is continuous through the excretory duct with the epithelium of the sinus and is transformed in the recesses into many-layered glandular epithelium (Fig. 399,*II*). The marginal cells are low, but the more central ones become polygonal. Fat globules appear in the protoplasm. The nuclei undergo shrinkage, followed by disintegration of the cells, which form fatlike spheroid droplets. Numerous smooth muscle fibers are present in the papilla. They run circularly around the excretory ducts or follow a longitudinal course. Small feathers (*c*) are found next to the excretory ducts. The uropygial gland is a branched, alveolar holocrine gland, resembling the sebaceous glands. The secretion is utilized in oiling the feathers. The gland is more highly developed in aquatic birds.

F. THE MUSCLES, VESSELS, AND NERVES OF THE SKIN

In various portions of the body striated muscle fibers and bundles radiate from the cutaneous muscle into the corium and, in carnivores, attach to the follicles of the tactile hairs. Many striated muscles are present at the natural body openings, at the mucocutaneous junctions.

Smooth muscle occurs in sheets and as muscles of hair follicles (arrectores pilorum). Smooth muscle in sheetlike expanses is found on the penis, scrotum, teats, and in the eyelid (m. tarsalis). The arrectores pilorum (Fig. 377,i) are rich in elastic tissues and extend obliquely from the lower third of the follicle to the epidermis, passing around the sebaceous glands, often by means of a bifurcation. They are always found on that side of the follicle which forms an obtuse angle with the skin surface. Their contraction erects the hair, and they usually pass into elastic tendons.

The mm. arrectores pilorum are perforated by the excretory ducts of the tubular glands, which, if large, are partially ensheathed in the muscles. They are also reflected on the body of the gland, sometimes in the form of a fan-shaped branch. The larger the glands, the thicker are the muscles. Arrectores pilorum are absent from tactile hairs (which have striated fibers), and from the vibrissae. They are conspicuously thick in the sheep and poodle, often double in the pig. They are thin on the bristles of the pig and the hairs of the mane of the horse.

The arterial branches arising from the small subcutaneous trunks at first give off twigs that supply the capillary nets of the fat deposits and tubular glands. Then they contribute branches to the capillary networks of the sebaceous glands and the arrectores pilorum and terminate finally in the subepidermal capillary nets. From these arise the radicles of the veins, which lie alongside the arteries and receive venous branches from the other two capillary areas. Thus there are three capillary areas in the skin: the superficial subepidermal, the intermediate one of the glands, and the deeper one of the fat deposits. The connective tissue between the glands and follicles lacks capillaries. The walls of the cutaneous vessels contain nets of reticular fibers. Arteriovenous anastomoses occur in the skin, but their significance and distribution are not yet sufficiently clear.

The lymphatics arise from capillary nets, some of which lie in the superficial part of the corium, while others surround the follicles and glands. The vessels arising from these nets drain into a subcutaneous lymphatic plexus.

The small nerve trunks lie within the subcutis. They are continued by a nerve plexus extending through the corium to the epidermis. Some of the branches arising from this plexus enter the epidermis; others supply glands, muscles, and hairs; still others terminate in special nerve endings.

Every hair is equipped with a nerve ending. The sensory nerves penetrate the follicles immediately below the sebaceous gland ducts to the glassy membrane. There they divide and arrange themselves parallel to the longitudinal axis of the hair so that their straight terminal fibers (Fig. 400,d) surround the outer root sheath in the manner of a picket fence. There is a more peripheral plexus of circular ter-

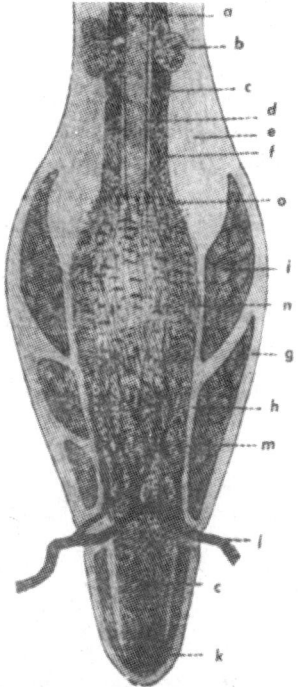

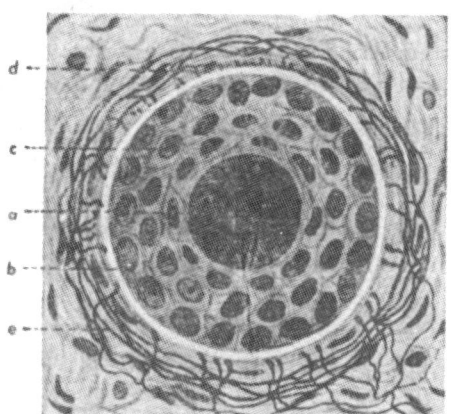

Figure 400 (left). Cross section through a facial hair of the cat below the sebaceous gland (400×). *a,* hair; *b,* glassy membrane; *c,* outer root sheath; *d,* cross sections of straight, and *e,* circular, terminal nerve fibers. (After Kadanoff.)

Figure 401 (right). Nerve endings in a sinus hair follicle of the pig; gold preparation (50×). *a,* hair; *b,* sebaceous glands; *c,* outer, *d,* inner, root sheath; *e,* hair follicle; *f,* glassy membrane; *g,* external layer of the dermal follicle; *h,* internal layer of the dermal follicle; *i,* sinus; *k,* hair papilla; *l,* small nerve trunks; *m,* superficial nerve plexus; *n,* layer of tactile cells, the menisci of which have been stained black by the gold treatment; *o,* spade-shaped nerve endings, over which a few fine unmyelinated circular fibers are shown.

minal nerve fibers. Some fibers end in tactile corpuscles inside the glassy membrane; others terminate a good distance from it. In the follicles of sinus hairs arborizations of nerve fibers are apposed to the glassy membrane. Other nerve fibers penetrate to the outer root sheath, where they terminate in tactile menisci. Between the glassy membrane and the stratum spinosum of the outer root sheath there is an actual coat of tactile nerves (Fig. 401). Sympathetic nerves at first form epilemmal nets around the tubular glands. These networks give rise to delicate plexuses, the fibers of which penetrate the glassy membrane and enter between the secretory cells as hypolemmal fibers.

A terminal network of autonomic fibers is associated with the sebaceous glands. It is derived mainly from the nerves that encircle the hair immediately below the opening of the sebaceous gland.

G. CORNIFIED EPIDERMAL STRUCTURES

The epidermis shows a high degree of specialization in the hoofs, claws, and horns. The underlying corium is characterized by an abundance of nerves and blood vessels and by a great increase in surface area. In many places it lacks a subcutis and the deeper layers blend with the periosteum. The papillary body is high and usually modified to form long macroscopic papillae or ridges or leaflike structures, the dermal laminae.

The deepest layer of stratum germinativum is the high columnar stratum cylindricum, as in the ordinary skin. It shows many tonofibrils. The stratum spinosum is made up of one or two cell layers, and gives rise to the heavy stratum corneum. On the papillae of the corium the stratum germinativum produces horn tubules; between the laminae of the corium it produces epidermal laminae.

1. The Hoof

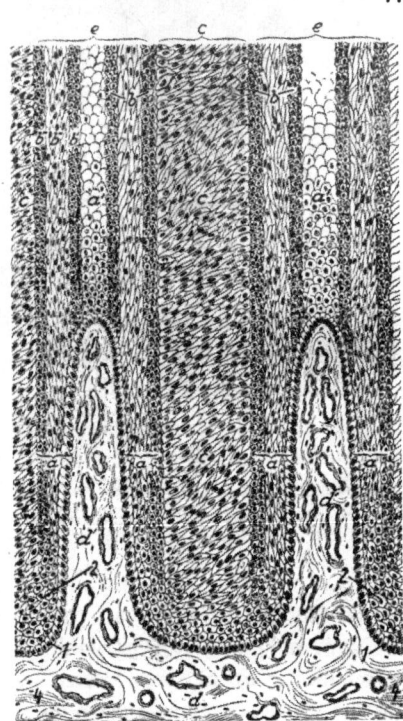

Figure 402. Sagittal section through corium and epidermis of the hoof, semidiagrammatic. *1*, stratum cylindricum; *2*, stratum spinosum; *4*, corium; *a*, peripapillary, *a'*, suprapapillary epithelium (=medulla of the tubule); *b*, cortex of the tubule, with three zones; *c*, interpapillary epithelium (intertubular horn); *d*, corium; *d'*, papillary body; *e*, an entire horny tubule. (After Nickel.)

The hoof proper is the cornified epidermis of the end of the digit. The integument here has the same layers as in other parts of the body.

(a) The subcutis is absent wherever the skin overlies bone. Where the skin covers tendons and cartilage, a generally tough subcutis with much elastic tissue is found. Such is the case over the extensor tendons and the lateral cartilages. In the region of the coronet the subcutis forms the perioplic and coronary cushion. It reaches its greatest thickness under the frog and the bulbs, where it forms the shock-absorbing digital cushion.

The tissue of the bulbs and frog consists of elastic and fibrous tracts, which interweave and form meshes that contain fat. The tissue of the bulbs encloses a thick pad of adipose tissue, which serves as an elastic filler. Toward the apex of the frog, elastic and adipose tissue decrease in quantity. The structure becomes tougher and firmer. Frog and bulbs contain packets of tubular glands (see p. 356).

(b) The corium of the hoof (pododerm) shows regional modifications which divide it into perioplic, coronary, laminar, sole, bulb, and frog corium. It is made up of collagenous tissue rich in elastic fibers

(Fig. 406,*d*). It consists of a stratum reticulare and a stratum papillare. The stratum reticulare, which corresponds to that of the rest of the integument, is a highly vascular layer. It is thickest in the coronary region and at the edge of the sole and thinnest at the frog. It blends into the subcutis or periosteum. The stratum papillare forms macroscopic elongated papillae everywhere except in the laminar corium, where the laminae take the place of papillae.

The perioplic corium is a narrow band that spreads out into the bulbar corium, and this is continuous with the corium of the frog and sole. The thin corium of the sole has long, frequently compound papillae and also shorter ones. The corium of the frog bears small papillae.

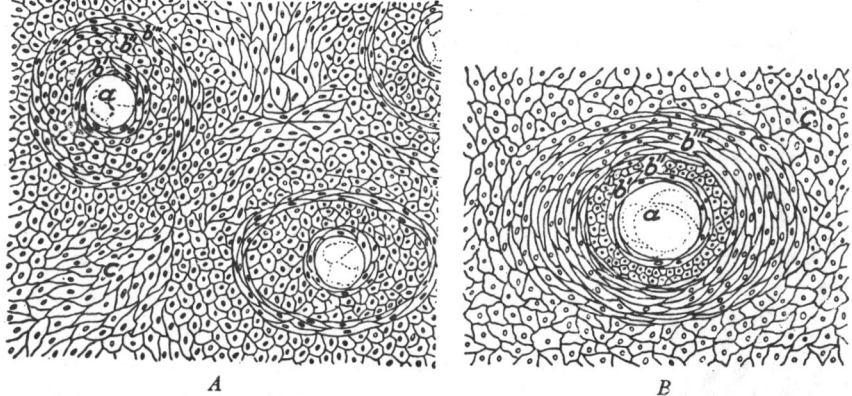

Figure 403. Horny epidermis showing transverse sections of horn tubules with predominantly steep (*A*) and flat (*B*) spirals, semidiagrammatic. *a*, medulla; *b*, cortex of horn tubules, with three zones; *c*, intertubular horn. (After Nickel.)

The coronary corium bears elongated papillae, which are longest over the coronary cushion (4–6 mm.) and become more slender and shorter (1–2 mm.) at the border with the laminar corium. The coronary papillae bear longitudinal ridges but are always unbranched. Near the laminae they are arranged in rows.

The corium of the wall and bars bears dermal laminae (Fig. 406,*d*), which are separated by deep furrows and are largest on the dorsal surface of the digit. On the sides of the foot, toward the bars, they decrease in length and height. The laminae are low at their origin from the distal border of the coronary cushion. They gain rapidly in height in the proximal third, then maintain a uniform height of about 4 mm. to the distal end, where they terminate in several long papillae. The dermal laminae become slightly thinner toward the distal end. About 600 primary laminae are present on the horse's foot. Their surface is increased by small secondary laminae (100–200), which cover the sides and free edge of the primary laminae and lend to them a feather-like appearance in cross section. The secondary laminae arise just below the proximal end of the primary lamina.

(c) **The epidermis** of the hoof is divided into the thin stratum germinativum and the heavy stratum corneum, or hoof proper. The horny hoof is composed of the horny wall, sole, bulbs, and frog.

The horny wall which corresponds to the human nail plate, is composed of three layers. The outer layer is formed in the region of the coronet by the *periople*, a band of soft tubular horn which passes through a keratohyaline stage in its cornification. It blends with the haired skin above the hoof. It scales off at a variable distance down the hoof wall, leaving only a thin layer of flat cells, the *stratum tectorium* (Fig. 406,*a*). This is often lacking in old horses.

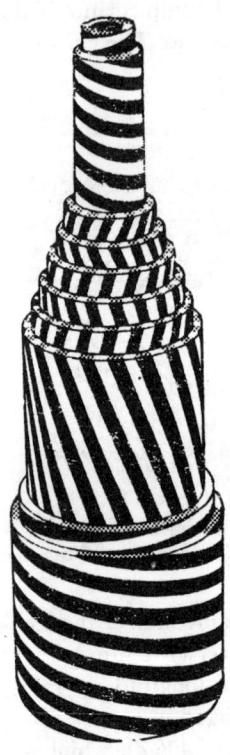

Figure 404. Scheme of a horn tubule with predominantly steep spirals. Note the thickness of the middle layer with the alternate spirals to right and left. The inner and outer zones are thin and arranged in flat coils. (From Nickel.)

The *stratum medium* (Fig. 405,*b*) is produced by the epithelium on the coronary corium. It is the thickest and toughest layer and consists of horn tubules that run distad parallel to the surface of the wall. The tubules are united by intertubular horn.

The horn tubules are round, oval, or wedge-shaped in cross section. They have a cortex and a medulla which are formed from the sides and the tip of a dermal papilla much like the cortex and medulla of a hair (compare Figs. 402 and 378). The cells of the stratum cylindricum that are attached to the sides of the papilla form with the papillary axis an acute angle that opens distally. The new cells that are formed by proliferation are pushed outward and distad, and cornify progressively as they go. At the same time these cells of the tubal cortex become oriented with their long axes parallel in cords and form three cortical zones (Figs. 402; 403,*b*). The cell cords of the inner zone are wrapped around the medulla in flat spirals (Fig. 404). Those of the middle zone are steeply spiraled, while the outer zone is composed of flat spirals. On the basis of the comparative development of these zones two types of tubules may be differentiated: those showing predominantly steep spirals (with a thick middle zone; Fig. 403,*A*,*b''*) and those showing mainly flat spirals (with a thick outer zone, Fig. 403,*B*,*b'''*). The steep-spiraled tubules are found in the inner portion of the stratum medium of the hoof wall and are said to be more elastic under the stress of weight bearing.[7]

The cells of the medulla of the horn tubules are formed by the stratum germinativum on the tips of the papillae. The medullary cells perform no supporting function. They begin to shrink as they are pushed more and more distad, until finally they are merely a mass of loose debris, comparable to the medulla of a feather. They may even separate from the tubule, leaving it hollow. The degree of this degeneration varies in different tubules.

The interpapillary portions of the stratum germinativum give rise to the intertubular horn (Figs. 402; 403,c), the cells of which also line up to form cords. The direction of these cords is oblique to the tubules and varies in different parts of the epidermis. The intertubular horn is more or less pigmented, except for the inner zone next to the laminae, which is always white. There is no formation of keratohyaline in the cornification of the stratum medium. This is characteristic of hard horn.

The *stratum lamellatum* (Fig. 406,c) is the true epidermis of the wall and consists of nonpigmented horny laminae. It is present wherever dermal laminae are found. The horny laminae are softer near the coronary region. Both dermis and epidermis are characterized by primary and secondary laminae (Fig. 407). The cells of the primary laminae of the epidermis cornify as they move distad, but the secondary laminae do not cornify.

The primary epidermal laminae are formed and pushed distad by the coronary stratum germinativum located between the proximal ends of the dermal laminae.[8] This laminar horn is thus continuous with the interpapillary or intertubular horn of the stratum medium. Lamellar, tubular, and intertubular horn are united into a solid mass, probably by tonofibrils. As the horny laminae move distad, they increase in height but only very slightly in thickness. The close bond between the horny laminae and the laminae of the corium is maintained by the uncornified cells of the secondary epidermal laminae. These cells are directed obliquely distad and multiply throughout the length of the laminae, but only enough to keep up with the downgrowth of the horny laminae. The cells produced in the process are added to the sides and edges of the horny laminae and become cornified, but there is little increase in the height and thickness of the horny laminae below the proximal third. The stratum spinosum is only one or two cells thick and cornification occurs without the formation of keratohyaline.

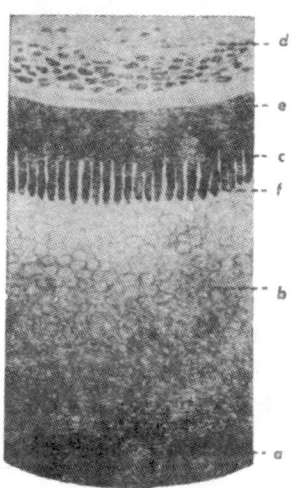

Figure 405. Transverse section through the horny wall and dermal laminae of the hoof of the horse (2×). *a*, periople; *b*, stratum medium; *c*, laminar horn (light); *d*, third phalanx; *e*, corium of the wall with *f*, its laminae (dark).

There is some confusion in the use of the terms *sensitive lamina* and *dermal lamina*. They are not synonymous. When the horny hoof is removed by maceration, the cornified and uncornified layers of the epidermis separate. The stratum germinativum is left on the dermal laminae, and the two tissues make up the sensitive laminae.[9]

Toward the distal border of the wall, where the dermal laminae end, the interstices between the horny laminae are filled in by tubular interlaminar horn. This

[8] Möller, Zur Anatomie und Physiologie der Huflederhaut, *Arch. Tierhlk. 3* (1877): 169–194.
[9] W. Baier, Über die Beziehungen zwischen Epidermis und Korium an Huf und Klaue, *Ber. tierärztl. Wschr.* (1950): 59–63.

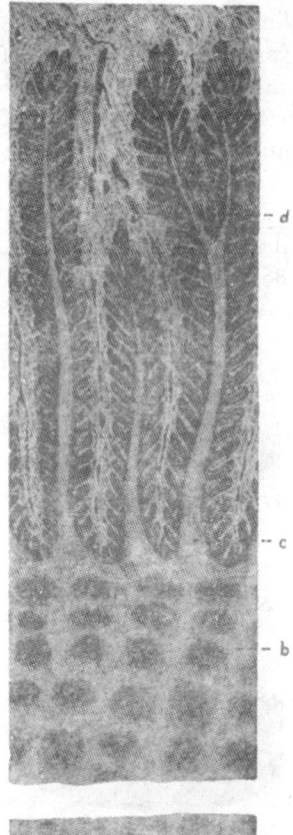

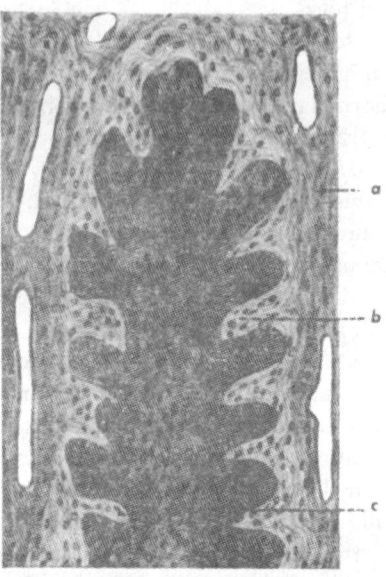

Figure 406 (*left*). Horizontal section through the horny wall and the corium of the wall of the equine hoof (45×). *a*, stratum tectorium; *b*, stratum medium; *c*, horny lamina; *d*, corium of the wall, showing its primary and secondary laminae and its rich vascular supply.

Figure 407. From a cross section through the bases of the dermal laminae of a newborn foal (200×). *a*, primary dermal lamina with vessels; *b*, secondary lamina; *c*, primary epidermal lamina with secondary laminae (right and left).

is produced by the epidermis of the papillae on the distal ends of the dermal laminae. The substance consisting of horny laminae and interlaminar horn forms the junction between the stratum medium of the wall and the edge of the horny sole. Together with the inner zone of the stratum medium it is called the *white line*.

The horny sole consists of firmly joined tubules and intertubular horn. Its superficial layers are easily peeled off in the form of flat scales. The horny bulbs and frog are composed of incompletely cornified horn tubules and intertubular horn. Together they represent the digital pad of carnivores.

2. The Claws of Ruminants and Swine

(a) **The corium** of the bovine claw resembles structurally the pododerm of the horse. The papillae of the perioplic and especially the coronary corium often possess longitudinal ridges and small secondary papillae. The coronary corium forms a very wide flat band. The corium of the sole is very thin and bears small, thickset papillae, which are curved and point craniad. The papillae of the bulb are larger (up to 1.5 mm.) and often compound. The sensitive laminae are not so high as

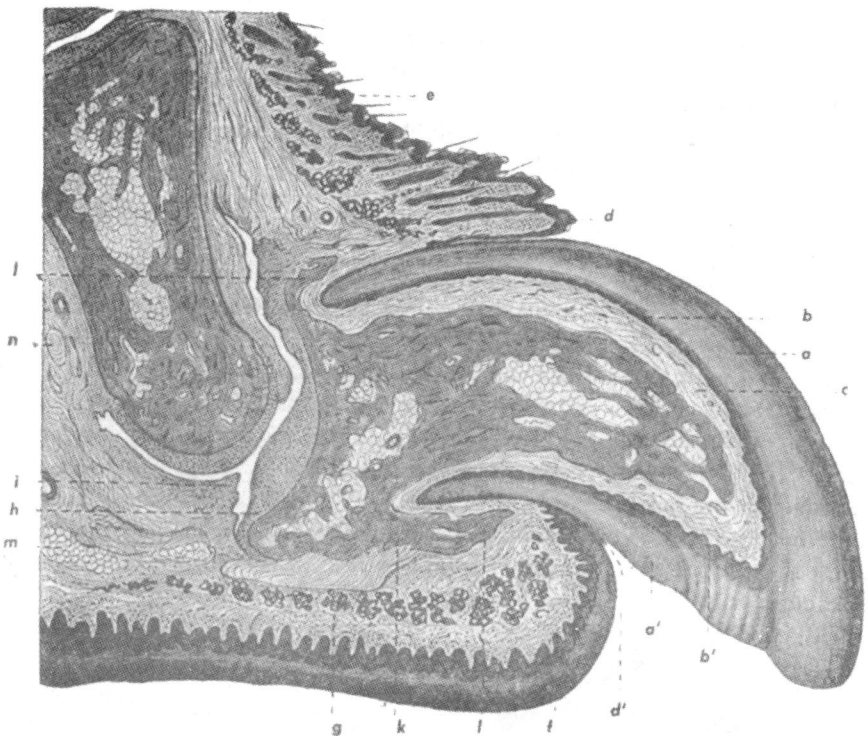

Figure 408. Mid-sagittal section through the claw of the dog. *a*, stratum corneum of the epidermis of the claw; *a'*, stratum corneum of the epidermis of the sole; *b,b'*, deep, non-cornified epidermal layers of the dorsum and sole of the claw; *c*, corium (papillated in the area of the sole); *d*, claw fold; *d'*, limiting furrow separating the sole from the digital pad; *e*, skin with hair and glands; *f*, epidermis of the digital pad with stratum granulosum and lucidum; *g*, tubular glands in the digital pad; *h*, articular cartilage of the third phalanx, bone shown in red; *i*, meniscus; *k*, Sharpey's fibers from a tendon insertion; *l*, ungual crest; *m*, fat cushion within the digital pad; *n*, lamellar corpuscle.

those of the horse. They lack secondary laminae and contain large veins. They curve around the edge of the sole and often end in several papillae.

(b) **The horny claw** of the ox is covered by a stratum tectorium produced by the periople, as in the horse. The middle and thickest layer of the horny wall consists of tough horn tubes bordered by intertubular horn. The innermost layer is made up of horny laminae, which lack secondary laminae. A large part of the ground surface of the claw is formed by a continuation of the horny bulb, which consists of tubular and intertubular horn and is often strongly fissured. Under the bulbar corium is the tough fibrous bulbar cushion (subcutis) containing elastic and adipose tissue. The true sole is restricted to a narrow zone next to the wall. It is difficult to distinguish from the bulbar portion externally but is characterized by harder horn, smaller papillae, the turned-under ends of the laminae, and the lack of a subcutis.[10]

The claws of the sheep and goat resemble those of the ox except that the thin,

[10] Ernst Wyssmann, Zur Anatomie der Klauenlederhaut, *Arch. Tierhlk.* **28** (1902): 577–625.

dense, elastic wall horn extends beyond the sole and both margins turn under. It is often fissured. Most of the ground surface is formed by the horny bulb, but the true sole is more apparent in these species than it is in the ox. The papillae of the sole corium are arranged in rows and fused basally. Similar conditions are found in the pig. The bulb is well differentiated from the sole.

The dewclaws resemble the main claws.

3. The Claws of Carnivores

(a) **The corium** of the claw is a continuation of the corium of the skin which has been reflected around the ungual crest of the third phalanx (Fig. 408,*l*) and covers the long ungual process. It is closely attached to the bone and forms its periosteum. The corium is divided into the coronary, wall, and sole corium.

The coronary corium begins down on the sides of the claw as a narrow flat band, becoming wider dorsally. On the dorsal surface it forms a beaklike thickening, the dorsal ridge (Fig. 409,*a*), which extends to the apex of the third phalanx. The dorsal ridge is more pronounced in the cat than in the dog. Its surface is smooth for the most part. Only on the proximal part of the coronary corium and, more rarely, on the dorsal ridge are rudimentary papillae seen. Most of the horny claw is formed on the coronary corium and dorsal ridge.

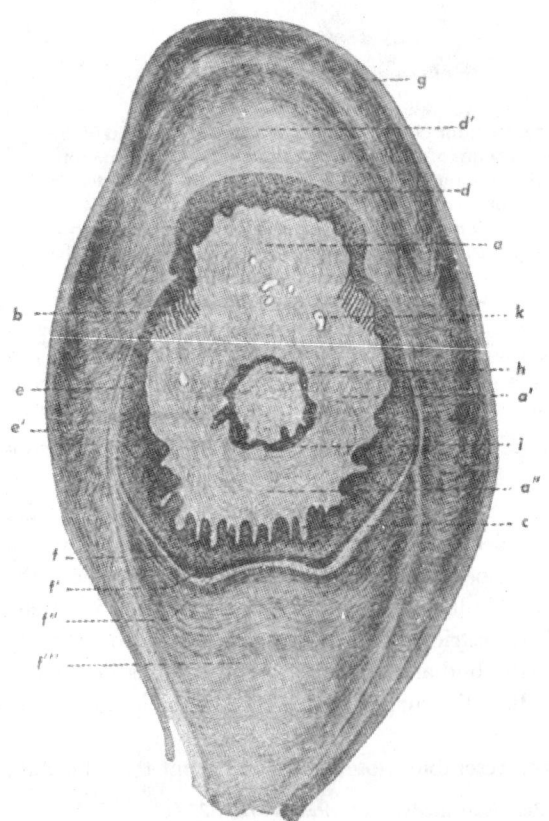

Figure 409. Cross section through the claw of the dog near the end of the third phalanx (37×). *a*, dorsal ridge; *a'*, wall corium; *a''*, corium of the sole; *b*, lamellae of the wall corium; *c*, papillae of the corium of the sole; *d*, epidermis of the dorsal ridge with *d'*, its stratum corneum; *e*, epidermis of the wall with *e'*, its stratum corneum; *f*, epidermis of the sole with *f'*, its stratum granulosum, *f''*, its stratum lucidum, and *f'''*, its stratum corneum; *g*, stratum tectorium; *h*, bone marrow; *i*, bone; *k*, blood vessel. *d'*, *e'*, and *f'''* constitute the horny claw; *d'* and *e'* make up the claw plate.

The corium of the wall (Fig. 409,*a'*) is separated into two parts by the dorsal ridge. It is applied to both sides of the third phalanx. Basally it has small, slender, distally pointing papillae. Toward the apex it bears delicate rudimentary lamellae, which are directed parallel to the dorsal ridge (Fig. 409,*b*).

The corium of the sole (Fig. 409,*a''*) of the dog bears numerous distally directed papillae. In the cat these are usually very low and extend for a short distance on the dorsal and lateral surfaces at the apex of the claw.

(b) The epidermis of the claw has a heavy stratum corneum, the horny claw. The curved *claw plate*, which covers the coronary corium and the corium of the wall (Fig. 409,*d'*,*e'*) is thicker in the area of the dorsal ridge. On the sides its thickness decreases, and its free horny margins extend beyond the horny sole and may sometimes meet each other. The strong stratum corneum of the claw plate consists of flat, cornified epidermal cells joined closely together and often strongly pigmented. They are usually parallel to the surface. The stratum germinativum is especially thick in the region of the dorsal ridge (*d*). The inner surface of the wall bears small, soft epidermal lamellae. The narrow, drawn-out epidermis of the *sole* also bears a heavy stratum corneum (Fig. 409,*f'''*), which contains only feeble vestiges of horn tubules or none at all. The more superficial layer is made up of loose, friable horn. The wall is sharply set off from the horny sole by its contrasting staining properties. The epidermis of the sole is characterized by the presence of a stratum granulosum and lucidum.

The *claw fold* (Fig. 408,*d*) is a fold of skin that covers the root of the plate dorsally and on the sides. Its inner surface is free from hair and fused to the horn of the plate. As the plate grows out it carries with it for a variable distance a thin stratum tectorium produced by the inner surface of the fold.

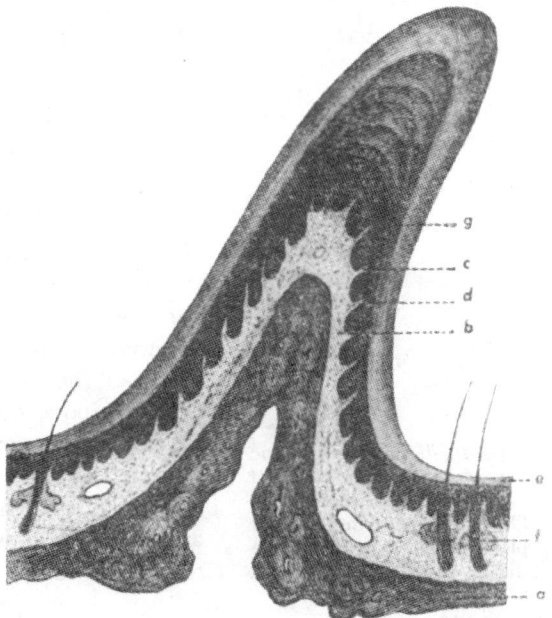

Figure 410. Longitudinal section through the horn and cornual process of the calf. *a*, cornual process of the frontal bone; *b*, corium covering *a; c*, dermal papillae; *d*, stratum germinativum; *e*, stratum corneum of the skin; *f*, hairs with sebaceous glands; *g*, stratum corneum of the cornual epidermis.

The claw fold is continuous with the *digital pad* on the volar surface (Figs. 376; 408,*f*). The pad is separated from the sole of the claw by a limiting furrow (*d'*). It has a subcutaneous cushion containing fat and tubular glands (*g*).

4. Chestnut and Ergot

Chestnut and ergot are structurally alike. They are free from hair and glands. The epidermis bears a heavy stratum corneum consisting of horn tubes and inter-tubular horn. The tough connective tissue corium forms a simple papillary body. The subcutis is thickened and heavily infiltrated with fatty tissue, especially in the region of the ergot.

5. The Horns

The cavity of the cornual process (Fig. 410,*a*), which forms the core of the horns, is a diverticulum of the frontal sinus and, like the sinus, is lined by a continuation of the respiratory mucosa, which also serves as periosteum. On the outside the cornual process is covered by the periosteum and the corium of the horn (*b*). The two are fused.

(a) **The corium** of the horn possesses filiform, apically directed papillae (*c*) or ridges (rudimentary dermal laminae) that bear papillae. Near the base of the process the papillae are larger and form something like a coronary band.

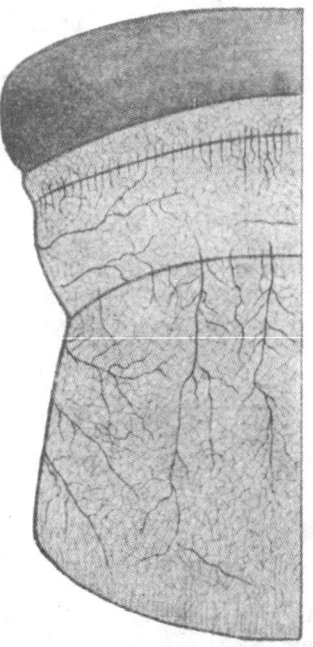

Figure 411. Diagrammatic representation of the course of the nerves in the pododerm. Only the larger nerves and plexuses in one plane are shown. (After Krawarik.)

(b) **The epidermis** of the horn, whose thick stratum corneum constitutes the horny sheath (*g*), forms at the root of the horn the soft epikeras. This projects only a short distance beyond the root of the horn and usually shows desquamation of horny scales. It corresponds to the periople of the hoof. The main substance of the horn is composed of fine tubules, which contain medullary substance in the central portion of the horn only. Otherwise they contain air. In some cases the tubules and especially their cortex are not so typical and easily recognized as in the wall of the hoof.

The horn tubules are connected by loose inter-tubular horn, which is very abundant in sheep, less abundant in the goat, and scarce in cattle. In particularly dense bovine horns it may be entirely lacking. The formation of rings around the horns is due to periodic changes in the rate of growth. Each ring visible on the surface is the basal margin of a cone of horn produced during a growth period (*g*).

VESSELS AND NERVES OF THE CORIUM OF HORNY STRUCTURES. The blood vessels are arranged in several layers of anastomosing plexuses, in which arteriovenous anastomoses occur. In the laminae the vessels course along the center of the lamina and form superficial capillary nets. In the papillae the vessels show a disposition similar to that in the intestinal villi. Venous plexuses are present in all parts of the pododerm. They are especially extensive in the region of the lateral cartilages. Dense venous plexuses are also present in the perioplic and coronary cushions. The veins lack valves.

The lymphatics show an arrangement similar to that in the rest of the skin. Underlying the papillae of the sensitive sole and frog is a large lymph vessel. There is also a large lymphatic in the base of each lamina. It drains the vessels of the lamina. In the stratum reticulare the lymphatics lie side by side with the blood vessels.

The nerves form interconnected networks in all parts of the pododerm of domestic mammals. The plexuses ascend from the deeper strata of the corium to the more superficial layers. Immediately below the papillae or laminae the nerve plexuses exhibit the smallest meshes and the finest fibers, but also the greatest density of fibers. Fine nerve fiber plexuses are continued into the papillae and laminae. The nerve endings in the pododerm are varied and many. In addition to arborizations of fibers, there are bulb and club-shaped terminal corpuscles as well as various forms of lamellar corpuscles.

XVIII

The Ear

A. THE EXTERNAL AND MIDDLE EAR

1. Auricle

THE basis of the auricle (pinna, concha) is a curved plate consisting largely of elastic cartilage. It is covered by skin, which on the concave surface contains large sebaceous glands and small tubular glands.

2. External Auditory Meatus

The wall of the external auditory meatus is partly cartilaginous (Fig. 412,*d*) and partly osseous. The cartilaginous portion is connected to the bony part by tough connective tissue. It is composed of the annular cartilage and the proximal end of the conchal cartilage, both of which are mainly elastic. The external auditory meatus is lined by a cutaneous membrane, which is a continuation of the skin and includes stratified squamous epithelium, hair, and sebaceous and tubular glands (Fig. 412). Some of the sebaceous glands are associated with hair follicles, but others occur independently. The tubular glands are a modification of the ordinary tubular glands of the body surface. They have a wide lumen. The simple columnar secretory epithelium elaborates a mucous fluid and yellowish pigment granules. The mixture of the secretions of both kinds of glands is the ear wax, or cerumen. The subcutaneous tissue in the osseous meatus is rich in vessels and resembles a corpus cavernosum.

In herbivores glands and hairs are present only in the cartilaginous portion. In the pig tubular glands are also found in the osseous section, while in carnivores hairs and both types of glands occur in the cartilaginous and osseous parts. The sebaceous glands in the osseous meatus are large and resemble the tarsal glands of the eyelid.

3. Tympanic Membrane

This membrane consists of a cutaneous layer, a lamina propria, and a mucous membrane. The cutaneous layer is loosely, the mucosa firmly, connected with the lamina propria. The cutaneous layer is the thin continuation of the skin of the external meatus and lacks papillary body, hairs, and glands. The collagenous lamina propria consists of a taut outer layer of radial collagenous fibers and a medial sheet of circular fibers. The two layers are not very firmly joined. At the point of insertion of the malleus, they become interwoven and pass into its periosteum. The mucosa lacks glands and bears simple squamous epithelium.

The blood vessels form cutaneous and mucosal capillary plexuses, which anastomose with each other as they spread out between the fibers of the lamina propria. The tissue spaces of the lamina propria communicate with the lymphatic

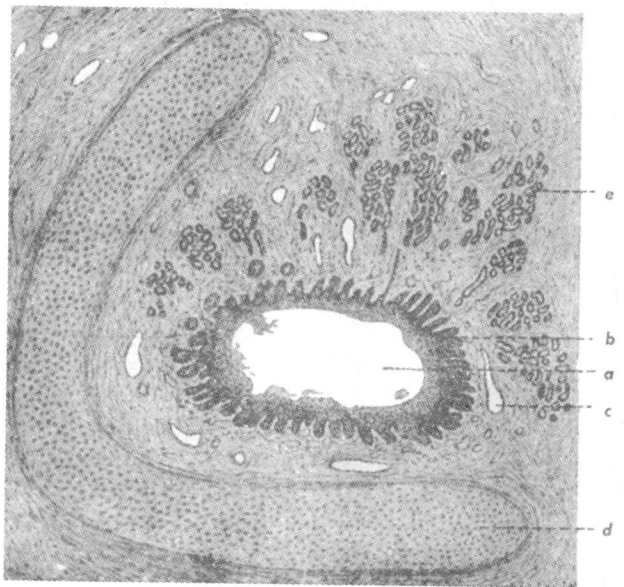

Figure 412. Cross section through the cartilaginous external auditory meatus of the pig. *a,* lumen; *b,* squamous epithelium; *c,* vein; *d,* cartilage; *e,* tubular glands. On the left, immediately below the epithelium, are sections of sebaceous glands.

networks in the cutaneous and mucosal layers. Dense nerve plexuses are present in all three layers.

4. Tympanic Cavity

This chamber is enclosed by bone. The osseous wall is spongy in the horse, ox, and pig, and compact in the sheep, goat and dog. In the cat it is double with a space between the two plates of bone. The lateral wall of the cavity is formed by the tympanic membrane, the medial wall by the osseous labyrinth of the inner ear (see p. 373). Extending across the cavity is a chain of three small bones, the auditory ossicles. They are named, beginning at the tympanic membrane, the malleus, incus, and stapes (hammer, anvil, and stirrup). The base of the stapes is fixed in the *fenestra ovalis* of the medial wall by a fibroelastic ligament. Another opening in the medial wall, the *fenestra rotunda*, is closed by the secondary tympanic membrane.

The periosteum of the tympanic cavity is covered by a thin mucosa bearing a usually two-layered ciliated columnar epithelium, which shows cryptlike diverticula. It is especially high in the region of the opening of the Eustachian tube. Simple squamous epithelium is found in the ventral portion of the tympanic cavity and on the tympanic membrane, the auditory ossicles, and the secondary tympanic membrane. In the nasal portion of the cavity of man, carnivores, and sheep a serous alveolar gland is found.

The external ear receives and conveys sounds. The vibrations of the air cause

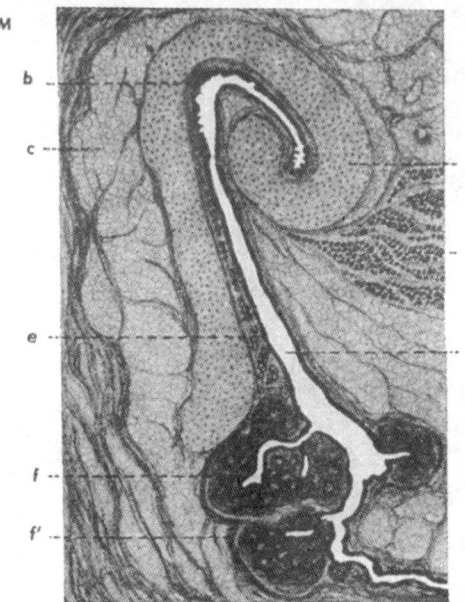

Figure 413. Cross section through the pharyngeal part of the Eustachian tube of the pig. *a*, cartilage; *b*, mucosa; *c*, adipose tissue; *d*, tubal muscle; *e*, glands; *f*, tubal tonsil showing crypts and *f'*, capsule; *g*, lumen; *L*, lateral; *M*, medial side.

the tympanic membrane to vibrate. The auditory ossicles relay these vibrations to the fibroelastic membrane covering the fenestra ovalis. An equalization of the air pressure in the cavity with that outside is necessary for the normal transmission of sound. This equalization is accomplished by the Eustachian tube, which opens during swallowing.

5. Eustachian Tube (Pharyngotympanic Tube)

The Eustachian tube consists of osseous and cartilaginous segments (Fig. 413). The cartilaginous portion is supported by a trough-shaped plate of cartilage, which is hyaline in newborn animals but later becomes elastic. The mucosa bears pseudostratified ciliated epithelium containing goblet cells. The propria contains flat nets of elastic fibers and deposits of lymphatic tissue. In some areas this occurs as nodules, and near the pharyngeal opening in ruminants and swine it forms the tubal tonsil (*f*). Mucous and mixed glands occur in the propria and submucosa and are especially numerous in sheep. Beneath the mucosa or cartilage a cushion of fat is present, especially laterally. It is invaded by the striated musculature of the tube.

The function of the *guttural pouches* of the horse (Fig. 414) is still unsettled. Their mucosa bears ciliated pseudostratified epithelium with goblet cells. Elastic and smooth muscle fibers are arranged in layers in the collagenous propria. The propria also contains mucous and serous glands and lymph nodules. The fibroelastic adventitia includes abundant adipose tissue, large blood vessels, and nerves.

B. THE INNER EAR

The inner ear, or labyrinth, is contained in a system of canals and cavities lined by periosteum and surrounded by bone containing islands of cartilage, the *osseous labyrinth.*

The *membranous labyrinth* (Fig. 415) is composed of the pars statica or vestibular organ, which includes two membranous sacs and the membranous semicircular canals, and the pars auditiva or cochlear duct. The two sacs, called the *sacculus* (*b*) and *utriculus* (*a*), are connected by ducts which join in a Y to form the endo-

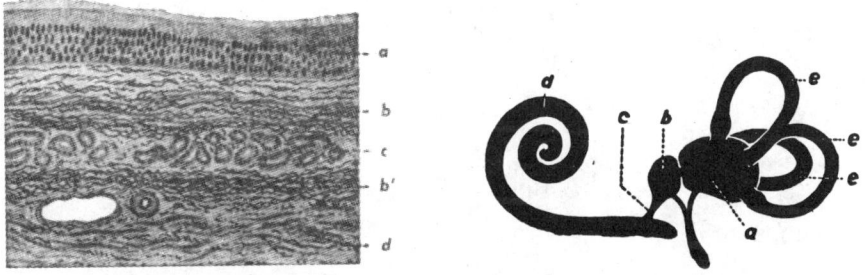

Figure 414 (left). Section through the wall of the guttural pouch of the horse. *a*, ciliated pseudostratified epithelium; *b*, propria mucosae with smooth muscle cells and a subepithelial layer of elastic fibers; *b'*, subglandular layer of elastic fibers; *c*, glands; *d*, adventitia.

Figure 415 (right). Diagram of the membranous labyrinth. *a*, utriculus; *b*, sacculus; *c*, ductus reuniens; *d*, cochlea; *e*, semicircular canals.

lymphatic duct. This passes through a canal in the bone, the vestibular aqueduct, and widens into the endolymphatic sac just outside the dura mater. From the sacculus the short ductus reuniens (*c*) leads into the ductus cochlearis (*d*). On the utriculus are situated the three membranous *semicircular canals,* the initial portions of which are enlarged into the *ampullae.*

1. Vestibular Organ

The wall of this structure is formed by a richly vascularized, lamellar stratum of connective tissue, lined by a simple squamous epithelium. On the concave surface of the semicircular canals a strip of columnar epithelium is present, which extends into the ampullae and forms the raphe.

The membranous structures are filled with endolymph. With the exception of the ampullae they are smaller than the corresponding spaces in the bone. Their walls touch the osseous wall with only one surface, namely the medial side of the sacculus and utriculus, and the convex side of the canals. At these points they are

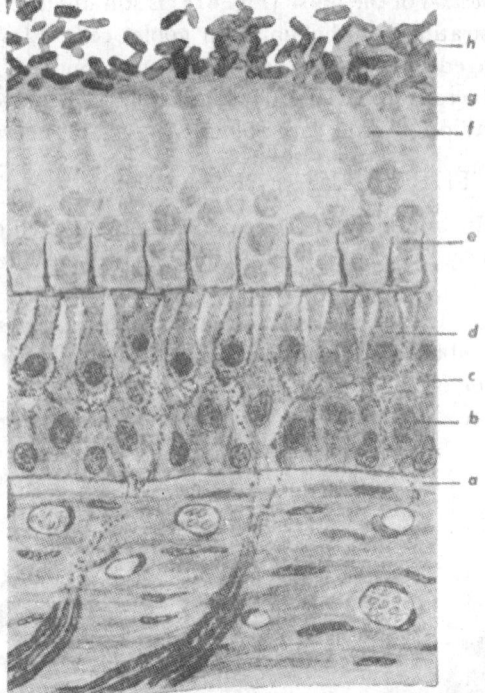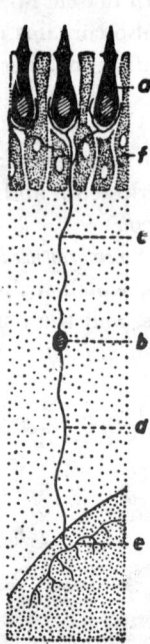

Figure 416 (left). Section from the macula sacculi of the horse (750×). *a*, basement membrane showing perforating unmyelinated nerve fibers; *b*, sustentacular cells; *c*, nerve plexus; *d*, hair cells; *e*, globules (artefacts?) in the endolymph around the hair tufts; *f*, otolithic membrane; *g*, cover layer; *h*, otoliths. (After Cohrs.)

Figure 417 (right). Diagram of the macula and crista statica. *a*, hair cells; *b*, nerve cell; *c*, nerve fiber conducting toward the cell body, its fibrils ending near the hair cells; *d*, nerve fiber conducting away from the cell body and, *e*, its ending in the brain; *f*, sustentacular cells.

fused with the periosteum. The unoccupied space contains the perilymph and is bridged in certain areas by collagenous trabeculae, which support the vessels and extend from the periosteum to the walls of the vestibular organ. The perilymphatic spaces are directly continuous with the scala vestibuli of the cochlea (see below). They are lined with a mesenchymal epithelium.

The areas to which the vestibular nerve is distributed can be recognized with the unaided eye: the *maculae utriculi* and *sacculi* are white oval spots, while on the ampullae of the semicircular canals they appear as transverse bars, called the *cristae ampullares.* Here all layers of the wall are thickened and the subepithelial layer contains many cells, including pigment cells. In the outer layer a plexus of myelinated nerves (Fig. 416) is present, which gives rise to numerous fibers that ascend toward the epithelium, lose their myelin sheaths, pass through the basement membrane, and enter the epithelium.

The simple neuroepithelium is composed of two types of cells: the hair cells and the sustentacular cells. The sustentacular cells (Figs. 416,b; 417,f) are slender supporting cells with oval nuclei. They are attached with wide or narrow bases to the basement membrane and extend to the free surface. Between their distal ends lie the short columnar hair cells. The rounded bulbous base of the hair cell contains a deeply staining nucleus. These cells extend only to the middle of the epithelial layer. The distal end of the hair cells is formed by a round plate. From this arises the sensory tuft, consisting of thin long cilia cemented together. In the area surrounding the maculae and cristae the squamous epithelium becomes simple columnar. Its cells bear a cuticle on their free surfaces, which is continued on the sustentacular cells of the neuroepithelium. Here it forms a continuous framework around the distal plates of the hair cells.

The fibers of the vestibular nerve (Fig. 416,c) lose their myelin upon entering the epithelium and continue between the sustentacular cells to the basis of the hair cells. Here the axis cylinders break up and form plexuses, from which numerous fine fibrils arise to end on the sides or in the superficial layer of cytoplasm of the hair cells.

The neuroepithelium of the maculae is covered by the otolithic membrane (Fig. 416,f), which is supported by the sensory hairs. There is an endolymphatic space between the cells and the membrane. In histological preparations acidophilic, albuminous globules are found between the hair tufts. The membrane itself is made up of a soft gelatinous layer, which shows alternate dark fibrillar and light structureless columns and is covered by a denser layer. The light columns are endolymphatic spaces around the hair tufts. On top of this membrane lies a stratum of minute prisms of calcium carbonate, called the otoliths (h). The neuroepithelium of the cristae ampullares is covered by the gelatinous cupula, which is bell-shaped in cross section and consists of dark fibrillar columns and light endolymphatic spaces around the hair tufts. The cupula, as well as the gelatinous portion of the otolithic membrane, is probably greatly altered by fixation.

The ductus reuniens and the endolymphatic duct consist of a thin collagenous lamina propria and flat polygonal epithelium.

The hair cells of the maculae and cristae are the sensory terminations of the vestibular nerve and register changes in the position of the head. Therefore they play a part in the maintenance of equilibrium. The hair cells of the maculae are stimulated by the pressure or traction of the otoliths, while those of the cristae are stimulated by a shifting of the endolymph within the semicircular canals.

2. Cochlea

This organ is composed of a number of structures, some of which are highly complex. Descriptions of the cochlea usually presume it to be in an upright position with its base downward. The terms inner or central are used in reference to the axis of the spiral.

The cochlea (Fig. 418) is divided into two compartments by a horizontal partition, the *spiral lamina*. The lamina is osseous near the bony axis of the cochlea

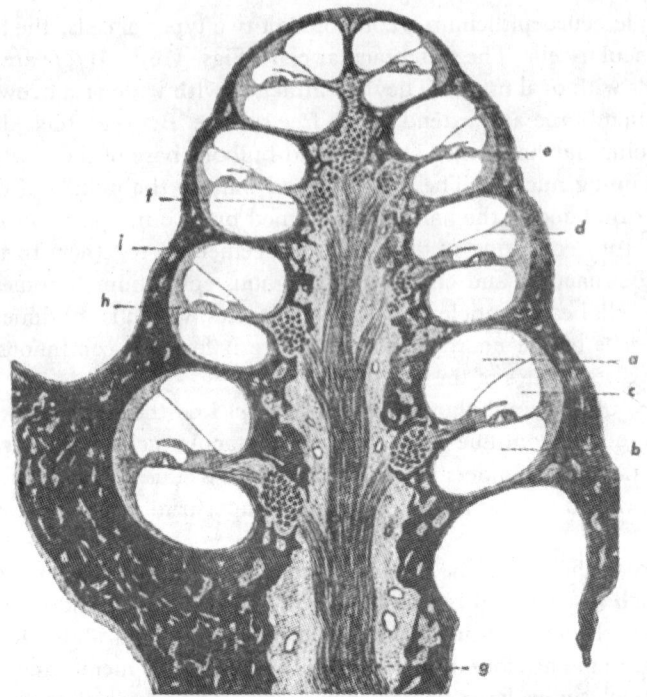

Figure 418. Axial section through the cochlea of the guinea pig
(16×). *a*, scala vestibuli; *b*, scala tympani; *c*, cochlear duct;
d, vestibular membrane; *e*, organ of Corti; *f*, spiral ganglion;
g, cochlear nerve; *h*, spiral ligament; *i*, osseous cochlea.

(modiolus) but is entirely membranous in the peripheral portion, which is called
the basilar membrane. Of the two compartments the upper one is called the *scala
vestibuli* (*a*), the lower one the *scala tympani* (*b*). The spiral lamina does not extend
to the blind end (apex) of the cochlea, so that the two compartments communicate
by a passage called the helicotrema.

Between the abaxial portions of the two scalae lies the *cochlear duct*, a trilateral
tube (*c*). The cochlear duct of the horse, sheep, and goat makes $2\frac{1}{4}$ turns, that of
carnivores 3, of the ox $3\frac{1}{2}$, and of swine 4. The scalae vestibuli and tympani are
perilymphatic spaces, which communicate with the perilymphatic space of the vestibule. They are lined by collagenous periosteum covered by flat mesenchymal epithelium. They communicate with the subarachnoid space through the cochlear
aqueduct from the scala tympani.

The cochlear duct, on the other hand, is an endolymphatic space. Its wall is a
continuation of the membranous walls of the sacculus and utriculus. Its lumen communicates by way of the ductus reuniens (Fig. 415,*c*) with the sacculus and thereby
with the utriculus. The cochlear duct (Fig. 419) is considered to have three walls:
peripheral, vestibular, and tympanic.

The peripheral wall is fused with the periosteum, which is at this point greatly

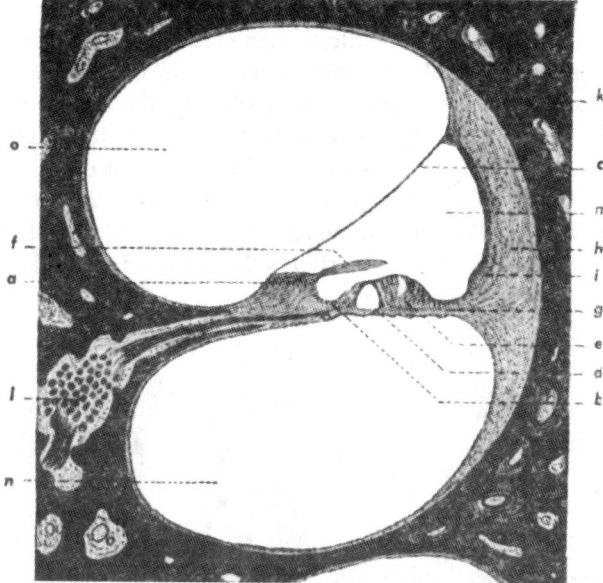

Figure 419. Cross section through the cochlea. *a*, labium vestibulare, *b*, labium tympanicum of the limbus spiralis; *c*, vestibular membrane; *d*, tunnel of Corti; *e*, organ of Corti; *f*, tectorial membrane; *g*, crista basilaris; *h*, ligamentum spirale; *i*, prominentia spiralis; *k*, osseous wall of the cochlea; *l*, spiral ganglion; *m*, cochlear duct; *n*, scala tympani; *o*, scala vestibuli.

thickened and covered by cuboidal epithelium. It is called the ligamentum spirale (*h*) and is thickest at the crista basilaris where the basilar membrane (*g*) is attached. The depression between the crista basilaris and the prominentia spiralis (*i*) is called the external spiral sulcus. From this area to the point of attachment of the vestibular membrane (*c*) extends the pigmented stria vascularis, a strip of cuboidal epithelium, which is invaded by capillaries from the connective tissue. The epithelial cells seem to secrete the endolymph.

The upper, vestibular wall consists of the thin, tightly stretched *vestibular membrane* (of Reissner), the cochlear surface of which bears a simple flat epithelium. The vestibular surface is covered by the mesenchymal epithelium of the scala vestibuli. The vestibular membrane, which in ruminants is richly vascularized, extends from the ligamentum spirale to the labium vestibulare. Most of the limbus spiralis (see below) is included in the cochlear duct.

The lower, tympanic wall of the cochlear duct (Figs. 419, 420) is divided into two parts. The axial part, called the limbus spiralis, arises by considerable thickening of the periosteum of the osseous lamina spiralis, while the peripheral part is formed by the basilar membrane. The line of demarcation between the two parts is the perforated zone, where the cochlear nerve fibers penetrate into the epithelium.

The limbus spiralis (Fig. 420,*a*) consists of very dense connective tissue fibers, which include many star- and spindle-shaped cells. It begins at the line of attachment of the vestibular membrane and terminates in two lips, which enclose the internal spiral sulcus (*b*). This is lined by cuboidal epithelium. One of the lips projects freely into the lumen of the cochlear duct. This is the labium vestibulare. The other one, which is continued by the basilar membrane, is called the labium tympanicum (Fig. 420,*c*). The surface of the limbus spiralis, when viewed from above, is seen to be covered with ridges which form projections at the labium vestibulare, called the auditory teeth (of Huschke). The hillocks, ridges, and furrows are covered by a single layer of flat epithelial cells.

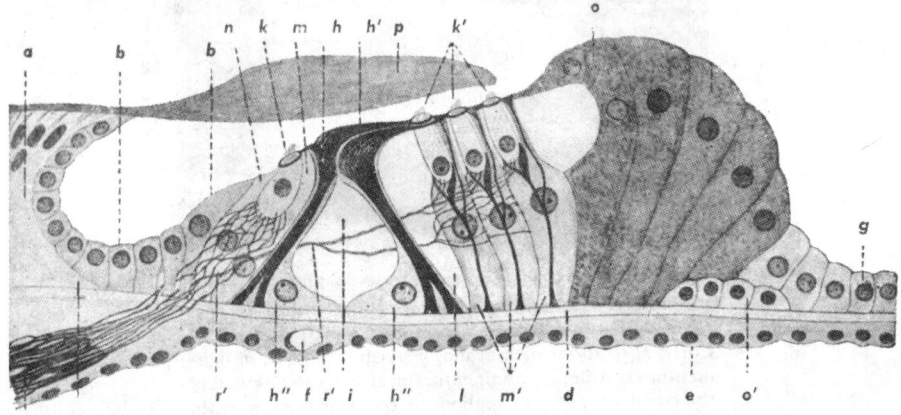

Figure 420. Diagram of the organ of Corti. *a*, limbus spiralis; *b*, epithelium of the internal sulcus; *c*, labium tympanicum; *d*, basilar membrane; *e*, tympanic covering layer; *f*, vas spirale; *g*, cells of Claudius; *h*, inner, *h'*, outer pillar cells; *h''*, basal nucleated part of pillar cells; *i*, tunnel of Corti; *k*, inner, *k'*, outer hair cells; *l*, space of Nuel; *m*, inner phalangeal cell; *m'*, outer phalangeal cells (supporting cells of Deiters); *n*, inner border cell; *o*, cell of Hensen; *o'*, germinal layer; *p*, tectorial membrane; *r*, myelinated nerve fibers of the cochlear nerve; *r'*, unmyelinated nerve fibers continued by *r*. (From Cohrs.)

The *basilar membrane* (Fig. 420,*d*) has a lamina propria known as the layer of basilar fibers. This layer contains in its homogeneous ground substance numerous fibers which extend from the labium tympanicum to the crista basilaris. These are very fine and interwoven in the axial part. In the peripheral half of the membrane, however, starting at the base of the outer pillar cell (see below), they become thicker, run a straight course, and are known in that part as auditory strings. They pass into the fibers of the spiral ligament. The tympanic side of the basilar membrane bears an extension of the periosteum lining the scala tympani, the tympanic covering layer. This is a thin layer of connective tissue which contains spindle cells and, slightly peripheral to the labium tympanicum, the vena spiralis. This blood vessel courses along the entire cochlear duct and may be double. On the cochlear side the vestibular covering layer contains radially arranged nuclei in a homogeneous ground substance. ·

The *organ of Corti* (basilar papilla, spiral organ; Figs. 419,*e;* 420) is located on the basilar membrane, where it appears in cross sections of the cochlea as a trapezoid elevation or papilla. It consists of sustentacular cells, hair cells, and the tectorial membrane and contains the endings of the cochlear nerve.

Among the sustentacular cells the *pillar cells* are the most conspicuous (Fig. 420,*h,h',h''*). They occur in two rows, the inner and outer pillars, which are slanted toward each other like the rafters of a roof. Together with the basilar membrane they form the tunnel of Corti, which is filled with a soft intercellular substance. The pillar cells are modified epithelial cells, the cytoplasm of which forms a thin sheath around the fibrils of the pillar, while the basal cell portion with the nucleus is wide where it attaches to the basilar membrane. The bodies of the pillars do not touch; clefts remain between them allowing for the circulation of fluids. The basal parts of the pillar cells, on the other hand, are in apposition.

The *hair cells* stand obliquely on either side of the tunnel of Corti (Fig. 420,*k,k'*). They are connected with the fibers of the cochlear nerve and number 16,000 to 20,000 in man.

We recognize inner and outer hair cells. They are flask-shaped and bear on their round cuticular plate a number (15 in the horse) of rodlike auditory hairs, which are arranged in a curved row. The spheroid nucleus is basal. The cells do not extend to the basilar membrane. Below them are Nuel's spaces (Fig. 420,*l*), which communicate with each other and with the tunnel of Corti. The inner hair cells (*k*) lie in a row along the inner pillars. The cuticular plates of the pillar cells give off horizontal processes, which extend between the distal ends of the inner hair cells. On the inner surface of the inner hair cells are the border cells (*n*). These are attached to the basilar membrane near the perforated zone. They are arranged in one (as in pig and carnivores) or several (in horse and ruminants) rows. Their nearly rectangular cuticular plates are apposed peripherally to the inner hair cells, while axially they border on slender columnar cells (*b*), which decrease in height until they pass into the cuboidal epithelium of the sulcus spiralis internus. The outer hair cells (*k'*) form three rows (4 in the dog) adjoining the tunnel of Corti. They differ from the inner hair cells in that their auditory hairs are shorter, more numerous, and arranged in a horseshoe pattern. The cytoplasm is more granular.

Between the inner pillar and hair cells is found a layer of inner *phalangeal cells* (*m*), which are difficult to fix and usually appear in sections as vacuolized masses. The outer hair cells are maintained in their position by the outer phalangeal cells (of Deiters; *m'*). The number of rows of outer phalangeal cells equals that of outer hair cells. The body of the phalangeal cell is attached to the basilar membrane. A slender process extends between the hair cells and expands at the surface to form a phalangeal plate. These plates are elongated radially and notched on the sides to receive the heads of the hair cells. The outer phalangeal plates are connected to form the reticular membrane. The cuticles of the outer hair cells are fixed in the holes of the membrane.

Outside the outer phalangeal cells, on the outer slope of the organ of Corti, lie the prismatic cells of Hensen (*o*), which become lower peripherally and finally pass into the cells of Claudius (*g*). The cells of Claudius are low, undifferentiated epithelial cells. They cover the remainder of the basilar membrane and often extend to the spiral prominence. In the basal turn of the cochlea four to six rows of cells are wedged between the cells of Hensen and those of Claudius. These cells do not extend to the surface and are characterized by their granular, strongly staining cytoplasm. They are presumably arrested in their development. All sustentacular cells contain a diplosome near their distal pole.

The *tectorial membrane* (Fig. 420,*p*) is a finely striated membrane, which arises on the upper surface of the labium vestibulare by a thin stalk. It thickens distally

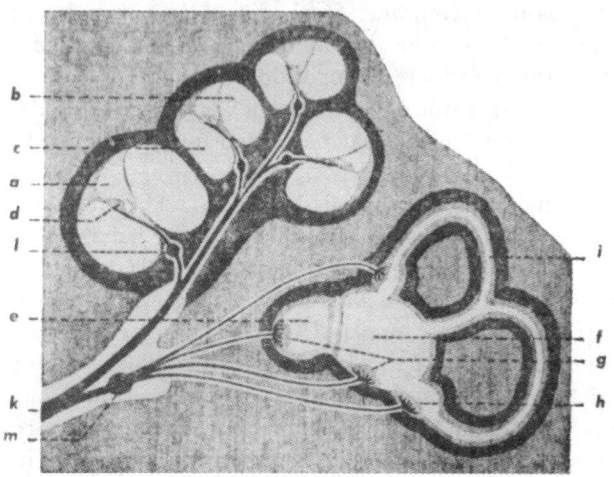

Figure 421. Diagram of nerve distribution in the labyrinth. *a*, cochlear duct; *b*, scala vestibuli; *c*, scala tympani; *d*, organ of Corti; *e*, sacculus; *f*, utriculus; *g*, maculae staticae; *h*, crista ampullaris in *i*, the semicircular canals (only two are shown); *k*, acoustic nerve; *l*, spiral ganglion; *m*, vestibular ganglion.

and covers the organ of Corti, extending to the most peripheral row of hair cells. It exhibits delicate fibers embedded in a weakly staining, homogeneous matrix.

The vibrations relayed by the auditory ossicles to the oval window are passed on to the perilymph of the scalae and thence to the organ of Corti. When the basilar membrane is set into vibration, the hairs of the sensory cells are stimulated rhythmically by contact with the tectorial membrane. This stimulus is transmitted to the nerve endings on the hair cells and is conveyed via the spiral ganglion and the cochlear nerve to the brain, where it is resolved into a sensation of sound.

VESSELS AND NERVES OF THE INNER EAR. The blood vessels are derived from the labyrinthine artery, which divides into vestibular and cochlear branches. Their capillary networks communicate with other vascular beds only in the internal acoustic meatus and at the openings of the two aqueducts. The veins of the cochlea are located in the wall of the scala tympani. The vena spiralis is found directly under the organ of Corti in the tympanic covering layer of the basilar membrane.

The endolymphatic and perilymphatic spaces serve as lymphatics in the inner ear. From the endolymphatic space arises the endolymphatic duct, located in the vestibular aqueduct. It leads into the endolymphatic sac, which is considered to be an organ of resorption for fluids and particulate matter from the membranous labyrinth. This sac is said to communicate with the extradural space by minute tubules. The perilymphatic spaces communicate with the subarachnoid space by the perilymphatic duct, which arises at the scala tympani and courses through the cochlear aqueduct.

The nerves of the labyrinth are derived from the acoustic nerve (eighth cranial). This nerve consists of a vestibular and cochlear branch, each of which arises from its own nucleus. The vestibular nerve divides into several branches supplying the hair cells of the maculae of the sacculus and utriculus and the cristae of the semicircular canals (Fig. 421). The cochlear nerve is located in the modiolus of the cochlea, extending to the tip. Along its course it receives many tufts of fibers (Fig. 418,*g;* 421). Each of these fibers is the axon of a bipolar nerve cell located in the spiral ganglion. The ganglion forms an uninterrupted chain along the line of origin of the osseous spiral lamina. The dendrites of the ganglion cells form a plexus which occupies the entire width of the osseous spiral lamina and splits the latter into two strata (Fig. 419). At the internal spiral sulcus the nerve fibers lose their sheaths and pass through slitlike openings (foramina nervorum) to the hair cells (Fig. 420,*r'*). Some fibers run a straight radial course to the cells. Others turn in the direction of the cochlear spiral, forming strands, the first of which courses inside the inner pillars, the second in the tunnel, and the remaining ones inside each row of the outer phalangeal cells. The strands give off fine fibers that end on the hair cells.

THE EAR OF THE CHICKEN. There is no auricle. The tympanic cavity is traversed by a thin cartilaginous rod, the columella. The cochlea is a tube shaped like the scabbard of a saber but with a slight spiral twist. The basilar membrane is stretched between two small cartilaginous bars. The cochlear duct is separated from the scala vestibuli by the highly vascular tegmentum vasculosum. The tectorial membrane is attached at both edges. The cells of the organ of Corti as well as the other components resemble the corresponding elements in mammals.

XIX

The Eye

THE eye consists of the eyeball, its protective organs (lids and lacrimal apparatus), and the oculomotor apparatus.

A. THE EYEBALL

The wall of the bulbus oculi is composed of the outer, middle, and inner tunics. The outer tunic consists of the cornea and sclera; the middle tunic, of the chorioid membrane, ciliary body, and iris; and the inner tunic, of the retina. The contents of the eyeball are the lens, the vitreous body, and the aqueous humor. In descriptions of the eyeball the terms anterior and posterior refer to the poles—the ends of the optic axis, which passes through the center of the cornea, lens, and vitreous body. The terms inner and outer refer to relative distances from the center of the eyeball.

1. The Fibrous (External) Tunic

The fibrous tunic is tough and firm, consists of fibrous connective tissue, and is poorly vascularized. The cornea is avascular.

(a) **The sclera** (Figs. 422,b; 433,e) is a highly resistant protective membrane covering the greater portion of the eyeball. It consists of dense fibrous connective tissue containing elastic fibers, flat fibroblasts, and pigment cells, which become more numerous near the chorioid and at the entrance of the optic nerve. At this point the sclera is perforated like a sieve and is called lamina cribrosa or cribriform area. The sclera is also penetrated by canals which convey vessels and nerves to the chorioid. Peripherally the sclera passes into the loose, vascular episcleral tissue. On its inner surface near the cornea the sclera shows a thickening, the *scleral roll* (Figs. 422; 428,b), which is especially well developed in carnivores. Inside the scleral roll and anterior to it is the *border ring* (Fig. 428,2) composed of predominantly circular elastic and collagenous fibers. It forms the posterior limit of the meshwork at the angle of the iris (p. 390). It is strong in the horse, poorly developed in swine, carnivores, and man. Between the border ring and the scleral roll lies the circular *plexus venosus sclerae* (Fig. 428,1), which corresponds to the canal of Schlemm in man.

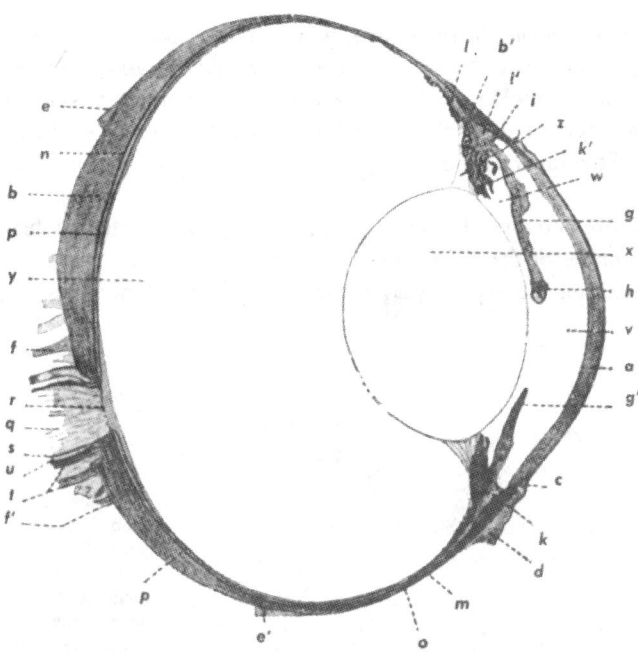

Figure 422. Sagittal section through the eyeball of the goat. *a*, cornea; *b*, sclera; *b'*, scleral roll; *c*, corneoscleral junction; *d*, bulbar conjunctiva; *e*, m. rectus dorsalis; *e'*. m. rectus ventralis; *f,f'*, m. retractor oculi; *g*, iris; *g'*, m. sphincter pupillae; *h*, granula iridis; *i*, iris process; *i'* spaces of Fontana; *k*, ciliary crown; *k'*, ciliary processes; *l*, ciliary muscle; *m*, ciliary ring; *n*, chorioid; *o*, ora serrata; *p*, retina; *q*, optic nerve; *r*, lamina cribrosa; *s*, pia mater; *t*, dura mater of the optic nerve; *u*, arachnoid space; *v*, anterior chamber; *w*, posterior chamber; *x*, lens; *y*, vitreous body; *z*, zonula ciliaris. (After Zietschmann.)

Blood vessels are few. They arise from the episcleral vascular plexus and form a wide-meshed net of fine capillaries. A system of tissue spaces is present in the sclera. It is an extensively branching network of clefts, which contain the interconnected fibroblasts. The nerves are derived from the trunks lying between the sclera and the tunica vasculosa and are mostly vasomotor. Sensory fibers are also present, especially near the corneoscleral junction.

(b) **The cornea** (Figs. 422,*a;* 423) is the site of entrance of the light rays. It is covered by five to twelve layers of squamous *corneal epithelium* (Fig. 423,*a*), the uppermost cell layers of which do not cornify but remain soft and nucleated. The adjoining *substantia propria* (*b*) consists of lamellae composed of parallel fibrils. The direction of the fibrils varies from one layer to the next. Firm cohesion of the lamellae is insured by the interweaving of their fibrils. In the soft cementing substance between lamellae there are spaces containing the flat, fixed corneal cells (Fig. 424). The cell processes are connected through canaliculi. Isolated wandering cells are also met with. Deep to the corneal epithelium lies the thin and nearly homogeneous *external limiting membrane* (of Bowman), which is not distinct in all species. The *internal limiting membrane* (of Descemet) is a fairly thick, glassy, homogeneous membrane, which is microchemically related to elastic tissue. Its posterior surface is covered by a single layer of flat, polygonal cells, the *corneal mesenchymal epithelium* (Fig. 423,*c*). This layer is the lining of the anterior wall of the anterior chamber (Fig. 422,*v*).

Aside from the network of marginal loops (Fig. 423,*h*), which is derived from the episcleral branches of the ciliary vessels, there are no blood vessels in the cornea. Lymphatics are represented only by the interlamellar system of tissue spaces, which

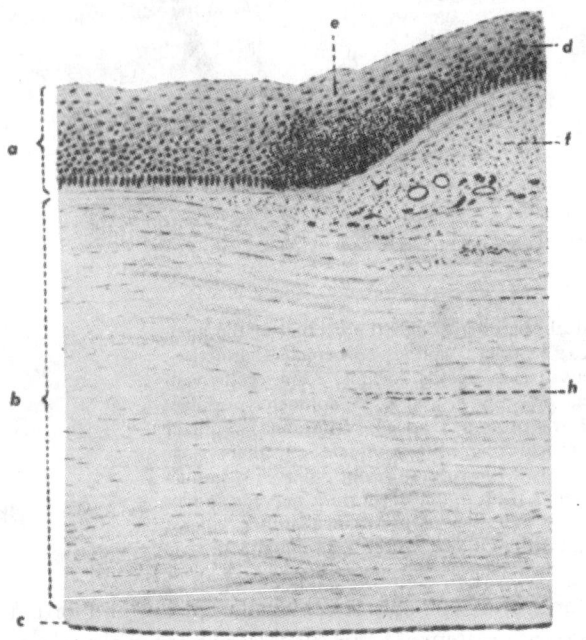

Figure 423. Meridional section through the corneoscleral junction of the donkey (90×). *a*, corneal epithelium; *b*, propria of the cornea; *c*, Descemet's membrane, white; the dark line below it, mesenchymal epithelium of the anterior chamber; *d*, conjunctival epithelium; *e*, transitional zone between *d* and *a*, with pigment deposits; *f*, propria of the bulbar conjunctiva; *h*, blood vessel (marginal loop in the propria of the cornea).

drain into the conjunctival lymph vessels. Most of the corneal nerves are branches of the ciliary nerves. They form the annular plexus at the corneal margin. Then they enter the substance of the cornea and form a plexus throughout all its layers. The processes of the intraepithelial plexus end between the epithelial cells.

(c) **The corneoscleral junction** (Fig. 428,*c*) is the zone in which the wavy opaque scleral bundles are continuous with the taut, transparent corneal bundles. In sections the indistinct border between the two tissues forms an oblique line, the angle of which differs in the various quadrants. The beveled edge of the sclera lies outside the margin of the cornea, or corneal limbus. Here the sclera contains many pigment cells, which, except in solipeds, are also found between the corneal lamellae for some distance beyond the junction. The corneal epithelium is continued by that of the bulbar conjunctiva (p. 405).

2. The Vascular (Middle) Tunic

The middle layer, also called the uvea,[1] is characterized by an abundance of blood vessels and pigment cells. It contains nerve fibers in all its parts and, except in the region of the iris, also nerve cells. Some portions have smooth muscle fibers.

(a) The chorioid membrane (Fig. 425) is composed of nets of elastic fibers, of pigmented connective tissue, and especially of blood vessels, which are arranged in two layers. One of these is made up of larger vessels and is therefore called the

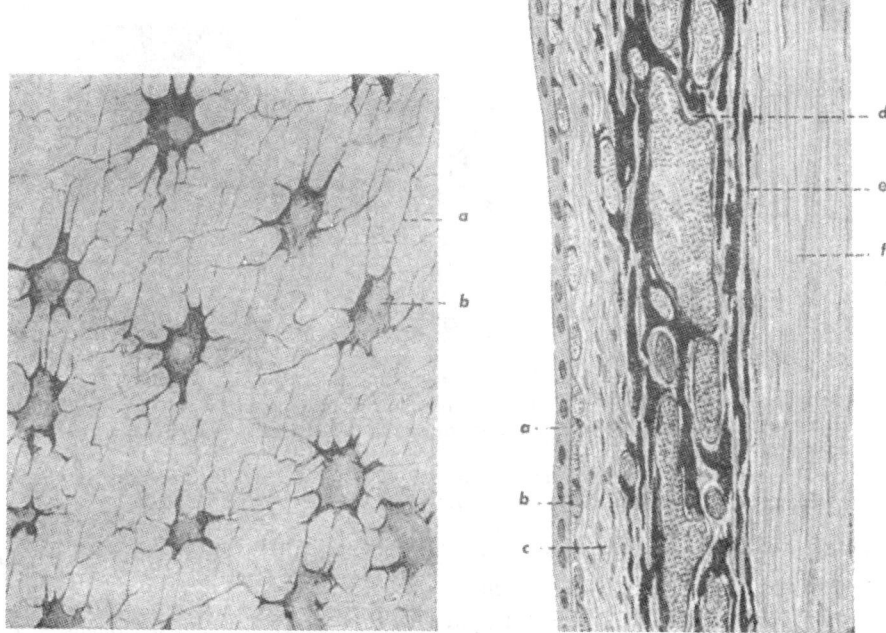

Figure 424 (left). Tangential section of the cornea of the ox (450×). *a*, canaliculi; *b*, corneal cell in an interlamellar space.

Figure 425 (right). Section through the chorioid with the tapetum fibrosum of the horse (315×). *a*, pigment epithelium of the retina (unpigmented at the level of the tapetum); *b*, glassy membrane with closely adjoining choriocapillary layer; *c*, tapetum fibrosum containing some pigment in its outer portion; *d*, vessel layer with many pigmented connective tissue cells; *e*, suprachorioid layer; *f*, sclera.

vessel layer, while the other one consists of capillaries and is called the choriocapillary layer. The two layers enclose the tapetum between them. The vessel layer is bordered peripherally by the suprachorioid layer, and the capillary layer is adjoined centrally by the glassy membrane of Bruch.

The *suprachorioid layer* (Fig. 425,*e*) connects the sclera with the chorioid. It is a loose black membrane, perforated by many vessels and nerves but otherwise avascular. It is composed of delicate, loosely connected lamellae consisting of a net-

---

[1] L. *uva* grape. When exposed by dissection the vascular layer resembles a grape skin.

work of elastic fibers and pigmented connective tissue cells. The pigment cells (Fig. 50) are flat, fusiform, or rounded, and characteristic for each species. The tissue spaces between lamellae intercommunicate and constitute the perichorioid lymph spaces.

The *vessel layer* (Fig. 425,*d*) is the thickest layer of the chorioid. It consists essentially of a dense vascular plexus. This is formed by arteries that ramify from the outside inward and by veins that converge from the inside outward. Its framework has a lamellar structure similar to that of the suprachorioid layer. The veins collect blood from the choriocapillary layer and converge at four to six vortices to form

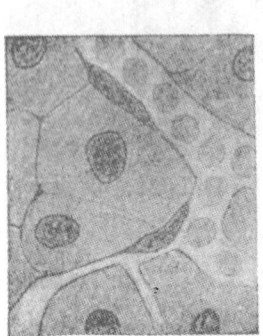 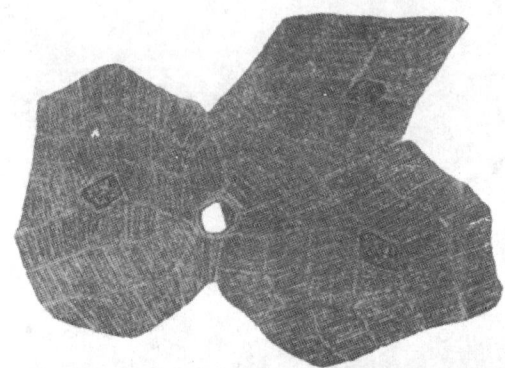

Figure 426 (left). Tapetum cells of the dog in a surface view (1000×). Between the cells is a system of grooves, containing the vessels of the choriocapillary layer. (After Zietzschmann.)

Figure 427 (right). Tapetum cells of the cat (1000×). A vessel is surrounded by the three cells, which are filled with crystalline needles. (After Zietzschmann.)

the vena vorticosae. The more superficial veins have a cellular connective tissue sheath that is absent from the arteries.

The avascular *tapetum*, which is responsible for the luster of the eyes of some species, is absent in man and swine. Its structure in the horse and ruminants is fibrous (tapetum fibrosum), while in the dog and cat it is cellular (tapetum cellulosum). The tapetum fibrosum consists of collagenous bundles only, which have a wavy course and a generally concentric arrangement (Fig. 425,*c*). Beween the bundles lie connective tissue cells and, in the peripheral layers, also pigment cells. The tapetum cellulosum of carnivores consists of ten to fifteen layers of flat, irregularly pentagonal or hexagonal cells (Figs. 426, 427). In the cat the cytoplasm of these cells contains regularly arranged bundles of crystalline needles. Both kinds of tapetum become thinner toward their margins. In man and swine the tapetum is replaced by a limiting layer of stroma made up of elastic fiber networks.

The *choriocapillary layer* (Figs. 425,*b;* 445,*m*) is a dense capillary plexus in an apparently homogeneous pigmented matrix. The glassy membrane is a thin, structureless membrane next to the retinal epithelium.

(b) The ciliary body (Fig. 428,*k*) is divided into a posterior, thinner, finely fluted portion, called the ciliary ring (orbiculus ciliaris) and an anterior, thicker portion, the ciliary crown, which has bigger folds.

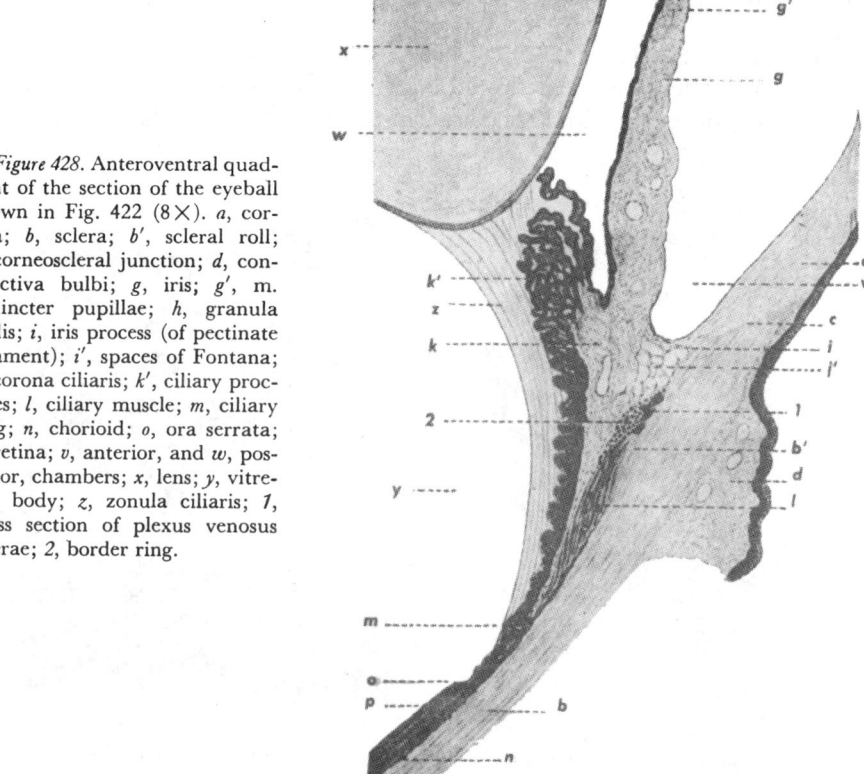

Figure 428. Anteroventral quadrant of the section of the eyeball shown in Fig. 422 (8×). *a*, cornea; *b*, sclera; *b'*, scleral roll; *c*, corneoscleral junction; *d*, conjunctiva bulbi; *g*, iris; *g'*, m. sphincter pupillae; *h*, granula iridis; *i*, iris process (of pectinate ligament); *i'*, spaces of Fontana; *k*, corona ciliaris; *k'*, ciliary processes; *l*, ciliary muscle; *m*, ciliary ring; *n*, chorioid; *o*, ora serrata; *p*, retina; *v*, anterior, and *w*, posterior, chambers; *x*, lens; *y*, vitreous body; *z*, zonula ciliaris; *1*, cross section of plexus venosus sclerae; *2*, border ring.

The ciliary ring (*m*) is the direct continuation of the chorioid and is distinguished from it by the lack of a choriocapillary layer, and by the meridional orientation of its collagenous bundles. The boundary between the chorioid and the ciliary ring is marked by the ora serrata (*o*). Fine folds on the surface become higher toward the lens to form the ciliary processes. The tissue of the ciliary ring passes into that of the ciliary crown without sharp demarcation.

The ciliary crown (Fig. 428,*k*) consists of the base plate and the ciliary processes. The base plate is a direct continuation of the ciliary ring. It is fibrillar and contains radially arranged blood vessels. Among the abundant collagenous fibers are many pigmented connective tissue cells. The ciliary crown is covered on its inner surface by a glassy membrane, which is a continuation of that of the chorioid but is more fibrous in this area. The ciliary processes (Figs. 428,*k'*; 429) gradually rise from the base plate. They are believed to secrete the aqueous humor. They are fibroelastic ridges which follow a meridional course toward the iris. They reach their greatest height at the margin of the iris, where they end abruptly. They enclose numerous blood vessels, and their surface bears small intersecting folds. Both the ring and the crown are covered by a double layer of epithelium, the pars ciliaris retinae. The pigmented outer cell layer is the continuation of the pigmented retinal epithelium (Fig. 429,*c*). The inner stratum consists of unpigmented columnar cells (*d*).

The *ciliary muscle* (Fig. 428,*l*) lies between the ciliary body and the sclera. Its smooth muscle fibers originate from the scleral roll, the fibers in the angle of the iris, and the base of the iris. They are inserted on the outer surface of the ciliary ring.

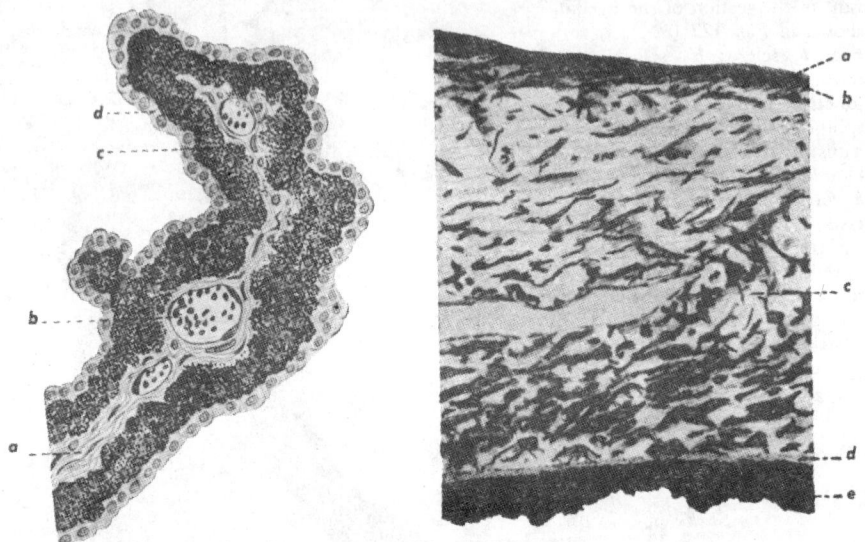

Figure 429 (left). Longitudinal section through the terminal portion of a ciliary process of the ox (290×). *a*, collagenous core; *b*, large caliber capillary; *c*, pigmented, and *d*, unpigmented, layers of epithelium belonging to the pars ciliaris retinae. (After Zietzschmann.)

Figure 430 (right). Radial section through the iris of the dog (180×). *a*, mesenchymal epithelium; *b*, anterior stromal lamella; *c*, stroma with a vessel sectioned longitudinally; *d*, m. dilatator pupillae; *e*, layer of pigmented epithelium; *a–c*, pars uvealis iridis; *d,e*, pars retinalis iridis. (After Zietzschmann.)

In the horse, pig, and carnivores the ciliary muscle also contains circular fibers. In the horse, which possesses the weakest ciliary muscle, the circular fibers are restricted to the nasal third. In the pig, dog, and cat, there are circular muscle fibers around the entire circumference. The ciliary muscle functions in the accommodation of the lens. In the resting state the zonular fibers (p. 399) exert traction on the capsule of the lens at the equator. When the ciliary muscle contracts, the chorioid is stretched and the ciliary body is drawn forward, allowing the zonular fibers and the lens capsule to relax. This permits the lens to become more convex as a result of its internal elasticity. Its refractive power is increased and an image of nearby objects is focused on the retina. Accommodation is poor in domestic mammals, excellent in birds.

(c) **The iris** (Figs. 428,*g;* 430–432) consists of uveal and retinal portions.

The uveal part (Fig. 430,*a–c*) bears a *mesenchymal epithelium* covering all of the anterior surface of the iris; i.e., the posterior wall of the anterior chamber of the eye. The adjoining *anterior stromal lamella* is a condensed layer of the iridic stroma, into which it blends without any sharp demarcation. It is composed almost exclusively of dense branched and anastomosing pigmented cells. The *vascular stroma* of the iris (Figs. 430,*c;* 432,*a*) contains many pigment cells, most of which are extensively branched. These are interconnected by their cytoplasmic processes forming a loose framework, which is interwoven with delicate collagenous bundles of

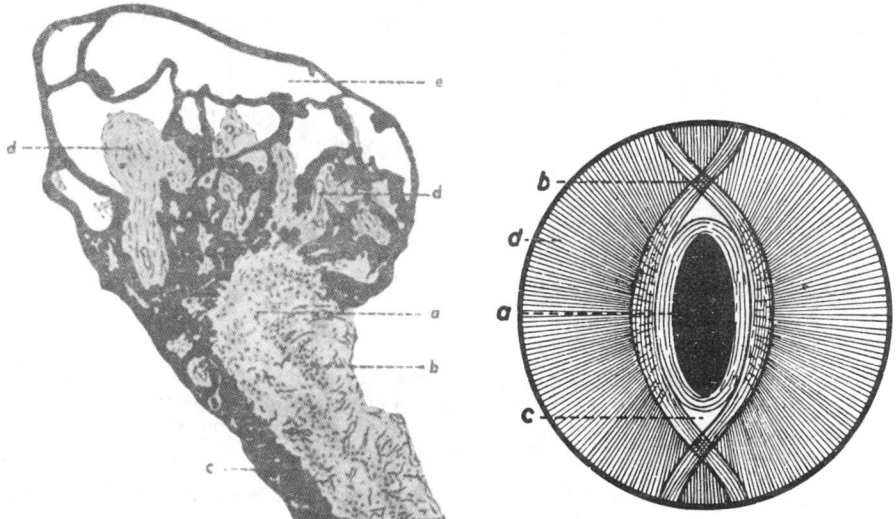

Figure 431 (left). Meridional section through the pupillary zone of the iris of the goat. *a*, pupillary margin of the iris; *b*, m. sphincter pupillae; *c*, pigmented epithelium of the iris (pars retinalis iridis); *d*, capillaries in the connective tissue that partially fills the spaces in the granulum iridis; *e*, peripheral space filled only with liquid. (After Zietzschmann.)

Figure 431A (right). Diagram of the course of the muscle fibers in the constricted feline pupil. *a*, pupil; *b*, intersection of peripheral sphincter fibers; *c*, space between the two parts of the sphincter; *d*, m. dilatator pupillae. (After Raselli.)

predominantly radial orientation. The iridic stroma is loose, except in the horse, ox, and pig. Its tissue spaces communicate by way of unlined crypts on the anterior surface with the anterior chamber. Vessels and nerves are ensheathed in a denser layer of stroma. The arteries of the iris form the circulus arteriosus iridis major and minor. The stroma also contains elastic fibers and the *m. sphincter pupillae* (Figs. 428,*g';* 431,*b*). This muscle is a flat circular band, which lies in the deepest part of the stroma near the pupillary margin and consists of smooth muscle fibers. In animals with oval pupils the sphincter pupillae also includes fibers that intersect at acute angles at both commissures of the iris (Fig. 431,A).

The retinal part of the iris (Figs. 430,*d,e;* 432,*b,c*) is composed of an anterior muscular layer and a stratum of pigmented epithelium. The former is the *m. dilatator pupillae*, a single layer of radial smooth muscle fibers. These fibers are peculiar in that the nucleated portion of the cell is pigmented and is applied to the posterior surface of the fiber. The unpigmented fibers are joined to form the radially striated posterior stromal lamella, while the nucleated, pigmented parts give the appearance of a separate layer of pigment cells. During pupillary constriction when the dilator is stretched, the nucleated parts of its muscle cells are drawn into the same plane with the fibers. There is an interchange of fibers between the sphincter and the dilator. The posterior surface of the iris is covered by the pigmented epithelium, composed of fairly high cells. The color of the eye is determined by the pigmentation of the iridic stroma. If it contains little pigment, the pigmented epithelium on the posterior surface shows through and gives a blue

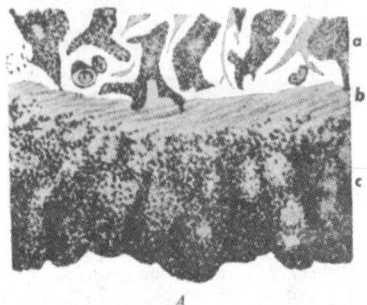 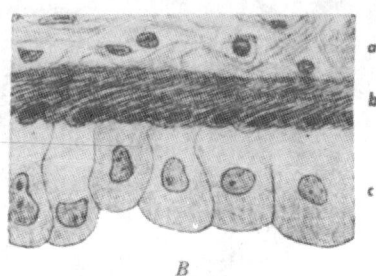

A   *B*

Figure 432. Radial section through the posterior layers of the canine iris. *A*, pigmented; *B*, pigment removed (550×). *a*, stroma of the iris; *b*, m. dilatator pupillae (the muscular layer in *A* is pigmented in its nucleated portion); *c*, pigmented epithelium of the pars retinalis iridis. (After Zietzschmann.)

coloration. The peculiar golden sheen of the feline pupil is caused by the diffuse yellow pigmentation of stromal cells.

The free edge of the iris of the horse, donkey, and ruminants often bear the granula iridis (corpora nigra; Figs. 428,*h;* 431). They are continuous with the pigmented layer of the iris and consist of a framework enclosed by strongly pigmented epithelial cells. They contain liquid-filled spaces, which represent an extension of those of the iris stroma and, as such, contain many vessels accompanied by delicate connective tissue. In the ox the granula iridis are small and actually only an eversion of the pigmented layer.

(d) The angle of the iris is the circular recess where cornea, sclera, the ciliary border of the iris, and the ciliary body meet. Here a peculiar framework of trabeculae with irregular spaces is found. It is called the pectinate ligament of the iris and is much better developed in domestic mammals than in man.

The *pectinate ligament* is an annular structure which assists in forming the peripheral wall of the anterior chamber. Its anterior part consists of wide-meshed tissue formed by the iris processes—several rows of pigmented, collagenous trabeculae, which curve across the iris angle to the corneoscleral junction (Fig. 428,*i*). They are firmly attached to the sclera and to the membrane of Descemet, which passes over from the cornea to the surfaces of the trabeculae. Some of the trabeculae penetrate Descemet's membrane and join the substantia propria of the cornea. The

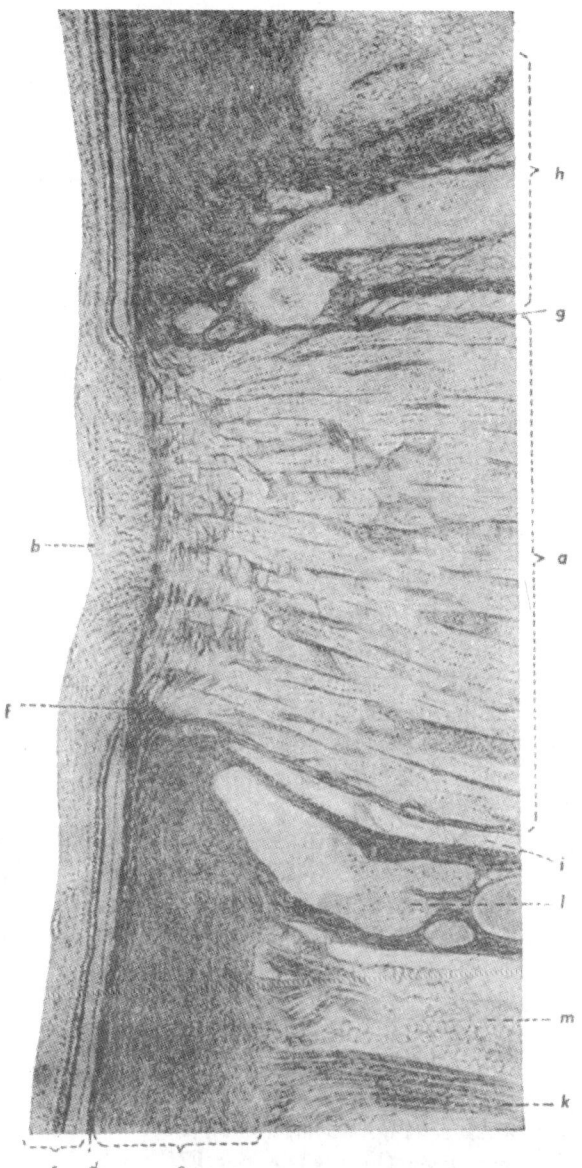

Figure 433. Sagittal section through the optic
papilla of the goat (20 ×). *a*, optic nerve; *b*, physiological excavation showing retinal vessels; *c*, retina;
d, chorioid; *e*, sclera; *f*, lamina cribrosa; *g*, pial
sheath of the optic nerve; *h*, dural sheath with large
blood vessels; *i*, arachnoid space; *k*, bundles of the
retractor oculi; *l*, blood vessels; *m*, intraorbital fat.
(After Zietzschmann.)

trabeculae are covered by the mesenchymal epithelium of the anterior chamber. Between them lie the *spaces of Fontana* (Fig. 428,*i'*), which play a major part in the drainage of fluids from the eye into the plexus venosus sclerae. Trabeculae that extend from the base plate of the ciliary body to the sclera also participate in the meshwork of the iris angle, which is deeper than in man. Toward the ciliary muscle the trabecular skeleton breaks up into a fine network, which is partly fibrillar but consists mainly of cells and their cytoplasmic processes.

3. The Retina and the Optic Nerve

(a) **The optic nerve** (Figs. 422,*q;* 433,*a*) is actually a tract of the central nervous system. It is divided into the myelinated, white, orbital segment and the unmyelinated gray intraocular segment.

The orbital segment is covered by sheaths continuous with the pia mater and dura mater (Fig. 433,*g,h*). Between them is a space traversed by arachnoid trabeculae (*i*). The pia sends processes into the optic nerve, which group the nerve fibers into bundles. Many glia cells are present between the fibers. The central retinal artery and vein, covered by a strand of connective tissue, enter the nerve close to the sclera and run along its axis. At the point where the nerve enters the eyeball, i.e., in the intraocular segment, the optic nerve fibers abruptly lose their myelin sheaths and penetrate the cribriform area (Fig. 433, *f*), which receives its collagenous bundles mainly from the sclera but also to some extent from the chorioid. The dura and pia pass into the sclera. The unmyelinated fibers spread radially over the inner surface of the retina. In the circular zone where the nerve fibers bend over the margin of the cribriform area, they form an elevation around the central retinal vessels, the optic papilla. This has a central depression, the physiological excavation of the optic nerve (Fig. 433,*b*).

(b) **The retina** is composed of optic, ciliary, and iridic portions.

The optic part of the retina occupies the entire posterior inner surface of the eyeball and extends to the vicinity of the ciliary body, where it ends in a jagged line, the ora serrata (Fig. 428,*o*). Starting from the innermost, the layers of the retina are as follows:

(1) Inner limiting membrane (Fig. 435,*li*)
(2) Layer of optic nerve fibers (Figs. 434,*a;* 435,*I*)
(3) Layer of ganglion cells (Figs. 434,*b;* 435,*II*)
(4) Inner plexiform layer (Figs. 434,*c;* 435,*III*)
(5) Inner nuclear layer (Figs. 434,*d;* 435,*IV–VI*)
(6) Outer plexiform layer (Figs. 434,*e;* 435,*VII*)
(7) Outer nuclear layer (Figs. 434,*f;* 435,*VIII*)
(8) Outer limiting membrane (Figs. 434,*g;* 435,*le*)
(9) Layer of rods and cones (Figs. 434,*h;* 435,*IX*)
(10) Pigment epithelium (Figs. 434,*i;* 435,*X*)

The supportive tissue is neuroglia, which is distributed throughout the retina. The radial fibers of Müller (Fig. 435,*m*) are special neuroglial cells. At the internal surface of the retina they have conical expansions, which join to form the glassy internal limiting membrane. The fibers run vertically through all layers, sending

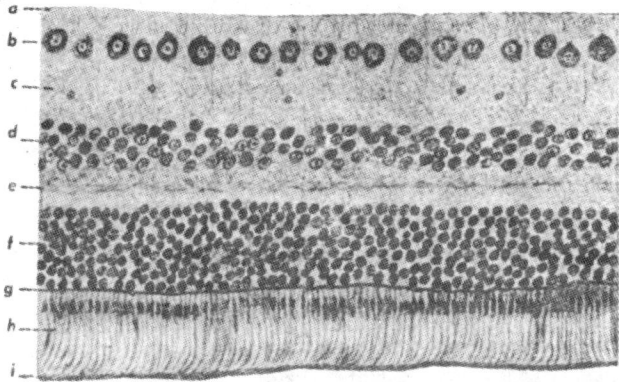

Figure 434. Section through the retina from the posterior portion of the eye of the sheep (135×). *a*, layer of optic nerve fibers; *b*, ganglion cell; *c*, inner plexiform layer with scattered cells; *d*, inner nuclear layer; *e*, outer plexiform layer; *f*, outer nuclear layer; *g*, outer limiting membrane; *h*, layer of rods and cones; *i*, pigment epithelium.

spinous, fibrous, or foliate processes between the nervous elements, and extend to the external limiting membrane. At the level of the inner nuclear layer (Fig. 435,*IV–VI*) the slender cell body shows an enlargement which houses the elongated nucleus. In both nuclear layers it has saclike recesses for the accommodation of the various cell bodies. On the outer surface of the outer nuclear layer the radial fibers unite to form the outer limiting membrane. This is a structureless membrane with many perforations, through which the processes of the rod and cone cells pass to

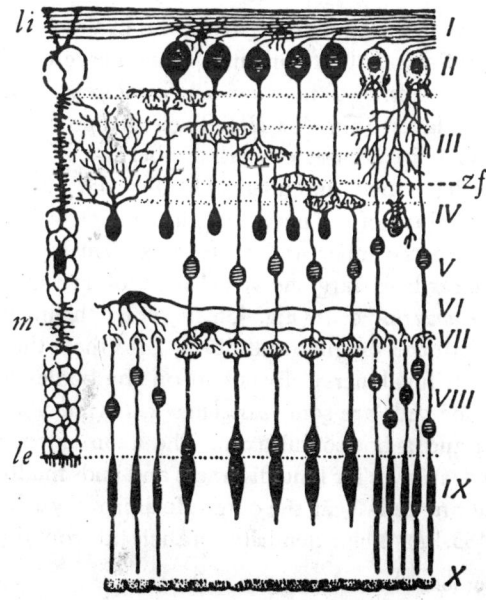

Figure 435. Diagram of the retina. *I*, layer of optic nerve fibers with glia cells; *II*, layer of ganglion cells; *III*, inner plexiform layer; *IV*, layer of amacrine cells (*left*, a diffuse amacrine cell; *right*, layer-forming cells); *V*, layer of bipolar nerve cells; *VI*, layer of horizontal cells; *IV–VI*, inner nuclear layer; *VII*, outer plexiform layer; *VIII*, outer nuclear layer; *IX*, layer of rods and cones; *X*, pigment epithelium; *le*, outer limiting membrane; *li*, inner limiting membrane; *m*, radial fibers of Müller; *zf*, centrifugal fiber. (After Greeff.)

the outer nuclear layer. The outer limiting membrane also gives rise to fibers that are directed toward the outside and surround the bases of the rods and cones. In addition to the radial fibers, there are also glia cells of the type of the fibrous astrocytes. These are located in the layer of optic nerve fibers and the layer of ganglion cells, where they give off long horizontal processes (Fig. 435,*I*).

The layers of the retina show the following structure: The fibers of the optic nerve spread radially from the papilla to the ora serrata, forming the *layer of optic nerve fibers*. On the way to the ora serrata, one fiber after another turns outward to the ganglion cells, so that the layer becomes thinner and thinner. Almost all the fibers of the optic nerve are axons of the *ganglion cells*. A few fibers extend to the inner

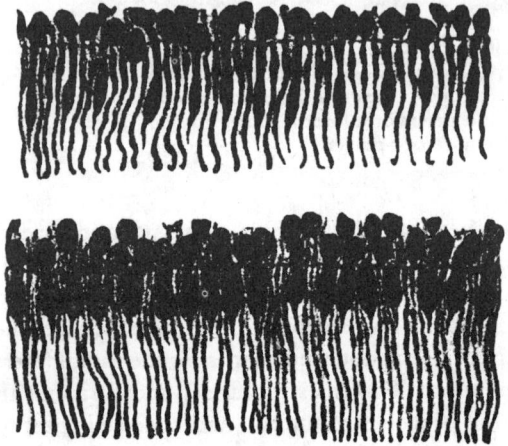

I

Figure 436. Rod and cone layer of the retina (635×). The parts shown come from a region about midway between the optic papilla and the ora serrata. *I*, horse—the cones have the shape of ears of corn; *II*, pig—the cones are short and thick. (After Zürn.)

II

nuclear layer; they represent centrifugal fibers conducting from the brain. Near the ganglion cells the axons give off collaterals that surround other nerve cells. Each ganglion cell gives off one or more dendrites to the *inner plexiform layer*. These may spread out diffusely or in horizontal layers (Fig. 435,*III*). Their fine processes along with those of other nerve cells make up a dense feltwork of fibers.

The *inner nuclear layer* contains the nuclei of the radial fibers of Müller and a large number of *bipolar nerve cells* (Fig. 435, *V*). Each of the nerve cells has a central and a peripheral process, which terminate in the inner and outer plexiform layers. Near the inner border of the inner nuclear layer large nerve cells are found which lack a true axon. The dendrites of these *amacrine*[2] cells (Fig. 435,*IV*) enter the inner plexiform layer and come in contact with the ganglion cell fibers. Like these they branch diffusely or in layers. The centrifugal nerve fibers end on the bodies of the amacrine cells. Among the amacrine cells are some *association cells* (not illustrated), which have stubby dendrites and a horizontal axon. The axon extends along the inner border of the inner nuclear layer for long distances and ends finally on the process of a layer-forming amacrine cell. Near the outer plexiform layer lie the *horizontal cells* of the retina (Fig. 435,*VI*). Their dendrites branch horizontally

---

[2] Gr. *a-* not, *makros* long, *inos* fiber: without long fibers.

and their axon takes a horizontal course and ends in the *outer plexiform layer*. This layer contains, in addition to the fibers of the bipolar cells, the inner ends of the visual cells.

The visual receptors are the highly differentiated rod and cone cells. The external limiting membrane, through which the visual cells project, divides each cell into an outer and an inner part. The inner part contains the nucleus. The densely packed nucleated inner portions of the visual cells make up the *outer nuclear layer* (*VIII*), while the nonnucleated outer parts constitute the *layer of rods and cones*. The portion of the rods and cones nearest the external limiting layer is surrounded by the processes of the radial fibers known as fiber baskets.

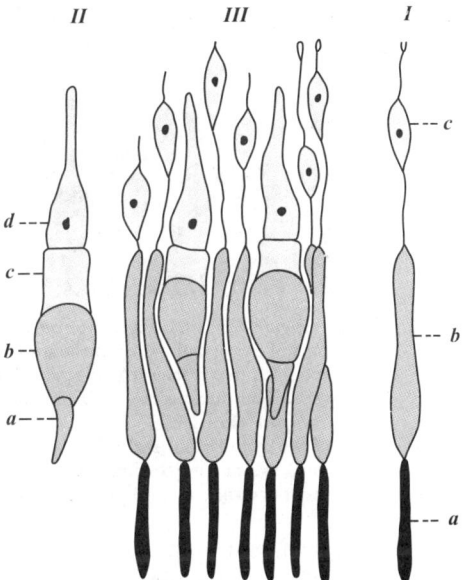

Figure 437. Rods and cones from the pig; teased preparation. *I*, isolated rod cell: *a*, outer segment; *b*, inner segment; *c*, rod fiber with rod body and rod spherule; *II*, isolated cone cell: *a*, outer segment; *b* and *c*, inner segment; *b*, fiber apparatus; *c*, cone myoid; *d*, cone fiber with cone body; *III*, group of rod and cone cells. The outer segment of the rods is only half as long as the inner segment. The inner segment adapts its shape to that of the neighboring rods and cones. (After Greeff.)

The rod proper is a slender cylinder. Its outer segment (Fig. 437,*I*,*a*) is homogeneous in life and contains the visual purple (rhodopsin). The inner segment (*I*,*b*) contains in its slightly enlarged outer third an oval, longitudinally striated particle, called the fiber apparatus (not illustrated). The inner part of the rod cell consists of the slender rod fiber and the rod body, a swelling that encloses the nucleus. In ruminants and swine the chromatin appears as several transversely arranged discs. The rod fiber continues to the outer plexiform layer, where it ends in a small rod spherule.

The cone proper has a shorter, conical outer segment (*II*,*a*), except in the cat, where it is long and narrow. The thick inner segment (*II*,*b*,*c*) also shows a fiber apparatus (*b*), which takes up about two-thirds of the inner segment. The inner third stains poorly and has been found to be contractile in some of the lower vertebrates. The inner segment varies in shape among the different species. It is slender in the horse and carnivores (Fig. 436,*I*) and short and plump in ruminants and swine (*II*). Inside the limiting membrane and usually close to it is the thick body of the cone cell, containing the nucleus. From the cell body a thick cone fiber extends to the outer plexiform layer, where it ends in a broad pedicle with fine radial processes.

Even in routine preparations the rod and cone fibers are visible in the outer plexiform layer as fine striations. This stratum has been named Henle's outer fiber layer. It is most distinct in carnivores. The spherules and pedicles of the rod and cone fibers are in contact with the peripheral branches of the bipolar nerve cells.

To reach the rods and cones, which are directed toward the sclera, the light rays must pass through eight of the other layers of the retina. These layers are almost

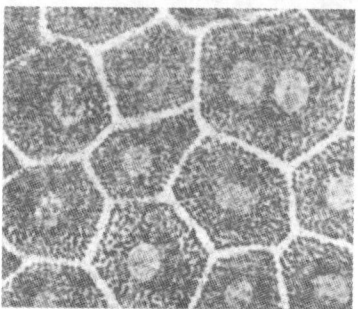 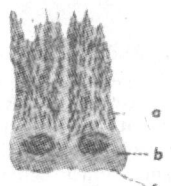

Figure 438 (left). Pigment epithelium of the retina from the posterior part of the eye of a dog; surface view (320×). On the right top, a large cell with two nuclei; the pigment is deposited in the form of crystalline rods. The nucleus is visible in most cells as a lighter spot.

Figure 439 (right). Vertical section through pigmented epithelial cells of the retina of an owl (550×). *a*, inner part of the cell with long processes, which project between the rods and contain long, pointed pigment crystals; *b*, unpigmented part with nucleus; *c*, cuticular cover.

perfectly transparent in life. The light stimuli received by the rods and cones are transmitted through the bipolar cells to the ganglion cells and thence to the brain via their axons. Thus the complex stratification of the retina may be boiled down to three layers of cells with synaptic zones (plexiform layers) between them. The retina is not a simple receptor organ, however. Its neurons perform many of the integrative functions usually associated with the central nervous system.

The cells of the *pigment epithelium* (Fig. 435,*X*; 438), adjoining the layer of rods and cones on the outside, contain rod-shaped crystalloids of the brown pigment fuscin. During illumination of the eye a portion of the pigment enters into the numerous filiform processes which project into the layer of rods and cones. In albino animals and in the portion of the retina overlying the tapetum the cells contain little or no pigment.

The area of keenest vision on the human retina has a yellow color and is called the macula lutea. The corresponding structure in the domestic animals is the *area retinae.* This is a round spot lateral to the optic papilla; in some animals it also includes a light streak that extends from the round spot across the retina above the papilla. It is recognizable with the unaided eye. In the round area the ganglion cells are stratified, and the bipolar cells as well as the cone cells are greatly increased in number at the expense of the rod cells. The rod cells may be absent from the round area in ratters and hunting dogs. In the streak there is an increase in the number of ganglion and bipolar cells. The round area serves in binocular vision and is found in all domestic mammals. The horse, ox, and pig also have a streak, which is employed in monocular vision.

There is a conspicuous reduction in the layers of the retina in the region of the macula lutea of man. In this way an excavation, the fovea centralis (interna), is formed. Only cone cells occur in it. The fovea centralis interna is absent in all domestic mammals. The dog and the cat, however, have a fovea externa (Fig. 440,*h'*); which is a slight depression on the outside of the retina.

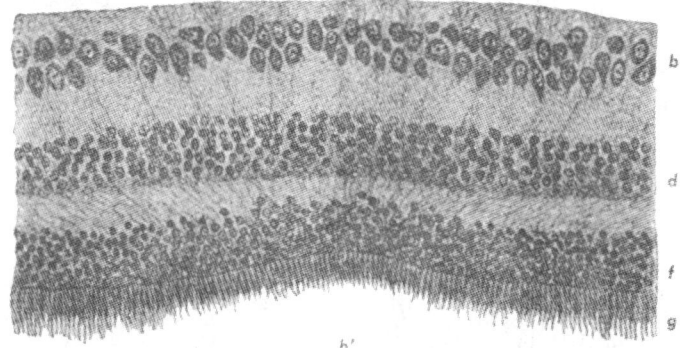

Figure 440. Area centralis from the retina of the dog, showing fovea externa (245×). *a*, layer of optic nerve fibers; *b*, layer of ganglion cells; *c*, inner plexiform layer; *d*, inner nuclear layer; *e*, Henle's fiber layer with the narrow outer plexiform layer above it; *f*, outer nuclear layer; *g*, layer of rods and cones, which appears indented into the fovea externa from the outside; *h*, outer limiting membrane; *h'*, fovea externa, containing cones, but no rods.

The *pars ciliaris retinae* is the thinned continuation of the retina, which loses its nervous elements abruptly at the ora serrata. It consists of an outer layer of pigmented cells, representing an extension of the pigment epithelium of the retina, and an inner layer of unpigmented columnar cells (Fig. 429,*c,d*). Their inner surface bears a thin membrane, the continuation of the inner limiting layer of the optic part.

The pars iridica retinae is described on p. 389.

BLOOD VESSELS OF THE RETINA. The arteries are derived from the central retinal artery. In the horse this artery breaks up inside the lamina cribrosa into thirty to forty branches, which emerge at the circumference of the optic papilla. In other species it divides in the papilla into two to four branches, which may either emerge in the center or, as in the cat, at the papillary margin. The vessels radiate from the papilla and break up into capillaries surrounded by extensive elastic nets. The veins arising from the capillary bed lead into the central vein of the retina. The vessels are distributed only to the inner layers of the retina; the rod and cone cells and the pigment epithelium are always avascular. The central artery of the retina anastomoses with branches of the posterior ciliary arteries and varies in caliber inversely with the extent and size of these anastomoses (Fig. 445).

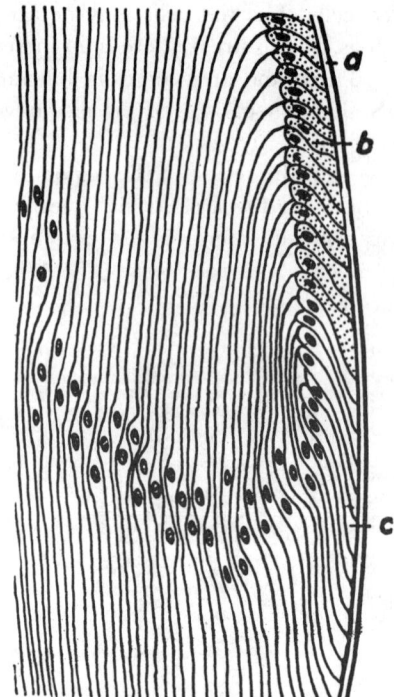

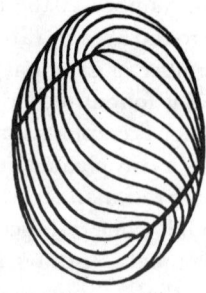

Figure 442. Diagram showing the course of lens fibers; side view. One main ray of a lens star is shown on each surface.

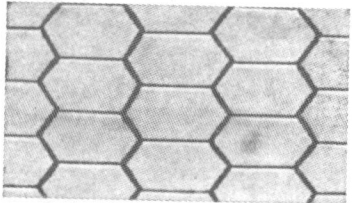

Figure 441 (left). Portion of a meridional section through the equator of the equine lens, showing the transformation of the epithelial cells of the lens into lens fibers. a, capsule of the lens; b, epithelium of the lens; c, nucleated lens fibers.

Figure 443 (right). Cross section through the fibers of a frozen lens, treated with silver nitrate. (After Arnold.)

4. The Refractive Media of the Eye

(a) **The lens** (Fig. 422,x) is surrounded by an elastic, homogeneous *capsule* (Fig. 441,a). This is loosely connected to the substance of the lens and is thicker on the anterior than on the posterior surface of the lens. Deep to the anterior sheet of the capsule is the simple cuboidal *epithelium of the lens*. Toward the equator of the lens the epithelial cells increase in height, become arranged in meridional rows, and form the *lens fibers*.

The substance of the lens is soft peripherally but becomes firmer interiorly with each successive layer. In the center it is hard (lens nucleus). It is composed of long, flat, transparent, hexagonal lens fibers (Fig. 443). The peripheral fibers, which make up most of the lens, are nucleated and have a semiliquid content. The central ones have serrated edges and are more slender, firmer, and nonnucleated. The fibers are joined together by cement. Toward the poles of the lens, where the ends of the fibers meet, accumulations of cementing substance form the lens stars, which usually consist of three main rays arranged in a Y-shaped pattern. The lens stars are clearly visible on both surfaces of the lens during maceration, just before the lens separates into laminae. Fibers coming from the center of one star terminate at the free ends of the rays of the other star and vice versa. Among the fibers attached to intermediate portions of the rays, the closer to one pole a fiber arises, the farther from the opposite pole will be its insertion. Therefore, no fiber passes around a full half of the lens (Fig. 442).

Vessels and nerves are lacking in the lens. Aided by the cornea, the lens refracts light rays in such a manner that a small inverted image of the object emitting or reflecting the rays is formed on the retina.

The lens is maintained in its position by a *suspensory apparatus*, also called the zonula ciliaris (Fig. 428,*z*). This consists of fine, homogeneous fibers, which arise from the pars ciliaris retinae. They extend between the ciliary processes and are inserted on the lens capsule both behind and in front of the equator. Some of the fibers cross. Between the zonular fibers all around the lens equator are the intercommunicating spaces of the suspensory apparatus.

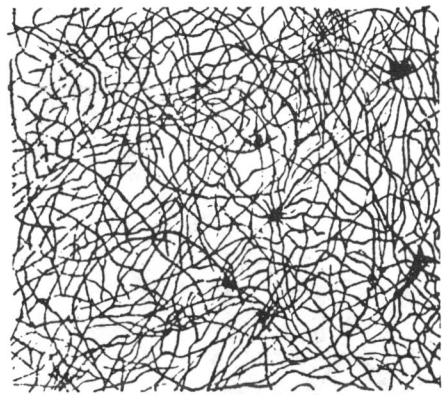

Figure 444. Meshwork of fibers from the vitreous body of man (500×). (After Retzius.)

(b) **The vitreous body** (Figs. 422,*y;* 444) is a gelatinous mass containing protein and a great deal of water. It has a framework of fine, granular, transparent fibers, the meshes of which contain fluid. Isolated leukocytes also occur in it. On the surface the fibers are condensed into the hyaloid membrane. In it the fibers of the vitreous body follow primarily an equatorial course. In the middle of the vitreous body lies the hyaloid canal containing remnants of the hyaloid artery (as in the ox, pig, and carnivores). It extends from the optic papilla to the posterior pole of the lens.

(c) **The anterior and posterior chambers** of the eye (Fig. 422,*v,w*) are filled with the aqueous humor. This fluid contains only a small amount of salts, among them mainly chlorides. Other constituents are traces of lipids and soluble proteins. Particulate matter and cells are absent.

The aqueous humor flows constantly from the posterior chamber around the pupillary margin into the anterior chamber and from there into the spaces of Fontana, whence it is absorbed by the scleral venous plexus.

(d) **The cornea,** an important refractive structure, is described on p. 383.

VESSELS AND NERVES OF THE EYEBALL. The blood vessels (Fig. 445) belong to the ciliary and retinal systems. The retinal system has already been discussed on p. 397. The ciliary system is derived from the external ophthalmic artery. It is distributed through the vascular tunic and sclera. The following vessels are recognized:

(1) **Four to six short posterior ciliary (chorioid) arteries (*a*)** which ramify within the chorioid.

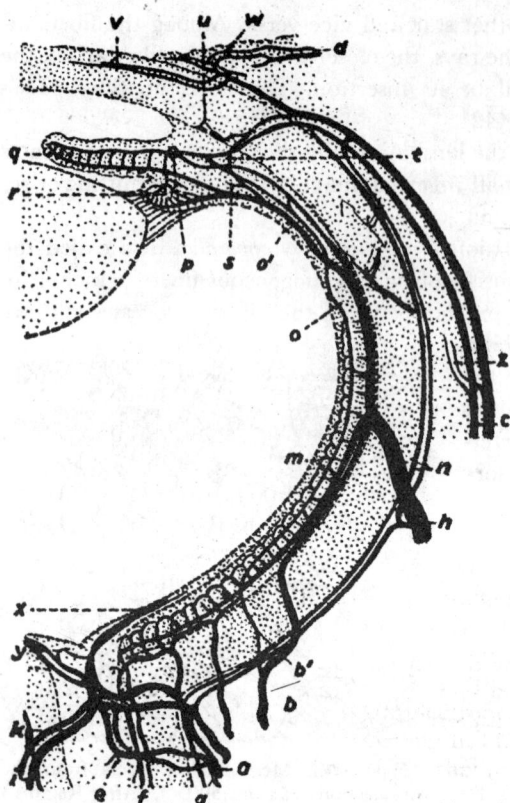

Figure 445. Vascular system of the eye of the horse, diagrammatic. Red: arteries. Black: veins. *a*, short posterior ciliary artery; *b*, long posterior ciliary artery; *b'*, branches from *b* to the chorioid; *c*, anterior ciliary arteries; *d*, posterior conjunctival artery and vein (from vessels of lids); *e*, central retinal artery and vein; *f*, vessels of the inner, and *g*, of the outer, sheath of the optic nerve; *h*, long posterior ciliary (vorticose) veins; *i*, short posterior ciliary veins; *k*, cilioretinal branch (artery and vein); *m*, capillary layer of the chorioid; *n*, episcleral vessels; *o*, recurrent artery of the chorioid; *o'*, veins of the ciliary body; *p*, circulus arteriosus ciliaris major in cross section; *q*, vessels of the iris; *r*, vessels of the ciliary processes; *s*, vein from the ciliary muscle, emptying into the vorticose vein; *t*, vein from the ciliary muscle, emptying into the anterior ciliary vein; *u*, plexus venosus sclerae; *v*, marginal plexus of the cornea; *w*, anterior conjunctival artery and vein (from anterior ciliary vessels); *x*, retinal vessels, which arise from *e* and in other species extend to the ora serrata; *y*, capillary loops in the region of the optic papilla; *z*, branches to the eye muscles, arising from *c*. (After Zietzschmann.)

(2) Two long posterior ciliary (iridic) arteries (*b,b'*) run between the sclera and chorioid toward the cornea, one of them medially, the other laterally. Along their way they give off a number of branches. In the region of the ciliary body these arteries divide into two branches each and anastomose with each other to form near the outer edge of the iris the circulus arteriosus iridis major (*p*). This contributes branches to the ciliary muscle, the ciliary processes (*r*), and the iris (*q*). The iridic branches course radially toward the pupillary margin and ramify mainly in the sphincter pupillae. Transverse anastomoses, which connect these radial vessels a short distance from the pupillary margin, may be considered as an incomplete circulus arteriosus iridis minor. In carnivores the two long posterior ciliary arteries give off anastomosing branches in the chorioid, forming an annular plexus, which communicates with the greater circle and also sends branches to the ciliary body.

(3) The anterior ciliary arteries (ramuli ciliares; *c*) communicate with the greater circle of the iris and with the chorioid arteries. This system of vessels also sends branches to the conjunctiva, which, however, receives most of its blood supply from the vessels supplying the lids. Other structures supplied by the anterior ciliary arteries are the sclera, the ciliary muscles, and the corneal limbus.

The venous tributaries converge toward the equator and unite into four (rarely five to six) long posterior ciliary, or vorticose, veins (*h*), which perforate the sclera and pass into the ophthalmic vein. The anterior radicles of the vorticose veins are united in the region of the ora serrata into an annular plexus, which receives the veins of the ciliary body with its iridic tributaries (*o'*). In addition, there are also the small short posterior ciliary veins (*i*) and the anterior ciliary veins (*c*). The anterior ciliary veins communicate with the plexus venosus sclerae (Schlemm's canal in man).

The eyeball has no lymph vessels but only lymph spaces, which may be divided into anterior and posterior lymph pathways. The anterior pathways include the chambers of the eye, the spaces of Fontana, and the spaces of the suspensory apparatus. The posterior pathways are those of the retina, chorioid, and sclera. The lymph spaces of the retina are perivascular clefts, which drain into the clefts of the sheath of the optic nerve. The main lymph space of chorioid and sclera is the perichorioid lymph space. This space communicates by way of the perivascular spaces of the vorticose veins with the peribulbar space of Tenon, which is continuous with a space surrounding the sheath of the optic nerve. This again communicates via perivascular spaces with the subarachnoid space of the optic nerve and brain.

The nerves of the eyeball course toward the cornea between the sclera and chorioid and form a plexus in the chorioid and then the plexus gangliosus ciliaris on the ciliary body, which gives rise to the nerves for the ciliary muscle, the iris, and the cornea.

THE EYE OF THE BIRD. Only the most important differences from the mammalian eye will be mentioned here. The orbital part of the sclera, behind the equator of the eyeball, consists of hyaline cartilage. The part adjoining it anteriorly is the collagenous scleral ring, which contains a shingle-like arrangement of plates of osseous tissue. The ciliary muscle is made up of three parts and, like the sphincter pupillae, consists of striated muscle. The yellow color of the iris of the chicken is due to fat enclosed in crypts. Around the equator of the lens is an annular pad formed of long narrow radial cells. On the back of the lens they are succeeded by the lens fibers. Between the lens pad and the nucleus formed by the lens fibers there is a cleft, the lens chamber. The pecten is a wedge-shaped structure that projects for a varying distance into the vitreous from the optic papilla, which it covers. It is formed by a sheet of tissue thrown into folds, and contains blood vessels, glia, nerve fibers, and many round pigmented cells in a dense capillary network. It probably has a nutritive function.[3]

B. THE PROTECTIVE APPARATUS OF THE EYE

1. The Lacrimal Apparatus

(a) **The lacrimal gland** (Fig. 446) is a lobulated, tubuloalveolar serous gland. It is mucous in swine, and cells giving a mucin reaction are also found in the sheep, goat, and dog. In all domestic mammals the secretory cells often contain fat drop-

[3] Gordon Lynn Walls, *The Vertebrate Eye* (Bloomfield Hills, Mich.: Cranbrook Press, 1942), p. 657.

lets. The long intercalated ducts pass into excretory ducts, of which the smaller have a simple, the larger ones a two-layered, cuboidal epithelium. In the pig the epithelium of the larger excretory ducts is of the high columnar type. Intercellular secretory capillaries are present in all species except the pig.

(b). **The lacrimal passages** are the lacrimal ducts, lacrimal sac, and the naso-lacrimal duct.

The lacrimal ducts consist of a fibroelastic stratified propria covered by squam-

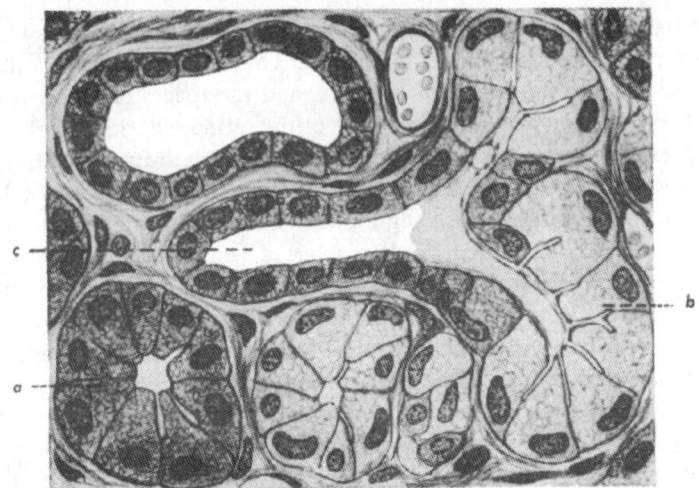

Figure 446. From the lacrimal gland of the sheep (550×).
a, cross section through a serous end-piece with intercellular secretory capillaries; *b*, mucous secretory end-piece; *c*, inter-calated duct below an excretory duct.

ous or, in the horse, columnar epithelium. The wall of the upper duct of swine contains cartilage.

The wall of the lacrimal sac is composed of a propria, which contains lymph cells, and even lymph nodules (in the horse), and a stratified epithelium. The epithelium may be columnar or transitional (in the pig) and passes into that of the nasolacrimal duct. The initial portion of this duct, the ampulla, is made up of an outer dense collagenous layer adjoined by a cavernous stratum, which is composed of a plexus of large veins. There follows a subepithelial layer, which is often lymphatic, and a layer of stratified columnar epithelium. In the middle segment the cavernous layer is replaced by isolated clefts lined by endothelium. In the terminal section the lymph nodules disappear and mucous glands are present. These, however occur along the entire nasolacrimal duct of the horse, as well as in its lacrimal sac and ducts.

The lacrimal fluid keeps the anterior surface of the eye moist and clean. In addition to salts (NaCl, about 1 percent), it contains a little protein. The lacrimal fluid also contains the bactericidal enzyme lysozyme and may therefore be considered part of the defense against infection.

2. The Eyelids

The eyelids (palpebrae; Fig. 447) contain a layer of tendinous connective tissue, the palpebral fascia. This fascia becomes thicker and denser toward the free palpebral margin to form the tarsus, which contains the tarsal glands. The fascial layer is covered on the outside by the middle layer (*II*), containing the striated muscle fibers of the m. orbicularis oculi. The middle layer is covered by skin (*I*), which bears several rows of eyelashes near the outer margin of the lid and at the inner margin passes into the conjunctiva (*III*). This membrane covers the inside of the lid (palpebral conjunctiva) and is reflected on the eyeball (bulbar conjunctiva).

The *tarsus* (*d*) is much less developed in domestic animals than in man. It is a dense collagenous plate, which is indistinctly set off from the surrounding tissue, and is formed by fusion of the collagenous capsules surrounding the tarsal glands. In the pig a secondary tarsus, consisting of collagenous tissue and fibrocartilage, is present toward the base of the lid. The *tarsal glands* (of Meibom; *e*) are better developed in the upper than in the lower lid. They are drained by excretory ducts, which open on the inner margin of the lid. A number of sebaceous gland lobules are clustered around each of these excretory ducts. The glands discharge a fatty secretion on the palpebral margin; this secretion prevents the overflow of tears. The glands are especially small in the pig.

The skin layer is rich in elastic fibers. It is covered by a dense coat of fine hair and is relatively poor in sebaceous and tubular glands. The sebaceous glands present are small, and the tubular glands show little coiling. Only in the pig does one find coarser and more widely scattered hair as well as highly developed tubular and sebaceous glands.

The eyelashes (cilia) are thick and deeply rooted hairs equipped with large sebaceous (*h*) and tubular (*i*) glands. Lashes are small in the lower lid, where they are lacking entirely in carnivores and swine. Sinus hairs also occur on the lids. Bundles of smooth muscle extend from the tarsus to the follicles of the eyelashes as arrectores ciliorum. They are absent in carnivores and man.

The transition to the conjunctiva takes place on the border between the outer and inner palpebral margin. Here the stratified squamous epithelium rests on a papillary body but lacks hairs. The pigmentation of the epithelium may extend for a certain distance on the conjunctiva.

The loose, fat-free subcutis passes without any sharp demarcation into the intermuscular tissue of the m. orbicularis oculi (*k*). Some fibers of this muscle are separated from the rest by the eyelashes to form the muscle of Riolan, which is especially distinct in the ox.

The palpebral fascia contains slips of the levator palpebrae superioris in the upper lid and of the ventral rectus in the lower lid. Both muscles are attached by tendon to the orbital edge of the tarsus. In addition to striated fibers, there are also smooth muscle fibers, which represent the tarsal muscle of Müller. The horse has exclusively smooth fibers in the upper lid.

EYELIDS OF THE CHICKEN. The upper lid is short and thick, and its free margin

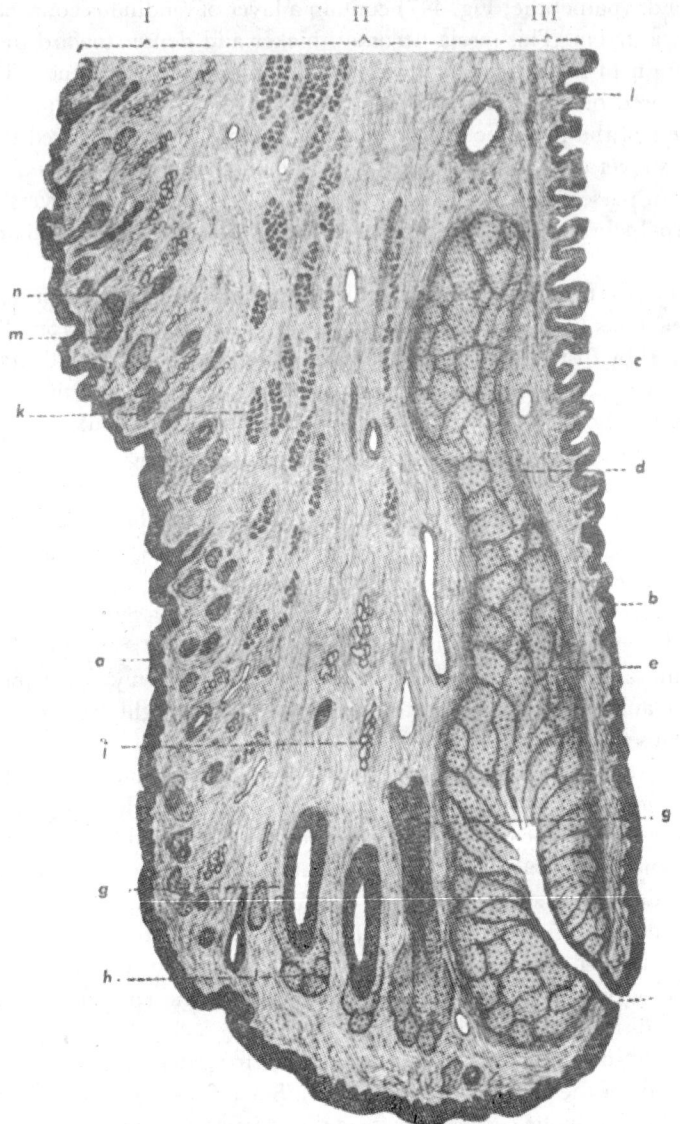

Figure 447. Sagittal section through the upper eyelid of a newborn foal (25 ✕).
I, skin; *II*, middle layer; *III*, conjunctival layer; *a*, epidermis; *b*, conjunctival
epithelium; *c*, grooves in the conjunctiva; *d*, tarsus; *e*, tarsal gland; *f*, opening of
the excretory duct of the tarsal gland; *g*, oblique sections through eyelashes;
h, their sebaceous glands; *i*, their tubular glands; *k*, bundle of the m. orbicularis
palpebrae; *l*, m. tarsalis; *m*, hairs; *n*, their sebaceous glands.

is split into two sheets. The inner one of these is overlapped by the longer and thinner lower lid when the lids are closed. On the superior conjunctiva the epithelium is two-layered cuboidal, while the inferior conjunctiva is lined by columnar epithelium. The propria contains an abundance of lymphocytes.

3. The Conjunctiva

The palpebral conjunctiva consists of a collagenous lamina propria and a stratified epithelium. The palpebral conjunctiva of the horse shows broad papillae separated by epithelial grooves (Fig. 447,c). At the fornix conjunctivae, the line of reflection between the palpebral and bulbar conjunctiva, the propria contains de-

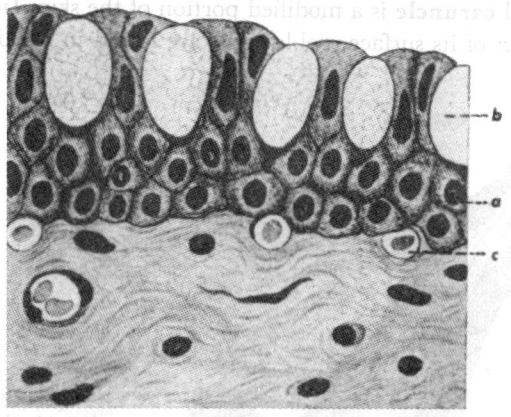

Figure 448. Section through the conjunctiva of the upper lid of the dog. *a*, stratified columnar epithelium; *b*, goblet cell; *c*, capillaries in the propria.

posits of lymphatic tissue. These give rise to ridgelike prominences separated by grooves. Only the horse has glands in this region.

At about the level of the tarsal glands the conjunctival epithelium (Fig. 448,a) changes from stratified squamous to stratified columnar in the horse and carnivores, or to transitional in ruminants and swine. Goblet cells are present. Its bulbar portion (Fig. 423) passes at some distance from the cornea into stratified squamous epithelium, its propria forming a papillary body. Near the corneal limbus the epithelium always contains pigment but finally passes into the unpigmented, corneal epithelium, which has no papillae. The propria is continued as a narrow strip along the corneal margin forming the conjunctival limbus (Fig. 423, near *f*).

The Third Eyelid (Nictitating Membrane)

The third eyelid (Fig. 449) is a fold of conjunctiva supported by a cartilage, which is hyaline or, in the horse, cat, and pig, elastic. The conjunctiva contains scattered lymphoid cells and numerous lymph nodules (*c,e*). Surrounding the cartilage is the *superficial gland of the third eyelid* (*g*), which resembles the lacrimal gland and is serous in the horse and cat; mixed in the ox, sheep and dog; and mucous in the pig. The third eyelid of birds lacks cartilaginous support. It may be drawn completely over the eyeball by means of two smooth muscles. Its bulbar surface bears the so-called feathered epithelium, composed of cells with many fine protoplasmic processes. It is supposed to keep the cornea polished.

The *deep gland of the third eyelid* (Harder's gland) is a mixed gland. The pig is the only domestic animal in which it occurs as a separate organ. It does not occur in the dog. The convex surface of the third eyelid also bears a gland in the pig, frequently in the ox, and more rarely in the horse. In the chicken the gland of the third eyelid is often larger than the lacrimal gland. These glands are extensively branching alveolar glands with columnar cells, which are filled with acidophilic granules.

The lacrimal caruncle is a modified portion of the skin. In the stratified squamous epithelium of its surface, goblet cells are found in the dog, pig, and horse.

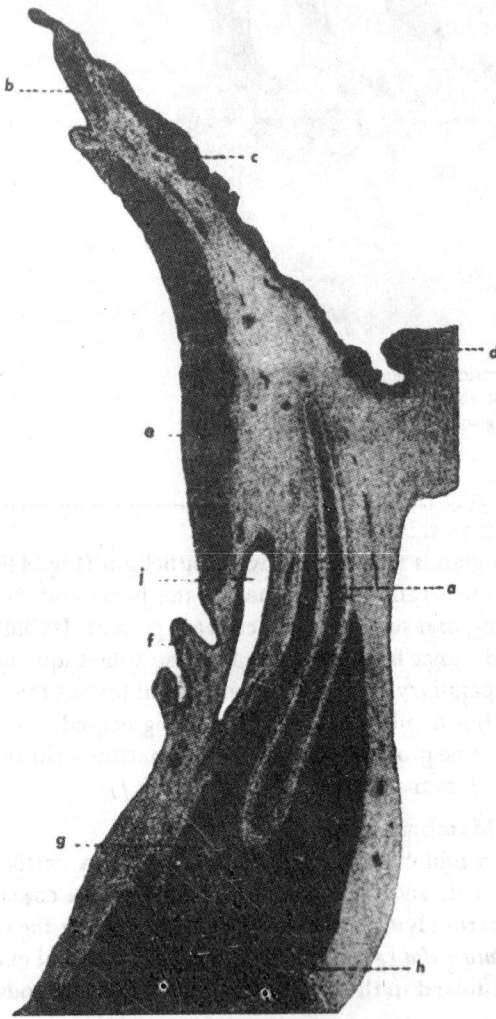

Figure 449. Longitudinal section through the third eyelid of the sheep (8.5×). *a*, cartilage; *b*, its peripheral portion in cross section; *c*, lymphatic tissue with germinal centers in the conjunctiva facing the true eyelid, which is reflected on the lid at *d*; *e*, lymphatic tissue with many germinal centers on the mucosa facing the eyeball, which is reflected on the eyeball at *f*; *g*, gland of the third eyelid; *h*, small interlobular excretory duct; *i*, large excretory duct of the gland. (After Zietschmann.)

The propria contains many leukocytes and, in the dog, horse, and ox, lymph nodules. The lacrimal caruncle bears small hairs with sebaceous and tubular glands the latter being absent in the dog. Horses and carnivores also have seromucous glands resembling the lacrimal gland in structure (accessory lacrimal glands).

C. THE MOTOR APPARATUS OF THE EYE

The extrinsic muscles which are inserted on the eyeball are striated. They are invested by a cover of delicate connective tissue, which condenses into a sheath at the entrance of the muscles into the orbital fat. The tendon bundles of the eye muscles are continued directly into the scleral connective tissue. The deep orbital fascia, which is continuous with the muscle sheaths, separates the orbital fat from the eyeball. The circumbulbar space of Tenon intervenes between the eyeball and this fascia (the capsule of Tenon).

General References

THE books listed here were found useful in the preparation of the American edition. They are recommended as guides to the extensive literature of animal histology. Works consulted in connection with special topics only have been cited in footnotes.

Arey, Leslie B. *Developmental Anatomy.* 5th ed. Philadelphia: Saunders, 1947. (This standard textbook of human embryology is supplemented by a laboratory guide to the study of the pig and chick.)

Asdell, S. A. *Patterns of Mammalian Reproduction.* Ithaca, N.Y.: Comstock, 1946. (A wide range of species is covered, in many cases with histological descriptions of the genital organs. A bibliography is included for each species.)

Best, Charles H., and N. B. Taylor. *The Physiological Basis of Medical Practice.* 5th ed. Baltimore: Williams and Wilkins, 1950. (Much of the evidence cited is from animal experimentation, and the references often include histological descriptions.)

Bremer, J. Lewis, and H. L. Weatherford. *A Textbook of Histology.* 6th ed. Philadelphia: Blakiston, 1944. (A great deal of space is devoted to the embryological introduction of each topic. No titles of papers are given in the bibliography.)

Cowdry, E. V. (ed.). *Special Cytology.* 2 vol. New York: Paul Hoeber, 1928. (Although the primary interest of the contributors is man, they have included some comparative cytology and histology. The bibliographies include the titles of the articles.)

De Robertis, E. P. D., W. W. Nowinsky, and F. A. Saez. *General Cytology.* Philadelphia: Saunders, 1948. (This book is recommended for descriptions of protoplasm, fibrillar structures, mitosis, meiosis, etc.)

Dukes, H. H. *The Physiology of the Domestic Animals.* 6th ed. Ithaca, N.Y.: Comstock, 1947. (Indispensable in its field, this book also contains a great deal of anatomy and histology.)

Ellenberger, Wilhelm (ed.). *Handbuch der vergleichenden mikroskopischen Anatomie der Haustiere.* 3 vol. Berlin: Paul Parey, 1906–1911. (This exhaustive reference work is the source of much of the material in the *Lehrbuch der Histologie und vergleichenden mikroskopischen Anatomie der Haustiere.* Detailed descriptions of each species are given. It is, of course, deficient in recent advances in cytology.)

Ellenberger, Wilhelm, and H. Baum. *Handbuch der vergleichenden Anatomie der Haustiere.* 18th ed. Berlin: Springer, 1943. (The bibliographies of this reference work on the gross anatomy of domestic animals include many histological publications.)

Kuntz, Albert. *A Textbook of Neuroanatomy.* 5th ed. Philadelphia: Lea and Febiger, 1950. (Human neurology.)

Maximow, A. A., and William Bloom. *A Textbook of Histology.* 5th ed. Philadelphia: Saunders, 1948. (The references in this well-illustrated textbook of human histology are complete with titles. Many descriptions of animal histology are cited.)

Möllendorff, Wilhelm von (ed.). *Handbuch der mikroskopischen Anatomie des Menschen.* 7 vol. Berlin: Springer, 1930. (The title is deceptive. A great deal of comparative histology is included. The bibliographies are extensive.)

Papez, J. W. *Comparative Neurology.* New York: T. Y. Crowell, 1929. (This book deserves a wider distribution among those who write on veterinary neurology.)

Ranson, Stephen W., and S. L. Clark. *The Anatomy of the Nervous System.* 8th ed. Philadelphia: Saunders, 1947. (Human neurology.)

Sisson, S., and J. D. Grossman. *The Anatomy of the Domestic Animals.* 3d ed. Philadelphia: Saunders, 1938. (This is another well-known textbook that contains more histology than it is generally given credit for.)

Smith, Philip E., and W. M. Copenhaver. *Bailey's Textbook of Histology.* 12th ed. Baltimore: Williams and Wilkins, 1948. (This is a standard textbook of human histology and a favorite with students.)

Zietzschmann, Otto. *Lehrbuch der Entwicklungsgeschichte der Haustiere.* Berlin: Richard Schoetz, 1924. (This is the most recent textbook of the embryology of domestic animals. It contains descriptions and illustrations of the development of such specialized structures as the hoof, colon, and ruminant stomach.)

Index